drug information

A GUIDE FOR PHARMACISTS

Notice

Medicine is an ever-changing science. As new research and clinical experience broaden our knowledge, changes in treatment and drug therapy are required. The authors and the publisher of this work have checked with sources believed to be reliable in their efforts to provide information that is complete and generally in accord with the standards accepted at the time of publication. However, in view of the possibility of human error or changes in medical sciences, neither the authors nor the publisher nor any other party who has been involved in the preparation or publication of this work warrants that the information contained herein is in every respect accurate or complete, and they disclaim all responsibility for any errors or omissions or for the results obtained from use of the information contained in this work. Readers are encouraged to confirm the information contained herein with other sources. For example, and in particular, readers are advised to check the product information sheet included in the package of each drug they plan to administer to be certain that the information contained in this work is accurate and that changes have not been made in the recommended dose or in the contraindications for administration. This recommendation is of particular importance in connection with new or infrequently used drugs.

drug
information
A GUIDE FOR PHARMACISTS

Patrick M. Malone, PharmD, FASHP
Associate Professor of Pharmacy Practice
Coordinator, Drug Informatics Services
Director, Asynchronous Pharmacy
  Pathway
School of Pharmacy and Allied Health
  Professions
Creighton University
Omaha, Nebraska

**Kristen Wilkinson Mosdell, PharmD,
  BCPS**
Director, Scientific Affairs
Professional Services Department
Immunex Corporation
Seattle, Washington

Karen L. Kier, PhD, MSc, RPh
Professor of Clinical Pharmacy
Director, Drug Information
College of Pharmacy
Ohio Northern University
Ada, Ohio

John E. Stanovich, RPh
Assistant Professor of Clinical Pharmacy
Assistant Dean
Ohio Northern University
Ada, Ohio

McGraw-Hill
Medical Publishing Division

New York • St. Louis • San Francisco • Auckland • Bogotá • Caracas • Lisbon • London
Madrid • Mexico City • Milan • Montreal • New Delhi • San Juan
Singapore • Sydney • Tokyo • Toronto

McGraw-Hill

A Division of The **McGraw·Hill** Companies

Drug Information: A Guide for Pharmacists, Second Edition

Previous edition © 1996 by Appleton & Lange

3 4 5 6 7 8 9 0 DOC DOC 0 9 8 7 6 5 4 3 2

ISBN 0-8385-1577-0

This book was set in Century Old Style by North Market Street Graphics.
The editor was Steve Zollo.
The production supervisor was Catherine H. Saggese.
Project management was performed by Jennsin Publishing Services.
The cover was designed by Mary Skudlarek.
R.R. Donnelley & Sons was the printer and binder.
This book is printed on acid-free paper.

Library of Congress Cataloging-in-Publication Data

Drug information : a guide for pharmacists / Patrick M. Malone . . . [et al.].—2nd ed.
    p. ; cm.
  Includes bibliographical references and index.
  ISBN 0-8385-1577-0 (alk. paper)
  1. Pharmacy—Information services. 2. Drugs. I. Malone, Patrick M., PharmD.
  [DNLM: 1. Drug Information Services. 2. Pharmacy Administration—methods. QV 737
  D793 2001]
  RS56.2 .D78 2001
615'.1—dc21   00-055919

ISBN: 0-07-118268-3 (international)

Contributors

Ann B. Amerson, PharmD
Professor
College of Pharmacy
University of Kentucky
Lexington, Kentucky

Karim Anton Calis, PharmD, MPH, BCPS, BCNSP, FASHP
Clinical Specialist, Endocrinology & Women's Health
Coordinator, Drug Information Service
Clinical Center Pharmacy Department
National Institutes of Health
Bethesda, Maryland
Clinical Associate Professor
School of Pharmacy
University of Maryland
Baltimore, Maryland
Associate Clinical Professor
School of Pharmacy
Virginia Commonwealth University
Richmond, Virginia

Mary Lea Gora-Harper, PharmD
Associate Professor and Director
Drug Information
College of Pharmacy and Hospital
University of Kentucky
Lexington, Kentucky

Philip J. Gregory, PharmD
Assistant Editor
Natural Medicines Comprehensive Database
Stockton, California

Bambi Grilley, RPh, CCRA, CCRC
Director, Clinical Protocol Research and Regulatory Affairs
Texas Children's Cancer Center
Center for Cell and Gene Therapy
Baylor College of Medicine
Houston, Texas

Amy Marie Heck, PharmD
Clinical Assistant Professor of Pharmacy Practice
Purdue Pharmacy Programs at Indianapolis
Indianapolis, Indiana
At the time of writing, she was:
Specialized Resident in Drug Information Practice and Pharmacotherapy
Warren G. Magnuson Clinical Center
National Institutes of Health
Bethesda, Maryland

Carrie J. Johnson, PharmD
Professional Services Manager
Immunex Corporation
Seattle, Washington

Craig F. Kirkwood, PharmD
Associate Professor of Pharmacy and
  Pharmaceutics
School of Pharmacy
Virginia Commonwealth University,
  Medical College of Virginia
Associate Director for Pharmacotherapy
  Services
Department of Pharmacy Services
Medical College of Virginia Hospitals
Richmond, Virginia

Kevin G. Moores, PharmD
Director, Iowa Drug Information Network
Clinical Assistant Professor
College of Pharmacy
University of Iowa
Iowa City, Iowa

Mark A. Ninno, PharmD
Clinical Coordinator, Drug Information
  Services
Orlando Regional Healthcare System
Orlando, Florida

Sharon Davis Ninno, PharmD
Clinical Projects Coordinator
Orlando Regional Healthcare System
Orlando, Florida

Linda K. Ohri, PharmD
Assistant Professor of Pharmacy Practice
School of Pharmacy & Allied Health
  Professions

Creighton University
Manager, Pediatric Drug Information
  Service
Children's Hospital Pharmacy
Omaha, Nebraska

Karen L. Rascati, PhD
Professor, Pharmacy Practice and
  Administration Division
University of Texas College of Pharmacy
Austin, Texas

**Martha M. Rumore, PharmD, JD,
  RAC, FAPhA**
Drug Regulatory Affairs Consultant
New York, New York

James P. Wilson, PharmD, PhD
Assistant Professor
Pharmacy Practice & Administration
  Division
University of Texas College of Pharmacy
Austin, Texas

Linda R. Young, PharmD
Director, Drug Information Center
Assistant Professor, Department of
  Pharmacy Practice and
  Pharmacoeconomics
College of Pharmacy
University of Tennessee Health Science
  Center
Memphis, Tennessee

Contents

Preface

Sit down and talk to a drug information specialist; you will find someone who is convinced that the future of pharmacy depends on improved information management. There is good reason for that conviction. Just look at the rapid advances in automation—machines that dispense products, laws that permit robots to deliver drugs without having pharmacists check their work[1] (after all, those machines may not make even a single error in a year or more[2]), robots that mix intravenous solutions, and computers that manage billing and other business functions. When you look at this list, it appears that one of the most important roles left for pharmacists is information management directed at improved patient outcomes.

Even then, all is not easy in information management. For years, computers have checked for drug interactions and printed out patient information sheets. Now, computers can even check for patient-specific issues, such as appropriate dose based on renal and/or hepatic function, appropriate route of administration (no more giving intravenous products to someone who has been eating for a week since their surgery), appropriate indications, and so on. Artificial intelligence may take over numerous pharmacy functions in the future. Such computerized functions, however, cannot replace the skills of a pharmacist trained in information management. A computer program may alert someone to the fact that a drug interaction is possible, but is the interaction clinically significant based on the profile of the patient? Pharmacists need to develop new and improved services that are grounded in information management, while utilizing the new technologies to free up time and streamline operations. If these value-added services are not developed, pharmacy will cease to exist, to be replaced by automation.

Patients still like to talk to humans, rather than machines, as do other health care professionals, which benefits the profession of pharmacy. Nonetheless, many pharmacists will need to develop new roles to justify their existence. All pharmacists are finding that they need to increasingly manage information, whether in clinical, business, or other arenas. For example, some drug information specialists are developing the information used by the computer programs mentioned.

Unfortunately, many pharmacists have not recognized the need for information management and have not developed skills in this area to improve patient care outcomes. Librarians recognized the need for better information management to assist physicians, suggesting a "clinical librarian" that sounded a great deal like a clinical pharmacist in the early 1980s.[3] Although pharmacists have the clinical knowledge that librarians do not possess, they often do not realize the need for greater skills in information management. Until the 1990s, schools of pharmacy often provided only rudimentary training in information management. Also, information resources have grown at an explosive rate over the last few years. As a result, many pharmacists, particularly in institutional practice, are finding the need to have skills that were possessed only by drug information specialists around 1980.

Unfortunately, pharmacists in practice may find it difficult to learn how to manage information because good, comprehensive resources to teach them proven methods for improving their skills are not readily available. Students also need a source to supplement the classroom and clerkship training they receive. It is to serve those populations that this book was originally written. In this second edition, the goal continues to be to educate both students and practitioners on how to efficiently research, interpret, collate, and disseminate information in the most usable form. While there is no one "right" method to do these things, proven methods are presented and demonstrated. Also, seldom-addressed issues are covered, such as the legal and ethical considerations of providing information.

The book begins by introducing the concept of drug information, including its history, and providing information on various places drug information specialists may be employed.

The book continues by describing the steps for obtaining, evaluating, and providing information. As with the first edition, the Modified Systematic Approach to answering a question is presented. A new chapter, "Formulating Effective Responses and Recommendations" (Chap. 3), further expands this topic by addressing problems that pharmacists experience when answering questions and providing techniques for overcoming these issues to reach appropriate conclusions. This section of the book is designed to teach pharmacists and students useful methods for determining what information is actually needed and how to adequately respond to requests.

Subsequent chapters allow readers to further expand their skills in these areas. Once the pharmacist determines what information is needed using the skills outlined in the initial chapters, resources must be consulted to formulate a response. As with the first edition, a chapter (Chap. 4) discussing various resources that may be used for specific types of information has been provided. Additionally, a chapter on electronic information management (Chap. 5) has been included. At the time the first edition was written, relatively few electronic sources of information were available to pharmacists.

This has changed tremendously, particularly with the rapid growth in the use of the Internet. This new chapter explores many aspects of obtaining and providing information using electronic resources. In addition, a number of useful Internet addresses are provided that will assist pharmacists and students in their pursuit of information.

Even when information is found, pharmacists must evaluate the literature for quality and usefulness. The first edition of this book concentrated on traditional methods for evaluation of clinical studies. Those evaluation techniques are again provided in this edition (Chap. 6); however, a new chapter (Chap. 7) provides techniques to evaluate most other types of literature that may be consulted by pharmacists.

Two specific types of literature have been identified for even greater examination in this edition—pharmacoeconomics and evidence-based clinical practice guidelines. Information is presented on how to both perform such functions and evaluate work prepared by others. Chapter 8 on pharmacoeconomics is entirely new and is particularly helpful for those pharmacists evaluating drug products based on pharmacoeconomic principles.

Evaluation of information resources often requires knowledge about statistical tests. Chapter 10, "Clinical Application of Statistical Analysis," is an expansion of information provided in the first edition. The reader will discover how to evaluate the appropriateness of statistical tests used in clinical studies.

Pharmacists may be asked to provide information in written form. Chapter 11 describes how this may be done. Additionally, new sections describing how to prepare materials for formal presentations (platform and poster) and develop web sites are also provided.

The legal and ethical aspects of providing information always must be considered. The chapters on these topics have been updated and improved to be even more useful than those of the first edition.

The remaining chapters deal with specialized functions that have often been the responsibility of drug information specialists, but may be addressed by other pharmacists. These chapters build on the first part of the book. Much of the information in these chapters was covered in the Pharmacy and Therapeutics (P&T) chapter of the first edition; however, that chapter is now mostly limited to formulary management and some minor P&T functions. In the first edition, information on drug usage evaluation and drug utilization review was contained in the P&T chapter, but this information has now been relocated to the chapter on quality assurance, which is expanded and improved. Similarly, the topic of adverse drug reactions has been separated into a new chapter that now includes the topic of medication errors.

Finally, Chap. 17, on investigational drugs has been updated to take into account new information and procedures.

With the veritable Niagara Falls of drug or pharmacy information available, much of which is complex, pharmacists have an increasing need for information management skills. This book will assist any pharmacist or student in the improvement of his or her skills in this area and allow individuals to evolve into new roles for the advancement of both the profession and care of patients. We hope you enjoy your journey toward expertise in information management.

REFERENCES

1. Smart robots? Hosp Pharm Rep 1995;9(4):1.
2. Blank C, Gannon K. More freedom for robots? Some states explore the idea. Hosp Pharm Rep 1997;11(10):68.
3. Matheson NW, Cooper JAD. Academic Health Sciences Center: roles for the library in information management. J Med Educ 1982;57.

Chapter One

Introduction to the Concept of Medication Information

Ann B. Amerson • Mary Lea Gora-Harper

Objectives

After completing this chapter, the reader will be able to

- Define the term *drug information,* use it in different contexts, and relate it to the term *medication information.*
- Describe the importance of drug information centers in the evolution of pharmacy practice.
- Identify the services provided by drug information centers.
- Identify medication information functions performed by individual pharmacists.
- Describe the skills needed by pharmacists' to perform medication information functions.
- Identify major factors that have influenced the ability of pharmacists to provide medication information.
- Describe practice opportunities for medication information specialists.

The provision of medication information is among the most fundamental responsibilities of pharmacists. The information may be either patient specific, as an integral part of pharmaceutical care, or relative to a group of patients, such as in the context of a disease management program or in publishing a newsletter. The pharmacist can serve as a resource for issues regarding cost-effective medication selection and use, medication policy decisions (drug benefits), medication information resource selection, or practice-related issues. Medication information opportunities are developing and expanding with changes in the health care environment. With national efforts to expand access to care

1

while reducing health care costs, the advent of consumerism, and the integration of new technologies, medication information opportunities are growing in several areas including managed care organizations, the pharmaceutical industry, ambulatory care, and the insurance industry.

The term *drug information* may have different meanings to different people depending on the context in which it is used. If asked to define this term, one could describe it as information printed in a reference or verbalized by an individual that pertains to drugs. In many cases individuals put this term in different contexts by associating it with other words, including

- Specialist/practitioner/pharmacist/provider
- Center/service/practice
- Functions/skills

The first group of words implies a specific individual, the second a place, and the third activities and abilities of individuals. The term *drug information* will be used in these different contexts to describe the beginnings and evolution of this area of practice. Relative to current practice, the term *medication information* is used in place of *drug information* to convey the management and use of information on medication therapy and to signify the broader role that all pharmacists take in information provision. Drug informatics is another term used to describe the evolving roles of the drug information specialist. The impact of new technologies and opportunities in drug informatics on current and future practice will be discussed later in this chapter.

The goals of this chapter are to describe how the role of the pharmacist has evolved in providing medication information, factors contributing to the evolution, and opportunities for use of medication information skills, either as a generalist or in a specialty practice. This chapter provides the foundation for understanding the pharmacist's need to have proficiency in the knowledge and skills discussed in this book.

The Beginning

The term drug information developed an identity in the early 1960s when used in conjunction with the words *center* and *specialist*. In 1962, the first drug information center was opened at the University of Kentucky Medical Center.[1] An area separated from the pharmacy was dedicated to provide drug information. The center was to be "a source of selected, comprehensive drug information for staff physicians and dentists to evaluate and compare drugs"[1] as well as provide for the drug information needs of nurses. The

TABLE 1–1. MEDICATION INFORMATION SERVICES

Support for clinical services
  Answering questions
  Developing criteria/guidelines for medication use
Pharmacy and therapeutics committee activity
  Development of medication use policies
  Formulary management
Publications—newsletter, journal columns
Education—inservices for health professionals, students
Medication usage evaluation/medication use evaluation
Investigational medication control
  Institutional Review Board activities
  Information for practitioners
Coordination of reporting programs—e.g., adverse medication reactions
Poison information

---

center was expected to take an active role in the education of health professional students including medicine, dentistry, nursing, and pharmacy. A stated goal was to influence pharmacy students in developing their role as drug consultants.

Several other drug information centers were established shortly thereafter. Different approaches to providing drug information services included decentralizing pharmacists in the hospital, offering a clinical consultation service, and providing services for a geographic area through a regional center. The first formal survey conducted in 1973 identified 54 pharmacist-operated centers in the United States.[2]

The individual responsible for operation of the center was called the *drug information specialist*. The expectation was that drug information would be stored in the center and retrieved, selected, evaluated, and disseminated by the specialist. Information would be disseminated to respond to specific questions, assist in the evaluation of drugs for use in the hospital, or inform through newsletters of current developments related to drugs. These and other functions as listed in Table 1–1 have evolved over a period of years but reflect the services provided in most drug information centers. More detail is provided on these functions in other chapters that will relate their applicability to current practice.

To develop some perspective for the reader on why development of drug information centers and specialists was important, consider 4 of the 15 summary points in a congressional review of a survey by the National Library of Medicine on "The Nature and Magnitude of Drug Literature" published in 1963.[3]

- "Drug literature is vast and complex. The very problem of defining what constitutes the literature is difficult."
- "Drug literature is growing rapidly in size. It is also increasingly complex, i.e., interdisciplinary and interprofessional in nature. Thus, drug information 'sprawls across' many professional journals of the most varied types."

- "Literature on clinical experience with drugs is sizable and is growing. Its effective use by the practitioner offers many difficulties."
- "Competent evaluation of masses of drug information is particularly necessary."

Interestingly, these statements still seem applicable even today when given the figures of more than 20,000 biomedical journals and approximately 17,000 new biomedical books published annually are considered.[4]

In the 1960s, the availability of new drugs (e.g., neuromuscular blockers, first-generation cephalosporins) provided challenges for practitioners to keep abreast and make appropriate decisions for their patients. Part of the problem was finding a way to effectively communicate the wealth of information to those needing it. The information environment relied heavily on the print medium for storage, retrieval, and dissemination of information. The Medical Literature Retrieval and Analysis System (MEDLARS) was developed by the National Library of Medicine in the early 1960s.[5] Although it provided a computerized form of searching, requests for searches were submitted by mail and results returned by mail. The ability to transmit such information over telephone lines (on-line technology) was not available until 1971 when MEDLINE was introduced and was limited to libraries. During this time, the drug information specialist was viewed as a person who could bridge the gap and effectively communicate drug information.[6,7]

In describing the training required for a drug information specialist, the following areas were identified to either need strengthening or addition to pharmacy school curricula: biochemistry, anatomy, physiology, pathology, and biostatistics and experimental design (with some histology, embryology, and endocrinology incorporated into other courses).[6] Such topics were either not incorporated or emphasized in pharmacy curricula of the 1960s. In today's curricula, most of these topics receive considerable emphasis.

The development of drug information centers and drug information specialists was the beginning of the clinical pharmacy concept. It laid the groundwork for pharmacists to demonstrate the ability to assume more responsibility in providing input on patient drug therapy. Pharmacists were provided the opportunity to extend their patient care contribution by taking a more active role in the clinical aspects of the decision making process as it related to drug therapy. By using their extensive drug knowledge and expanding their background in certain areas, pharmacists could offer their expertise as consultants on drug therapy. The tool the pharmacist uses to function in this capacity is the clinical drug literature. This role of consultant has expanded for all pharmacists and is discussed in more detail later.

The Evolution

It is useful to look at the evolution of drug information practice from the perspective of drug information centers as well as from the perspective of practicing pharmacists. Over the years, the number of drug information centers has increased. For example, in surveys of centers, 54 responded in 1973, 106 in 1980, and 130 in 1990.[2] In the two most recent surveys performed in 1992, 154 of 194 centers and 140 of 179 centers responded.[8,9] Although the *2000 Red Book* lists a total of 109 drug information centers, determining accurate numbers is difficult; the actual numbers are probably higher. These centers are identified through various listings that have developed over the years but no agency or organization is responsible for maintaining a list. Well-defined criteria are not established for using the titles of drug information center or service. Likewise, these lists only address drug information centers listed in the United States and not those that have been created internationally. They also exclude centers or services provided by the pharmaceutical industry. However, the numbers do indicate a continued increase. It is not clear whether this increase is due to the creation of centers that are used either locally or regionally.

According to the 1992 survey, the large majority of centers (>80%) are located in hospitals or medical centers and interface with the pharmacy services provided.[9] A few (7%) are located in colleges of pharmacy. Seventy-five percent have an affiliation with a college of pharmacy primarily for educational purposes. Over half provide a rotation site to do experiential training for pharmacy students. Many are involved in training of pharmacy practice residents and some offer specialty residencies in drug information. The number of personnel employed in drug information centers has increased. Many of the services listed in Table 1–1 still continue as the major responsibilities of drug information centers. The scope and depth have changed largely because of a number of factors that have influenced all of pharmacy practice. Drug information centers continue to be providers of information to individual health professionals and groups (pharmacy and therapeutics committee) but in a more sophisticated way. With many pharmacists providing medication information, the problems referred to drug information centers tend to be more complex, require use of specialized resources, or require more in-depth analysis. Many centers have increased revenue with new clients. For example, 36% and 23% of drug information centers provide services for either law firms or pharmaceutical companies, respectively.[9] Other clients include hospital pharmacies, health maintenance organizations, hospital pharmacy management companies, and insurance companies. The types of services offered through these agreements include expert testimony, drug information for professionals or consumers, drug evaluations for pharmacy and therapeutics committees, newsletters, evidence-based guidelines, and medication use evaluation criteria or outcomes analyses.[10]

DRUG INFORMATION—FROM CENTERS TO PRACTITIONERS

The responsibilities of individual pharmacists regarding the provision of drug information have changed substantially over the years. Impetus for this change was provided not only by the development of drug information centers and the clinical pharmacy concept, but also by the Study Commission on Pharmacy.[11] This external group was established to review the state of the practice and education of pharmacists and report its findings. One of the findings and recommendations stated that

> . . . among deficiencies in the health care system, one is the unavailability of adequate information for those who consume, prescribe, dispense and administer drugs. This deficiency has resulted in inappropriate drug use and an unacceptable frequency of drug-induced disease. Pharmacists are seen as health professionals who could make an important contribution to the health care system of the future by providing information about drugs to consumers and health professionals. Education and training of pharmacists now and in the future must be developed to meet these important responsibilities.[11]

The report of the Commission was issued in 1975 and since that time drug information practice has changed both for drug information centers and individual pharmacists. The development of clinical pharmacy has helped move pharmacy forward in recognizing its capabilities to contribute to the care of patients. Clinical pharmacy was thought of primarily as an institutional patient care process and did not gain widespread acceptance outside of hospitals. The advent of the term pharmaceutical care broadens the scope of applicability with a focus on the patient in any environment. *Pharmaceutical care* is defined as "the responsible provision of drug therapy for the purpose of achieving definite outcomes that improve a patient's quality of life."[12] Pharmacists who actively participate in delivering pharmaceutical care use the medication literature as one of the tools. As a provider of pharmaceutical care, the pharmacist is the primary professional responsible for provision of medication information.[13]

Pharmacists involved in patient care areas (e.g., hospitals, clinics, long-term care, home health care) now frequently answer drug information questions, participate in evaluating a patient's drug therapy, and conduct medication usage evaluation activities. The provision of medication information may be on a one-on-one basis or may occur using a more structured approach, such as a presentation to a class of diabetic patients or a group of nurses in the practice facility. In either case, the pharmacist educates those who are the beneficiaries of the medication information. Pharmacists may also participate in precepting students in patient care or pharmacy environments. In any of these roles as a teacher, the pharmacist must use appropriate information retrieval and evaluation skills to make sure that the most current and accurate information is provided to make decisions about medication use for those they are serving. Opportunities continue to grow for pharmacist participation in home health care and long-term care that require a solid therapeutic knowledge base, an understanding of the medical literature, and the ability to communicate the information via either verbal or written consultation. Pharmacists in community settings counsel patients, answer drug information questions, review patient medication regimens for potential problems, and participate in helping patients manage their chronic diseases.

FACTORS INFLUENCING THE EVOLUTION OF THE PHARMACIST'S ROLE AS A MEDICATION INFORMATION PROVIDER

In addition to the changing philosophy of practice, several other factors are influential in the evolution of the pharmacist's role as a medication information provider. These include the growth of information technology, changes in the health care environment with focus on evidence-based medicine and evaluation of outcomes, the sophistication of medication therapy, and a more knowledgeable patient.

Integration of New Technologies

Computer technology has changed drastically, but positively, the ability to store and to access information. Even though the literature is vaster today than earlier, it is more manageable. The Internet has grown into a vast network of computers that millions of users can access in most countries. The World Wide Web, a method of sharing information over the Internet, allows the user to easily access the scientific literature, government publications, items in the news, and many other things. The information may be purely in textual form, or include graphics, video, or sound. A pharmacist in a local community pharmacy or rural hospital can communicate with health care professionals or their patients locally, or can obtain information about a medication found only in another country. Although drug information centers may have ready access to the Internet, and the specialist uses information from this resource on a daily basis, businesses have yet to take full advantage of this technology.[14] In a recent study, only 21% of community and 10% of corporate pharmacists have access to the Internet at their practice site, and of these, only about one third of pharmacists access this information on a daily basis.[15] This will likely change in the near future. Local area networks are frequently used to connect computers within a drug information center, building, or neighboring areas. The use of wide area networks will grow as institutions merge and interconnect data management functions.[16] Likewise, the use of palm top computers has grown. These systems can offer the convenience of collecting and accessing information using a unit that can be retrieved from a user's pocket. These systems can be used more conveniently than a desktop computer for online searching, to provide medication profiles, to set appointments and search drug information databases (e.g., *Physician's Desk Reference* [*PDR*]). Although technology affords remote-site access of medication information sources, it is critical that pharmacists have the skills to perceive, assess, and evaluate the information, and apply the information to the situation. One of the most rapidly changing technologies in health care is information technology. It is important that pharmacists not only keep up with medication use concepts, but that they also stay abreast of developments in the area of information technology in an effort to integrate new and valuable systems in a timely and efficient manner.

Future technology developments are likely to further enhance access and use of information. The medical record, including administrative information, laboratory data, and pharmaceutical information, is amenable to access by computer in patient care areas. A properly configured medical record provides decision support, facilitates workflow, and enables the routine collection of data for performance feedback.[17] This offers opportunities for pharmacists, and in particular medication information specialists, to take a leadership role in planning and implementing computerized intervention programs that automatically educate at the point of prescribing. Although the Internet has been used to transfer information instantaneously to clinicians and researchers, its value as a patient care resource and professional education tool is only starting to be explored. One of the concerns in using the Internet for transfer of patient information is patient confidentiality.[18,19] The use of virtual private networks (VPN) should eliminate many of the technical issues surrounding security of information.

Focus on Evidence-Based Medicine and Drug Policy Development

The pharmacist's ability to apply medication information skills to drug policy decisions by identifying trends of inappropriate medication use in groups of patients, and providing supporting scientific evidence to help change behaviors will be of growing importance in this changing health care environment. Continued growth in national health expenditures has raised the concerns of government, insurance agencies, health care providers, and the public in identifying strategies to control spending while maintaining access to quality health care. With a projected $184 billion to be spent on pharmaceuticals in 2008, increased from $62.2 billion in 1996, questions inevitably arise about the value of services received.[20] In recent years, there has been a shift from a fee-for-service, inpatient focus, to a capitated, managed care, ambulatory care focus.[21] Managed care— a process seeking to manage the delivery of high-quality health care to improve cost effectiveness—is consuming an ever-increasing portion of health care delivery. Providers are relying less on impressions and more on data than they did in the past.

Evidence-based medicine is an approach to practice and teaching that integrates current clinical research evidence with pathophysiologic rationale, professional expertise, and patient preferences.[22] This has strengthened the need for pharmacists to have a solid understanding of drug information concepts and skills. Pharmacists need to be able to evaluate the medication use issues for a group of patients, be able to search, retrieve, and critically evaluate the scientific literature, and apply the information to the targeted group of patients. Evidence-based medicine techniques are used in managed care organizations in the development and implementation of therapeutic guidelines, clinical pathways, medication use evaluations, and disease state management. All of these situations require pharmacists to use medication information skills and to have various kinds of medication information support at the practice site or easily accessible at a remote site. The process of evidence-based medicine requires that systems be developed to measure and report processes and outcomes that can be used to drive quality improvement efforts. Data can be collected and analyzed by a drug information specialist using scientific methods to support the decision making process in a managed care organization. Outcomes research can be used to identify the effectiveness of pharmaceutical products and services in achieving desired health outcomes. Likewise, the branch of outcomes research, pharmacoeconomics, provides tools to assess cost, consequences, and efficiency. For more information refer to Chaps. 8 and 9.

Sophistication of Medication Therapy

The sophisticated level of medication therapy that occurs today provides pharmacists much more opportunity to lend their expertise in assessing the medication information needs of professionals, patients, or family members. Pharmacists can provide literature to differentiate the choice of medications within a class, convey the appropriate information to help patients correctly and safely use the more potent medications, and address administration and delivery problems. It is increasingly difficult for physicians and other health professionals to keep up with all of the developments in medication therapy as well as keep abreast of the other information required for their practice. The pharmacist, whose focus is medications, can work effectively with other health professionals to resolve and often avoid medication therapy problems. The pharmacist often needs to use the literature to do this effectively.

Consumerism

Finally, consumers have a continually growing desire for information about their medications. The growth of the self-care movement, the increase in focus on health care costs, and the improved accessibility of health information are some of the factors that have influenced patients to participate more fully in health care decisions, including the selection and use of medications. Based on these needs, direct-to-consumer advertising (DTCA) campaigns have appeared in virtually all mediums including magazines, television, and radio. In 1996 for the first time ever, the amount spent on DTCA exceeded the amount spent on direct-to-physician advertising.[23] In 1997, the pharmaceutical industry spent over $1 billion on DTCA, up 61% from 1996.[24] One of the reasons for this increase may be secondary to the success of the program.[25] Likewise, it has been estimated that over 9 million individuals in the United States and Canada use the World Wide Web on a daily basis, one-third of them to find information on health. Because a single individual is able to serve as author, editor, and publisher of information on the Internet, there is no safeguard on the quality of information provided. The end result is a potentially misinformed consumer.[26,27] A pharmacist can help consumers critically assess the medication information that they find in the lay press or through pharmaceutical manufacturer advertisements, and add to the information based on specific patient-related needs. This is particularly important for information on complementary and alternative medicine, with an estimated one of three Americans choosing this option.[28] This area presents a challenging situation for pharmacists because of the lack of relevant outcomes data from well-designed clinical trials.

Groups like the National Council on Patient Information and Education (NCPIE) encourage patients to seek information when they have questions. The experience with some "medication information hotlines" that have been established for public access indicates the public's desire and need for information.[29] Such hotlines, often established by pharmacists, are intended to enhance the relationships between pharmacists, physicians, and patients.

The changing environment affords the pharmacist many opportunities to use the full spectrum of medication information skills. Factors such as integration of new technologies, focus on evidence-based medicine and drug policy development, sophistication of medication therapy, and advent of consumerism require that all pharmacists have a strong foundation in drug information concepts.

EDUCATING FOR THE NEED

The education of pharmacists continues to evolve in scope and depth. Many of the areas identified as needed by the drug (medication) information specialist are now incorporated into pharmacy curricula and taught to all pharmacists. In 1991, a consensus conference was held in New Mexico to define a set of objectives for didactic and experiential training in drug information for 2000.[30] Twenty-three educators and practitioners participated in the conference. There were several key concepts that were developed, including the following.

1. Drug information should be a required component of the pharmacy curriculum and include both didactic and competency-based experiential components.

2. Drug information concepts and skills should be spread throughout the curriculum, beginning the day the students enter pharmacy school.
3. Problem solving should be a major technique in drug information education, with the goal of developing self-directed learners.

Developing these skills should provide the foundation for the pharmacist to be a lifelong learner and problem solver. Based on the work of this conference, as well as changes in the health care system and the movement toward outcome-based education, colleges of pharmacy have begun to redesign their curricula to provide a more comprehensive and integrated approach to teaching medication information concepts and skills.[31,32] Communication skills are taught formally to facilitate the pharmacist's ability to transmit information to both health professionals and patients. Medication information and policy development are two of the key areas addressed in the pharmacy practice residency standards. Specialty practice residencies in medication information are also available in a variety of practice sites.[33]

Opportunities in Specialty Practice

As the role of the practicing pharmacist has changed regarding medication information activities, so has the role of the specialist. The role of the drug information specialist has changed from an individual who specifically answers questions to one who focuses on medication policies and provides information on complex medication information questions. A specialist in medication information can provide leadership in medical informatics, medication policy development, poison control, the pharmaceutical industry, and academia. A specialist in medication information can be involved in one or all of the activities listed below. The role of the drug information specialist in these areas will be discussed in the next subsection.

MEDICAL INFORMATICS

With the growth and development of new technologies (e.g., information systems), there are tremendous opportunities for an informatics specialist—an individual that has advanced medication information skills with a keen understanding of computer technology. This individual can help to support the concepts of pharmaceutical care by improving the efficiency of workflow and increasing access to patient-specific information and the medical literature through technology by remote site availability. This individual may also be involved in the area of institutional drug policy management. As more information is computerized (e.g., medical records), data that were only accessible through a paper record will be available for those professionals that understand the type of data that is needed for quality improvement efforts, and are able to get information efficiently out of the system.[34] As database designs evolve and become more user friendly, and computer systems become more sophisticated, there are increasing opportunities for applying computer technology using clinical decision support systems to enhance many aspects of the medication use process. Clinical decision support systems can integrate patient-specific information, perform complex evaluations, and present this information to a clinician in a timely manner. These systems can be used to support initiatives with adverse drug reaction reporting and analysis programs, formulary management, and continuous quality improvement efforts.

HEALTH MAINTENANCE ORGANIZATIONS, PHARMACY BENEFIT MANAGEMENT ORGANIZATIONS, AND MANAGED CARE ORGANIZATIONS

In 1994, the Consortium for the Advancement of Medication Information, Policy and Research (CAMIPR) met to initiate a strategic plan for the future of medication information practice.[35] A key opportunity identified was the growing role for medication information specialists in the area of medication policy development/research and technology. Because pharmaceuticals account for approximately 10% of health care dollars, up from 7% 5 years ago, this offers tremendous opportunities for the medication information specialist to provide leadership in the development and implementation of mechanisms to support the cost-effective selection and use of medications.[36] The specialist may coordinate activities relating to formulary development and implementation, adverse drug event reporting and analysis, and therapeutic guideline development. Medical and pharmaceutical outcomes research has been an increasing interest among health care providers, payers, and regulatory agencies. With the appropriate training (e.g., specialized residency in medication information practice or managed care experience) and expertise, there are growing opportunities for the medication information specialist in the insurance industry, health maintenance organizations, managed care organizations, pharmacy benefits management companies, state and national government agencies (e.g., Medicaid, Medicare) as well as others interested in the cost-efficient use of medications.

CONTRACT DRUG INFORMATION SERVICES

The need for accurate information pertaining to drug therapy is more acute today than ever before in the history of health care. Within the next decade health care costs will increase at an alarming rate with expenditures reaching the $2.1 trillion mark. A majority of these costs will be shouldered by the private sector with a significant increase in prescription drug costs. Drug information practitioners are in an enviable position as health care professionals to provide a service that will improve patient outcomes and decrease health care costs through the provision of unbiased information that supports rational, cost-effective, patient- and disease-specific drug therapy.

The best way to deliver such information is through a formalized drug information service. It is well established in the literature that the most cost-effective method to deliver quality unbiased information is through a health care practitioner, formally trained and practicing in an information center. Contracting with a formalized drug information center has recently evolved as the preferred method for obtaining these services.

Examples of contracted drug information services include contracts between formalized centers and managed care groups, contract pharmacy services, pharmacy benefits managers, buying groups, small rural hospitals, chain pharmacies, and independent pharmacies. Several different arrangements have been developed for providing these services, from a simple fee per question to a detailed proposal that offers a menu of services that can be selected, with the final cost dependent on the number of services chosen by the contracting party.

Drug information services provided within these contracts may include providing answers to drug information requests, preparation of new drug monographs, formulary drug class reviews, development of medication utilization evaluation criteria, providing journal reprints, pharmacoeconomic evaluations, writing a pharmacotherapy newsletter, and providing continuing education programming. Additional services the center may make available are access to on-line resources, access to in-house question files for sharing of information on commonly asked questions, and direct access to the center's Internet home page for review of medical use evaluations, formulary reviews, and newsletters.

POISON CONTROL

Poison information is a specialized area of medication information with the practitioner typically practicing in an accredited poison information center or an emergency room. Similar to the mission of traditional drug information centers, poison information centers exist to provide accurate and timely information to enhance the quality of care of patients. There are, however, several differences between a traditional drug information center and poison control center. Health professionals generate most consultations received in drug information centers, whereas in a poison control center most are generated from the public. Poison information centers must be prepared to provide information on management of any poison situation including household products, medications, and other chemicals. Because of the type of information that the specialist provides, nearly all requests for information to a poison control center are urgent, with an average response time of 5 minutes, compared to anywhere from 30 minutes to days for drug information centers, depending on the urgency of the call and complexity of information required. A specialist in poison information therefore requires expertise in clinical toxicology, as well as an ability to obtain a complete history that correctly assesses the potential severity of exposure, an understanding of where to search for this type of information, and the ability to communicate the information and plan in a comprehensive, concise, and accurate manner to a consumer at all levels of education. Because of the unique expertise of this type of specialist, a national certification examination is offered through the American Association of Poison Control Specialists (AAPCC). In addition to a poison control center providing information regarding individual patients, centers in the United States also contribute data to a larger program through the Toxic Exposure Surveillance System (TESS), which is coordinated by the AAPCC. The data can be used to compare safety profiles for similar products, develop risk assessment guidelines for specific substances, target national prevention programs, and conduct postmarketing surveillance on products (e.g., chemicals).

Despite the impact that regional poison control centers have on reducing morbidity and mortality with poison exposures, they are also facing increasing emphasis on economic justification. One study used a decision analysis to compare the cost effectiveness of treatment of poison exposures with the services of a regional poison control center and treatment without access to any poison control center.[37] The average cost per patient treated with the services of a poison control center was almost half of that achieved without the services of a poison control center. These results were consistent regardless of exposure type, average inpatient and emergency department costs, and clinical outcome probabilities.

PHARMACEUTICAL INDUSTRY

The pharmaceutical industry provides many career opportunities for pharmacists including sales, marketing, product formulation, quality control, regulatory affairs, professional affairs, medical information services, and clinical research.[38] Within the area of medical information services, the pharmacist participates in traditional drug information activities, such as answering drug information questions, reporting and monitoring adverse drug reactions, and providing information support to other departments. Pharmacists providing medication information in the pharmaceutical industry may also provide support for individuals responsible for drug formularies or participate in quality improvement efforts with the medication use process. In addition to providing written information on the drug produced by the manufacturer, there are opportunities to provide additional information at pharmacy and therapeutics committees or state drug use review (DUR) boards. Pharmaceutical companies have extensive scientific data on their products, some of which are not available through other published sources or may require a formal freedom of information (FOI) request. Medication information specialists may also serve as reviewers for journal articles, evidence-based guidelines, and published drug monographs. Medication information specialists may interact with sales and marketing, participate with regulatory affairs issues, and handle product complaints. As the sophistication of drug products and information management (e.g., electronic new drug applications [NDAs]) has increased, so have the opportunities for pharmacists to practice in the pharmaceutical industry and focus on using the skills of a medication information specialist.

ACADEMIA

The medication information specialist has the opportunity to provide leadership in the pharmacy curriculum, including both didactic and experiential training. In addition to teaching medication information skills that are required across practice sites, the specialist also serves as collaborator with other faculty on cases and activity design to reinforce drug information skills for students. Approximately one-third of drug information centers are funded by a college of pharmacy. This environment allows the student to be prepared to efficiently and accurately provide information to the appropriate audience, while emphasizing both didactic and competency-based experiential training.[9]

Summary and Direction for the Future

All pharmacists must be effective medication information providers regardless of their practice. As defined by the New Mexico Conference, an effective provider perceives, assesses, and evaluates medication information needs and retrieves, evaluates, communicates, and applies data from the published literature and other sources as an integral component of pharmaceutical care.[30] If the profession is to be successful in adopting and implementing the philosophy of pharmaceutical care, all pharmacists must achieve a certain minimum level of skill to survive in the changing practice environment. Developing the skills of an effective medication information provider is the foundation for the pharmacist to be a life-long learner and problem solver. The literature is a valuable component of both of these processes and will allow the individual pharmacist to adapt to the needs of a rapidly changing health care system.

Opportunities abound for pharmacists to use medication information skills in all practice settings, either as a generalist or a specialist practitioner. There is still the need for the practitioner to have support from drug information centers to meet special information needs, serve as a resource on effective medication use, and assist pharmacy practitioners as well as others in solving medication therapy situations. Individuals with special training as medication information specialists will be needed to operate the centers, and provide leadership in the area of drug informatics, institutional drug policy, poison control, pharmaceutical industry, and academia.

Study Questions

1. How has computer technology changed the ability of a user to store and access information regarding patients and their medications?

2. How can the process of evidence-based medicine be integrated into drug policy development?

3. How has consumerism changed the practice of medication information?

4. What are the differences between the functions of a traditional medication information center and a poison control center?

5. What are the skills needed by pharmacists to perform medication information functions?

REFERENCES

1. Parker PF. The University of Kentucky drug information center. Am J Hosp Pharm 1965;22:42–7.
2. Amerson AB, Wallingford DM. Twenty years' experience with drug information centers. Am J Hosp Pharm 1983;40:1172–8.
3. Walton CA. The problem of communicating clinical drug information. Am J Hosp Pharm 1965;22:458–63.
4. Lowe HJ, Barnett GO. Understanding and using the Medical Subject Headings (MeSH) vocabulary to perform literature searches. JAMA 1994;271:1103–8.
5. Mehnert RB. A world of knowledge for the nation's health: The U.S. National Library of Medicine. Am J Hosp Pharm 1986;43:2991–7.
6. Walton CA. Education and training of the drug information specialist. Drug Intelli Clin Pharm 1967;1:133–7.
7. Francke DE. The role of the pharmacist as a drug information specialist. Am J Hosp Pharm 1966;23:49.

8. Beaird SL, Coley RMR, Crea KA. Current status of drug information centers. Am J Hosp Pharm 1992;49:103–6.

9. Rosenburg JM, Ruentes RJ, Starr CH, Kirschenbaum HL, McGuire H. Pharmacist-operated medication information centers in the United States. Am J Health-Syst Pharm 1995;52:991–6.

10. Forrester LP, Scoggin JA, Valle RD. Pharmacy management company-negotiated contract for drug information services. Am J Health-Syst Pharm 1995;52:1074–7.

11. Study Commission on Pharmacy. Pharmacists for the future. Ann Arbor: Health Administration Press; 1975. p. 139.

12. Hepler CD, Strand LM. Opportunities and responsibilities in pharmaceutical care. Am J Hosp Pharm 1990;47:533–50.

13. American Society of Health-System Pharmacists. ASHP Guidelines on the provision of medication information by pharmacists. Am J Health-Syst Pharm 1996;53:1843–5.

14. Johnson ST, Wordell CJ. Internet utilization among medical information specialists in the pharmaceutical industry and academia. Drug Information Journal 1998;32:547–54.

15. Ukens C, Vecchione A. How pharmacists are riding the technology tidal wave. Hosp Pharm Rep 1997;22S–23S.

16. Malone PM, Young WW, Malesker MA. Wide area network connecting a hospital drug informatics center with a university. Am J Health-Syst Pharm 1998;55:1146–50.

17. Elson RB, Connelly DP. Computerized medical records in primary care. Their role in mediating guideline-driven physician behavior change. Arch Fam Med 1995;4:698–705.

18. Rind DM, Kohane IS, Szolovits P, Safran C, Chueh HC, Barnett GO. Maintaining the confidentiality of medical records shared over the Internet and world wide web. Ann Intern Med 1997;127:138–44.

19. Frisse ME. What is the Internet learning about you while you are learning about the Internet? Acad Med 1996;71:1064–107.

20. Blank C. Spending on pharmaceuticals will pass $180 billion by 2008. Hosp Pharma Rep 1998; 12:54.

21. Opportunities for the community pharmacist in managed care. Special Report. American Pharmaceutical Association, 1994.

22. Ellrodt G, Cook DJ, Lee J, Cho M, Hunt D, Weingarten S. Evidence-based disease management. JAMA 1997;278:1687–92.

23. Special Feature: direct-to-consumer advertising. Medical Marketing and Media 1996;15:8.

24. Piturro M. D-T-C thrives. Managed Healthcare News 1998;14:1.

25. Basara LR. The impact of a direct-to-consumer prescription medication advertising campaign on new prescription volume. Drug Information Journal 1996;30:715–29.

26. Silberg W, Lundberg GD, Musacchio RA. Assessing, controlling, and assuring the quality of medical information on the Internet. JAMA 1997;277:1244–5.

27. Wyatt J. Measuring quality and impact on the world wide web. Br Med J 1997;314:1879–81.

28. Practice and Policy Guidelines Panel, National Institutes of Health Office of Alternative Medicine. Clinical Practice Guidelines in complementary and alternative medicine: an analysis of opportunities and obstacles. Arch Fam Med 1997;6:149–54.

29. Meade V. Patient medication information hotlines multiply. Am Pharm 1991;NS31:569–71.

30. Troutman WG. Consensus-derived objectives for medication information education. Drug Information Journal 1994;28:791–6.

31. Ferrill MJ, Norton LL. Drug information to biomedical informatics: a three tier approach to building a university system for the twenty-first century. Am J Pharm Educ 1997;61:81–6.

32. Gora-Harper ML, Brandt B. An educational design to teach drug information across the curriculum. Am J Pharm Educ 1997;61:296–302.

33. American Society of Health-System Pharmacists. Residency Directory. Vol 2. Bethesda (MD): American Society of Health-System Pharmacists Inc.; 1998. pp. 59–64.

34. Woodruff AE, Hunt CA. Involvement in medical informatics may enable pharmacists to expand their consultation potential and improve the quality of healthcare. Ann Pharmacother 1992; 26:100–4.

35. Vanscoy GJ, Gajewski LK, Tyler LS, Gora-Harper ML, Grant KL, May JR. The future of medication information practices: a consensus. Ann Pharmacother 1996;30:876–81.

36. Warren PN. Pharmacists to the fore. Managed Healthcare News 1997;13:20H–20I.

37. Harrison MAJ, Draugalis JR, Slack MK, Langley PC. Cost-effectiveness of regional poison control centers. Arch Intern Med 1996;156:2601–8.

38. Gong SD, Millares M, VanRiper KB. Drug information pharmacists at health-care facilities, universities, and pharmaceutical companies. Am J Hosp Pharm 1992;49:1121–30.

2

Chapter Two

Modified Systematic Approach to Answering Questions

Craig F. Kirkwood

Objectives

After completing this chapter, the reader will be able to

- Determine pertinent background information when presented with a drug information question and given requestor demographics.
- Categorize the ultimate question and develop an efficient search strategy upon determining and soliciting the most important background information.
- Formulate a response appropriate for the sophistication of the requestor after evaluating the drug information and literature obtained from a search.
- List the categories of drug information questions that are appropriate for follow-up.
- Identify one potential question that would benefit from using the modified systematic approach and describe the advantages of the approach for each potential question identified, given three different practice settings.

"Ask a silly question, get a silly answer" is a common expression, and several cartoonists have capitalized on the humor of the customer service schedule that includes "Answers $10; Correct Answers $15." Regarding the scientific method, a similar phrase is "How you word your question determines your answer." A common expression overheard within many pharmacy practices, as a pharmacist responds to another health care provider, is "Why didn't he tell me that's what he really wanted in the first place?" The scenario may be a pharmacist responding to an interaction with a physician, manager, or

TABLE 2–1. SYSTEMATIC APPROACH (1975)

Step I.	Classification of the request
Step II.	Obtaining background information
Step III.	Systematic search
Step IV.	Response
Step V.	Reclassification

SOURCE: Watanabe et al.[1]

patient. An alternative scenario may be a technician or assistant responding to an interaction with a pharmacist. In any language, the information a person requests (i.e., what is asked) may not be what a person desires, and health care practices are not exempt from this problem.

In 1975, Watanabe et al.[1] presented a systematic approach for responding to drug information requests. The systematic approach was comprised of five steps (Table 2–1) and was developed to provide instruction for pharmacy students. These concepts were expanded and embellished to produce a textbook on the subject of drug information services.[2] For several years, the original article and subsequent textbook served as the core for training pharmacy students and practitioners about responding to drug information requests.[3] The systematic approach principles were used in assuring quality for drug information service responses, training in drug information skills, and developing and enhancing programs[4–6] (see Appendix 2–1, Drug Information Response Quality Assurance Evaluation). New technologies have facilitated the labor-intensive teaching of the systematic approach to students and practitioners, either in a modified version as the subject of a computer program[7] or as a module of a more complete drug information computer program.[8] The modified systematic approach has been adapted by others and used for the combined purposes of quality assurance and student evaluation in drug information clerkships.[9] The subsequent chapters of this book follow the modified systematic approach.

Modified Systematic Approach

Drug information services may use the systematic approach, or an adaptation of it, as the basis for responding to drug information inquiries (see Appendix 2–2, Drug Information Request/Response Form); however, the utility of this approach is not limited to the confines of a drug information center. These approaches have application in any pharmacy practice area, including community pharmacy, the pharmaceutical industry, and institutional pharmacy management, as well as general application in any type of professional consultation. The steps to the modified systematic approach (Table 2–2) will be reviewed in this chapter.

TABLE 2–2. MODIFIED SYSTEMATIC APPROACH (1987)

Step I.	Secure demographics of requestor.
Step II.	Obtain background information.
Step III.	Determine and categorize ultimate question.
Step IV.	Develop strategy and conduct search.
Step V.	Perform evaluation, analysis, and synthesis.
Step VI.	Formulate and provide response.
Step VII.	Conduct follow-up and documentation.

Source: From Host and Kirkwood.[7]

REQUESTOR DEMOGRAPHICS

The first step in the modified systematic approach is to accept the initial question and secure requestor demographics. Although the presentation of the initial question provides insight to the requestor's sophistication and knowledge regarding the subject matter, it is important to more directly determine the requestor's position, training, and anticipated knowledge. For example, an elderly patient and cardiovascular specialist may each inquire about the availability of an investigational medication; however, each brings a different frame of reference to the request, and the approach and final response to the request will differ for each requestor. In addition to information regarding the requestor's background, it is imperative to secure a mechanism for delivery of the response, regardless of the medium (e.g., verbal, written, e-mail). Therefore, telephone number(s), fax number, pager number, and/or address (mail or e-mail) or location, and so on, are important facts to obtain from the requestor.

BACKGROUND QUESTIONS

The ability to obtain background information, to develop a more complete picture of the question, is essential for effectively using the modified systematic approach. Historically, this step is the most difficult for both students and practicing pharmacists. If an individual can truly answer the question "Why is the requestor asking for this information?" then adequate background information has been obtained. To answer this question, the background information must be sufficiently comprehensive. This places the responder in a conflict: the quantity of background information must be sufficient, but the requestor's and responder's time are at a premium—if the responder is perceived as inefficient, it will alienate the requestor, a productive exchange may not occur, and an opportunity will be lost.

Background questions, therefore, must be appropriate for the circumstances. Some general information should always be obtained; for example, whether the request is concerning a specific patient's condition or is truly academic. Other background questions should be specific for the nature of the request. Examples of general background questions are provided in Table 2–3; examples of specific background questions are provided in Appendix 2–3. Background question inquiry and reply, when performed optimally, should be a dialogue. During this dialogue the sequence and exact wording of each background question must depend on the flow of the verbal interaction. Rarely will one obtain adequate background information by forcibly demanding such information. An interrogation style will perhaps be effective only in a superior-to-subordinate relationship.

On occasion one may discover, while researching a request, that inadequate background information was obtained. This predicament may result when either the wrong questions were asked or the background assessment was insufficient (e.g., the responder was not adequately familiar with the subject matter). If one consumed considerable time in obtaining background information originally, exhausting the time and confidence of the requestor is a possible risk to returning with more background questions. In this setting, a technique of "bait and hook" may be applied and achieve satisfactory results. This method involves providing a portion of the response and linking it to an important background question. Based on the background information obtained, more response or questions would follow. Be forewarned that the risk of the requestor "running" with the portion of the response is real, and the outcome of the exchange may be more detrimental than the outcome of losing a requestor who received no response. Given these risks, the "bait and hook" technique should be limited to cases in which the original collection of background information was unfinished and incomplete.

Although often neglected, it is commonly useful to ascertain which resource(s) the requestor has checked or used. This information is useful to avoid duplication of effort; however, often individuals do not know how to effectively use the resource(s) available to them. The responder may need to double-check the used resources to verify the information present or better appreciate the requestor's understanding of the subject. Knowledge of resources used is also helpful in determining the baseline sophistication of requestor. For example, one would consider the user of the primary literature to be more sophisticated than the requestor who only used a general reference.

TABLE 2–3. GENERAL QUESTIONS FOR OBTAINING BACKGROUND INFORMATION

Requestor's name
Requestor's location and/or pager number
Requestor's affiliation (institution or practice), if a health care professional
Requestor's frame of reference (i.e., title, profession or occupation, rank)
Resources that the requestor already consulted
Whether the request is patient specific or academic
Patient's diagnosis, other medications, and pertinent medical information
Urgency of the request (i.e., negotiate the time response)

Source: Standard Questions for Obtaining Background Information from Requestors. *Drug Information Service, Department of Pharmacy Services, Medical College of Virginia Hospitals, ca. 1990.*

Requestors who are intermediaries in the transfer of information present a special challenge for obtaining background. Intermediaries may include medical students, nurses, pharmacists, and administrators' assistants—generally anyone involved in the process that is not truly the end-user of the response. In some situations, the intermediary may not have sufficient information to satisfy background questions. In other cases, the intermediary may put an incomplete "twist" on the background information according to their frame of reference. (Most students by high school have played a game of story sharing: the student in one corner of the classroom tells the student immediately behind her a multifaceted "secret," and the second student in turn tells a third and so on, until the "secret" has been told to the last student. Generally, the final data are significantly different from the original "secret" as everyone lends their own frame of reference to the information.) When dealing with intermediaries, one must decide to work with them (i.e., educate them concerning the information needed, and why it's needed) or bypass them (i.e., interact with the end-user of the information directly). Each option has its strengths and weaknesses, and the decision must be made on a case-by-case basis. One should not allow an intermediary with incomplete or inaccurate background information to drive the consultative process.

With practice, the process of obtaining background information can become an admirable skill. When background questions are utilized appropriately, the response to information requests or inquiries is very efficient. Like other skills, however, obtaining background information requires practice to maintain competence. An anecdotal observation from the Medical College of Virginia Hospitals' Drug Information Service is that a substantial loss of skill regarding the gathering of background information occurs if one stops the practice for more than 8 consecutive weeks. When done correctly and efficiently as a result of continuous application, all parties involved (requestor, responder, and patient or health care system) benefit.

ULTIMATE QUESTION/CATEGORIZATION OF QUESTION

After a precursor of the modified systematic approach was instituted, a survey of drug information questions answered by the Drug Information Service at the Medical College of Virginia Hospitals over a 6-month period was performed. In 85% of the questions, the subject researched (termed the ultimate question) was significantly different than the original question, such that provision of the final response would not have agreed with the initial question. For these questions (i.e., disagreement between original question and response provided), the requestor was satisfied with the response provided (i.e., the answer to the ultimate question). This disparity demonstrates that refocusing the requestors' question was useful for most of the drug information requests in the survey.

The determination of the ultimate question is important for effective use of the modified systematic approach. If background information is obtained in an open, productive exchange, the ultimate question is easily unveiled; if adequate background information is not obtained, the determination of the ultimate question may not be possible. The ultimate question may essentially be the same as the original question, particularly if the question is truly not patient specific. An example of the difference between an original question and the ultimate question (which was researched) is provided in Appendix 2–4. In this case, responding to the original question possibly would have precluded two therapeutic options—one because the original drug may not have been readily available for the specific patient's disease, and the other because an equally effective, unrestricted alternative may not have been fully considered. Occasionally, the pursuit of the ultimate question provides an opportunity for injection of another professional's perspective, and this process alone may lead to consideration of other useful therapeutic approaches.

It is imperative that the requestor confirm the ultimate question prior to categorization and the development of a search strategy. To avoid having the requestor interpret the response to a different (the ultimate) question as condescending, the discussion must be tactful and oriented toward the attainment of the common goal of both requestor and responder.

Although perhaps best described as a requestor demographic, the expected time of response should be discussed at this juncture. This time should be negotiated based on the requestor's needs and the responder's realistic assessment of the information or literature, as well as other factors (e.g., other competing responsibilities, resource limitations). If a realistic agreement cannot be met, mutually acceptable alternative plans may be made. Because one is essentially serving in the role of a consultant, the responder should not accept an insufficient completion time for the appeasement of the requestor.

Once the ultimate question has been decided and acknowledged, the question is categorized. Categorization is useful not only for the initial development of the search strategy, but also for the determination of resources and staff training to be maintained. Categorization schemes vary among drug information services; the best scheme is the one that is closest to meeting the service needs. An example of a categorization scheme, with the selection of a category for an ultimate question, is shown in Appendix 2–2. Once an ultimate question is categorized, the development of a search strategy has been initiated.

SEARCH STRATEGY

The categorization of the ultimate question prompts the resource selection process. For example, the categorization of a question as "adverse effect" suggests the use of adverse effect–oriented resources. Once resources have been selected, they are prioritized based on probability of containing the information or data desired. Without prioritization, resources may be utilized based on ease of access or degree of comfort, instead of probable efficiency. The resources are thoroughly characterized in Chap. 4.

To assist in mapping the search process and developing a response, the utility of all selected references and secondary resources is noted on the request/response form. A simple method is to use a nominal scale (e.g., notation of "+, ~, or –" for useful, somewhat useful, and not useful reference), and place the notation immediately after the name of the resource utilized on the request/response form. Although this process may seem obsessive, the benefit regarding the rebuilding of available information is substantial, and the process will facilitate the preparation of the practice's budget, as the utility of resources compared to the practice's needs is objectively (rather than subjectively) demonstrated.

DATA EVALUATION, ANALYSIS, AND SYNTHESIS

At this step in the modified systematic approach, the information retrieved must be objectively critiqued. The techniques and skills for literature evaluation and clinical application of statistical analysis, as discussed in detail in Chaps 6 through 10, are applied at this juncture. Application of these skills at this step is one of the opportunities to differentiate the professional from the technician through using the modified systematic approach. The analysis and synthesis must be performed with consideration of the background information obtained previously for the response to be pertinent and useful to the requestor.

FORMULATION AND PROVISION OF RESPONSE

Although one cannot absolutely know how another individual will use information provided, a responder should think about how the soon-to-be-provided information may be used. This thought process should reference the background information received when formulating the search question. Although it would be unethical to misrepresent results of the analysis and synthesis of the literature evaluated, one may formulate a response that discourages a reaction that the responder believes is not supported by the interpretation of the literature. As a consultant, one has a professional responsibility to clearly inform the requestor when one course of action is clearly more desirable than an alternate action. This consideration is not an issue when the analysis and synthesis of literature or information leads to an unequivocal conclusion concerning two mutually exclusive courses of action.

TABLE 2–4. FORMAT FOR LOGICAL ARGUMENT IN RESPONSE FORMULATION

Step I.	Present the competing viewpoints or considerations.
Step II.	State the assessment of the literature or information reviewed and claim the superior viewpoint.
Step III.	Succinctly refute the major strengths and present weaknesses of the inferior viewpoint.
Step IV.	Defend the major weaknesses and promote the strengths of the superior viewpoint.
Step V.	Reiterate the final assessment in support of the superior viewpoint.

If the literature includes conflicting data that must be presented to the requestor, one may need to use a logical argument. Should only one side of the conflict be presented, the requestor may not benefit from the complete picture or may mistrust the responder upon later learning that another aspect of the conflict was not represented. The steps to follow in this scenario, after restatement of the ultimate question, are presented in Table 2–4. Despite the setting or circumstances, the formulated response must be succinct and adequately comprehensive.

The provision of a response is essential in the modified systematic approach. If the response is not provided in a timely manner or is delivered at an inappropriate level of sophistication, conceivably the effort expended would be wasted. The subject of written communications will be considered in Chap. 11. Verbal communications, however, are more frequently used within most practice settings. The utilization of good verbal communication skills, from confident delivery to correct pronunciation of all terms, is imperative for ideal response provision. Often the delivery of a complete response is analogous to the delivery of a presentation or lecture—one must be prepared for additional questions. Therefore, the information presented is only part of the responder's total knowledge and preparation on the subject. The remnants from the process of preparing a succinct response are typically the material used for addressing additional minor questions.

FOLLOW-UP, FOLLOW-THROUGH, AND DOCUMENTATION

Follow-up is the process of verifying the appropriateness, correctness, and completeness of a response following the communication. Not only is follow-up "good business," it presents a professional approach to consultative assistance. Certain circumstances command follow-up. Patient-specific requests, especially if judgmental (i.e., therapeutic assistance or dosing recommendations), are outstanding opportunities for follow-up. Any situation in which a therapeutic decision depended on assumptions or "soft" data is also a candidate for follow-up. Pharmacy services and practices, in addition to patients and health care providers, may benefit substantially through the provision of follow-up assistance. Providing follow-up assistance for responses that subsequently led to dependent administrative decisions can enhance the perception of service delivery and the quality of the complete response.

Follow-through is the process of readdressing a request based on the availability of new data or a change in the situation or circumstances that were decisive factors in the synthesis of a response. For example, the basis of a decision to use a novel therapy in a patient may be confirmed or refuted according to a new article. In the same scenario, the development of renal failure (as a comorbidity) in this patient may prompt an update of the original response. In most circumstances, the provision of follow-through may also be perceived as good practice. Providing an update, when new information becomes available supports the responder's expertise and command of the literature. The update of current information would be particularly useful in chronic patients or administrative problems.

Thorough documentation is essential for reducing one's liability, and potentially promoting the development of a continual service. The method of documentation may be a simple form or an extensive review and summation of all processes completed. At a minimum, the ultimate question (as verified by the requestor), the materials searched (with pertinent findings noted), the response, and follow-up (or follow-through, if applicable) should be documented. For reimbursement of services and credit of service delivery, it may be necessary to record the achievement of the objectives in service provision. Regarding professional liability concerns, an attorney familiar with the requirements of the specific locality may be consulted. The documentation of improved patient outcomes subsequent to a response for information would be an optimal method for justification of practices.[10]

Summary

More than 20 years ago, Watanabe and colleagues presented a systematic approach for responding to drug information requests. The systematic approach, which consisted of five steps as outlined in Table 2-1, was developed to provide instruction for pharmacy students. Modifications of the systematic approach (an example is outlined in Table 2-2) have been utilized by others in service provision, practice quality assurance, and student evaluation. The enhancements, relative to the original systematic approach, are reasonable when one considers the explosion of drug information in the last 20 years; the expansion, sophistication, and patient orientation of pharmacy services today; and the growth and advancement of drug information resources over the past two decades. The modified systematic approach preludes the retrieval of drug literature or information with the securing of requestor's demographics, determination of related background information, and probable reformulation (with classification) of the original search question. Following the development of an efficient search strategy, the completion of the search, and evaluation, analysis, and synthesis of the information retrieved, a response is formulated and provided to the requestor. When indicated, follow-up and/or follow-through assistance is provided and the process is well documented. As a result of this approach, questions that appear more difficult and complex, as presented by the requestor, are therefore more amenable to response; questions that appear easy or simple upon initial presentation often require greater effort and consideration than was first apparent. Although the use of the modified systematic approach to significantly improve patient outcomes or administrative decisions has not been demonstrated, several quality assurance programs for drug information responses consider the adherence of the modified systematic approach as cornerstone to ideal practice.

The modified systematic approach has its proponents and opponents. From the opponents, the most frequently cited disadvantage is the substantial energy expenditure in documentation. This documentation, however, is useful for the defense of a response or a recommendation, whether it be in a legal or consultative scenario. If the practice site is a drug information center, the documentation available from completed responses may be utilized for the development of a database of requests/responses (as discussed in Chap. 5, considering placing this material on a web server for easy access by practitioners in an institution). Documentation may also be utilized for the justification of pharmaceutical care services, or enhancement of practice-related responsibilities or compensation.

Use of the modified systematic approach offers practice-related advantages. First, the responder is prompted to practice in a consultative capacity (i.e., engage the requestor and garner important background information), rather than in a technical manner (i.e., passively responding to each question without insight). Second, the responder will perform efficiently. For example, using the modified systematic approach, the requestor will determine the ultimate question early in the exchange, rather than after work has been expended to answer an incomplete or incorrect original question. Selection of resources may be more efficient through use of the modified systematic approach, rather than using the most familiar or readily available resource, the best resource would be utilized first. As stated, the additional effort expended in documentation could be very useful for the practitioner. These advantages are generally pertinent to the use of the modified systematic approach regardless of the practice setting or responsibilities.

Study Questions

1. A caller requests information regarding the use of aspirin for the prevention of preeclampsia.

   a. List the steps involved in the modified systematic approach to answering questions. What is the importance of each of these steps?

   b. What specifics regarding caller demographics should be secured?

   c. What questions should be asked to obtain background information from the caller? Consider different questions that could be asked depending on the focus of the request (e.g., general information, dosage, method of administration, drug interactions, drug of choice, adverse effects, teratogenicity).

   d. Depending on its focus, the request could be categorized in several ways. Considering the possible focuses listed in Part c, categorize the question and develop possible search strategies.

   e. Considering the possible focuses listed in Part c and various caller backgrounds (e.g., consumer, pharmacist, physician), evaluate, analyze, and synthesize data to be used for answering the request.

   f. For the possible scenarios listed in Part e, formulate oral and written responses to the request.

   g. For the possible scenarios listed in Part e, consider follow-up questions that should be asked of the caller.

2. Considering three different practice settings (i.e., hospital, community pharmacy, pharmaceutical manufacturer, ambulatory clinic, insurance company) identify potential questions that would benefit by using the modified systematic approach in formulating a response in each of those settings, and describe the advantages of the approach for each potential question identified.

REFERENCES

1. Watanabe AS, McCart G, Shimomura S, Kayser S. Systematic approach to drug information requests. Am J Hosp Pharm 1975;32(12):1282–5.
2. Watanabe AS, Conner CS. Principles of Drug Information Services. A syllabus of systematic concepts. Hamilton (IL): Drug Intelligence Publications, Inc.; 1978.
3. Limon L, Kirkwood CF, Moore AO, Mullins PM. Evaluating drug information performance of staff pharmacists. Paper presented at the 22nd Annual ASHP Midyear Clinical Meeting. December 1987; Atlanta. Abstract.
4. Kirkwood CF, Jackson D. Effect of implementation of a quality assurance program on performance of a drug information service. Paper presented at the 20th Annual ASHP Midyear Clinical Meeting. December 1985; New Orleans. Abstract.
5. Kirkwood CF. Quality assurance in drug information at the Medical College of Virginia Hospitals. Paper presented at the 22nd Annual ASHP Midyear Clinical Meeting. December 1987; Atlanta. Abstract.
6. Kirkwood CF, Kessler JM. Influencing physician use of a drug information service. Paper presented at the 19th Annual ASHP Midyear Clinical Meeting. December 1984; Dallas. Abstract.

7. Host TR, Kirkwood CF. Computer-assisted instruction for responding to drug information requests. Paper presented at the 22nd Annual ASHP Midyear Clinical Meeting. December 1987; Atlanta. Abstract.

8. Tunget CL, Smith GH, Lipsy RJ, Schumacher RJ. Evaluation of DILearn: An interactive computer-assisted learning program for drug information. Am J Pharm Educ 1993;57(4):340–3.

9. Restino MSR, Knodel LC. Drug information quality assurance program used to appraise students' performance. Am J Hosp Pharm 1992;49(6):1425–9.

10. Hermes ER, Kirkwood CF, Mullins PM, Pugh MC, Memmott HL. Evaluation of impact of drug information responses on patient care. Paper presented at the 27th Annual ASHP Midyear Clinical Meeting. December 1992; Orlando. Abstract.

3

Chapter Three

Formulating Effective Responses and Recommendations: A Structured Approach

Karim Anton Calis • Amy Marie Heck

Objectives

After completing this chapter, the reader will be able to

- Develop strategies to overcome the impediments that prevent pharmacists from providing effective responses and recommendations.
- Outline the procedures that are necessary to identify the true drug information needs of the requester.
- List the four critical factors that should be considered and systematically evaluated when formulating a response.
- Define analysis and synthesis and explain how they are employed in the process of formulating responses and recommendations.
- List the elements and characteristics of effective responses to drug information queries.

Pharmacists are asked to provide responses to a variety of drug information questions every day. While the type of requester, query, and setting can vary, the process of formulating responses remains consistent. This chapter elaborates on the basic concepts and principles presented in preceding chapters, and introduces an organized, structured approach for formulating effective responses and recommendations.

As the medical literature expands, access to drug information resources by health care professionals and the public continues to grow. Yet many professionals and consumers lack the necessary skills to use this information effectively. This presents an opportunity and a challenge for pharmacists who wish to become bonafide drug therapy experts and assume a broader role in health care.

Regardless of specialty or practice site, pharmacists must strive to become pharmacotherapy specialists. Whether in a community pharmacy, outpatient clinic, or at the hospital bedside, pharmacists can apply their knowledge to the care of patients. The role of the pharmacist should not be limited to that of information dispenser or gatekeeper. Pharmacists must extend their knowledge of drugs and therapeutics to the clinical management of individual patients or the care of large populations, and promote rational pharmacotherapy by ensuring that drug information is appropriately interpreted and correctly applied.

Accepting Responsibility and Eliminating Barriers

Pharmacists should recognize that their responsibility extends beyond simply providing an answer to a question. Rather, it is to assist in resolving therapeutic dilemmas or managing patients' medication regimens. Knowledge of pharmacotherapy alone does not ensure success. Moreover, isolated data or information do not provide answers to questions or ensure proper patient management. In fact, it is uncommon to find comprehensive answers in the literature that completely and effectively address specific situations or circumstances that clinicians face in their daily practices. Responses and recommendations must often be thoughtfully synthesized using information and knowledge gathered from a number of diverse sources. To effectively manage the care of patients and resolve complex situations, pharmacists also need added skills and competence in problem solving and direct patient care.

For pharmacists to provide meaningful responses and effective recommendations to drug information questions, real or perceived impediments must first be overcome. One such impediment is the false perception that most drug information questions do not pertain to specific patients. Another is the perception that the seemingly casual interactions with requesters and the lack of formal, written consultation requests preclude the need for in-depth analysis and extensive involvement in patient management. Pharmacists sometimes oversimplify their interactions with requesters and fail to identify the context of the question or recognize its significance. Absence of sufficient background information and pertinent patient data greatly diminish the ability of pharmacists to provide effective responses.

Identifying the Genuine Need

Most queries that pharmacists receive are not purely academic or general in nature. They often involve specific patients and unique circumstances. For example, a physician who asks about the association of lovastatin and liver toxicity is probably not asking this question whimsically or out of curiosity. He or she most likely has a patient who has developed hepatic impairment that may be associated with the use of this medication. Other reasonable scenarios, albeit less likely, could also have prompted such a question. Even questions that are not related to patient care must be viewed in their proper context. Requesters of information are typically vague in verbalizing their needs and provide specific information only when asked. Although these requesters may seem confident about their perceived needs, they may be less certain after further probing by the pharmacist. Requesters, regardless of background, are often uncertain about what the pharmacist needs to know to assist them optimally. Therefore, critical information that defines the problem and elucidates the context of the question is not readily volunteered, but must be expertly elicited by the pharmacist using questioning strategies (asking logical questions in a logical sequence) and other means. Such information may be essential for formulating informed responses. Failure of the requester to disclose critical information or clarify the question does not obviate the need for such information or relieve the pharmacist of the responsibility to collect it. Although it is easy to assign the blame on the requester for failing to provide needed information, pharmacists must understand that it is their responsibility to obtain it completely and efficiently. Good communication skills (both listening and questioning) are essential for enabling the pharmacist to gather relevant information and understand the "real" question and the genuine needs of the requester. Providing responses and offering recommendations without knowledge of pertinent patient information, the context of the request, or how the information will be applied is irresponsible and potentially dangerous.

Before attempting to formulate responses, pharmacists must consider several important questions to ensure that they understand the context of the query and the scope of the issue or problem (Table 3–1). Without this information, pharmacists risk providing general responses that do not address the needs of the requester. More concerning, however, is that the information provided can be misinterpreted or misapplied. This not only compromises the pharmacist's credibility but also can jeopardize patient care.

Pharmacists must recognize the value and potential benefits of their contributions as members of the health care team. Lack of confidence in communicating with requesters can be a limiting factor. Because a telephone call or visit from a physician may not be perceived as a formal request for a consult, the significance of such apparently informal daily interactions can be easily overlooked. Pharmacists should understand that interactions

TABLE 3–1. QUESTIONS TO CONSIDER BEFORE FORMULATING A RESPONSE

- Do I know the requester's name, profession, and affiliation?
- Does the question pertain to a specific patient?
- Do I have a clear understanding of the question or problem?
- Do I know if the correct question is being asked?
- Do I know why the question is being asked?
- Do I understand the requester's expectations?
- Do I know pertinent patient history and background information?
- Do I know about the unique circumstances that generated the question?
- Do I know what information is really needed?
- Do I know when the information is needed and in what format?
- Do I have insight about how the information I provide will actually be used?
- Do I know how the problem or situation has been managed to date?
- Do I know about alternative explanations or management options that have been considered or should be further explored?

with physicians and other clinicians present valuable opportunities for direct involvement in patient care. The lesson often missed is that there is a fine line between a simple, seemingly general drug information question and a meaningful pharmacotherapy consult. Knowing the context of the question, obtaining the pertinent patient data and background information, and understanding the true needs of the requester can often be the difference.

Some pharmacists are quick to attempt to answer questions without adequately understanding the context or unique circumstances from which they evolved. They focus exclusively on the answer and ignore or fail to obtain key information needed to establish the framework of the question. For example, in a question about the dose of an antibiotic, an incorrect response can be formulated and inappropriate recommendations made if one fails to consider such factors as the patient's age, gender, condition being treated, end-organ function, weight and body composition, concomitant diseases (e.g., cystic fibrosis), possible drug interactions, site of infection, spectrum of activity of the antimicrobial, resistance patterns, and other factors such as pregnancy, dialysis, or other extracorporeal procedures.

In the absence of information that provides the proper context, a question about the half-life of a medication appears rather simple. However, if the question were posed for the purpose of assisting the requester in determining a sufficient washout period for a crossover study, one would be remiss if factors other than the half-life of the parent compound were not considered. Proper determination of a washout period would mandate consideration of such factors as the activity and half-lives of known metabolites; the presence of potentially interacting medications; the effects of age, illness, or end-organ dysfunction; the persistence of pharmacodynamic effects of the medication beyond its detection in the plasma (e.g., omeprazole); and the effect of administration route on the apparent half-life (e.g., transdermally administered fentanyl).

TABLE 3–2. IMPORTANT QUESTIONS NOT POSED BY THE REQUESTER

Initial query posed by requester: Can ranitidine cause thrombocytopenia?

- What is the incidence of ranitidine-induced thrombocytopenia?
- Are there any known predisposing factors?
- Is the pathogenesis of this adverse effect understood?
- How does the thrombocytopenia typically present?
- Are there any characteristic subjective or objective findings?
- Does thrombocytopenia due to ranitidine differ from that caused by other histamine-2 receptor antagonists, other medications, or other etiologies?
- Is the thrombocytopenia dose related?
- How severe can it become?
- How soon after discontinuing the drug does it reverse?
- How is it usually managed?
- What is the likelihood of cross reactivity with other histamine-2 receptor antagonists?
- How risky is rechallenge with ranitidine?
- Are there available treatments that can be used in place of ranitidine?
- Are there alternative explanations for the thrombocytopenia in this patient (including other medications, medication combinations, or underlying medical conditions)?
- What complications, if any, can be expected?

It is very important to look beyond the initial question and recognize that the requester's needs often go beyond a superficial answer to the primary question. Pharmacists should always anticipate additional questions or concerns, including those that are not directly asked or addressed by the requester. These questions must nonetheless be considered if a clinical situation is to be managed optimally. In Case Study 4, a question is posed about ranitidine as a possible cause of thrombocytopenia. Although the requester may neglect to ask additional questions, the pharmacist must anticipate and consider related issues and questions (Table 3–2). Failure to address these concerns will undoubtedly result in an incorrect or inadequate response.

Finally, pharmacists must learn to rely on their patient care skills, problem solving skills, insight, and common sense. Computer data bases and other specialized information resources can assist the pharmacist in identifying critical data, but over reliance on such resources without careful attention to pertinent background information and patient data can mislead even the most experienced clinician.

Formulating the Response

BUILDING A DATABASE AND ASSESSING CRITICAL FACTORS

Formulating a response involves a series of steps that must be performed completely, objectively, and in a logical sequence. This mandates the use of a structured, organized approach whereby critical factors are systematically considered and thoroughly evaluated. The steps in this process include assembling and organizing a patient database, gathering information about relevant disease states, collecting medication information, obtaining pertinent background information, and identifying other relevant factors and special circumstances. Table 3–3 outlines in detail the specific types of information that should be considered for each factor. It should be noted that only some of this information might be pertinent for a given query or case scenario.

For patient-related questions, development of a pharmaceutical care patient data base is one of the first steps in preparing a response. This requires collection of pertinent information from the patient, caregivers, health care providers, medical chart, and other patient records. A comprehensive medication history obtained by a pharmacist is also essential. This data base invariably includes information common to the medical and nursing data bases. Because physicians, nurses, patients, and others often lack a

TABLE 3–3. FACTORS TO BE CONSIDERED WHEN FORMULATING A RESPONSE

Patient Factors

- Demographics (e.g., name, age, height, weight, gender, race/ethnic group, setting)
- Primary diagnosis and medical problem list
- Allergies/intolerances
- End-organ function, immune function, nutritional status
- Chief complaint
- History of present illness
- Past medical history (including surgeries, radiation exposure, immunizations, psychiatric illnesses, etc.)
- Family history
- Social history (e.g., alcohol intake, smoking, substance abuse, exposure to environmental or occupational toxins, employment, income, education, religion, travel, diet, physical activity, stress, risky behavior, compliance with treatment regimen)
- Review of body systems
- Medications (prescribed, over-the-counter, and complementary/alternative)
- Physical examination
- Laboratory tests
- Diagnostic studies or procedures

Disease Factors

- Definition
- Epidemiology (including incidence and prevalence)
- Etiology
- Pathophysiology (for infectious diseases, consider site of infection, organism susceptibility, resistance patterns, etc.)
- Clinical findings (signs & symptoms, laboratory tests, diagnostic studies) [*Note:* Factors such as disease or symptom onset, duration, frequency, severity, etc. must always be carefully assessed]
- Diagnosis
- Treatment (medical, surgical, radiation, biological and gene therapies, other)
- Prevention and control
- Risk factors
- Complications
- Prognosis *continued*

TABLE 3–3. FACTORS TO BE CONSIDERED WHEN FORMULATING A RESPONSE (*Continued*)

Medication Factors

- Name of medication or substance (proprietary, nonproprietary, other)
- Status and availability (investigational, over-the-counter, prescription, orphan, foreign, complementary/alternative)
- Physicochemical properties
- Pharmacology and pharmacodynamics
- Pharmacokinetics (liberation, absorption, distribution, metabolism, and elimination)
- Uses (FDA approved and unlabeled)
- Adverse effects
- Allergy/cross reactivity
- Contraindications and precautions
- Effects of age, organ system function, disease, pregnancy, extracorporeal circulation, or other conditions or environments
- Mutagenicity and carcinogenicity
- Effect on fertility, pregnancy, and lactation
- Acute or chronic toxicity
- Drug interactions (drug–drug or drug–food)
- Laboratory test interference (analytical or physiologic effects)
- Administration (routes, methods)
- Dosage and schedule
- Dosage forms, formulations, preservatives, excipients, product appearance, delivery systems
- Monitoring parameters (therapeutic or toxic)
- Product preparation (procedures, methods)
- Compatibility and stability

Pertinent Background Information, Special Circumstances, and Other Factors

- Setting
- Context
- Sequence and timeframe of events
- Rationale for the question
- Event(s) prompting the question
- Unusual or special circumstances
- Acuity and time constraints
- Scope of question
- Desired detail or depth of response
- Limitations of available information or resources
- Completeness, sufficiency, and quality of the information
- Applicability and generalizability of the information

clear understanding of the type of information needed for effective pharmacotherapy consultations, pharmacists must be able to identify and efficiently extract pivotal patient information from diverse sources.

Once these data are collected and carefully assembled, they must be critically analyzed and evaluated in the proper context before final responses and recommendations are synthesized. Background reading on topics related to the query (diseases, medications, laboratory tests, etc.) is often essential. To effectively perform the steps outlined above, one must begin with a broad perspective (i.e., see the "big picture") to avoid losing sight of important information. Approaching the problem haphazardly or with tunnel vision, and prematurely focusing on isolated details, can misdirect even the most skilled pharmacist.

ANALYSIS AND SYNTHESIS

Analysis and synthesis of information are the most critical steps in formulating responses and recommendations. Together they assist in forming opinions, arriving at judgments, and ultimately drawing conclusions. *Analysis* is the critical assessment of the nature, merit, and significance of individual elements, ideas, or factors. Functionally, it involves separating the information into its isolated parts so that each can be critically assessed. Analysis requires thoughtful review and evaluation of the weight of available evidence.

Once the information has been carefully analyzed, synthesis can begin. *Synthesis* is the careful, systematic, and orderly process of combining or blending varied and diverse elements, ideas, or factors into a coherent response through the use of logic and deductive reasoning. This process relies not only on the type and quality of the data gathered, but also on how it is organized, viewed, and evaluated. Synthesis as it relates to pharmacotherapy involves the careful integration of critical information about the patient, disease, and medication along with pertinent background information to arrive at a judgment or conclusion. Synthesis can give existing information new meaning and, in effect, create new knowledge. Use of analysis and synthesis to formulate a response is much like assembling a jigsaw puzzle. If the pieces are identified and then grouped, organized, and assembled correctly, the picture will be comprehensible. However, if too many of the pieces are missing or are not arranged logically, it may be altogether impossible to clearly discern the image.

RESPONSES AND RECOMMENDATIONS

An effective response must obviously answer the question. Other characteristics of effective responses and recommendations are outlined in Table 3–4. The response to a question must include a restatement of the request and clear identification of the problems, issues, and circumstances. The response should begin with an introduction to the topic and systematically present the specific findings. Pertinent background information and patient data should be succinctly addressed. Conclusions and recommendations are also included in the response along with pertinent reference citations from the literature. The format of responses (verbal or written) is discussed in Chap. 11. In formulating responses, pharmacists should disclose all available information that is relevant to the question. They should also present all reasonable options and explanations along with an evaluation of each. Specific recommendations must be scientifically sound and clearly justified.

TABLE 3–4. DESIRED CHARACTERISTICS OF A RESPONSE

- Timely
- Current
- Accurate
- Complete
- Concise
- Well referenced
- Clear and logical
- Objective and balanced
- Free of bias or flaws
- Applicable and appropriate for specific circumstances
- Answers important related questions
- Addresses management of patients or situations

FOLLOW-UP

When recommendations are made, follow-up should always be provided in a timely manner. Follow-up allows pharmacists to know if their recommendations were accepted and promptly implemented. It is also a hallmark of a true professional and demonstrates the pharmacist's commitment to patient care. Furthermore, follow-up is required for outcomes assessment and, when necessary, to reevaluate the recommendations and make appropriate modifications. Finally, follow-up allows pharmacists to receive valuable feedback and learn from the experience.

Case Study 1

■ INITIAL QUESTION

What is the molecular weight of enalapril?

■ PERTINENT BACKGROUND INFORMATION OR SPECIAL CIRCUMSTANCES

The requester is a basic scientist who is conducting an in vitro experiment to evaluate the pharmacologic effects of enalapril. She would like to know the molecular weight of enalapril so that she can perform appropriate calculations specified for this experiment.

■ PERTINENT PATIENT FACTORS

N/A

■ PERTINENT DISEASE FACTORS

N/A

■ PERTINENT MEDICATION FACTORS

Enalapril is a prodrug that is converted in vivo to the active form, enalaprilat.[1,2] Both enalapril and enalaprilat are commercially available for use in the United States.

■ ANALYSIS AND SYNTHESIS

Considering that enalapril is a prodrug that must be converted to a pharmacologically active compound in vivo, and given that this researcher wishes to conduct an in vitro study, the researcher should use the active form of the drug in her experiment. She should, therefore, have requested the molecular weight of enalaprilat.

■ RESPONSE AND RECOMMENDATIONS

Enalapril is an oral angiotensin-converting enzyme inhibitor that is indicated for the management of hypertension, symptomatic congestive heart failure, and asymptomatic left ventricular dysfunction. Because enalapril is a prodrug that requires conversion to the active form, the requester was advised to consider using enalaprilat in the experiment. The molecular weight of enalaprilat is 384.43.[1,2]

■ CASE MESSAGE

This example illustrates the importance of collecting pertinent background information, even for seemingly uncomplicated questions. Failure to understand exactly how the information that you provide will be used could result in an inaccurate or misleading response. In this case, providing the molecular weight of enalapril would have resulted in wasted time and money, and the results of the experiment would likely have been invalid.

Case Study 2

■ INITIAL QUESTION

What is the maximum dose of oprelvekin (Neumega) that can be used for the treatment of thrombocytopenia?

■ PERTINENT BACKGROUND INFORMATION OR SPECIAL CIRCUMSTANCES

The requester is a physician who is managing a patient with HTLV-1–associated adult T-cell leukemia. The patient received myelosuppressive chemotherapy and subsequently developed prolonged and severe thrombocytopenia. Oprelvekin (interleukin 11) was prescribed in an attempt to improve the patient's platelet count and allow continuation of therapy. After 4 days of oprelvekin therapy (50 µg/kg/d), the platelet count did not increase substantially. The physician would like to know if doses greater than 50 µg/kg/d of oprelvekin have been studied. She plans to increase the patient's dose to 100 µg/kg/d to achieve a better response.

■ PERTINENT PATIENT FACTORS

R.R. is a 44-year-old man with HTLV-1–associated adult T-cell leukemia who has been treated with zidovudine plus interferon alpha-2b, three cycles of CHOP, and three cycles of ^{90}yttrium-labeled humanized anti-Tac (investigational regimen at the time of this case) with calcium DTPA. After these treatments, R.R. developed severe and protracted thrombocytopenia, which has prevented further treatment.

Past Medical History

- HTLV-1 adult T-cell leukemia
- Cardiomegaly (ejection fraction 0.28) secondary to AZT + INF alpha-2b treatment
- Peptic ulcer disease
- Thrombocytopenia

Social History

- Ø alcohol
- Ø tobacco

Current Medications

- Oprelvekin 50 µg/kg/d SQ
- Sucralfate oral suspension (1 g/10 mL) 20 mL bid
- Dexamethasone 40 mg po qd
- Loperamide 4 mg po prn diarrhea
- Acetaminophen 325 mg po prn headache
- ∅ complementary/alternative or other OTC medications

Allergies/Intolerances

No known drug allergies

Laboratory Results

Sodium 135 mmol/L, potassium 4.9 mmol/L, chloride 103 mmol/L, CO_2 22 mmol/L, creatinine 0.6 mg/dL, glucose 91 mg/dL, BUN 15 mg/dL, albumin 3 g/dL, calcium (total) 2.49 mmol/L, magnesium, 0.75 mmol/L, phosphorus 3.4 mg/dL, LFTs wnl, WBC 28.3×10^9/L, Hgb 10.1 g/dL, Hct 28.1%

Date	Platelet count
7/13	25 K/mm^3
7/14[a]	21 K/mm^3
7/15	26 K/mm^3
7/16	29 K/mm^3
7/17	28 K/mm^3

[a]Day 1 of oprelvekin therapy

■ PERTINENT DISEASE FACTORS

It is not known whether patients with adult T-cell leukemia respond differently to oprelvekin than those with other types of nonmyeloid malignancies.

■ PERTINENT MEDICATION FACTORS

Oprelvekin (Neumega), or recombinant interleukin-11, is indicated for the prevention of severe thrombocytopenia induced by chemotherapy. The FDA-approved dose of oprelvekin is 50 µg/kg/d for up to 21 days.[3] Platelet counts usually begin to increase between 5 to 9 days after initiation of therapy, with peak counts occurring after about 14 to 19 days of therapy.[3,4] Larger doses of oprelvekin (75 to 100 µg/kg/d) have been studied in patients with breast cancer.[5] Constitutional symptoms associated with oprelvekin therapy, such as myalgias, arthralgias, and fatigue, were noted to increase in a dose-dependent fashion. One patient who received 100 μg/kg/d of oprelvekin experienced a cerebrovascular event after the third dose. Dose escalation greater than 75 μg/kg/d was discontinued in this study, and the maximum tolerated dose of oprelvekin was determined to be 75 μg/kg/d.

■ ANALYSIS AND SYNTHESIS

Because R.R. has only received 4 days of oprelvekin treatment and platelet counts are expected to increase between 5 to 9 days after the initiation of therapy, adequate time for an optimal response to oprelvekin therapy has not been reached. In addition, oprelvekin doses higher than 75 μg/kg/d have been associated with serious adverse effects. Therefore, increasing the dose of oprelvekin in this patient is probably not necessary, and may increase the risk of serious adverse effects without providing additional therapeutic benefits.

■ RESPONSE AND RECOMMENDATIONS

Oprelvekin (Neumega), or recombinant human interleukin-11, is a thrombopoietic growth factor that stimulates the proliferation of hematopoietic stem cells and megakaryocyte progenitor cells, resulting in increased platelet production. Oprelvekin is indicated for the prevention of severe thrombocytopenia in patients with nonmyeloid malignancies who are at high risk for severe thrombocytopenia following chemotherapy.[3] Platelet counts usually begin to increase between 5 to 9 days after initiation of oprelvekin, with peak platelet counts occurring after 14 to 19 days of therapy.[3,4] R.R. has only received 4 days of oprelvekin treatment, which is insufficient for an optimal response. In addition, the adverse effects of oprelvekin therapy (e.g., myalgias, arthralgias, fatigue) are dose dependent, and the maximum tolerated dose of oprelvekin is 75 μg/kg/d.[5] Therefore, increasing the oprelvekin dose at this time is not warranted. In fact, doing so may predispose the patient to an increased risk of adverse effects without the prospect of added therapeutic benefit.

■ CASE MESSAGE

This example demonstrates the importance of understanding the proper context of the question. In this case, the physician is asking the wrong question. The pharmacist must collect critical background information to determine the actual drug information needed. Had the pharmacist failed to collect pertinent patient information, the physician would likely have increased the dose of the medication after being told that doses of 75 µg/kg/d of oprelvekin have been used. This would have been inappropriate, given that this patient had not received the medication for a sufficient duration to achieve optimal response. Moreover, larger doses of this medication are associated with a higher incidence of adverse effects.

Case Study 3

■ INITIAL QUESTION

Are there any drug interactions between labetalol, clonidine, amlodipine, lorazepam, and minoxidil?

■ PERTINENT BACKGROUND INFORMATION OR SPECIAL CIRCUMSTANCES

The requester is a physician who is caring for a patient with severe hypertension. The physician plans to add minoxidil to the antihypertensive regimen because the patient's morning blood pressure is not optimally controlled. He would like to make sure that there are no drug interactions between minoxidil and the patient's other medications.

■ PERTINENT PATIENT FACTORS

S.L. is a 40-year-old, HIV-infected man with severe hypertension and renal dysfunction.

Past Medical History

- HIV infection (1998)
- Hepatitis C (1997)
- Hypertension × 4 years
- Renal dysfunction

Social History

- 1 to 2 pints of vodka daily × 12 years
- 1 PPD of cigarettes × 25 years
- History of intravenous drug abuse

Current Medications

- Labetalol 400 mg po qd (@ 9 AM)
- Clonidine transdermal patch 0.3 mg/d
- Amlodipine 10 mg po qd (@ 9 AM)
- Lorazepam 1 mg po prn anxiety
- Multiple vitamin tablet po qd
- ∅ complementary/alternative or other OTC medications

Allergies/Intolerances

Lisinopril (angioedema)

Laboratory Results

- Sodium 136 mmol/L, potassium 4.7 mmol/L, chloride 102 mmol/L, CO_2 24 mmol/L, creatinine 2.9 mg/dL, glucose 98 mg/dL, BUN 14 mg/dL
- Viral DNA < 500 copies/mL
- CD_4 count 900 cells/mm^3

Blood Pressure Measurements

4/15		4/16		4/17	
@ 6 AM	172/116	@ 6 AM	168/110	@ 6 AM	178/114
@ noon	121/81	@ noon	116/86	@ noon	119/84
@ 8 PM	158/100	@ 8 PM	150/104	@ 8 PM	166/100

■ PERTINENT DISEASE FACTORS

None

■ PERTINENT MEDICATION FACTORS

There are no reports in the tertiary literature of drug interactions between minoxidil and any of R.L.'s current medications.[1,2,6,7] A review of the patient's current antihypertensive medications indicates that the dose of each agent is appropriate for achieving adequate blood pressure control in the face of significant renal compromise.[8] However, the duration of action of labetalol is 8 to 12 hours, and this agent is typically dosed twice daily. R.L. is receiving 400 mg of labetalol qd at 9 AM.

■ ANALYSIS AND SYNTHESIS

R.L.'s blood pressure appears to be highest in the morning, just before the daily doses of labetalol and amlodipine are administered. He is receiving 400 mg of labetalol qd at 9 AM. Because the duration of action of labetalol is 8 to 12 hours, and the usual maintenance dose is 200 to 400 mg bid, the increase in blood pressure observed in the morning could be due, at least in part, to inappropriate dosing of labetalol. This medication should generally be administered twice daily to achieve maximal benefit. Adjustment of the labetalol dose should precede the addition of other antihypertensive agents to this patient's medication regimen. Although long-term cigarette smoking can increase the cardiovascular risk associated with hypertension, there is no indication that smoking or alcohol ingestion are contributing to this patient's present problem.

■ RESPONSE AND RECOMMENDATIONS

There do not appear to be any significant drug interactions between any of R.L.'s current medications and minoxidil.[1,2,6,7] However, a review of the patient's current antihypertensive regimen indicates that the dosing of labetalol may be inadequate. The duration of action of labetalol is 8 to 12 hours, and the usual maintenance dose is 200 to 400 mg bid. Because R.L. is receiving 400 mg of labetalol once daily at 9 AM, the increase in blood pressure observed in the morning could be due to inadequate labetalol dosing. The physician was directed to optimize labetalol therapy before the addition of another antihypertensive agent. If the patient's blood pressure is not controlled with proper dosing of labetalol and minoxidil therapy is required, the physician should be advised that minoxidil is usually administered with a diuretic to prevent fluid retention.

■ CASE MESSAGE

This is another example emphasizing the importance of the proper context of the question. In this case, the pharmacist was able to recommend appropriate drug therapy management, even though the initial question posed by the physician was not related to dosage and administration of labetalol.

Case Study 4

■ INITIAL QUESTION

Can ranitidine cause thrombocytopenia?

■ PERTINENT BACKGROUND INFORMATION OR SPECIAL CIRCUMSTANCES

The requester is a physician who is evaluating a patient for suspected Cushing's disease. The patient has been hospitalized for 8 days and has undergone extensive diagnostic tests including serial blood sampling to establish the diagnosis. Over the last 4 days, the patient has experienced a rapid decline in her platelet count. The physician is aware that cimetidine can cause thrombocytopenia. Her patient is taking ranitidine, and she would like to know if the thrombocytopenia could be induced by this medication.

■ PERTINENT PATIENT FACTORS

L.B. is a 38-year-old obese woman with Type 2 diabetes who is being evaluated for Cushing's disease.

Past Medical History
- Gastroesophageal reflux disease (GERD) × 6 years
- Type 2 diabetes × 1 year

Social History
- Ø alcohol
- Ø tobacco

Current Medications
- Ranitidine 150 mg po bid (intermittently for 6 years)
- Metformin 500 mg po tid (for about 8 months)
- Heparin 100 USP U/mL (prn for flushing heparin lock)
- Ø complementary/alternative or OTC medications

Allergies/Intolerances

Penicillin (rash)

Laboratory Results

Sodium 137 mmol/L, potassium 4.9 mmol/L, chloride 102 mmol/L, CO_2 24 mmol/L, creatinine 0.9 mg/dL, glucose 133 mg/dL, BUN 12 mg/dL, albumin 3.4 G/dL, calcium 2.35 mmol/L, magnesium, 0.81 mmol/L, phosphorus 3.8 mg/dL, LFT's wnl, WBC 5.6×10^9/L

Date	Platelet count
4/20[a]	230 K/mm^3
4/24	212 K/mm^3
4/25	159 K/mm^3
4/26	114 K/mm^3
4/27	97 K/mm^3
4/28	81 K/mm^3

[a]Day of admission

■ PERTINENT DISEASE FACTORS

L.B.'s thrombocytopenia is of new onset and is characterized by a rapid decline in the platelet counts over a few days. This patient does not appear to have a readily identifiable medical condition as a likely cause of the thrombocytopenia.

■ PERTINENT MEDICATION FACTORS

Metformin has not been reported as a cause of thrombocytopenia.[1,2] Ranitidine, however, has been infrequently associated with thrombocytopenia.[1,2,9,10] This is a relatively rare but readily reversible complication of ranitidine therapy.[1,10] Ranitidine-induced thrombocytopenia usually develops within the first 30 days of therapy, but its pathogenesis remains unclear.[1,10] Most hematologic toxicities reported with the H_2 receptor antagonists appear to occur in patients with serious concomitant diseases or in those receiving other treatments more commonly associated with hematologic adverse effects.[9,10] Thrombocytopenia has been reported in about 5% of patients treated with heparin.[1] Heparin-induced thrombocytopenia does not appear to be dose dependent and has been reported in patients receiving less than 500 units of heparin per day. This condition typically develops within 5 to 9 days after initiation of therapy and reverses readily after discontinuation of the drug.

■ ANALYSIS AND SYNTHESIS

Although both ranitidine and heparin have been reported to cause thrombocytopenia, heparin appears to be the most likely culprit in this case. L.B. has been taking ranitidine intermittently for nearly 6 years. Thrombocytopenia induced by H_2 receptor antagonists usually develops within the first 30 days of therapy. Moreover, heparin-induced thrombocytopenia is a more common adverse effect and has been reported in patients receiving very small daily doses of heparin (including heparin lock flush solution). It usually develops within 5 to 9 days after initiation of therapy. Based on the presentation and temporal sequence of events, heparin-induced thrombocytopenia is the most likely explanation for L.B.'s acute drop in platelet count.

■ RESPONSE AND RECOMMENDATIONS

A review of L.B.'s current medications reveals two agents, ranitidine and heparin, that have been reported to cause thrombocytopenia.[1,2,9] Ranitidine-induced thrombocytopenia is most likely to occur within the first 30 days of therapy.[1,2] Because L.B. has been taking ranitidine intermittently for GERD for approximately 6 years, it is unlikely that ranitidine is responsible for the acute decrement in platelet count. Ranitidine, however, cannot be immediately ruled out as a possible cause. Heparin-induced thrombocytopenia is a more common adverse effect that has been reported even with very small daily doses of heparin (e.g., heparin lock flush solution). The thrombocytopenia is acute and usually develops within 5 to 9 days after initiation of therapy.[1] Based on the presentation and temporal relationship, heparin appears to be the most likely cause of thrombocytopenia in this patient. The physician was advised to discontinue the heparin lock flush solution and closely monitor the patient's platelet count. If the counts do not return to normal within several days after discontinuation of heparin, other potential causes of thrombocytopenia should be considered. However, if the platelet counts recover after discontinuation of heparin, testing for heparin antibodies (using a commercial laboratory) is advised to confirm the diagnosis of an immune-mediated reaction and guide future therapy.

■ CASE MESSAGE

This question highlights the importance of skillful problem solving. As always, collecting appropriate background information and patient data is critical. Analyzing this information before synthesizing a logical response is paramount for effective patient management. In this case, failure to recognize that the patient was receiving heparin lock flush solution could have inappropriately excluded heparin as a possible cause of the thrombocytopenia.

Conclusion

Formulating effective responses and recommendations requires use of a structured, organized approach whereby critical factors are systematically considered and thoroughly evaluated. The steps in this process include organizing a patient data base, gathering information about relevant disease states, collecting medication information, obtaining pertinent background information, and identifying other relevant factors and special circumstances. Once these data are collected and carefully assembled, they must be critically analyzed and evaluated in the proper context. Responses and recommendations are synthesized by integrating data from these diverse sources through the use of logic and deductive reasoning.

Study Questions

1. Why is it necessary to gather background information and patient data? Why do pharmacists often fail to obtain this information?

2. What factors should be considered in making a recommendation regarding dosage and administration of an antibiotic? Provide a justification for each factor.

3. Given the question "Can naproxen cause nephrotoxicity?", list at least five related questions that should also be considered.

4. List three patient-related factors that should be considered for a question pertaining to potential drug interactions.

BIBLIOGRAPHY

Watanabe AS, Conner CS. Principles of drug information services. Hamilton (IL): Drug Intelligence Publications Inc; 1978.

Galt KA, Calis KA, Turcasso NM. Clinical skills program: Module 3 drug information. Bethesda (MD): American Society of Health-System Pharmacists Inc; 1995.

REFERENCES

1. McEvoy GK, ed. AHFS drug information 98. Bethesda (MD): American Society of Health-System Pharmacists; 1998.
2. Physicians' desk reference. 52nd ed. Montvale (NJ): Medical Economics; 1998.
3. Neumega [package insert]. Cambridge (MA): Genetics Institute; 1997.
4. Gelman CR, Rumack BH, Hutchison TA, eds. DRUGDEX® system. Englewood (CO): MICRO-MEDEX, Inc.; 1998.
5. Gordon MS, McCaskill-Stevens WJ, Battiato LA, Loewy J, Loesch D, Breeden E, et al. A phase I trial of recombinant human interleukin-11 (Neumega® rhIL-11 growth factor) in women with breast cancer receiving chemotherapy. Blood 1996;87(9):3615–3624.
6. Hansten PD, Horne JR. Hansten & Horn's drug interactions analysis and management. Vol 2. Vancouver (WA): Applied Therapeutics, Inc.; 1998.
7. Tatro DS, ed. Drug interaction facts. St. Louis: Facts and Comparisons; 1998.
8. Bennett WM, Aronoff GR, Golper TA, Morrison G, Brater DC, Singer I, eds. Drug prescribing in renal failure. 3rd ed. Philadelphia: American College of Physicians; 1994.
9. Dukes MNG, ed. Meyler's side effects of drugs. 13th ed. Amsterdam: Elsevier Science; 1996.
10. Yim JM, Frazier JL. Ranitidine and thrombocytopenia. j Pharm Technol 1995;11:263–266.

4

Chapter Four

Drug Information Resources

Karen L. Kier • Patrick M. Malone • Kristen W. Mosdell

Objectives

After completing this chapter, the reader will be able to

- Describe how the exponential growth of drug information challenges the practice of drug information.
- Describe the attributes of and the differences between tertiary, secondary, and primary resources.
- Critique primary, secondary, and tertiary resources.
- Identify the most appropriate resources for a given drug information inquiry and use them effectively.
- Recognize that primary, secondary, and tertiary resources may be available in hard copy, CD-ROM, on-line, and/or other formats.
- Describe how to search computerized data bases.
- Describe the role of the Internet as a drug information resource.
- Recognize that professional organizations, pharmaceutical manufacturers, drug information centers, and poison control centers are alternate sources of drug information.

For centuries, management of vast quantities of medical information has challenged the disciplines of pharmacy and medicine.[1] Given the exponential rate at which information is increasing, this represents one of the greatest challenges faced by these professions today. Technology for storage and retrieval of medical information will continue to advance to meet these demands, resulting in a greater dependence on electronic information management. Today, medical information is stored in a variety of media—textbooks, journals, newsletters, microfiche, optical disks, computer systems, and so on. Proficiency in strategies for searching this medical information is of vital importance to pharmacists striving to meet the demands of pharmaceutical care.

Recognizing the most appropriate resources to consult in a given clinical situation and how to apply these resources increases the likelihood of locating relevant medical information and, therefore, improves the level of patient care. The purpose of this chapter is to introduce the various resources available to pharmacists, highlight their attributes, and provide information to help the reader learn how to best use these resources.

Modified Systematic Approach to Drug Information

As presented in Chap. 2, the modified systematic approach to answering drug information questions consists of the following steps: (1) secure demographics of requestor, (2) obtain background information, (3) determine and categorize the ultimate question, (4) develop a search strategy and conduct search, (5) perform evaluation, analysis, and synthesis, (6) formulate and provide response, and (7) conduct follow-up and documentation.[2] To perform Step 4 appropriately and efficiently, an understanding of the numerous resources available is needed. When a question is asked, resources need to be prioritized on the basis of their likelihood for containing the requested information. This requires knowledge of the content of the resources, as well as proficiency in searching the resource.

Generally, a stepwise approach is used for searching drug information resources, which involves consulting tertiary and secondary (e.g., indexing and abstracting services, which can be computer based or hard copy) sources followed by primary (e.g., research articles from biomedical journals) resources. Tertiary references provide rapid access to information and familiarize the reader with the topic; however, they are often several years out of date and may not reflect current standards of practice. Further information, when necessary, can be obtained by searching the biomedical literature through use of an indexing and abstracting service. Indexing and abstracting services reference both review articles and primary research articles from various journals and can provide further insight into a topic. Primary articles can be used for obtaining more in-depth, current information and allow the reader to critique study methodology to determine whether the results and conclusions are valid. It should also be mentioned that a valid resource is an expert in the field. Such an expert can be consulted before, during, or after any of the above steps, although it should be noted that such an expert will not always be available or willing to help. Also, it is becoming increasingly common that questions are derived from news reports, thus news web sites may need to be regularly consulted for background information before proceeding with further searching. These and other potential sources of information will be covered in more detail in the later sections of this chapter and in Chap. 5.

Oftentimes, a search does not require use of all three types of resources. For example, information to be provided to a patient as part of a consultation will likely be found in tertiary resources. Likewise, simple questions such as those pertaining to availability of dosage strengths and forms, active ingredients of preparations, or FDA-approved indications may be easily located in tertiary references. If an adequate answer is found in tertiary resources, it is possible to conclude the search at that point; however, sometimes the information found in tertiary resources needs to be validated, more in-depth information is required to address the question, or an answer cannot be located in tertiary resources. Consultation with secondary and primary resources is then necessary.

The type of requester may also dictate which resources are used when answering drug information questions.[3] As stated, information to be provided to a patient probably can be located in tertiary resources, which provide drug information in lay language. Nurses may be interested in questions pertaining to administration of drugs or compatibility of medications that also may be located in tertiary resources. Physicians, on the other hand, may require more in-depth information related to pharmacotherapeutic management of disease states. In these situations, primary research that the physician can critique and discuss with colleagues may be useful or specifically requested.

Tertiary Literature

The *tertiary literature*,[3–6] sometimes referred to as general literature, consists of textbooks (e.g., *Goodman and Gilman's The Pharmacological Basis of Therapeutics*), compendia (e.g., *American Hospital Formulary Service, Drug Information, Drug Facts and Comparisons*), and full-text computer data bases (e.g., *MICROMEDEX Computerized Clinical Information System* [CCIS], CliniSphere). In addition, review articles in biomedical journals are sometimes classified as tertiary literature, as is much of the information found on the Internet (Table 4–1). These references are the most commonly used sources of information because they are easy to use, convenient, concise, and compact. Often they provide a review of the literature by an acknowledged expert in the field. A great majority of the information that a practitioner needs can be found in these resources.

TABLE 4–1. TYPES OF TERTIARY LITERATURE

- Textbooks
- Compendia
- Full-text computer databases (including the Internet)
- Review articles

There are, however, some disadvantages associated with use of tertiary literature. First, the information may not be complete. Topics may be presented in insufficient detail due to space limitations of the textbook or the degree of importance placed on the topic by the author. Authors also may conduct incomplete literature searches prior to writing a textbook, thus failing to include all pertinent information on a topic. Second, information may not be timely. "New" textbooks may be several years out of date owing to lag time that occurs from the time a book is written until the time it is published. Because standards of medical practice may change during this lag time, a new textbook may not contain all of the relevant or important information in a field. Finally, various other problems may occur in tertiary literature such as human bias, errors in transcription, incorrect interpretation of research, and lack of expertise by the author. In general, the reader should judge a tertiary reference as carefully as a journal article (see Chaps 6 and 7). Several issues that should be considered when evaluating tertiary literature are addressed below.

- Does the author have sufficient experience and expertise to be writing on the topic? Despite experience and credentials, however, some authors may promote information not supported in the biomedical literature.
- Is this the most recent edition of the tertiary reference? Is the information contained in the most recent edition likely to be timely based on the date of publication of the textbook? Occasionally, it is necessary to use older editions (e.g., to identify a product removed from the market years ago), but typically the most recent information available is sought.
- Are statements of fact appropriately supported by citations? While handbooks, by necessity, leave out references, this is not desirable in any larger or computerized reference. As discussed in Chap. 11, any statement of fact is, for all practical purposes, worthless unless it is supported by the primary literature. Citations allow the reader to refer back to the original source for additional information and to verify the author's interpretation of the literature.
- Is the reference likely to contain information relevant to the subject being researched? This is based on selection of the appropriate category as part of the modified systematic approach. For example, it would be inappropriate to use a textbook focused on drug interactions to identify the active and inactive ingredients present in an unidentified tablet.

- Is the reference clear, concise, and easy to use? Time and efficiency is wasted using references that are difficult to use when friendlier alternatives are available.

Compiling a list of tertiary resources useful to the practice of pharmacy is a formidable task. The clinical setting, types of patients serviced, and budgetary constraints will all dictate the resources available at a given practice site. Minimal standards for textbooks required by law to be available at every practice site vary by state.

The following list is the authors' selection of resources found to be most beneficial in the practice of drug information. Most of these resources relate to either drug therapy or disease state management.[3] Resources related to drug therapy are organized either by individual agent or therapeutic drug class.[3] Those references that are updated yearly or more frequently are indicated. Such resources are more likely to be current than publications that are only published every 3 to 5 years. Another source of suggested references can be found at <<http://www.aacp.org/Resources/Reference/Basic_Resources/basic_resources.html>>.

Pharmacists should become familiar with this list to make knowledgeable decisions when selecting resources for various practice settings. Rarely will the texts required by state law or OBRA '90 be sufficient to meet the resource needs of pharmacists and a more comprehensive library should be developed for any practice site.

Resources are available in many formats, including hard copy, microfiche, and computerized versions. Computerized resources may be available on floppy disks or CD-ROMs for use on a single personal computer, a computer network, a mainframe system, or via the Internet. In most instances electronic forms of resources are preferable because they are easy to use, allow information to be accessed quickly, and provide the capability to search multiple resources at the same time. It is also becoming more common that references may be available for palmtop computers, allowing practitioners to carry very compact electronic references in their personal data assistant (PDA).

Networked versions of resources offer the advantage of resource availability at multiple locations concurrently. In the future, it will become more common for pharmacists to have access to resources in patient care areas or other practice sites via wireless network connections from their personal notebook computers to the Internet (see Chap. 5) or other networked resources. Due to increased access to computerized resources via network systems, or the Internet, pharmacists are able to conduct information searches previously only possible in centralized drug information centers. Drug information services are moving on to other functions (e.g., training staff on use of computerized resources, exploring and creating new resources, and coordination of extensive projects involving information management).

ADVERSE EVENT OR ADVERSE DRUG REACTIONS RESOURCES

Clin-Alert 2000

Technomic Publishing Co., Inc., Lancaster, PA. A new source of adverse drug reaction and drug interaction information, including interactions with alternative medicines. Published annually.

Meyler's Side Effects of Drugs

Elsevier Publishing Company, Amsterdam, The Netherlands. The most comprehensive resource for information on adverse reactions associated with drug therapy. Extremely well-referenced. Published every 4 years. Complemented between issues by *Side Effects of Drugs Annual*. Also available in CD-ROM format (SEDBASE).

Textbook of Adverse Drug Reactions

Chapman & Hall Medical, New York. A good compilation of adverse reaction information. Not as comprehensive as Meyler's, but often easier to use.

BIOEQUIVALENCE RESOURCES

Approved Bioequivalency Codes

Facts and Comparisons, St. Louis, MO. A listing of FDA bioequivalence ratings for drug products. Also contains orphan drug status of medications, patent information, and manufacturers' addresses. Published annually with monthly updates.

USPDI, Volume III

United States Pharmacopeial Convention, Inc., published by MICROMEDEX, Inc., Englewood, CO. Approved Drug Products and Legal Requirements. Includes information found in the FDA Orange Book that indicates products that are A/B rated and, therefore, considered bioequivalent. Also provides a list of discontinued drug products and other documents from the United States Pharmacopeial Convention. Published annually with monthly updates. Also available through various computer systems, including the Internet at <<http://www.fda.gov/cder/ob/default.htm>>.

DRUG INTERACTION RESOURCES

Drug Interaction Facts

Facts and Comparisons, St. Louis, MO. A resource for information on drug–drug and drug–food interactions. Well-referenced, providing details on mechanisms, clinical significance, and management of drug interactions. This is also one of the clearest and easiest to use publications. Updated quarterly. Also available as a computer program (as part of the CliniSphere) that is updated on the same schedule as the book.

Drug Interactions Analysis Management

Facts and Comparisons, St. Louis, MO. A well-referenced guide to drug–drug, and some drug–food, interactions that includes information on mechanisms, clinical significance, and management. Published annually with quarterly updates.

DRUG-REAX

MICROMEDEX, Inc., Englewood, CO. Lists adverse drug reactions by drug name and occurrence. Available for numerous platforms (i.e., floppy disk, CD stand alone, CD network, mainframe, Intranet, Internet).

Evaluations of Drug Interactions

PDS Publishing Co., St. Louis, MO. Textbook that provides information on mechanisms, clinical significance, and management of drug interactions. This reference is endorsed by the American Pharmaceutical Association, which once published it, and contains some of the most comprehensive information. Updated bimonthly.

Food Medication Interactions Handbook and HIV Medications Food Interactions

Food-Medication Interactions, Pottstown, PA. Two separate handbooks of interactions between foods and medications, the latter specifically addressing medications used in the treatment of HIV infections. Also available in computerized format.

Handbook on Drug & Nutrient Interactions

The American Dietetic Association, Chicago. A well-referenced guide to drug–nutrient interactions subdivided by disease states.

Medi-Span Drug Therapy Screening System

Medi-Span, Inc., Indianapolis. A computerized information system that allows the user to screen a number of drugs a particular patient is receiving for drug–drug and drug–food interactions. In addition, the user can enter information about prior adverse reactions experienced by patients (e.g., allergies) and the list of drugs will be screened for cross-reactions. Updated quarterly.

Pocket Guide to Evaluation of Drug Interactions

American Pharmaceutical Association, Washington, D.C. A condensed version of *Evaluations of Drug Interactions* that provides concise monographs for the busy practitioner. Contains drug interaction monographs organized by drug class.

DRUG USE IN RENAL FAILURE RESOURCES

Drug Prescribing in Renal Failure. Dosing Guidelines for Adults

The American College of Physicians, American Society of Internal Medicine, Philadelphia. A guide to drug dosage in patients with diminished renal function. Contains recommendations for patients undergoing hemodialysis and continuous ambulatory peritoneal dialysis.

Pocket Reference to Renal Dialysis

Petroc Press, Plymouth, United Kingdom. A good overall discussion of dialysis including drugs whose pharmacokinetics are altered by dialysis.

Clinical Nephrotoxins & Renal Injury from Drugs and Chemicals

Kluwer Academic Publishers, Boston. Information on nephrology, toxicology, and general medicine. Includes information on medications that can be nephrotoxic and treatment of drug-induced nephrotoxicity.

EXTEMPORANEOUS COMPOUNDING RESOURCES

Extemporaneous Ophthalmic Preparations

Applied Therapeutics, Inc., Vancouver, WA. A handbook on extemporaneous preparation of ophthalmic products.

Pediatric Drug Formulations

Harvey Whitney Books Company, Cincinnati, OH. A referenced recipe manual of formulations commonly compounded for pediatric patients.

Remington's Pharmaceutical Sciences

Mack Publishing Co., Easton, PA. Contains useful information for prescription compounding. Some older editions, particularly 1960 or before, are particularly good sources of compounding information. Also available in a CD-ROM format.

Stability of Compounded Formulations

American Pharmaceutical Association, Washington, D.C. A well-referenced textbook authored by Lawrence Trissel containing common compounded formulations and their known stability.

Trissel's Tables of Physical Compatibility

Multi Matrix, Inc., Lake Forest, IL. A compilation of physical compatibility test results.

USP-NF

United States Pharmacopeial Convention, Inc., Rockville, MD. Some older editions, particularly 1960 or before, are particularly good sources of compounding information.

IDENTIFICATION RESOURCES FOR TABLET AND CAPSULE IMPRINT CODES

Clinical Reference Library

Lexi-Comp, Inc. Hudson, OH. A CD-ROM compilation of handbooks related to drug therapy such as the *Drug Information Handbook* that includes a search engine to identify tablets and capsules and shows a picture of the product. This feature is only available with the CD-ROM or Internet (<<http://www.lexi.com>>) versions.

IDENTIDEX

MICROMEDEX, Inc., Englewood, CO. A resource for identifying capsules and tablets by imprint code or visual characteristics. Product imprint codes are listed both alphabetically and numerically. Also, provides directory of slang terms for street drugs. Available for numerous platforms (i.e., floppy disk, CD stand alone, CD network, mainframe, Intranet, Internet). Updated quarterly.

Ident-A-Drug Reference

Therapeutic Research Center, Stockton, CA. List of imprint codes on United States tablets and capsules. Updated annually.

DOMESTIC DRUG IDENTIFICATION RESOURCES

American Drug Index

Facts and Comparisons, St. Louis, MO. A dictionary of drug products available in the United States cross-referenced by trade, generic, and chemical name. Manufacturer, chemical, or generic name, package size, dosage form, strengths, and therapeutic category are provided for each trade name entry. Also contains many useful charts. Published annually.

Merck Index

Merck Research Labs, Merck & Co., Inc., Rahway, NJ. A listing of over 10,000 chemical compounds. Useful for locating information on the physical and chemical properties (molecular weight, solubility, melting point, etc.) of drugs and other chemicals. Also lists trade names, including foreign products. CD-ROM version also available.

PRICE-CHEK PC

Medi-Span, Inc., Indianapolis, IN. A computerized list of strengths, sizes, and prices of products available in the United States. Also, can be used to prepare your own formulary. Updated monthly.

Red Book

Medical Economics Data, Montvale, NJ. Resource for information relevant to ordering drug products. Products are listed by trade name. Each entry contains manufacturer, package sizes available, dosage forms, and average wholesale cost. Lists manufacturers addresses and phone numbers. Provides information on durable medical equipment, information on manufacturers of herbal and vitamin supplements, lists products that cannot be crushed, products that are alcohol-free and sugar-free, and lists the top 200 drugs by generic and brand name. Also contains many useful charts including lists of drug and poison control centers, state and national pharmaceutical associations, state boards of pharmacy, federal government offices, and state Medicaid drug program administrators. Published annually with monthly updates of average wholesale prices.

USP Dictionary of USAN & International Drug Names

United States Pharmacopeial Convention, Inc., Rockville, MD. A directory of drug names registered in the United States. Most entries contain pronunciation, chemical name, structure, CAS registry number, therapeutic category, and manufacturer. Cross-referenced to trade names and synonyms.

FOREIGN DRUG IDENTIFICATION RESOURCES

British National Formulary

BMJ Publishing, London, United Kingdom. The standard reference for prescribing and dispensing drugs in Britain. Included are notes on the different drug groups to help in the choice of appropriate treatment. The BNF is updated in March and September of each year and is also available on disk and CD-ROM as the *Electronic British National Formulary.* An electronic web-based format is also available.

Diccionario De Especialidades Farmaceuticas

Medical Economics Data, Montvale, NJ. A guide to over 2000 Mexican pharmaceutical products that have been approved by the Secretary of Health. Published in Spanish.

DRUGDEX Information System

MICROMEDEX, Inc., Englewood, CO. A well-referenced drug resource in monograph format. Often will include foreign drug names. Available for numerous platforms (i.e., floppy disk, CD stand alone, CD network, mainframe, Intranet, Internet). Updated quarterly.

European Drug Index

European Society of Clinical Pharmacy, Noordwijk, The Netherlands. A directory of drug products available in Europe by trade and generic name. Each entry lists product ingredients, dosage strengths, and manufacturer.

<<home.intekom.com/pharm>>

A web site list of drugs with package inserts that are available in South Africa.

Index Nominum

Medpharm Scientific Publishers, Stuttgart, Germany. A compilation of domestic and foreign drug products by generic and trade names. Each generic name entry lists international trade names, manufacturers, and therapeutic use category. Updated biannually. Also available as part of MICROMEDEX CCIS system.

Martindale: The Complete Drug Reference

(Formerly Martindale: The Extra Pharmacopeia) Pharmaceutical Press, London, United Kingdom. Extensive information on 4000 domestic and foreign drug products in monograph format. An excellent resource for foreign drug identification and information on herbal and homeopathic medications. Also available on CD-ROM and as part of the MICROMEDEX CCIS.

GENERAL DRUG INFORMATION RESOURCES

AHFS Drug Information

American Society of Health-System Pharmacists, Bethesda, MD. An informative drug information resource in monograph format that includes information on both FDA-approved and nonlabeled indications. Updated annually with quarterly supplements. Also available in full-text format (e.g., with references) on CD-ROM and on-line systems.

Clinical Pharmacology

Gold Standard Multimedia Inc., Tampa, FL. A computerized information system providing brief monographs on a variety of drugs via a graphical user interface. Useful for maintaining patient information that can be analyzed for problems such as additive adverse effects, drug interactions, and mismatches between diagnoses and drug therapies. Designed to be usable by the clinician on a notebook computer in a clinical situation. Updated 4 times a year. Available free on the Internet at <<http://cp.gsm.com>>.

Clinical Reference Library

Lexi-Comp, Inc., Hudson, OH. A compilation of tertiary references that includes the *Drug Information Handbook, Pediatric Dosage Handbook, Geriatric Dosage Handbook, Infectious Disease Handbook, Poisoning & Toxicology Handbook, Laboratory Test Handbook,* and the *Diagnostic Procedure Handbook.* These textbooks can be purchased in hard copy separately or purchased as a clinical reference library (CRL) on CD-ROM or the Internet. This system is easy to search by using individual terms or strings of text. When initiating a search in the CRL, all texts can be selected and searched by categories, such as disease state, drug name (brand or generic), identification of medication, adverse effects, toxicity, patient symptoms, dosages, and compatibility/stability. The authors have made a specific point to have extensive information on dosing changes required in renal and hepatic dysfunction. This system allows individuals or institutions to personalize their information by placing "sticky notes" at certain points in the system. A version of the *Drug Information Handbook* is also available for Palm Pilots.

DRUGDEX Information System

MICROMEDEX, Inc., Englewood, CO. A well-referenced, expansive drug resource in monograph format. Also contains a drug consult section that provides responses to drug information questions written by drug information specialists. Available for numerous platforms (i.e., floppy disk, CD stand alone, CD network, mainframe, Intranet, and Internet). Updated quarterly.

Drug Facts and Comparisons

Facts and Comparisons, St. Louis, MO. A comprehensive reference containing comparative information, including relative cost, of individual drugs in specific drug classes. Indicates products that are sugar and alcohol free. Also contains many useful charts including manufacturers' addresses and phone numbers, FDA pregnancy categories, basic life support for acute overdosage, management of acute hypersensitivity reactions, basic pharmaceutical calculations, normal laboratory values, and standard pharmaceutical abbreviations. Monthly updates contain a "Keeping Up" section of investigational agents pending FDA approval. Loose-leaf edition updated monthly. Hardbound edition updated annually and also available on CD-ROM, as CliniSphere.

Drug Information Handbook

Lexi-Comp, Inc., Hudson, OH. A pocketsized handbook of drug information. Includes referenced drug monographs including indications, adverse reactions, drug interactions, nursing implications, dosing and administration, and dosing in renal failure, hepatic failure, pediatrics, and geriatrics. Also includes appropriate pronunciations of the drug names. Hardbound edition is updated annually. Also available on CD-ROM and web-based versions as part of the CRL, which is updated quarterly. A version of the *Drug Information Handbook* is also available for Palm Pilots.

Handbook of Clinical Drug Data

McGraw-Hill, New York. A pocketsized handbook that provides brief monographs for drug classes and individual agents, including several pending FDA approval. Useful for medical rounds and other situations where quick reference is needed.

Martindale: The Complete Drug Reference

(Formerly *Martindale: The Extra Pharmacopeia*) Pharmaceutical Press, London, United Kingdom. Extensive information on 4000 domestic and foreign drug products in monograph format. An excellent resource for foreign drug identification and information on herbal and homeopathic medications. Also available on CD-ROM and as part of MICROMEDEX CCIS.

MICROMEDEX Computerized Clinical Information System (CCIS)

MICROMEDEX, Inc, Englewood, CO. A combination of a variety of information sources that are mentioned elsewhere in this list. Some of the publications contained in this system include: DRUGDEX, POISINDEX, IDENTIDEX, *Martindale: The Complete Drug Ref-*

erence, P&T Quik (a compilation of Pharmacy & Therapeutics Committee drug evaluation monographs) and the *Physicians' Desk Reference.* Available for numerous platforms (i.e., floppy disk, CD stand alone, CD network, mainframe, Intranet, and Internet).

Mosby's GenRx

Mosby, St. Louis, MO. Monographs of frequently used brand and generic products. Additional information includes a drug identification guide, manufacturer information, normal laboratory guides, FDA pregnancy categories, DEA controlled substance schedules, discontinued products, look-alike and sound-alike drugs, poison control centers, and phone numbers to AIDS drug assistance programs. Available in CD-ROM format and accessible via the Internet for a fee. Updated annually.

Physicians' Desk Reference (PDR)

Medical Economics Data, Montvale, NJ. A compilation of package inserts for prescription drug products from pharmaceutical manufacturers. Both active and inactive ingredients are listed for most drug products. Companies who wish to place their package inserts in this textbook pay a fee, so some products are not covered by this reference. Also contains approximately 1000 photographs of drug products useful for identification. Addresses and phone numbers for pharmaceutical manufacturers provided. Also available in CD-ROM and hand-held computer formats. Updated annually. CD-ROM version updated quarterly.

PDR Generics

Medical Economics Data, Montvale, NJ. Monographs of frequently used brand and generic names. Additional information includes product category index, indications index including off-label uses, manufacturer directory, product identification imprint codes, pregnancy categories, poison control centers, drug information centers, newly approved drugs, and ADR reporting forms.

USPDI

United States Pharmacopeial Convention, Inc., published by Micromedex, Inc., Englewood, CO. Three-set volume. *Volume 1—Drug Information for the Health Care Provider.* Information on drug products in monograph format, including both FDA-approved and off-label indications. Includes information on veterinary drugs and OTC diagnostic agents. *Volume 2—Advice for the Patient.* Drug information for the patient in lay language grouped by drug class. *Volume 3—Approved Drug Products and Legal Requirements.* Includes information found in the FDA Orange Book that indicates products that are A/B rated and, therefore, considered bioequivalent. Also provides a list of discontinued drug products and other documents from the United States Pharmacopeial Convention. Published annually with monthly updates. Also available on various computer systems.

GERIATRIC DOSING RESOURCES

Geriatric Dosage Handbook

Lexi-Comp, Inc., Hudson, OH. A guide to drug dosage in geriatric patients including dosage recommendations for patients with renal and hepatic failure. Includes appendices on OBRA guidelines, immunization schedules, medications that cannot be crushed, drugs that are affected by dialysis, wound care, asthma guidelines, list of drugs that cause some common ADRs, normal laboratory values, medical abbreviations, HCFA guidelines for long-term care facilities, antipsychotic and antidepressant charts, and anticoagulation guidelines. Published annually and available as part of the CRL on CD-ROM.

Geriatric Pharmacology

McGraw-Hill, New York. A good review of geriatric drug therapy by disease state and medication related groups.

The Merck Manual of Geriatrics

Merck & Co., Rahway, NJ. A comprehensive review of clinical management of the elderly. Includes information on legal, ethical, social, and financial issues, including the older driver, elder abuse, Medicare, and nursing home and home care insurance. Web site at <<http://www.merck.com>>.

LABORATORY TESTS

Basic Skills in Interpreting Laboratory Data

American Society of Health-System Pharmacists, Bethesda, MD. A manual to learn how to interpret laboratory test information.

Clinical Guide to Laboratory Tests

W.B. Saunders, Philadelphia. A useful guide to laboratory tests. Contains information on normal laboratory values, clinical utility of each test, and substances (including drugs) that can interfere with test results.

Laboratory Tests and Diagnostic Procedures

W.B. Saunders, Philadelphia. A useful guide to laboratory tests listed by both disease state and by test name. Provides information on normal laboratory values, clinical utility of each test, and substances that can interfere with results.

Laboratory Test Handbook

Lexi-Comp, Inc. Hudson, OH. A well-referenced, useful guide to laboratory tests. Contains information on normal laboratory values and lists disease and drug entities that can alter laboratory test results. Provides information on appropriate tubes for collecting specimens as well as substances that can interfere with test results. Available as part of CRL.

MEDICAL RESOURCES

American Hospital Association Guide to the Health Care Field

American Hospital Association, Chicago. A listing of hospitals in the United States by city and state. Useful for locating peers and experts when consultations are desired. Also useful for patient referrals.

Cecil Textbook of Medicine

W.B. Saunders, Philadelphia. A well-respected medical textbook useful for researching diagnosis, symptomatology, and treatment of disease states. CD-ROM version also available.

Current Medical Diagnosis & Treatment

McGraw-Hill, New York. Ambulatory and inpatient medicine reference. Updated annually.

Dorland's Illustrated Medical Dictionary

W.B. Saunders, Philadelphia. A resource for definitions of medical terms.

Harrison's Principles of Internal Medicine

McGraw-Hill, New York. One of the most comprehensive medical textbooks useful for researching diagnosis, symptomatology, and treatment of disease states. Available in one- or two-volume sets and CD-ROM formats.

MAXX

Little Brown and Co., Boston. A full-text data base featuring titles from the collection of Little Brown Books. A special drug information component is optional. Updated three times per year.

The Merck Manual

Merck & Co., Inc., Rahway, NJ. A handbook on disease states and their management in easy-to-read format. Also available in microcomputer format, CD-ROM, and on the Internet at <<http://www.merck.com>>.

Scientific American Medicine

Scientific American, New York. An easy-to-read resource for disease state information. Contains a useful table to assist in dosing drugs in patients with renal failure. Monthly updates keep information current. Loose-leaf format, monthly updates, annual renewal. Also available in CD-ROM format.

STAT!-Ref

Teton Data Systems, Jackson, WY. A collection of up to 30 textbooks, drug compendia, journals, and Clinical MEDLINE on CD-ROM that allows detailed searching for biomedical information. Updated quarterly. Subscribers pay for and receive only the references they want.

Stedman's Medical Dictionary

Lippincott Williams & Wilkins, Philadelphia. A resource for definitions of medical terms. Available on CD-ROM as part of the Clinical Reference Library provided by Lexi-Comp, Inc., Hudson, Ohio. Also available in computer format that is compatible with some word processing programs.

Washington University Manual of Medical Therapeutics

Lippincott Williams & Wilkins, Philadelphia. A clinical guide to current management of common medical disorders. Updated every 1 to 2 years.

NATURAL PRODUCT RESOURCES

A Clinical Guide to Chinese Herbs and Formulae

Churchill Livingstone, Edinburgh, Scotland. A review of traditional Chinese herbs by action, indications, combinations, disease states, and formulas.

The Complete German Commission E Monographs: Therapeutic Guide to Herbal Medicines

IntegrativMedicine, American Botanical Council, Boston. A comprehensive source of the Commission E monographs as published in Germany listed by herbal product.

Herbal Drugs and Phytopharmaceuticals

CRC Press, Boca Raton, FL. A good review of the fundamentals of herbal therapy including information on preparing plants. The textbook is organized by plant monographs including pictures, growing conditions, and therapeutic uses of the plant.

The Honest Herbal: A Sensible Guide to the Use of Herbs and Related Remedies

Pharmaceutical Products Press, Haworth Press, Inc., Binghamton, NY. A good review of herbal products. Primarily focuses on pharmacognosy with some clinical application.

The Information Sourcebook of Herbal Medicine

The Crossing Press, Freedom, CA. A source book of Medline citations of published herbal papers, herbal pharmacology, herbal terminology, and a guide to computer databases.

Natural Medicines Comprehensive Database

Therapeutic Research Faculty, Stockton, CA. A well-researched set of monographs on natural products. Also available for subscription over the Internet at <<http://www. NaturalDatabase.com>>.

PDR for Herbal Medicines

Medical Economics Data, Montvale, NJ. Information taken from the German Commission E Monographs and supplemented with additional information. Published annually.

Professional's Handbook of Complementary & Alternative Medicines

Springhouse Corporation, Springhouse, PA. Monographs organized by natural products. Includes helpful information related to reported uses, doses, adverse reactions, drug interactions, and points of interest. See web site at <<http://www.springnet.com>>.

Review of Natural Products

Facts and Comparisons, Inc., St. Louis, MO. A well-referenced monthly newsletter (formerly known as the *Lawrence Review of Natural Products*) that focuses on natural products and herbal remedies. Listed in alphabetical order by natural product and includes information on chemistry, botany, toxicology, pharmacology, and clinical applications.

Tyler's Herbs of Choice: The Therapeutic Use of Phytomedicinals

Haworth Herbal Press, Haworth Press, Inc., Binghamton, NY. An authoritative reference on basic herbal principles, herbal regulatory history, and a list of herbal therapies by disease states.

OVER-THE-COUNTER DRUG RESOURCES

Handbook of Nonprescription Drugs

American Pharmaceutical Association, Washington, D.C. A comprehensive resource for information on nonprescription products.

Nonprescription Drug Therapy

Facts and Comparisons, St. Louis, MO. A comprehensive resource for information on treatment by nonprescription medications. Organized by disease state. Updated quarterly.

Nonprescription Products: Formulations and Features

American Pharmaceutical Association, Washington, D.C. Companion to the *Handbook of Nonprescription Drugs* that is updated and lists the current United States over-the-counter formulations by active and inactive ingredients and gives a comparison of products by therapeutic class.

Nonprescription Product Therapeutics

Lippincott Williams & Wilkins, Philadelphia. Good therapeutic monographs for a pharmacist to provide help to patients for over-the-counter therapies. Excellent algorithms to provide tools for assessment, therapy, and monitoring. Provides specific product information with comparisons between active ingredients. Lists poison control centers in the United States.

Physicians' Desk Reference for Non-Prescription Drugs

Medical Economics Data, Montvale, NJ. Information on over-the-counter drugs and products. Published annually.

PATIENT COUNSELING RESOURCES

AfterCare

MICROMEDEX, Englewood, CO. A system that contains drug information from the United States Pharmacopeial Convention Advice for the Patient. Available for numerous platforms (i.e., floppy disk, CD stand alone, CD network, mainframe, Intranet, and Internet). Contains standard English, Spanish, and easy-to-read formats. Updated quarterly.

Dr. Schueler's Home Medical Advisor

Pixel Perfect Inc, Merritt Island, FL. A multimedia computer software product intended for patients themselves, but useful for patient teaching.

Medication Teaching Manual

American Society of Health-System Pharmacists, Bethesda, MD. Drug information in lay language. Information on each drug is presented on a single page in question/answer format ideal for copying for patient use. A Spanish version is available. Also available as a computer program for single use or network installation.

Patient Counseling Handbook

American Pharmaceutical Association, Washington, D.C. Information on drug therapy relevant to patient counseling such as proper use of medications and adverse effects. Updated annually.

Patient Drug Facts

Facts and Comparisons, St. Louis, MO. Drug information in lay language. Monographs are published in English and Spanish. Published annually with quarterly updates. Computerized version also available.

USP-DI Volume II

See *AfterCare* above and *USP-DI* under General Drug Information Resources.

PEDIATRIC DOSING RESOURCES

Current Pediatric Diagnosis and Treatment

McGraw-Hill, New York. A general pediatrics textbook with emphasis on ambulatory care, acute critical care, and the practical approach to pediatric disorders. Updated every 2 years.

Harriet Lane Handbook

Mosby-Year Book, Inc., St. Louis, MO. A classic and well-respected manual on drug use in pediatric patients. CD-ROM version is available.

Nelson Textbook of Pediatrics

W.B. Saunders Company, Philadelphia. A general pediatrics therapeutics reference that also contains a table of pediatric doses. CD-ROM version is available.

Pediatric Dosage Handbook

Lexi-Comp, Inc., Hudson, OH. A guide to drug dosage in infants and children. Also provides recipes for extemporaneously compounding oral medications for pediatric use. Published annually. Also available on CD-ROM as part of the CRL.

Problems in Pediatric Drug Therapy

Drug Intelligence Publications, Inc., Hamilton, IL. A general pediatric pocket reference.

PHARMACOKINETICS RESOURCES

Applied Pharmacokinetics: Principles of Therapeutic Drug Monitoring

Applied Therapeutics, Inc., Vancouver, WA. A complete resource on the theory and practice of therapeutic drug monitoring and pharmacokinetics. Each chapter is devoted to a commonly monitored drug or drug class.

Basic Clinical Pharmacokinetics

Applied Therapeutics, Inc., Vancouver, WA. An easy-to-read primer on clinical pharmacokinetics and therapeutic drug monitoring.

Handbook of Basic Pharmacokinetics

American Pharmaceutical Association, Washington, D.C. A pocket-sized overview of bioequivalence and clinical pharmacokinetics.

PHARMACOLOGY RESOURCES

EMBASE Drugs and Pharmacology

Elsevier Science Publishers, Amsterdam, The Netherlands. A data base specializing in drug pharmacology, referenced to the literature. Available on CD-ROM.

Goodman and Gilman's Pharmacological Basis of Therapeutics

McGraw-Hill, New York. Often considered the premier textbook on pharmacology. CD-ROM version also available.

Human Pharmacology: Molecular to Clinical

Mosby, St. Louis, MO. A good overview of pharmacology. Excellent tables, graphs, charts, and explanations.

Principles of Pharmacology. Basic Concepts & Clinical Applications

Arnold Publishers, London, United Kingdom. A treatise on pharmacology compiled by an ad hoc group of experts.

PHARMACOTHERAPY RESOURCES (ALSO SEE REFERENCES LISTED UNDER MEDICAL RESOURCES)

Applied Therapeutics

Lippincott Williams & Wilkins, Philadelphia. A unique textbook that presents pathophysiology and treatment of disease states in case study format. A pocket-sized handbook is also available with summarized information and condensed tables and charts.

Avery's Drug Treatment

Adis International, Auckland, New Zealand. A textbook that provides drug therapy information as it relates to clinical pharmacology and therapeutics. Information is provided by disease states.

Conn's Current Therapy

W.B. Saunders, Philadelphia. Detailed information on treatment of commonly diagnosed disease states. Updated annually.

Pharmacotherapy—A Pathophysiologic Approach

McGraw-Hill, New York. An excellent reference for information related to pathophysiology of disease states and pharmacotherapeutic interventions. A pocket-sized handbook is also available with condensed information with tables and charts.

Pharmacotherapy Complete

McGraw-Hill, New York. A CD-ROM resource that includes *Pharmacotherapy: A Pathophysiologic Approach, Handbook of Clinical Drug Data, Pharmacotherapy: A Patient-Focused Approach,* and *Instructor's Guide to Accompany Pharmacotherapy.*

Textbook of Therapeutics

(Formerly known as *Clinical Pharmacy and Therapeutics*). Lippincott Williams & Wilkins, Philadelphia. A comprehensive resource on disease states and their treatments. A case book is available that accompanies this text.

PHARMACY PRACTICE RESOURCES

The Art, Science, and Technology of Pharmaceutical Compounding

American Pharmaceutical Association, Washington, D.C. Covers all aspects of compounding including legal/regulatory issues, facilities, equipment, step-by-step instruction, flavoring, packaging, stability, and veterinary medications.

Clinical Skills for Pharmacists: A Patient-focused Approach

Mosby, St. Louis, MO. A good guide for all aspects of skills useful for patient care including communication, medication histories, drug information, drug literature evaluation, laboratory monitoring, patient monitoring, physical assessment, patient case presentation, development of a therapeutic plan, and ethics.

FDA

<<http://www.fda.gov>>. Contains regulatory information on food, drugs, medical devices, cosmetics, and biologicals. Updated continuously.

Handbook of Drug Therapy Monitoring

Lippincott Williams & Wilkins, Philadelphia. A good reference with information pertaining to the medical chart, drug therapy monitoring and assessment, adverse effects, laboratory data, common medical terminology and abbreviations, and drugs that should not be crushed.

Handbook of Institutional Pharmacy Practice

American Society of Health-System Pharmacists, Bethesda, MD. A well-referenced compilation of issues that affect institutional pharmacy practice. Includes ASHP practice guidelines.

HCFA (Health Care Financing Administration)

<<http://www.hcfa.gov>>. Contains information on reimbursement issues and functions as a Medicare/Medicaid library. Updated monthly.

Pharmacy Law Digest

Facts and Comparisons, St. Louis, MO. A compilation of federal drug laws pertaining to the practice of pharmacy. Published annually with one update.

Physical Assessment: A Guide for Evaluating Drug Therapy

Applied Therapeutics, Inc., Vancouver, WA. An introduction to physical assessment of patients relevant to the provision of pharmaceutical care.

Practical Guide to Contemporary Pharmacy Practice

Lippincott Williams & Wilkins, Philadelphia. An excellent reference that provides guidelines for compounding various types of drug preparations. Information on solvents, preservatives, buffers, surfactants, vehicles, and bases is provided. In addition, information is included on professional guidelines and federal law.

Remington's Pharmaceutical Sciences

Mack Publishing Co., Easton, PA. A dissertation on the practice of pharmacy. Contains useful information for prescription compounding. Some older editions, particularly 1960 or before, are particularly good sources of compounding information.

POISON CONTROL INFORMATION RESOURCES

Clinical Management of Poisoning and Drug Overdose

W.B. Saunders, Philadelphia. Covers diagnosis and treatment of toxic emergencies.

Ellenhorn's Medical Toxicology: Diagnosis and Treatment of Human Poisoning

Lippincott Williams & Wilkins, Philadelphia. A general overview of toxicology and poisoning with a review of treatment by drug classifications.

POISINDEX Information System

MICROMEDEX, Inc., Englewood, CO. One of the most comprehensive, well-referenced resources for poison control information. Chemical composition of both drug products and household chemicals listed, and information on management of poisonings related to these products provided. Provides documentation on active and inactive ingredients for many medications. This reference can also be checked when trying to identify a discontinued or reformulated product. Available for numerous platforms (floppy disk, CD stand alone, CD network, mainframe, Intranet, and Internet). Updated quarterly.

Poisoning & Toxicology Handbook

Lexi-Comp, Inc., Hudson, OH. Monographs of poisonings by drug products, nonmedicinal agents, and biologicals. Antidote drugs used in the treatment, diagnostic tests and procedures, toxic ranges, dosages for pediatrics, and symptoms index are provided. Updated annually in a pocket-sized version and updated quarterly as a CD-ROM version.

Principles of Clinical Toxicology

Lippincott-Raven, Hagerstown, MD. Clinical guide to common poisonings.

Goldfrank's Toxicologic Emergencies

McGraw-Hill, New York. Clinical application of toxicology and poisonings. Guides for antidotes and supportive therapy. CD-ROM version available.

STERILE DRUG PRODUCT RESOURCES

Guide to Parenteral Admixtures

King Guide Publications, Napa, CA. A resource for information on stability and compatibility of injectable drug products in loose-leaf format. Updated quarterly. CD-ROM and Internet versions also available.

Handbook on Injectable Drugs

American Society of Health-System Pharmacists, Bethesda, MD. Comprehensive information on stability and compatibility of injectable drug products. Also available in a pocket-sized handbook, and a full-text format (with references), on CD-ROM and on-line systems.

DRUGS IN PREGNANCY AND LACTATION RESOURCES

Drugs in Pregnancy and Lactation

Lippincott William & Wilkins, Philadelphia. The most complete resource for information on use of drugs in pregnant and breast-feeding women. Well-referenced, containing summaries of available clinical studies. Unlike many other references in this category, this book concentrates on human data and is not a compilation of animal studies. Published every few years with an update newsletter published quarterly.

Reprorisk

MICROMEDEX, Inc., Englewood, CO. A collection of information on teratogenicity and reproduction effects of drugs and chemicals. Available for numerous platforms (i.e., floppy disk, CD stand alone, CD network, mainframe, Intranet, and Internet). Updated quarterly.

VETERINARY INFORMATION

The Merck Veterinary Manual

Merck & Co., Rahway, NJ. Contains veterinary information. Also available on CD-ROM. Updated annually.

Small Animal Medicine Therapeutics

Lippincott Williams & Wilkins, Philadelphia. A good guide to understanding therapeutic and drug therapy management in the small animal.

Veterinary Drug Handbook

Iowa State University Press, Ames, IA. A good text of drug monographs for veterinary use.

Veterinary Drug Therapy

Lea & Febiger, Philadelphia. A good guide to understanding drug therapy in a veterinary practice.

Veterinary Pharmaceuticals and Biologicals (VPB) (Veterinarian's PDR)

Medical Economics Data, Montvale, NJ. Biennially updated prescribing information for more than 4300 veterinary products.

Also see *USP-DI*, Volume I.

Secondary Literature

Secondary literature[4,5,7,8] consists of indexing and abstracting services of the primary literature. An indexing system provides only bibliographic information that is indexed by topic, whereas an abstracting service also provides a brief description (abstract) of information contained in a specific citation. Although most of these resources provide access to primary literature, each covers different biomedical journals, meeting abstracts, newsletters, textbooks, and other publications; therefore, use of more than one of these resources often allows for more thorough information retrieval.

Cost of these systems vary, but have been estimated to range from $150 to $5000.[7] Many of these systems are also available via on-line vendors or in CD-ROM format. Some systems are now available over the Internet, such as Grateful Med or PubMed from the National Library of Medicine (<<http://www.nlm.nih.gov>>). Electronic formats are preferable for ease and speed of search, in addition to providing a greater variety of indexed terms. Each vendor will provide access to numerous databases focused on a variety of areas such as current affairs, business and economics, social sciences and humanities, applied sciences, and biosciences.[9] Vendors typically provide training on use of their systems.[9] Cost of on-line access to secondary resources depends on the vendor, time of day the search is conducted, data base searched, citations printed, and other factors that vary with the service accessed.[7] For a fee, some vendors will send the complete journal article when requested.[10] For example, the National Library of Medicine provides the service Loansome DOC. The decision to purchase a data base or access via on-line vendors will depend on the frequency of use and number of users of the database in the clinical practice setting.[7] For systems that are used often by numerous individuals, CD-ROM formats may be preferable. With CD-ROM formats, a set fee is paid for the system and unlimited searching is available. Network and Internet versions, including web versions, of many CD-ROMS are available that allow numerous individuals to access the system simultaneously. This is in comparison to on-line services whose fees vary according to the factors listed above. It is often preferable to begin on-line searching with the least expensive databases (usually MEDLARS databases) and proceed to alternative databases if appropriate information is not located. On-line searching is particularly beneficial for searching databases that are seldom used, to access information from remote locations without networking capabilities, and for use by single users.

Anti-infectives Today

Adis International, Inc., Langhorne, PA. An indexing and abstracting service that summarizes current literature on drug therapy and management of infections. Available in newsletter and a variety of electronic formats. Published monthly.

BIOSIS Previews

BIOSIS, Philadelphia. A major comprehensive resource that covers all areas of biological research, including the biomedical sciences. Meeting and conference citations include the basic sciences; may be more comprehensive than MEDLINE.

Cancer Today

Adis International, Inc., Langhorne, PA. An indexing and abstracting service that summarizes current literature on the use of drugs in the management of cancer. Available in newsletter and a variety of electronic formats. Published monthly.

ClinAlert

Technomic Publishing Company, Lancaster, PA. A secondary system of adverse drug reaction case reports including herbal products and literature citations including herbal products. Available as a newsletter, CD-ROM, and on the Internet. Published semimonthly.

CNS Disorders Today

Adis International, Inc., Langhorne, PA. An indexing and abstracting service that summarizes current literature on all aspects of drug therapy and disease management of psychiatric and neurologic disorders. Available in newsletter and a variety of electronic formats. Published monthly.

Current Contents

Institute for Scientific Information, Philadelphia. A system that provides tables of contents for numerous medical and life science publications. Two versions useful to pharmacists, *Current Contents Life Sciences* and *Current Contents Clinical Medicine,* are available. Abstracts and author reprint addresses for journal articles also provided. Use of search terms enables specific information retrieval. Available in index, CD-ROM, online, and Internet formats. Published weekly.

Embase

Elsevier, Amsterdam, The Netherlands. A very complete abstracting source for the medical literature. Covers approximately 4500 periodicals. This publication is in many ways similar to Medline, however, it covers more international journals and meeting abstracts. Available in CD-ROM, network, and on-line formats. (Printed version is called *Excerpta Medica.*) *Drugs and Pharmacology,* a subset of this database, is of particular interest to pharmacists.

Index Medicus

U.S. Government Printing Office, Washington, D.C. An index to the biomedical literature that references over 3000 journals. Note that this is a printed subset of MEDLINE.

InPharma Weekly

Adis International, Inc., Langhorne, PA. An indexing and abstracting service that summarizes current literature related to pharmacotherapy. Available in newsletter, CD-ROM, on-line, Intranet, and Internet formats. Published weekly.

International Pharmaceutical Abstracts

American Society of Health-System Pharmacists, Bethesda, MD. The most comprehensive abstracting service for international information relevant to pharmacy and pharmaceutical sciences. Most other systems listed in this section cover only a very limited amount of the pharmacy literature, whereas the philosophy of this system is to cover all pharmacy periodicals, both domestic and international. Provides access to both journal articles and pharmacy meeting abstracts. Available as a print index, CD-ROM formats, and as an on-line service. Published twice a month or updated monthly.

Iowa Drug Information System (IDIS)

College of Pharmacy, The University of Iowa, Iowa City. An indexing service that allows retrieval of complete articles from over 180 biomedical journals. Information can be searched by keywords, generic drug name, disease classification, journal of publication, year of publication, authors, title, and type of study design. Available in microfiche, CD-ROM, and on-line formats. Articles published prior to 1998 are only available in microfiche format. After 1998, the articles are available in a microfiche format and a CD-ROM full-text version. Updated monthly.

Journal Watch

Massachusetts Medical Society, Waltham, MA. An abstracting service by the publishers of *New England Journal of Medicine* that includes recent citations from general medicine literature. This newsletter is published semimonthly. Additional newsletters are available in specialty areas such as psychiatry, infectious disease, women's health, and AIDS.

LEXIS-NEXIS

Academic Universe, Dayton, OH. This indexing/abstracting service with some full-text features provides access to a wide range of news, business, legal, and reference information. This service includes coverage of government, business, communications, law, finance, health care and medical information news, medical and health care journals, Joint Commission for Accreditation of Healthcare Organization publications, and FDC publications including *The Tan Sheets, The Pink Sheets,* and *Pharmaceutical Approvals Monthly.* Available for a fee at <<http://web.lexis-nexis.com/universe>>.

MEDLINE

National Library of Medicine, Bethesda, MD. One of the most expansive databases of biomedical information containing approximately 370,000 references. Citations from 1966 to the present can be searched for approximately 3500 journals. Available on CD-

ROM or via on-line services including the Internet as Grateful Med or part of PubMed <<http://www.nlm.nih.gov>>.

Paediatrics Today

Adis International, Inc., Langhorne, PA. An indexing and abstracting service that summarizes current literature on the use of drugs in children. Available in newsletter and a variety of electronic formats. Published monthly.

PharmacoEconomics & Outcomes News Weekly

Adis International, Inc., Langhorne, PA. An indexing and abstracting service that summarizes current literature on economic issues related to medicine, pharmacy, and health care. Available in newsletter, CD-ROM, and on-line formats. Published weekly.

Reactions Weekly

Adis International, Inc., Langhorne, PA. An indexing and abstracting service that summarizes current literature on adverse drug reactions, drug interactions, herbal products, drug dependence, and toxicology. Available in newsletter, CD-ROM, on-line, Intranet, and Internet formats. Published weekly. An annual compilation is also published.

Science Citation Index

Institute for Scientific Information, Philadelphia. An index that notes citation frequency of authors and journal articles. Available in network, CD-ROM, on-line, and Internet formats.

Searching Computerized Databases

Although search techniques for various CD-ROM systems and on-line vendors may vary, most follow a basic strategy. To begin a search, users must consider the question to be researched.[10] For example, consider the following inquiry: "Has diazepam been used rectally in pediatric patients for the management of status epilepticus?" The question emphasizes four major points: (1) diazepam, (2) pediatric usage, (3) rectal administration, and (4) status epilepticus. Thus, the question contains four search terms. The problem arises when the database does not recognize the search term selected by the user resulting in incomplete or inaccurate searches. Successful use of the database requires identification of the correct index terms for the data base.[10] As an example, users searching for information on total parenteral nutrition may consider using total parenteral nutrition, intravenous nutrition, parenteral hyperalimentation, or a variety of other terms for their search strategy. Only one term, however, may be recognized by the database. For databases available through National Library of Medicine, index terms are called Medical Subject Headings or MeSH terms.[10] Other indexing or abstracting services may call the list of terms a thesaurus. It is important to consult the index provided by the data base when searching for information, including the definition given for the term. For example, the term "pediatrics" may refer to the specialty area, and the term "child" may need to be used. Some of these indexes are available as part of the CD-ROM, web version, or computer software. Others are available in printed format.

Some computerized data bases also allow free-text searching.[10] With free-text searching, any word can be searched regardless of whether it is an index term. A citation will be identified if the word is located in the title, abstract, index terms or, possibly, other database fields for the journal article. Such techniques are helpful when a search using index terms is unsuccessful or provides only limited information, or when index terms are not available for the topic. Users usually must specify whether the search is a free-text or index-term search. Depending on the vendor or database, default for the system may be either free-text or index-term searching.

Boolean operators are used to combine search terms.[10] Three Boolean operators are used routinely—AND, OR, and NOT.[10] A symbolic representation of each of these as Venn diagrams is presented in Fig. 4–1. For the example above regarding rectal administration of diazepam, the four search terms would be combined with the operator AND. Such a search would identify all citations that contain *all* four search terms (i.e., the reference must contain all of the terms and will not be found if one or more terms is/are not applicable to the article). However, consider the situation where information on either rectal use of diazepam or paraldehyde for the treatment of status epilepticus in pediatric patients is desired. In this situation, the operator OR is used. The first step of the search would be to combine the terms diazepam OR paraldehyde. The results of this search would then be combined with the remaining three terms using the operator AND. Such a search would identify all articles that discuss rectal administration of either or both diazepam and paraldehyde for the management of status epilepticus in pediatric patients. A search using the operator OR is always equal or larger than one using only AND.[10] The operator OR is useful for searching synonyms.[10] Sometimes, users want to exclude certain topics. For instance, in the example above, information on status epilepticus related to febrile seizures may not be desired. In this case, the operator NOT is useful. The first step of the search process would be to com-

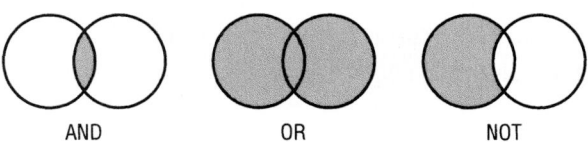

AND   OR   NOT

Figure 4–1. Venn diagram of logical operations.

bine the term status epilepticus NOT febrile seizures. The results of this search would then be combined with the remaining three terms using the operator AND. This search would identify citations that discuss rectal administration of diazepam in pediatric patients for the management of status epilepticus, but would eliminate all citations pertaining to febrile seizures. Use of the operator NOT decreases the results of a search and, therefore, should be used with caution to avoid incomplete access of information (e.g., an article that was otherwise perfect for the needs of the searcher, but happened to mention febrile seizures would have been eliminated by the above search strategy).[11] In addition, some data bases have Boolean operators known as WITH and NEAR. These logical operators are similar to AND; however, they require the terms to be within a certain number of words of each other. They are useful to search for phrases or in searches where a large number of articles happen to mention the desired terms, but not in conjunction with one another (e.g., they mention the drug in the introduction, but the disease state is only mentioned in the conclusion in a way unrelated to the drug).

Other ways to make a search more specific by using specialized search terms (e.g., chemical structure, chemical registry number) or by using other limiting factors or terms (e.g., age ranges, language, human studies only, review articles) are also available, depending on the data base.

Primary Literature

Primary literature consists of research studies published in biomedical journals, although there are now some Internet-only journals and many journals are becoming available electronically. Primary literature is usually the most current resource for information. Unlike tertiary or secondary resources, primary literature provides details of research methodology and scientific results that lead to therapeutic conclusions. Users of primary literature are, therefore, able to determine whether the study conclusions are sound based on the strength of the research techniques and scientific results of the study (see Chaps 6 and 7). Tertiary and secondary resources, on the other hand, consist of a review of published primary literature that may be biased or inaccurate. It is not unusual to formulate a different conclusion than that found in tertiary or secondary resources after analyzing the primary literature.

The primary literature is growing at an exponential rate. Over 20,000 biomedical journals are published annually.[13] An abbreviated list of journals useful to the practice of pharmacy is provided below. Most of these journals publish a combination of primary research studies and secondary review articles. The journals available in a particular practice setting will depend on the focus of the practice and the interests of the practitioners. In-depth descriptions of research designs commonly encountered in the biomedical literature are provided in Chaps 6 and 7.

Alternative Medicine Alert

American Health Consultants, Atlanta, GA. A newsletter dealing with alternative medicines. Published monthly.

American Druggist

The Hearst Corporation, New York. A pharmacy magazine with a community pharmacy focus that provides information on issues relevant to this practice setting. Rarely are primary research articles published in this journal. Published monthly.

American Journal of Cardiology

Excerpta Medica, Inc., Riverton, NJ. A journal dedicated to the specialty of cardiology. Published weekly. Internet access available for a fee at <<http://www.cardiosource.com>>.

American Journal of Health-System Pharmacy

American Society of Health-System Pharmacists, Bethesda, MD. A journal focused on clinical and managerial aspects of pharmacy practice in health systems. Published twice monthly. This journal previously was known as the *American Journal of Hospital Pharmacy* and incorporates the contents of a previously published journal known as *Clinical Pharmacy*. Available on the Internet at <<http://www.ashp.org>>.

American Journal of Pharmaceutical Education

American Association of Colleges of Pharmacy, Alexandria, VA. The official publication of the American Association of Colleges of Pharmacy that is dedicated to the documentation and advancement of pharmaceutical education. Published quarterly.

American Journal of Therapeutics

Lippincott Williams & Wilkins, Philadelphia. A journal that provides clinical and pharmacoeconomic perspectives on pharmacotherapeutic advances.

America's Pharmacist

National Community Pharmacists Association, Alexandria, VA. The official journal of the National Community Pharmacists Association (formerly known as National Association of Retail Druggists [NARD]). Published monthly.

Annals of Internal Medicine

American College of Physicians, Philadelphia. A highly regarded medical journal of the American College of Physicians that focuses on internal medicine, including pharmacotherapeutic management of disease states. Published twice monthly. Available on the Internet at <<http://www.acponline.org/journals/annals/annaltoc.htm?wni>>.

The Annals of Pharmacotherapy

Harvey Whitney Books Company, Cincinnati, OH. A well-respected journal pertaining to safe, effective, and economical use of pharmacotherapeutic agents. Published monthly. Previously known as *Drug Intelligence and Clinical Pharmacy* and later as *DICP The Annals of Pharmacotherapy.*

Archives of Internal Medicine

American Medical Association, Chicago. A journal specializing in the practice of internal medicine, including diagnosis and treatment of diseases. Published monthly. Available on the Internet at <<http://www.ama-assn.org/>>.

BioDrugs

Adis International, Ltd., Auckland, New Zealand. A journal that publishes review articles on clinical immunotherapeutics, biopharmaceuticals, and gene therapy. Published monthly.

Cancer

An Interdisciplinary International Journal of the American Cancer Society. John Wiley & Sons, Inc., New York. A journal that publishes research and information from all disciplines of oncology and supports the mission of the American Cancer Society. Published 30 times a year. Internet access available for a fee at <<http://www.cancer.org>>.

Chest. The Cardiopulmonary and Critical Care Journal

The American College of Chest Physicians, Northbrook, IL. The official publication of The American College of Chest Physicians that focuses on pulmonology, cardiology, critical care, and other related areas. Published monthly.

Clinical Drug Investigation

Adis International, Ltd., Auckland, New Zealand. A journal that publishes primary literature related to pharmacoeconomic and outcomes research. Published monthly. Internet access available for a fee.

Clinical Infectious Diseases

The University of Chicago Press, Chicago. The official publication of the Infectious Diseases Society of America. Published monthly.

Clinical Pharmacokinetics

Adis International, Ltd., Auckland, New Zealand. A journal that provides review articles relating to the following areas of clinical pharmacokinetics: pharmacokinetic–pharmacodynamic relationships, pharmacokinetic properties of drugs, therapeutic drug monitoring, the effect of age and disease states on pharmacokinetics, pharmacokinetic optimization of drug therapy, pharmacokinetic principles of drug interactions, bioavailability, and regulatory aspects of pharmacokinetics. Published monthly. Internet access available for a fee.

Clinical Pharmacology and Therapeutics

Mosby, St. Louis, MO. The official publication of the American Society for Clinical Pharmacology and Therapeutics and the American Society for Pharmacology and Experimental Therapeutics that publishes articles describing actions of drugs on the human body. Published monthly.

Clinical Therapeutics

Elsevier Science, New York. An international journal of drug therapy including review articles, new drug therapy, clinical studies, and pharmaceutical economics and health policy. Published six times per year.

CNS Drugs

Adis International, Ltd., Auckland, New Zealand. A journal that publishes review articles on pharmacotherapeutic aspects in the management of psychiatric and neurological disease. Published monthly.

Community Pharmacist

E.L.F. Publications, Inc. Lakewood, CO. A journal published to meet the professional and educational needs of today's practitioner. Published bimonthly. Internet access available for a fee.

The Consultant Pharmacist

American Society of Consultant Pharmacists (ASCP), Alexandria, VA. The official journal of the ASCP devoted to pharmacists who provide consultative services in various environments, including nursing home facilities. Published monthly. Available on the Internet at <<http://www.ascp.com>>.

Critical Care Medicine

Lippincott Williams & Wilkins, Philadelphia. The official journal of the Society of Critical Care Medicine. Published monthly.

Current Therapeutic Research

Elsevier Science, New York. This journal provides rapid publication of original reports of recent developments in drug therapy. Published monthly.

Disease Management & Health Outcomes

Adis International, Ltd., Auckland, New Zealand. A journal that publishes review articles on optimizing clinical outcomes and their economic consequences. Published monthly. Internet access available for a fee.

Drug Information Journal

Drug Information Association, Inc., Fort Washington, PA. The official publication of the Drug Information Association that focuses on technology related to information dissemination and data processing. The journal promotes cooperation between academia, pharmaceutical industry, and government. Published quarterly. Available on the Internet at <<http://www.diahome.org>>.

Drugs

Adis International, Ltd., Auckland, New Zealand. A journal that publishes review articles on pharmacotherapeutic aspects of both new and established drugs. Published monthly. Internet access available for a fee.

Drugs and Aging

Adis International, Ltd., Auckland, New Zealand. A journal that publishes review articles on pharmacotherapeutic aspects as it relates to the elderly. Published monthly. Internet access available for a fee.

Drugs in R & D

Adis International, Ltd., Auckland, New Zealand. A journal that publishes review articles on the therapeutic potential and impact of pharmaceutical compounds in development. Published monthly. Internet access available for a fee.

Drug Safety

Adis International, Ltd., Auckland, New Zealand. A journal that provides review articles related to epidemiology, diagnosis, management, and prevention of acute poisonings and adverse drug reactions. Published monthly. Internet access available for a fee.

Drug Topics

Medical Economics, Co., Montvale, NJ. A pharmacy news magazine with a community pharmacy focus useful for keeping up on new drug therapies and issues relevant to community pharmacy practice. Rarely are primary research articles published in this journal. Published twice a month. Available on the Internet at <<http://www.drugtopics.com>>.

FDA Medical Bulletin

Department of Health, Education and Welfare, Public Health Service, Food and Drug Administration, Rockville, MD. A publication of the Food and Drug Administration (FDA) that provides information on the safe and effective use of drugs and summarizes FDA rulings concerning drug products. Published irregularly. Available on the Internet at <<http://www.fda.gov>>.

F-D-C Reports ("The Pink Sheet")

F-D-C Reports, Inc., Chevy Chase, MD. A newsletter aimed at executives in the pharmaceutical industry that provides information pertinent to the pharmaceutical industry such as FDA rulings, new drug approvals, drug withdrawals, ongoing clinical trials and financial information. Published weekly. Available on the Internet at <<http://www.fdc reports.com>>.

F-D-C Reports ("The Tan Sheet")

F-D-C Reports, Inc., Chevy Chase, MD. A newsletter aimed at executives in the pharmaceutical industry that provides information pertinent to the over-the-counter and herbal products. Published weekly. Available on the Internet at <<http://www.fdcreports.com>>.

Food and Drug Law Journal

The Food and Drug Law Institute, Washington D.C. A journal dedicated to legislative, regulatory, legal, and public policy issues regarding the use of foods, drugs, biologics, cosmetics, and medical devices. Published quarterly.

Formulary

(Formerly known as *Hospital Formulary*). Advanstar Communications, Inc., Cleveland, OH. A journal directed at hospital and managed care decision makers that focuses on current issues in pharmacotherapy and drug policy management. Published monthly.

HerbalGram

American Botanical Council, Austin, TX. The official journal of the American Botanical Council and the Herb Research Foundation, which is published quarterly. The mission is to educate the public on the use of herbs and phytomedicines. Available on the Internet at <<http://www.healthy.net/hwlibraryjournals/HerbalGram/index.html>>.

The Herb and Dietary Supplement Report

Interpretive Medicine Communications, Newton, MA. A newsletter that provides news and commentary on herbs and supplements. Published monthly.

Hospital Pharmacy

Facts and Comparisons, St. Louis, MO. A journal devoted to the practice of pharmacy in institutional settings. Published monthly.

International Journal of Pharmaceutical Compounding

IFPC, Edmond, OK. The official journal of the International Federation of Pharmaceutical Compounding. Published bimonthly.

JAMA. The Journal of the American Medical Association

American Medical Association, Chicago. One of the premier medical journals that publishes investigations and review information of key importance to health care. Published weekly. Available on the Internet at <<http://jama.ama-assn.org>>.

Journal of the American Medical Informatics Association (JAMIA)

Hanley & Belfus, Inc., Philadelphia. The official publication of the American Medical Informatics Association that covers electronic management of medical information.

Published every 2 months. Also available on the Internet at <<http://www.amia.org/pubs/jamia/default.html>>.

Journal of the American Pharmaceutical Association

(Formerly known as *American Pharmacy*). American Pharmaceutical Association, Washington, DC. The official journal of the American Pharmaceutical Association that publishes news, information, and research in the areas of pharmacotherapeutic management of diseases, trends in pharmacy practice, and the provision of pharmaceutical care. Published monthly.

Journal of Applied Therapeutic Research

Harwood Academic Publishers, Gardia and Breach Publishing Group, Newark, NJ. A journal that focuses on the efficacy, safety, and rational use of drugs following approval by regulatory authorities for general marketing. Published monthly.

Journal of Clinical Oncology

Lippincott Williams & Wilkins, Philadelphia. The official journal of the American Society of Clinical Oncology. Published monthly.

The Journal of Clinical Pharmacology

Sage Science Press, Thousand Oaks, CA. The official journal of the American College of Clinical Pharmacology. Published monthly.

Journal of Herbs, Spices, & Medicinal Plants

Haworth Food Products Press, Binghamton, NY. Information on medicinal uses of plants. Published quarterly.

Journal of Managed Care Pharmacy

Academy of Managed Care Pharmacy, Alexandria, VA. The official journal of the Academy of Managed Care Pharmacy, which is published bimonthly. Available on the Internet at <<http://www.amcp.org>>.

The Journal of the National Cancer Institute

Oxford University Press, New York. A journal that publishes news, information, and research pertaining to cancer treatment, prevention, and control. Published twice monthly. Available on the Internet at <<http://www.jnci.oupjournals.org>>.

Journal of Parenteral and Enteral Nutrition

ASPEN, Silver Spring, MD. The official journal of the American Society for Parenteral and Enteral Nutrition. Published bimonthly.

The Journal of Pediatric Pharmacy Practice

Pediatric Pharmacy Concepts, Inc., St. Petersburg, FL. The official bimonthly journal of the Pediatric Pharmacy Advocacy Group, Inc.

Journal of Pharmaceutical Care in Pain & Symptom Control

Pharmaceutical Products Press, The Haworth Press, Inc., Binghamton, NY. This journal is an interdisciplinary publication focusing on rational drug therapy in the management of pain and related symptoms. Published quarterly.

Journal of Pharmaceutical Sciences

John Wiley & Sons, Inc. and American Pharmaceutical Association, Washington, D.C. A journal that focuses on the application of physical and analytical chemistry to the pharmaceutical sciences and technologies. Internet access available for a fee at <<http://www.interscience.wiley.com/jpages/0022-3549/>>. Published monthly.

Journal of Pharmacy Practice

Technomic Publishing Company, Inc. Lancaster, PA. A journal dedicated to providing practicing pharmacists with topical, important, and useful information to support pharmacy practice and pharmaceutical care, and to expand the pharmacist's professional horizons.

Journal of Pharmacy Teaching

Pharmaceutical Products Press, Binghamton, NY. A journal dedicated to issues relevant to pharmaceutical education. Published quarterly.

The Journal of Pharmacy Technology

Harvey Whitney Books Company, Cincinnati, OH. A journal that accepts publications related to pharmacy practice and pharmacy technology. Published bimonthly.

Journal of Social and Administrative Pharmacy

Swedish Pharmaceutical Press, Stockholm, Sweden. A publication focusing on issues of importance to pharmacy practice in all settings. Published quarterly.

The Medical Letter on Drugs and Therapeutics

The Medical Letter, Inc., New Rochelle, NY. A newsletter that provides review information on new drug therapies and lists drugs of choice for various disease states. Published biweekly. Also available as part of STAT!-Ref CD-ROM. Internet access available for a fee at <<http://www.medletter.com>>.

Morbidity and Mortality Weekly Report

U.S. Department of Health and Human Services, Centers for Disease Control, Atlanta, GA. A publication of the Centers for Disease Control (CDC) that provides statistics and recommendations for treatment of infectious diseases. Also available free on the Internet from the CDC's World Wide Web server at <<http://www2.cdc.gov/mmwr>>; the CDC will e-mail the table of contents when requested on the web site.

The New England Journal of Medicine

Massachusetts Medical Society, Boston. One of the premier medical journals that publishes original investigations and review information considered of significant importance to physicians and other health care professionals. Published weekly. Internet access available for a fee at <<http://www.nejm.org>>.

Paediatric Drugs

Adis International, Ltd., Auckland, New Zealand. A journal that publishes review articles on the evaluation of drug therapy and disease management in children. Published quarterly. Internet access available for a fee.

Pediatrics

American Academy of Pediatrics, Elk Grove Village, IL. Official publication of the American Academy of Pediatrics. Published monthly. An on-line version also available on the Internet at <<http://www.pediatrics.org>>.

Pharmacist's Letter

Pharmacist's Letter, Stockton, CA. A newsletter that briefly covers a number of new therapeutic issues that may be of interest to pharmacists. Published monthly.

PharmacoEconomics

Adis International Limited, Auckland, New Zealand. A publication focused on economic aspects of rational drug therapy and drug development. Published monthly. Internet access available for a fee.

Pharmacotherapy. The Journal of Human Pharmacology and Drug Therapy

Pharmacotherapy Publications, Inc., Boston. A publication of the American College of Clinical Pharmacy focused on pharmacotherapeutic aspects of disease state management including pharmacokinetics, bioavailability, drug interactions, clinical trials, and pharmacology. Published every 2 months. *Pharmacotherapy: A One Shot Dose of Information* is also available via fax/e-mail for a fee that provides information on clinical developments in a concise one page format.

Pharmacy Practice Management Quarterly

(Formerly called *Topics in Hospital Pharmacy Management*). Aspen Publishers, Frederick, MD. A journal focused on management issues pertinent to pharmacy departments in hospitals. Published quarterly.

Pharmacy Times

Romaine Pierson Publishers, Inc., Jamesburg, NJ. A pharmacy magazine with a community practice focus that provides information on new drug therapies, patient counseling and management, and issues relevant to pharmacy practice. Original investigations are not commonly published in this journal. Published monthly. Available on the Internet at <<http://www.pharmacytimes.com>>.

Psychopharmacology Bulletin

Division of Clinical and Treatment Research, National Institute of Mental Health, Rockville, MD. A journal dedicated to dissemination of research and information related to pharmacotherapy of mental illnesses. Published quarterly.

The Scientific Review of Alternative Medicine

Prometheus Books, Amherst, NY. A journal dedicated to the scientific review of alternative medical practices. Published biannually.

Scrip. World Pharmaceutical News

PJB Publications, Ltd., Richmond, Surrey, England. A newsletter that provides updates on worldwide news regarding the pharmaceutical industry. Published twice weekly. Available on the Internet at <<http://www.pjbpubs.co.uk/scrip/>>.

Sports Medicine

Adis International, Ltd., Auckland, New Zealand. A journal that publishes practical reviews of exercise science and sports medicine. Published monthly. Internet access available for a fee.

Therapeutic Drug Monitoring: A Journal Devoted to Therapeutic Drug Monitoring and Clinical Drug Toxicology

Lippincott Williams & Wilkins, Philadelphia. An official journal of the International Association of Therapeutic Drug Monitoring and Clinical Toxicology.

U.S. Pharmacist

Jobson Publishing L.L.C., New York. A pharmacy magazine focused on the practice of community pharmacy and issues pertinent to this setting. Original investigations are not commonly published in this journal. Published monthly. Also available on the Internet at <<http://www.uspharmacist.com>>.

Alternate Sources of Drug Information

On occasion, drug information inquiries cannot be answered using tertiary, secondary, or primary resources. In such cases, alternate sources of drug information can be used (Table 4–2). Efficient use of alternate sources of drug information requires some inge-

TABLE 4–2. ALTERNATE SOURCES OF DRUG INFORMATION

- Internet, list servers, and USENET news
- Telnet and file transfer protocol (FTP) programs
- Local and national professional organizations
- Pharmaceutical manufacturers
- Drug information and poison control centers

nuity and a little common sense. When a roadblock is reached and information has not been located, the question "Who may know the answer to this question?" needs to be asked. Experts in the area, professional associations, pharmaceutical manufacturers, and others may be consulted.

Searching the Internet is a viable and valuable source of information as technology for accessing the Internet improves and more users become proficient in its use. Refer to Chap. 5 for further information about the Internet.

Conclusion

Information technology is exploding at an unprecedented rate. The ability to rapidly access large quantities of information has become easier with the introduction of computers, CD-ROMs, and the Internet. New technologies and resources for locating drug information are likely to become available in the near future. Texts, journals, newsletters, and other printed media are not only available to traditional drug information centers, but to virtually every pharmacist, regardless of practice setting. Such ease of information access will enhance the ability of pharmacists to provide comprehensive patient care. As pharmacists develop a comprehensive knowledge of available resources and the necessary skills to use these resources efficiently, pharmacy will continue to move toward its goal as an information-based profession, which will be absolutely vital for the existence of the profession as automation takes over the more mechanical aspects that many pharmacists have concentrated on in the past. A list of topics, which are commonly inquired of pharmacists and useful tertiary and secondary resources for answering these questions, is provided in Appendix 4–1.

Understanding resources and technology, however, is only the first step. Slawson and associates stated: "Information is not *knowledge.* Knowledge comes from the interpretation of information. While we are constantly bombarded with *data* and *information,* what we want is *knowledge* and *wisdom,* i.e., the ability to understand and apply the facts."[14] Many of the chapters in this textbook are devoted to analyzing and applying the information located in the multitude of resources available to pharmacists.

Study Questions

1. P.T. is a 26-year-old white female who is admitted to the emergency department with elevated temperature (103°F), increased respiratory rate (45 per minute), and hypotension (90/45). The patient's husband informs the intern on-call that his wife is not taking any prescription or over-the-counter drug products. The patient, however, routinely uses an herbal remedy containing willow bark for menstrual cramps. The husband states that his wife has used the product excessively over the past week. The intern contacts the pharmacy department for information regarding whether willow bark may be contributing to the patient's current symptomatology.

   a. What is the role of tertiary, secondary, and primary literature in the provision of drug information? List the advantages and disadvantages of each of these types of resources.

   b. Is it necessary to provide all types of resources (tertiary, secondary, and primary) for this question?

   c. What tertiary resources would be useful for answering this question?

   d. What secondary resources would be useful for answering this question?

   e. (For after completing the next chapter) Where could you find information on the Internet that would be useful in answering this question?

2. Consider tertiary, secondary, and primary resources that would be useful in answering the following drug information questions:

   a. Identify a red and tan capsule with the imprint code CIBA 154.

   b. What is the dose of gentamicin for suspected meningitis in a 1.5-kg neonate?

   c. A hospital pharmacist receives an order for cefazolin 1 g intravenously every 8 hours in a 70-kg male with a serum creatinine of 7.8 mg/dL. Is this dosage appropriate?

   d. A 55-kg white female is receiving lidocaine at a dosage of 50 µg/kg/min. A serum level drawn 6 hours after initiation of the infusion is 5.7 µg/mL. Is a dosage adjustment needed, and if so, what changes should be made?

   e. A 32-year-old female patient who is HIV positive asks for information on the use of thalidomide for the treatment of aphthous ulcers. The patient is also wondering about special legal requirements that she has heard about the use of the drug.

   f. A mother asks a pharmacist to recommend a cold preparation that is sugar free and alcohol free for her 12-year-old son who is diabetic.

   g. A 56-year-old patient with a history of hypertension and atrial fibrillation comes into a community pharmacy with prescriptions for warfarin 5 mg daily, hydrochlorothiazide 25 mg daily, and atenolol 25 mg daily. She also wishes to purchase ibuprofen over the counter for treatment of minor arthritis pain. Should the pharmacist be concerned about any potential drug interactions?

h. On a recent trip to Europe, a patient purchased paracetamol for headache pain. He returns home and asks the pharmacist whether an equivalent product is available in the United States.

i. A surgeon is interested in using octreotide for the management of an enterocutaneous fistula in a postsurgical patient. She asks the pharmacist for further information.

j. A patient is given a routine urine test during an employee screening for drug abuse. The employer informs the patient that the test was positive for amphetamines. The patient is not abusing drugs and has only been taking pseudoephedrine over the past week for cold symptoms. The patient asks the pharmacist whether pseudoephedrine could interfere with the urine drug screen for amphetamines.

k. A patient with a prescription for acyclovir asks for written information on the product.

REFERENCES

1. Kirkpatrick BA. History of the development of medical information. Bull NY Acad Med 1985;61:230–9.
2. Host TR, Kirkwood CF. Computer-assisted instruction for responding to drug information requests. Presented at the Twenty-Second Annual Midyear Clinical Meeting, American Society of Hospital Pharmacists; December 1987; Atlanta. Abstract.
3. Price KO, Goldwire MA. Drug information resources. Am Pharm 1994;NS34:30–9.
4. Mazza JJ. A library for internists VIII. Recommendations from the American College of Physicians. Ann Intern Med 1994;120:699–720.
5. Collins GE. Searching and organizing the professional literature. In: Brown TR, Smith MC, editors. Handbook of institutional pharmacy practice. Baltimore: Williams & Wilkins; 1986. pp. 249–54.
6. Murdoch LL. Foreign drug identification. Drug Intell Clin Pharm 1989;23:501–6.
7. Baker DE, Smith GH, Abate MA. Selected topics in drug information access and practice: an update. Ann Pharmacotherapy 1994;28:1389–94.
8. Williams AL. Meet the matrix: information technology for consultant pharmacists. Consult Pharm 1993;8:847–54.
9. Tousignaut DR. Online literature-retrieval systems: How to get started. Am J Hosp Pharm 1983;40:230–9.
10. Anderson PO. How to get started with computerized literature searches. Am J Hosp Pharm 1994;51:2303–7.
11. Oxman AD, Cook DJ, Guyatt GH. Users' guides to the medical literature. VI. How to use an overview. JAMA 1994;272:1367–71.

12. Oxman AD, Guyatt GH. Guidelines for reading literature reviews. Can Med Assoc J 1988;138:697–703.

13. Lowe HJ, Barnett GO. Understanding and using the medical subject headings (MeSH) vocabulary to perform literature searches. JAMA 1994;271:1103–8.

14. Slawson DC, Shaughnessy AF, Bennett JH. Becoming a medical information master: feeling good about not knowing everything. J Fam Pract 1994;38:505–13.

5

Chapter Five

Electronic Information Management

Patrick M. Malone

Objectives

After completing this chapter, the reader will be able to:

- Explain how to integrate the following into his or her personal practice philosophy:
    - Searching the Internet for information necessary for pharmacy practice.
    - Providing pharmacy and drug information to others over the Internet.
    - Gathering input from health care practitioners and patients via web sites.
    - Using e-mail, including personal distribution lists and listservers.
    - USENET News.
    - Push technology.
    - Internet collaboration.
    - WebTV.
- Evaluate the credibility of Internet resources.
- Efficiently manage personal e-mail, both outgoing and incoming.

In 1981 drug information was revolutionized when it suddenly became possible for non-librarians to access MEDLINE directly. Those who first had access were required to participate in a weeklong training class given in only three locations in the country and then could only access the information via dumb-terminals using a 300 bits-per-second (bps) modem. Little did practitioners realize that they were starting down a technologic road that would quickly accelerate. A few years later some of the first pharmacy uses of what was to become the Internet were seen. At that time, some users of the Iowa Drug Information Service (IDIS) could e-mail search requests, via ARPANET (a predecessor of the Internet), to the University of Iowa, and would receive a reply with citations to the IDIS microfiche. Unfortunately, although the sender's computer might indicate the message was received in seconds, in reality it might take several days to make its way across the country. It would then take additional time for the reply. Certainly, this was a vast improvement over the very first MEDLINE searches that were requested and sent via the postal system, but still was not close to what practitioners take for granted today.

Today, pharmacists can access vast amounts of data locally or from computer systems around the world in seconds, using a powerful microcomputer system that costs less than $1000, at speeds of up to 100 million bps or more! These data can even be obtained at home at those speeds across cable TV lines. In addition to increases in amounts of data and speed, the ways data can be communicated have increased greatly and include graphics, sound, and video. These capabilities are seen around the world to some extent or another, with an estimated 72,398,092 host computers attached to the Internet as of January 2000, up from 19,540,000 in July 1997.[1] The speed of the computers will also increase, with IBM aiming to have a computer working at 1 quadrillion operations per second within 5 years, which would be 2 million times the speed of a 1999 computer.[2]

The overwhelming amount of information, and its hazards, has been recognized by pharmacy organizations as an area that needs to be addressed.[3] Also, the lack of training and lack of use of resources, particularly electronic, by health care practitioners must be recognized,[4] and is now beginning to be addressed in some schools of pharmacy.[5] Initially a way to communicate data, the Internet is fast becoming a way to simply communicate. E-mail is widely used in business and as a means of personal communication, but may be replaced by real-time video conversations in the future. Use of the Internet to provide telepresence may become one of its most important uses.

This chapter describes how pharmacists can access the Internet, the methods of communicating information over the Internet, some good sources of data, and how pharmacists can integrate these resources and the new information management and communication methods into their practices.

Technology—The First Step

Any microcomputer capable of running a current operating system (e.g., the current version of Windows) and web browser (e.g., Microsoft Internet Explorer, Netscape Navigator) is an appropriate choice for connecting to the Internet. Notebook computers are practical for the clinician moving from place to place; however, that often makes connection to the Internet more difficult, although wireless connections are rapidly becoming more common. That connection to the local area network (LAN) in the institution, clinic, or pharmacy, along with connection to the Internet, is vital. Pharmacists' computers must be set up to give the easiest, most transparent access to information. It should be no more difficult to switch from a local copy of MEDLINE to the Centers for Disease Control (CDC) web site than it is to switch from a word processing program to a spreadsheet program. In the future, it will even be possible to stay within the same program while accessing data from a variety of sources, using a universal search engine. For example, the beginning of such a system has been implemented at the University of Washington with the Willow Project.[6]

A possible replacement for personal computers, at least in some settings, is a palmtop computer (i.e., a tiny computer that can fit into a pocket), which contains a subset of the functions, programs, and data available on a normal desktop machine.[7] It has been noted that some physicians already use such equipment to perform searches of MEDLINE or other databases, retrieve patient information, set appointments, or other activities.[8] Many digital cellular phones also have web-browsing functions available,[9,10] but they do not yet seem practical for most practitioners, if for no other reason than the extremely small screen. They may also have some of the functions of a palmtop computer and even video phone capabilities.

The connection to the network should not be a problem for the practitioner because of security risks; however, some institutions are reluctant to provide practitioners easy connection from a personal computer to the Internet, or sometimes even to the hospital's network. There are a variety of methods for an institution to strike an appropriate balance between security and access. Cheryl Currid, the former head of computing at Coca-Cola, stated a number of years ago, "PCs go on networks, period. Stand-alone computing is worthless to an organization. Demand a LAN."[11] That should be taken a step further today—demand quality access to the Internet![12]

It has been estimated that 80% of Windows-based PCs have some sort of Internet connection.[13] Unfortunately, this was not the case in pharmacy in the late 1990s when only 21% of community pharmacists (29% independents, 13% chain), 57% of hospital pharmacists, and 10% of corporate pharmacists had access to the Internet at work (although about 60% of all pharmacists had access from home) and only about one-third to one-half of those pharmacists used that access daily.[14,15]

In cases where the concern of an institution or clinic is the cost of an Internet connection, it should be pointed out that the Telecommunications Act of 1996 or later funding might help to offset costs.[16] A third reason that Internet connections may be absent is the concern about abuse of web surfing by the employees. This is a valid concern, but should be addressed by clear, well-known web surfing policies that are enforced, rather than preventing Internet use altogether.[17]

Pharmacists practicing in a location where an institutional connection to the Internet is not possible or practical (e.g., a remote ambulatory clinic, community pharmacy) can still access the Internet. Perhaps the easiest will be a simple modem connection to an Internet Service Provider (ISP), requiring the extra step of connecting to the ISP each time the Internet connection is accessed. Other possibilities for connection, which may or may not be available in a particular location are listed in Table 5–1.[18–20]

There may be concerns about data security when operating over one of the listed commercial links; however, virtual private network (VPN) software allows secure transmission of confidential data over such links.[21,22] A VPN has been implemented by Carondelet Health Systems in St. Louis to provide physicians with secure access to patient data.[23] Once the computer is connected to the network, appropriate software is required. Typically, the newer operating systems provide simple telnet and file transfer protocol (FTP) programs. *Telnet* essentially turns a computer into a dumb terminal to access mainframe-like programs. *FTP* allows transfer of files to or from another computer. The functions provided by these programs are relatively limited to text material or very simple functions, and are now often superceded by web browsers.

The most popular web browsers are Microsoft Internet Explorer and Netscape Navigator/Communicator (both are currently available free of charge or for a small fee to cover distribution costs). The latter was at one time the most popular; however, the former has rapidly gained in popularity and has been rated as the better product.[24–27] Both have strengths and weaknesses, but either is likely to serve most needs of the average user. Web browsers also provide other functions, such as electronic mail (e-mail), USENET News Reader, live collaboration tools, live software updates, and web page authoring tools. In addition, other programs can work in conjunction to the web browser. For example, if a word processing file is downloaded with the web browser, the browser may start the copy of Word for Windows residing on the computer and display the document in the browser window. Also, there are a variety of free "Reader" programs that are available on the Internet to display data that is downloaded, whether or not the full version of the program has been purchased. For example, Adobe Acrobat Reader can be downloaded (<<http://www.adobe.com>>), to allow review of copies of *Morbidity and Mortality Weekly Report* (MMWR) from the CDC, and Microsoft provides reader programs for some of its Office programs. Often, web sites will alert a user to the need for these extra "plug-in" programs, and will give directions for obtaining them or provide an automatic method for installation.

Before ending this section, it is important to note that any personal computer should have antiviral protection that is updated regularly.[28] It may also be desirable to have other forms of software protection for web browsers, e-mail, and so on, which can be separately investigated.[29] Protection provided by each of these programs is becoming better and updating is often automatic. Finally, any organization with networked com-

TABLE 5–1. INTERNET CONNECTIONS

Connection	Advantages	Disadvantages
Cable TV modem	Up to 30 Mbps downstream and 4 Mbps upstream; may be inexpensive; provides a permanent, fast connection.[151–154]	Not available in all locations and may cost more than telephone modem connections.
DSL (digital subscriber line)—A major competitor to cable modems, because it uses phone lines and provides fast Internet access.[155–157] There are variations on this referred to by similar acronyms, such as ADSL (the most popular), EDSL, IDSL, SDSL, or VDSL, which may be the forms of this technology that are ultimately available due to capabilities or price.	Speeds of up to 8 Mbps downstream and 1.7 Mbps upstream are currently available.	Not available in all locations and may cost more than telephone modem connections.
ISDN (Integrated Services Digital Network) modems	Up to 1.536 Mbps.	Expensive.
Direct Broadcast Satellite (DBS) (also referred to as Digital Satellite Service [DSS])	Useful in rural areas. Two-way satellite communication is expected to be available around 2002, although the time lag for transmission to and from orbit may limit its usefulness in some ways.[158]	Download only (~400 Kbps) and requires a normal phone modem connection for uploading. May cost more than telephone modem connections.
Local Multipoint Distribution Service (LMDS)	A version of MMDS that uses higher frequencies that increase speeds (~1500 Kbps, but possibly much faster).	Decreases the possible distance between sender and receiver. Currently not very available. May cost more than telephone modem connections.
Multichannel Multipoint Distribution Service (MMDS)	Uses microwaves to beam signals at up to 800 Kbps to users receivers.	Limited to about 35 miles distance for download only and uses standard modems for upload. May cost more than telephone modem connections.
Frame relay connection	Effectively, a permanent connection leased from the telephone company between remote clinics and a central location, which can also be used for an Internet connection.	Expensive. Requires more technical support.

puters must make efforts to protect data integrity and confidential information through the use of protection procedures, such as firewalls, cryptography, and file server security software. There have been documented cases where patient record information has been altered as a prank, causing needless patient suffering. There is the potential for much greater harm in the future.[30]

Information via the Internet

Information can be communicated over the Internet many ways. This section describes the most common methods, provides examples of the information obtained and some likely sources of information, and provides information on how pharmacists can incorporate these capabilities into their actual practice.

THE PAST

People who used the Internet a few years ago will remember such terms as Telnet, FTP, Gopher, Archie, Veronica, and Jughead. The latter terms referred to methods of retrieving information and programs, but have disappeared over time. Gophers are still sometimes used as data or software repositories; however, they are rapidly being replaced by web servers. Telnet and FTP still remain to some extent, but are rapidly being superceded by web browsers. Telnet may still be seen in an institutional pharmacy to allow connection to a hospital's mainframe computer information system. If there is a need for those programs, it is possible to buy more powerful or easier to use versions of the programs that might even operate in such a way that is difficult to tell where the operating system software ends and the program starts.[31] Those people needing to know more about them are referred to other sources.[32]

THE PRESENT

It is nearly impossible to live in the United States these days without having heard of the World Wide Web (WWW). It is a very popular source of information, including health information. It was estimated in 1997 that 43% of U.S. adults with Internet access used it to obtain health information, and that there were at least 10,000 health and medical sites.[33] There has been a rapid increase in both of those figures, which is likely to continue. It has been proposed that there should be universal access to the Internet for health-related information to help improve the information reaching underserved populations.[34]

The quality and presentation of information retrieved from the Internet has progressed from simple, text-based information seen with telnet programs, to multimedia extravaganzas that can be accessed with web browsers. Much of the information currently available consists of text and simple graphics, but more sophisticated presentation of information is rapidly appearing. Reasons for the simpler material include lack of more advanced information in computer format (after all, good material takes time and effort to produce), lack of power in older computers, and a concern about the time that it takes to access material. Retrieval speed is particularly important to those who access the Internet via modem, where the slower speed can result in rather long waits before information can be downloaded to a computer. Even with direct connections to the Internet, the download time can be long during certain times of the day (e.g., mid-afternoon). Both of these problems are being addressed, but the growth of Internet usage often seems to counteract speed improvements. To best address the current situation, the various features available in the current web browsers will be covered.

Incorporating Web Browsing into the Systematic Search Process

The most common use for a web browser is its original purpose—to present information from WWW servers. However, before using a browser, the first step is to recognize the need to access the Internet and the value of the information it makes available. After all, to use the Internet, a pharmacist does need special equipment and some knowledge about how to use it. Often a simple look at a common textbook (e.g., *Drug Facts and Comparisons, AHFS—Drug Information*) may answer a question simply and efficiently. The key is to create an efficient search strategy. A full discussion of a systematic approach to answering a drug information question and preparing a search strategy is presented in Chap. 2. However, a few general rules can be stated. First, if a pharmacist is familiar with references that are likely to contain the information necessary to answer a question, those references should be consulted first. For example, to check for drug interactions, a drug interaction reference would be a logical choice. Second, there is no one "right" way to search.[35] Sometimes a person will know precisely where a piece of information is located from experience, even if it is obscure. In other cases, the searcher will realize that it is so unusual a topic that an immediate jump to Internet metasearch engines is warranted. Generally, Internet WWW browsing is likely to be farther down the list after books or other resources—perhaps even after MEDLINE searching, except in certain circumstances, such as:

- When a reference to the Internet is found (e.g., advertisement, citation).
- Situations where company-specific information is necessary (e.g., product package inserts). *Note:* some drug companies put only business information on the Internet because of their interpretation of FDA regulations concerning provision of clinical information. Others are beginning to put clinical information on the Internet (e.g., via searchable databases) that answer common drug information questions about their products.
- Items currently in the news (e.g., check sites listed in Appendix 5–9). As a side issue, this is becoming a much more important step that needs to be pursued in any situation where the origin of the question is vague (e.g., a patient heard about something and asked a physician, who then asked the pharmacist).
- When U.S. government information is required (e.g., Food and Drug Administration [FDA] or CDC specific subjects, including clinical information and new

drug approvals). The U.S. government has been very active in putting a great deal of information on the web (see Appendix 5–7).

- When the information is not likely to be contained in other available sources of information (e.g., alternative medicine [see Appendix 5–1] tropical diseases).
- When computer-related information or software updates are needed.

Why is there so much emphasis on web browsing versus some other form of obtaining information? Quite likely the reason is that web protocols allow easy access of various types of information on disparate computer systems—they are very flexible and powerful.[36] Also, it should be pointed out that it is predicted that all periodicals and many textbook publications will become web based over the next few years, due to ease of availability and use.[37] Most indexing or abstracting services are already available in network formats. Additionally, patient information will be increasingly available through web interfaces, due to ease of use, security, and the ability to transparently tie together information residing on separate, somewhat incompatible, computer systems.[38]

Web Addresses

Once the decision to search the web is made, the pharmacist needs to log onto a computer attached to the Internet and run the web browser. To obtain information, the user simply needs to put the address (referred to as a Uniform Resource Locator [URL]) of that information in the browser, which will then find it automatically. An example of an address is <<http://druginfo.creighton.edu>>, which is the address of the author's main web site. The first term in an address, which will be followed by a //, indicates the type of information provided at that site. In this case, http stands for hypertext transfer protocol, which is the technical term for the information generally contained by a site accessed with a web browser. Common types of information are[39]:

- http: hypertext transfer protocol—normal web information
- https: a secure form of http, used for confidential information (e.g., credit card numbers)
- telnet: a site that requires your computer to act like a "dumb terminal"
- ftp: file transfer protocol—allows you to transfer software or a file of information in various formats
- gopher: gopher link
- news: USENET News group
- mailto: Internet e-mail address

Soon, another version of hypertext markup language (HTML), refered to as eXtensible Hypertext Markup Language (XHTML), is expected to replace HTML. This is a reformulation of HTML as an application of eXtensible Markup Language (XML), and is felt to offer more capabilities.[40] For example, it is designed to separately provide content, presentation (how it looks—addressed by eXtensible Style Language [XSL]) and semantics (what it means).[41] That last capability should make it easier to find relevant information than is currently possible with many search engines.

The second term in the address ("druginfo") is often the name of the web server that you are accessing. Typically, the main web server for a particular organization will have an address name of "www." In actuality, one computer can host multiple addresses, through a process called multihoming. For example, http://druginfo.creighton.edu runs on the same computer as <<http://pharmacy.creighton.edu>> and several other web sites. The next item in this address is the organization's general address name. These servers are at Creighton University. Finally, you will notice a three-letter extension on the end of the URL. In this case, it is .edu, which indicates the address is to an educational institution. Common three-letter extensions seen in the United States include:

- .com—commercial (e.g., <<http://www.microsoft.com>> or <<http://www.netscape.com>>)
- .edu—education
- .gov—government (e.g., <<http://www.cdc.gov>> for the CDC)
- .mil—military
- .org—organization (e.g., <<http://www.ashp.org>> for American Society of Health-System Pharmacists)
- .net—network (network provider)

In foreign countries, addresses tend to end in a two-letter code that indicates the country (e.g., .fr = France). The country code for the United States is .us, but it is seldom used.

In addition, there can be a slash (/) followed by one or more names added onto the end of the address. These indicate the file name, including the server subdirectory. For example, <<http://druginfo.creighton.edu/Clerkships/HSL-DIC/duedates.htm>> on our server indicates that you are accessing a file called duedates in the Clerkships/HSL-DIC subdirectory (note long file names are permitted). The .htm indicates that the file is in hypertext markup language format (also sometimes abbreviated .html). That format is standard for much of the information available on the web; however, other file formats are occasionally used. For example, the .ppt in the address <<http://druginfo.creighton.edu/PHA458/NewsletterLec/Newsletter%20Lecture.ppt>> indicates that the file is actually in Microsoft PowerPoint format. More frequently, the extension .asp (active server page) is seen instead of .htm, but to the casual user they appear the same. The .asp simply gives some additional abilities to the file. A somewhat common extension that pharmacists may run across is .pdf, which stands for portable data file. This is the format used by the Adobe Acrobat Reader. A variety of information, such as MMWR from the CDC's web site, is available in this format. Other commonly seen extensions[39] are .gif (graphic image), .jpeg or .jpg (graphic image), .mov (movie/animation), .avi (movie/animation), .au (sound), .wav (sound), and .ra (RealAudio/sound).

Links to Internet Sites

In many cases, the URL of a company or organization's web site may be known; after all, such addresses seem to be on everything now. If the URL is unknown, often a correct guess may be made. For example, the American Society of Health-System Pharmacists is commonly known as ASHP and it is an organization. Therefore, <<http://www.ashp. org>> would be a logical guess of its web address, which happens to be correct.

A second easy way to find sites is to find cross references from similar sites or sites that would have an interest in the site. For example, a logical guess of the web address for the American Pharmaceutical Association would be <<http://www.apha.org>>, but this produces the web site for the American Public Health Association. However, by going to the ASHP web site, it is possible to easily find a link to the APhA web site at http://www.aphanet.org. Links are text or graphics on a web page that, when clicked on with a mouse or other pointing device, will take the user to another web page. That page may simply be another page on the same web site, but could also be located on another computer halfway around the world; that is one of the major advantages to web browsing—the ease with which a user can connect from one piece of information to another without having to worry about where that information is actually located. It is also possible to find links to a variety of other useful web sites at either the ASHP or APhA web sites. Lists of other useful web sites for pharmacists are presented in the appendices of this chapter. In particular, the Virtual Pharmacy Library (<<http://www.pharmacy. org>>), PharmWeb (<<http://www.pharmweb.net>>), or Drug InfoNet (<<http://www. druginfonet.com>>) can provide many leads for information. It is important to note that links on web sites are often shown in different colors than surrounding text or may be "boxed" by a different color. Usually, the mouse pointer will change into a different shape when passed over a link (e.g., a hand with the forefinger extended, as if to push a button), which also allows for easy identification of a link.

Using Search Engines

In many cases, the URL of a likely source of information is not known and a method of searching for the information is necessary. Fortunately, a variety of search engines have been developed for this purpose; some are general and some are specific to medically related topics, even medical specialties. A new term for these search engines is web portal, because a user might use one of them as his or her entrance to the Internet.[42] Once the decision is made to use one of these portals, it is then up to the user to decide which search engine is most appropriate for his or her needs. Unfortunately, there does not yet seem to be a truly excellent search engine specific to pharmacy. There are some search engines, such as Drug InfoNet (<<http://www.druginfonet.com>>), that provide some capabilities; however, those databases currently do not seem adequate for many searches.

When a pharmacist needs general medical information, there are a variety of medical search engines listed in Appendix 5–18. Even these search engines are not all encompassing, and it may be necessary to search several of them to find any information. It has been shown that MedBot, MedHunt, Medical World Search, and OMNI all tend to return a reasonably good number of items on a medically related search; however, none of that group seem to stand out as the best or most comprehensive (e.g., Medical World Search returned 828 "hits" on one specific search and 9 on another, whereas OMNI returned 15 and 158 hits, respectively, when the same searches were performed).[43] Part of this is the coverage of material and how it is created. The material may be compiled manually, MediS indexes only medical papers and abstracts, or material may even be indexed by Medical Subject Headings (MeSH, e.g., CliniWeb[44] and Medical World Search[43,45]).

Each search engine uses different methods for conducting Internet searches. An in-depth explanation of the ways to use each individual service is beyond the scope of this chapter; however, some general information can be provided. The first step is to pick the search engine that seems most likely to produce information. If a specific legitimate medical subject is to be searched, one of the medical search engines would probably be good. However, if the need is for information that might not be supported by the medical literature (e.g., finding what is being claimed by alternate medicine marketers, finding "street information" about illegal medications), it might be better to go to one of the general search engines listed in Appendix 5–18.

Those general search engines attempt to index as much of the WWW as possible. Some are referred to as web crawlers because they use intelligent software agents (termed "spiders") to crawl through sites across the Internet by exploring links on other web sites.[46] Because it is virtually impossible to do this and keep entirely up to date, the various web crawlers have a specific logic as to how often a site is "crawled." More important or common sites (e.g., CNN, Microsoft) and those known to change frequently are "crawled" more often. However, by indexing everything, a search on these general engines may produce too many "hits." It is not unusual for a vague or general search on a common term to produce thousands of hits. Needless to say, this amount of information is unmanageable and means that the search needs to be narrowed.

Even though the general search engines index a great number of web sites, they are not all inclusive. A study found that no single search engine indexes more than about one-third of the Internet web pages.[47] A more recent publication was even less optimistic, showing that the best search engine only indexed approximately 16% of the web.[48] Also, the frequency of adding new pages and deleting "dead links" should be at least once a month,[49] with some engines being rather dated. Other web technology, such as dynamically prepared pages and frames (screens on a web browser may consist of several "frames") may not be appropriately indexed by search engines.

Techniques to narrow a search are discussed in Chap. 4, under the secondary references section. These techniques may include the use of logical operators (i.e., AND, OR, and NOT) or other methods (e.g., putting a phrase in quotations). Unfortunately, the various search engines implement these search methods differently. For example, in some you might put in the word "and," in others it will need to be "AND" ("and" is just treated as a text word), and in some you might have to use "+" or "&." Also, features such as truncation, phrase searching, field searching (e.g., date, URL, language),[50] case-sensitivity (e.g., finding AIDS instead of aids),[51] and additional logical operators (e.g., "NEAR," "WITH," "BEFORE") may be available. On some search engines it is possible to search for nontextual information, such as graphic images or sounds (see Appendix 5–20).[52]

Many search engines may restrict certain words or short words from searches (e.g., Vitamin B will not be found because the "B" is too short). Because of these problems, the next rule of searching is to read the directions for using a search engine, before performing anything but a very simple search on an unusual topic (i.e., one that isn't likely to produce many hits).

The differences in search commands and capabilities can drastically change the quality of the search results, making more traditional secondary search programs (e.g., MEDLINE, International Pharmaceutical Abstracts) more likely to produce useful results with a number of searches.[53] Perhaps the easiest procedure for pharmacists is to become familiar with a couple of medical and general search engines and learn the directions for those. If those "favorites" do not produce an answer, the searcher can then pick others to try and read their help file while preparing a search strategy. In the future, there may be a standard set of search engine techniques; a project is underway at Search Engine Watch (<<http://searchenginewatch.com/standards>>), but for now the best that can be offered is a set of directions that is continually updated as search engines develop (see <<http://searchenginewatch.com/facts/powersearch.html>>).[54]

If the search covers a topic that is very unusual and it is expected that several general search engines will need to be consulted, it may be appropriate to use a multiple-web search engine, also referred to as a meta-search engine, which will search multiple search engines concurrently. Several of these are found in Appendix 5–18; the highest rated of these is MetaCrawler.[55] It may be tempting to hop directly to these multiple-web search engines, but two major problems are possible—information overload and slow speeds—so it might be best to save them until other search strategies have failed. Also, depending on the specific multiple-web search engine used, there are several other possible problems. These include the inability to use all logical operators (e.g., NEAR), a limit on the number of hits to be reported from the other search engines, and possible incompatibilities between the multiple-web search engine and the general search engine (i.e., the general search engine may have changed its format and the multiple-web search engine might have not yet noted and adjusted for that change).[56]

A related, but perhaps better, alternative to meta-search engines are programs residing on a user's computer that perform many of the same functions. For example, Copernic 2000 (<<http://www.copernic.com>>) provides a program that can search for a variety of types of information. This program gives a common interface and is automatically updated to best know how to interface with other search engines each time it is run.

Portal software provides a new means to search the Internet.[57] Portals were mentioned in this chapter as another name for some of the search engines; however, portal software may go much further. Some of the new portal software acts as a universal interface to allow searching of not only the Internet, but also an institution's intranet for documents, including databases, word processing documents, spreadsheets, slide presentations, and e-mail messages. In addition, this software may use logic to aid in identifying material by context, filtering out irrelevent information, based on the needs of the individual and his or her job description. The software may also be fault-tolerant, using fuzzy logic to identify documents when search terms are misspelled, or will even actively search out information on a prospective basis in the background. Portal software providers are investigating many new and innovative methods to help searchers find the most appropriate, high-quality information, such as the use of natural language processing for search terms.[58] The most successful of those methods will be available in the future.[59]

Besides using the above search engines, a version of a classic database is available on the Internet. PubMed and Grateful Med are versions of MEDLINE from the National Library of Medicine (NLM) that is available free on the Internet. Besides some of the well-known features of MEDLINE, it provides natural language searching and even links to some of the articles that might be found in other databases.[60] Further research is also being indexed as part of a new service that is called PubMed Central (<<http://www.pubmedcentral.nih.gov/>>). Electronic library card catalogs are also starting to provide such direct browser links to actual publications. Although this information might make it tempting to drop subscriptions to the MEDLINE database from other vendors to save money, pharmacists should take into account that the other vendors may provide value-added features and their products may be more easily accessible at a much faster speed.[61] Also, although the different vendors use the same MEDLINE database, results of querying the data base may vary from one vendor's system to another, because of different search engine capabilities and different rates of updating the database.[62] For example, some versions of MEDLINE available on the Internet do not allow normal use of logical operators. A search of "diazepam AND seizures" might result in a listing of citations that deal with either diazepam or with seizures; in other words, it would end up giving results normally found with a search of "diazepam OR seizures." Be sure to evaluate the quality of MEDLINE search engines before settling on one, to make sure that it meets the users' needs.[63]

It should also be mentioned that many full text publications are available on the Internet (see Appendix 5–14 for examples). These are likely to increase in number over the coming years and it is likely that users will be charged in some way for access to these sites, with advertising if not a more direct charge. Similarly, forms of some other references (e.g., MICROMEDEX, STAT!-Ref) may be placed on an institution's network and be searched using web browsers, even from remote sites, as long as licensing restrictions are observed through the use of passwords, proxy servers, or other means.

Evaluating Information on the Web

Finding the information is only part of the battle. Essentially anyone can put any information on the web, whether valuable, worthless, disgusting, or even dangerous.[64–66] It is necessary for pharmacists to use the skills discussed in Chaps 4, 6, and 7 on Drug Literature Evaluation. In particular, a web source should be evaluated for believability, the source (author), supporting evidence, logic, timeliness, and other factors.[67–69]

In classic literature evaluation, one of the first things that a person is taught to evaluate is the source of the information. In this case it would be the Internet web site, which should disclose its name, location, and sponsorship (which can be important in determining conflicts of interest). Sometimes the user will know the site. For example, it might be supported by a pharmaceutical manufacturer (whose information is regulated by the FDA[70]), university, or pharmacy organization, all of which generally provide good, high-quality information. However, even if the searcher does not know the source of information or the web site, there is a method for evaluating its overall quality. The Health on the Net Foundation has established an HONcode, which contains eight principles (see <<http://www.hon.ch>>). These principles, if met, support the quality of the information provided by a particular web site.[71] A webmaster for a particular site can apply to the Health on the Net Foundation to display their HONcode logo on a web site. The webmaster is required to abide by the eight principles and the Health on the Net Foundation does check to see that they do so. There are also many other site rating services that might be noted on the Internet; however, not all of them are known to have acceptable criteria for rating web sites.[72] It should also be pointed out that none of these site-rating services are considered to have a completely comprehensive method of doing so.[72]

A second way to evaluate the overall site is to use a piece of software that gives you information on how other people evaluate the site. One such program is called Alexa, a freeware program available at <<http://www.alexa.com/download>>.[73] This program provides such information on a web site as the name, address, and phone number of the site's owner, the number of hits the site receives; and a number of votes received from Alexa users on whether they do or do not like the site.[13] Actually, the information about who owns the site should be prominent on a site's home page—if not, beware. Another program is available from uTOK Users' Tree of Knowledge at <<http://www.utok. com>>, which allows users to prepare sticky notes that evaluate web sites.

Once at a particular site, the author of the information being evaluated should be considered. Unfortunately, there is great potential for problems here. There have been instances on the Internet of a person writing some piece of information claiming to be someone else, perhaps a well-known and respected individual. So, evaluation of the author's name and credentials should probably be coupled with evaluation of the source of the site itself—if the site is not trusted, do not trust that the supposed author really was the author.

Next, a mark of a good site is that it looks good and makes it easy to get to information and give feedback.[74] This includes not having huge graphics or other files that will take extended times to download, but do not add to the quality of the information. Also, good indexing and ease of navigation are necessary. This certainly is not an absolute in either the good or bad directions, but can be used as one of the factors in evaluating a site.

It is also important to see how recent the information actually is. A good site will list on each page the date it was last updated. In addition, check in other ways to see if the information itself, not just the web page, is up to date.

It is worthwhile noting that some web sites seem to only be a listing of other web sites with links to those sites. If that is their purpose, that is fine. But if the purpose of the site is to supposedly provide good information to the user, the overwhelming number of links should be considered to be a mark against them.[75]

If the above criteria are met, the reader should use traditional literature evaluation skills to determine whether the information is clear, concise, easy to use, fully presented, unbiased, relevant, well organized, and appropriately referenced. Just as there is no perfect study or perfect printed article, there is no perfect web page. Any page is likely to have some deficiencies, and it is up to the user to determine whether those deficiencies are fatal to the usefulness of the information.

If a web site is found that provides good and valuable information, it would be worthwhile to consider saving the URL. Web browsers allow saving such things as "bookmarks" or "favorites," to allow the user to get back to those addresses quickly.

Providing Information on the Web

Besides using the web to obtain information, pharmacists can use it to provide information.[76] Anyone with a connection to the Internet can have a personal web site (e.g.,

Microsoft offers personal web server software for various versions of Windows; software is also available for other operating systems). The software to host a web site is often available free or at little cost, at least for web sites that will not be requiring specialized functions (e.g., secure financial transactions) and those with relatively light use. More powerful and capable web servers can be purchased from a variety of vendors. It is also possible for people to lease a web site from a commercial provider. Just having the web address and some storage space for material may only cost a few dollars a month or be available as part of a subscription to an ISP. Commercial vendors can also prepare and publish the web pages themselves, for a fee. A pharmacy or institution should have available commercial web services, by contract or internally, with adequate support, to allow best interchange of information, although individual pharmacists may use their own web sites for small projects, committees, and so on.

Preparing the material to be placed on the web site can be accomplished using a variety of free or low-cost software, which can be specific for web page development or be part of other software (e.g., word processor, web browser, desktop publisher).

It has been suggested that there are four general uses for computer-based hypertext systems[77]:

- Macro literary systems—large libraries with computerized interdocument links
- Problem exploration systems—support for early unstructured thinking on a particular problem
- Structured browsing systems—can be used for reference or teaching; similar to macro literary systems, but are easier to use.
- General hypertext systems—general systems for experimentation with a wide range of hypertext applications

So, how can a pharmacist use these capabilities? Actually, he or she can do a variety of things. First, a web site can be used to provide information, just like any reference. For example, an institution's drug formulary, policies and procedures, IV guidelines, antimicrobial sensitivities, drug information, investigational drug protocols, and other institution-specific items can be placed on a web site.[78] These pieces of information should be interlinked to allow the user to go to other information. For example, an entry in the drug formulary system might be linked to a policy and procedure on who can use the medication, how it can be used, and/or where it can be used. Although there may be concern about making information available outside the institution, that is not a problem because web sites can have restricted access, by either location or by login name and password. When access is limited to users within an institution, it is called an Intranet. Kaiser Permanente has had such a system for several years,[79] and it has been suggested that such systems will have a strong future in managed care to improve information availability.[80] Intranets are also used in the pharmaceutical industry with Eli Lilly

& Co. even winning an excellence award for ELVIS (Eli Lilly Virtual Information System).[81] The initial expenses may be great in health care, but it is expected that the costs would be made up quickly by savings and improved patient care.[82]

The use of dynamic html allows the preparation of informational web pages that are specific to the user. For example, it might be possible to set things up so that when a physician accesses information on a drug, he or she might be presented first with information about indications, dosing, side effects and interactions, whereas, a nurse might be first presented with information on how to administer the drug and monitor the patient. A pharmacist in the IV room might be first given information on how to prepare the drug. Although the other information could be available to each of these individuals, the web site can, through the dynamic html, try to best serve the likely needs of the user.

Pharmacists can also provide education to patients and health care professionals via the web, within or outside the institution.[83-85] This might be purely textual material, but can also include slides,[86] pictures, video,[87-89] and sound. Right now network bandwidth often restricts at least the quality of such material, but that is improving. For example, there is video patient education material available at RxTV (<<http://www.rxtv.com>>). Some pharmacists do on-line consultations (<<http://www.rx.com>>). There can even be an on-line testing service for classes or continuing education programs. This can have advantages over traditional examinations because the testing system may provide immediate feedback to the user—not just a grade, but also an explanation of what the user answered wrong on the test and why it was wrong.

A web site can also be used to provide a place for on-line discussions, using such software as Expressions Interaction Suite, Microsoft Exchange, or WebBoard.[90] The author of this chapter has used this feature to conduct discussions among nontraditional PharmD students scattered all over the world for several years. The results have been quite good because the students can provide their input to the discussion when it is convenient to them over a period of time, allowing them adequate time to think about what they want to say. This type of software could also be used in patient groups to improve patient education and communication between the pharmacist and the patient.

Overall, the benefits of web publishing include[91]:

- Documents may be made available to anyone in the world with a computer and Internet access very quickly.
- Documents can be updated as often as necessary. For example, a few minutes work will update the drug formulary for everyone in the institution for practically no expense.
- Paper may be saved, although computer use has been shown to actually increase paper use.
- Everyone can publish web documents.

Besides providing information, web sites can also be used by the pharmacist to obtain information. For example, a web site could have input forms to be used as a way for health care professionals on the floor to easily report adverse drug reactions or request addition of drugs to the formulary. Information and prescriptions can be obtained from patients. As a matter of fact, some Internet pharmacies currently allow patients to manage their own medical information on the pharmacy web site (e.g., <<http://www.rx.com>>, <<http://www.webmd.com>>). Internationally, similar Internet data reporting systems have been used for epidemiologic research (e.g., FluNet).[92] These are suggestions and others will likely have other ideas; however, the main thing is that it is necessary to have an objective.[93] The objective(s) will likely grow, and regular updating and maintenance is necessary, but at least one good, useful reason for being on the web is necessary.

How a pharmacist puts together a web site can be compared to how he or she would put together a newsletter. The concepts and skills are much the same and are dealt with in greater detail in Chap. 11, Professional Writing; however, specific points are made in Table 5–2.[94-98] Also, it can be helpful to look at more detailed suggestion lists that are available on the Internet.

As a final thought in this section, Every document a pharmacist creates (with the possible exceptions of personal communications, confidential information, and material that will be submitted for journal publication[99]) should be considered for possible inclusion in web site information—share that information with others who need it; do not hoard it!

E-Mail

The ability to send brief, simple messages around the world in seconds is wonderful and efficient for both the sender and recipient. E-mail programs have proliferated and many are available at little or not cost (e.g., Eudora Lite, Pegasus Mail), or as part of web browsers, computer operating systems or office software suites. Free e-mail accounts are even available (e.g., Juno, HotMail), and e-mail accounts are often given out as part of a subscription to an ISP's services. As a side note, everyone should have their own business and personal e-mail addresses, and use them for those separate purposes for legal and ethical reasons. It is still possible to use a single e-mail program to process messages from multiple accounts concurrently, but separate accounts should exist.

Think about it—a pharmacist working at a computer remembers that he or she needs to let someone know about something or needs to get some information about a situation. If there was a need to have a record of communicating with that other person, in the past a person would have written a memo or a letter, which might have taken several days to be written, dictated, typed, and/or proofed. It would then be sent and might take several more days to work its way through the institution's mail system and, possibly, the postal system. Another possibility is to call and then jot down the information. Of course calling might require an extended period of "phone tag." Voice mail may make things simpler, although it certainly does not easily leave a permanent record of the information and many people do not like using it. The caller might actually get the person on the phone, but that could lead to spending a lot of time on irrelevant subjects, which sometimes leads people to hope they get the voice mail box instead.[100] An e-mail program running in the background can be quickly brought up and the person's address is typed in. The address is often much easier to remember than a postal address and is in a similar format to web addresses. Also, the user generally puts in a subject and can indicate whether the message is of high priority. When it is necessary to send other information, a computer file may be attached to the message before it is sent. Whether the addressee is in the next office or the next country, the message may be received in

TABLE 5–2. WEB SITE CREATION POINTS

- Know the mission and goals of the web site and regularly consider whether they are being addressed.
- Make sure the site has useful, timely, and, preferably, original information.
- Make sure the web site looks good—if it does not, it will be shunned.
- Use graphics, but only if they add something worthwhile to a page. Be sure to keep graphics small, so that downloads of pages will be quick.
- Keep the information to a reasonable length on each page (preferably just a screenfull).
- Make it easy to use and easy to move through and around the web site. That includes providing a good search engine. A great deal of effort should be placed into interlinking data to make it more accessible and useful. Also, a consistent and clear method to present information to navigate around the web site is necessary.
- Custom tailor information presented to each user.
- Use self-generating content, if appropriate. For example, information about formulary material may be in a data base format that is dynamically prepared in the format requested by the web user at the time of access.
- Test out the web site to make sure things work. That includes trying all web browsers and all versions of web browsers likely to be used by people looking at the site. This can include access by rather nontraditional browsers, such as those now found on cellular telephones. If the site requires a specific web browser or version of a browser, make that very clear.
- Remove broken links to other pages or web sites.
- Test out various methods of access for acceptability. For example, see whether the site is usable via modem—if not, remove big graphics, etc.
- Provide contact information (i.e., names, addresses, and phone numbers).
- Keep material up to date. Also, each page should indicate the date it was last changed.
- Leave out unnecessary information. Huge biographies of each of the pharmacists might be good for their ego, but otherwise useless.
- Consider the technical support needed by the web site users.
- Consider the costs involved for both you and the intended user.
- Consider the level of security needed. Such things as virtual private networks (VPNs) and firewalls may be needed.
- Register the site with search engines, if high traffic is desired (e.g., community pharmacy). Also, advertise the site, perhaps at other Internet sites that may be consulted by patients.
- Remember to assess what the users think about the web site—what is valuable and what needs to be improved or eliminated.
- Considered the disabled. Do you need to make the site accessible to the blind?

seconds or minutes. The person can then reply when he or she has the opportunity (quite often the reply may be received in minutes). One other advantage is that the recipient may be able to obtain the message from wherever he or she happens to be, including at long distances, as long as a computer is available. Overall, e-mail can greatly improve the speed and efficiency of brief communications and should be considered whenever a short memo or phone call would have been used in the past.

It should also be noted that by using e-mail it is possible to send information to personal distribution lists previously set up on the e-mail system. For example, the chairman of a committee with members scattered throughout the institution may need to regularly send short messages to all of them (e.g., the next meeting is on Friday at 10 AM in Room XXX). An e-mail user can use the name of the mailing list as the address and have it sent to the whole group.

Depending on the set up of the e-mail system, automated routing of forms, documents (e.g., for comments), and other items may be possible. For example, filling out a request for vacation time may be as simple as filling out an e-mail form that is automatically routed to an employee's supervisor.[82]

E-mail also gives the sender the option to automatically receive a message from the recipient's computer confirming he or she has read the message, which can sometimes be important when establishing whether lack of action is due to lack of communication or other reasons. Please note, however, it can be possible for such automated messages to be disabled or incompatibilities between e-mail programs can occasionally result in the "return-receipt" message being sent when the computer receives the message, rather than when it is actually read.

Using e-mail to communicate with patients may be an important tool in the future. Guidelines for doing so have been published,[101–103] and revolve around the ability to keep information confidential (encryption or informed consent may be necessary) and making a clear agreement with the patient as to what can be transmitted via e-mail and to what e-mail address (home vs. employer). Note that signed informed consent is suggested.[104] For example, would it be acceptable to e-mail a refill reminder to an HIV-positive patient for antiviral medications? A record of all e-mail communications should be kept as a part of the medical record and some method of assuring the identity of the medical professional (e.g., "cyber notaries") may be necessary.[104] A medicolegal problem to be resolved is the provision of advice via e-mail, or other electronic means, across state lines.

Although a health care practitioner cannot assume that the e-mail is read promptly or at all by the patient, the practitioner must make sure all e-mail communications receive an appropriate response quickly and that the patients know clearly how to contact them directly for more information or in an urgent situation.[101] A problem recently noted has been the possibility of patients sending unsolicited requests for information.

In such a case, the recipient may have legal, ethical, and other problems to overcome, and it will be necessary for such troubles to be addressed in the future.[105,106]

E-mail can now be used for physicians to send prescriptions to pharmacists in some places,[107] and the volume of such prescriptions is likely to increase in the future. There is even a company that has created a palm-top computer application to allow transmission of electronic prescriptions to pharmacists (<<http://www.pocketscript.com>>).

Whether used for patient communications or other functions, e-mail is "discoverable" in court and employers may have permanent records of e-mail messages that the sender and recipient thought were long ago deleted. Therefore, be as careful with e-mail as is necessary with written communications.[108] Jobs have been lost due to improper use of e-mail communications. Some suggestions for companies to protect against legal problems include[109,110]:

- Develop a written e-mail policy. Make it clear and usable, and then enforce it.
- Define who owns the contents of the e-mail system.
- Inform employees that old mail may be saved (e.g., backups) even if it was supposedly deleted.
- Teach employees e-mail appropriate conduct, including the avoidance of discrimination, harassment, or other misconduct.

Listservers

Listservers are similar to the distribution lists mentioned above. However, a server on the e-mail computer keeps the list, to which people can apply to be a member. Once the list is established, any messages sent to the list are automatically sent to all members of the list, making it easy to communicate within a group. To better explain the concept of listservers, an example will be used.

The Consortium for the Advancement of Medication Information Policy and Research (CAMIPR) is a group of drug information specialists originally brought together by Gordon Vanscoy, PharmD, at the University of Pittsburgh. To facilitate communications between members of the group, a listserver was established at Creighton University, with the address <<camipr@creighton.edu>>. To become members of the group, people send a message to <<majordomo@creighton.edu>>, which controls the listservers at the institution (note: majordomo is the usual address name for joining any listserver). The body of the message must have in it the phrase "subscribe camipr <<yourname@your-address.xxx>>" where <<yourname@youraddress.xxx>> is the prospective subscriber's own e-mail address (to leave the list at a later time, the same procedure is followed, substituting the word "unsubscribe" for "subscribe"). If this was a public listserver, the person would be automatically added to the e-mail address list and would receive both an automated message acknowledging joining the list (and usually providing directions on special functions of the list) and any future messages sent to the list. However, in this situation, CAMIPR has a private listserver. This means that all applicants must be approved for addition to the list. While the application procedure is the same as previously described, the result is an automated message to the listserver owner (the author), who must then send a message approving the addition of the new listserver member back to <<majordomo@creighton.edu>>. Other commands are available for the users of the listserver, including one that will provide a list of the addresses of current members. Once becoming a member of the listserver, a person can then send messages to the other members by addressing their e-mail to the listserver address, which in this case is <<camipr@creighton.edu>>.

Listservers act as a good conduit for discussions. For example, one member can pose a question or problem to the listserver. Others can then reply to the original message or to the other replies to the message. In addition to sending each of the messages in the discussion to the members' e-mail addresses, the listserver may keep a record of the discussion, which can later be posted on a web site to allow someone to read a continuous account of how a discussion proceeded. Also, a listserver can be moderated,[111] meaning that all messages are first approved by the "owner" of the list before other members receive them. That allows for elimination of inappropriate material.

Pharmacists can use the listservers to facilitate discussion between any group. Besides the use mentioned, it may be of value for committees, classes, or other groups. Various pharmacy organizations and special interest groups currently use listservers. The advantage of listservers over distribution lists is that the listserver is available to all members of the group (a distribution list is normally developed by an individual for his or her own use) and the listserver is dynamically changed for all members as others join or leave the group.

Pharmacists often get information on listerservers from acquaintances or publications; however, a rather massive list of available listservers is available on <<http://www.liszt.com>>.[112] Of particular interest to some pharmacists is the listserver from the CDC (<<http://www.cdc.gov/subscribe.html>>), which automatically sends a table of contents for the *MMWR* publications.

Extensions to the capabilities of listservers can be seen at such places as <<http://www.egroups.com>> (a free service on the Internet) or through the use of groupware (e.g., Team Folders in Microsoft Outlook), which cannot only facilitate communications within a group, but also provide a group calendar, task list, document storage site, and other functions.

Electronic Faxes

The ability to send and receive faxes via a fax/modem has been available for years. Recently, however, it has become possible to send or receive faxes via e-mail. In some cases the e-mail program acts like it is sending traditional e-mail, but then accesses the fax/modem. One interesting twist is the ability to have a fax number where the fax itself is turned into an e-mail message automatically and is then forwarded to the user's e-mail address to be read and/or printed. Similar to the free e-mail addresses mentioned previously, individuals can also sign up for a free fax phone number, where the message is delivered to his or her e-mail address (e.g., contact <<http://www.efax.com>>).[113] Sending faxes without charge is also possible (e.g., contact <<http://www.fax4free.com/>>). These services also may offer additional services for a fee. For example, an 800 fax phone number may be available.

How to Manage E-Mail

E-mail is a wonderful tool, but there is definitely something to be said about having too much of a good thing. It has been estimated that a total of 2.7 trillion e-mail messages were sent in 1997 and that total is expected to rise to 6.9 trillion messages for approximately 107 million users by the year 2000, which would mean nearly 65,000 messages a year per user![114] Although this may be worrisome, there are ways that people can handle numerous messages. The first rule, however, is to avoid adding to everyone else's e-mail inbox. Yes, it is easy to send messages to groups, but do not do so unless it is really necessary. Related to that, keep what is sent short, perhaps providing a longer version for those who need it, and do not bother with colored fonts and clip art.[115] Next, remember that programs do have filter features that will allow certain mail to be handled automatically.[116] For example, unsolicited mail from certain addresses can be automatically deleted, or an automatic reply can be sent to those messages. More important messages can be filtered to a common location for review as soon as possible. Also, e-mail program may display a few lines of all new messages allowing the user to scan, highlight, and delete unimportant messages within seconds. Finally, be sure to review e-mail regularly, probably several times a day. That way, it will not build up to unmanageable levels, and the efficiency of e-mail will be increased. This may seem like a big chore, but it does not have to be. Modern computer operating systems allow several programs to run concurrently. An e-mail program can be set to always be running in the background, so that a user going from one thing to another can quickly check for any e-mail.

Personal Information Managers

An item that can be covered with e-mail is the use of personal information managers (PIMs), because e-mail acts as a basis of many PIM functions. This can be taken to be specific pocket devices, but in this section will only refer to the functions, not the equipment the software resides on.

Many individuals carry pocket calendars or one of a number of notebooks designed to improve their productivity by expanding the calendar with to-do lists, contact information, and other items. For some people, such hard copy resources will continue to function; however, most people should be using the electronic versions of these items.

Many versions of PIM software are available to perform a variety of tasks. In particular, it should combine e-mail, calendar, to-do lists, contacts (e.g., address, phone number), and the innumerable notes that people commonly carry (e.g., budget numbers, directions, purchase lists). If at all possible, an institution should have a common system that allows people better interaction and easy access by individuals from multiple locations. For example, a person wanting to schedule a meeting should be able to use the software to find out when everyone is available, and then "penciling" the meeting in on the calendar of all the prospective attendees. Also, project software may send specific action items to appropriate individuals, and then monitor progress and due dates. In addition, having the institution's system track reporting and organizational structure allows specific messages to be automatically routed to the appropriate individuals. For example, an individual filling out a vacation or reimbursement request on his or her PIM will know that the request will automatically be sent to the appropriate people for review and approval, regardless of whether the usual person is on vacation or has left the company and someone else is covering the function.

For individuals who need to have a calendar immediately available (e.g., a clinician who is all over the institution, rather than setting at a desk), synchronization with a handheld device is certainly available. That way, when at his or her desk, the person has the ease of use of the keyboard and screen, but can keep both the PIM and him/herself up to date at all times. The PIM can also be used to carry other information, including reference manuals and books. Various health-care-related references for PIMS (some free) are available from <<http://www.memoware.com>>, <<http://www.palmgear.com>>, <<http://www.handheldmed.com>>, and <<http://www.skyscape.com>>. There is really very little excuse for a practicing clinical pharmacist not to have such capabilities available when practicing outside of the office (e.g., medical floor, clinic).

In the case of a small organization or individuals, there are web-based services on the Internet that will perform the services mentioned in this section.[117]

USENET News

USENET News can be considered a group of discussion areas on the Internet that resemble electronic bulletin board services, with areas for discussion of a wide variety of topics from the serious (e.g., adverse drug reactions) to the absurd (e.g., McDonald's ketchup). These newsgroups can be compared to "chat rooms" available from some services, such as America Online; however, in this case the discussions are asynchronous (i.e., the messages are available to people logging on later, perhaps for days or weeks) and may occur over an extended period of time.

USENET News servers are available from a number of locations. To access the servers it is necessary to have the appropriate software. Both Microsoft Internet Explorer and Netscape Communicator do provide such features, as do a variety of other programs. When the software is installed and an address of an available USENET News server is input, the user will be presented with a list of available discussion group topics. This list may contain thousands of topics. Not all news servers have all of the discussion areas, because of limitations in storage or other reasons. These topics are broken down into a number of areas, such as sci (science), comp (computer related), rec (recreation), and misc (miscellaneous). A common discussion group for pharmacists is sci.med.pharmacy.

Once in a particular discussion area, the pharmacist will be presented with a list of recent "postings." These resemble a list of e-mail messages, which in many ways they are. Users of the newsgroup have posted what they want to say, talk, or ask about on the newsgroup. The user will see the subject and who posted it (often the users will use very vague names or nicknames, similar to CB radio "handles"). For example, at the time this is being written, a current message is titled "Aricept and Alzheimer's Disease." It is a request for information. The person requesting information posted this message to the news server and it was then replicated to all other news servers carrying this discussion group around the world. By clicking on the listing, anybody can read it and reply. It is also possible to follow the "thread" of replies to a particular original posting over time. Therefore, a newsgroup can be used to obtain and give information. However, caution is advised. The quality of the postings varies widely. People in a particular discussion group may be world-renowned experts or crackpots. They may even be posing as someone else. Therefore, particular caution is advised—even more than is necessary with web sites. Studies have found that approximately 70% of the information given on USENET News is erroneous.[118,119] That is not to say there are not good groups or that they are not valuable. Some patient groups regularly exchange good and valuable information on their disease state (e.g., cancer, panic disorders, incontinence, impotence, alcohol and drug abuse, domestic violence, sexually transmitted diseases) using USENET News[120] and USENET News has been successfully used for disease research,[121] but it is necessary to be very careful.

It is also possible to search newsgroups for information using DejaNews (<<http://www.deja.com/usenet>>).

Chat

Chat rooms are a feature on the Internet that allow multiple people to concurrently (synchronously) discuss a topic. Chat rooms are only useful for the people in the chat room at any one time; once the information that was just typed scrolls off the screen, it is gone. It is possible to set up private chat rooms for patients, classes, and so on, but there does not seem to be much use in pharmacy at this time. Sometimes chat rooms may be used for distance learning classes, so that the instructor can hold virtual office hours.

Internet Collaboration

It is now possible for pharmacists to communicate directly over the Internet (i.e., voice and video pictures of themselves in real time) with other pharmacists while working together on a document. Collaboration with other pharmacists over the Internet has been available for a while, but there has not really been any evidence that it has been used to any extent. Reasons for this may include the possible use has not yet become widely known, pharmacists do not know what software to use (even though it might even already be on their computers as part of Microsoft Internet Explorer or Netscape Communicator), their network connection may be too slow, or even that they have not yet figured out how to integrate the use into their practice philosophy.

In the past such communication might have been through Internet Relay Chat (IRC); however, now it is more likely to be through CU-SeeMe (from Cornell University), Microsoft NetMeeting, or a commercially available product. In the future collaboration capabilities will be built into office software suites (e.g., word processors).[122] In general, the only equipment necessary for collaboration is a video camera for the computer, and then only if video is needed. Such equipment may be purchased for well under $100. The software is often free. Simpler methods of communicating that might fall under this topic are the "instant messenger" type products, such as those available from America On-Line (AOL), Microsoft, and Yahoo. These run on the desktop and pop up when someone wants to type a message back and forth. These can also be used to replace e-mail in some cases.

WebTV

It is now possible to use TV tuner cards in computers to receive typical television programs either through the Internet or via a local cable feed, with the pictures being projected on the computer monitor. An interesting innovation with this is that the software will "read" the closed captioning on the signal in the background, immediately popping up the viewer if a particular word or phrase is mentioned in a program. This allows users to keep up to date with late breaking news on a news network. Pharmacists need to take advantage of this technology to provide information to patients.

Related to that, pharmacists can prepare video or audio presentations that may be "streamed" to the Internet for patients, students, or other health care professionals. This would use software such as RealVideo or Microsoft's Windows Media.

Telepharmacy

Related to many of the above items, pharmacists are starting to use a variety of forms of communication over the Internet. For example, it is currently possible to make phone calls over the web, although such calls tend to sound like CB radios did 20 years ago. New ways of sending phone applets[123] (maybe as part of a refill reminder) might allow pharmacists to let patients contact them directly (both broadcast quality audio and visual) for some service via the Internet. This will be an expansion on televideo technology that is already being used for patient counseling.[124]

Pharmacists are also able to receive monitoring data from patients, for example, blood sugar readings from diabetics, peak flow and expiratory volume readings from asthmatics, or blood pressures and lipid profiles from cardiac patients.[125] It is expected that houses will be able to monitor their occupants in the future, even calling for help when necessary.

Expansion of these capabilities and education of pharmacists to use them is being promoted by pharmacy organizations.[126] Because many of the details of telepharmacy go beyond the scope of this book, the reader is referred to other sources on the topic.[127]

Push Technology

Push technology involves software that actually sends information to users' desktops. In many ways, this can be thought of as a marriage of web browsing, e-mail, and a screen saver, in that the information may resemble that found on a web site (e.g., text, graphics, audio, video), but it is delivered directly to the desk and may be displayed by the screen saver. Optionally, it may be set up to "pop up" when specific news is available (users set their preferences), as is seen with MSNBC News Alert (<<http://www.msnbc.com/>>), or as a window at the bottom of the screen, as seen with EntryPoint (<<http://www.entrypoint.com>>).[128] This was considered to be a concept with a great future in 1997, but the enthusiasm for it seems to have died down. The great advantage was that the user did not have to take much of an active role in getting information (other than perhaps setting up a list of preferences for their computer when the push technology was added). In addition to using commercial information feeds, this software also allowed companies to create their own information stream to the desktop,[129,130] perhaps to better inform employees about a variety of institution-related topics. The software to do this is available as part of either Microsoft Internet Explorer or Netscape Communicator, and is also available from companies that provide the server software.

Very closely related to push technology is a customizable news feed.[131] This service, which is provided by a variety of vendors including Yahoo!, Lycos, Microsoft, and Netscape, allows individuals to indicate what types of news that they would like to get (including local weather), which will be downloaded to their computer. It requires no special software. It can even be integrated into a person's calendar and task list, such as in Microsoft Outlook.

Push technology does have some possible use for pharmacists. First it can be used to inform pharmacists, even about news events (perhaps filtering medically related news from a news organization) and can be used within an institution for institution-related news (e.g., new formulary additions, new policies and procedures—essentially what would have previously been provided in a newsletter). The problems with push technology include that the information is often only being displayed when people are not using their computers (i.e., their screensaver starts up when they left their office) and that people may find it annoying.[132]

Outside of pharmacy, push technology is already being used in health care. For example, ambulances en route to an emergency may already be receiving information about the patient from the dispatcher, via a computer link, which also displays related information about what the paramedics need to do once they get there (e.g., diagnostic equipment they need to get ready, how to treat a patient with a poisoning).[82]

On a related topic, it should also be pointed out that some software allows automatic updates over the Internet (e.g., antiviral programs, newer versions of Microsoft Windows). In the future, push technology may even drive the updates and bug fixes to the desktop. The cost of doing this might be paid for by subscription or may even be free (due to advertising embedded in the updates).

Classified Advertisements

It is worth mentioning that classified advertisements are available on the Internet. Pharmacists may be interested in them for such things as personnel placement, or may even put advertisements in their web sites to obtain revenue to support the site.

THE FUTURE

In many ways, most people have seen much of the near future of information technology whenever they tune into their favorite science fiction program. Just as *Star Trek* in the mid-1960s anticipated today's sliding doors and personal communicators (i.e., cellular phones), current science fiction programs anticipate how information will be widely available in many forms.

To begin with, it can be assumed that there will be more computers, greater availability of information (reference, bibliography, electronic drug product labeling,[133] clinical decision support systems, and clinical information systems [standardized patient data], which will be a financial bonanza for the owners of that data[134]), and a huge increase in the speed and capabilities of computers. For example, it has been stated that a computer capable of similar processing power as the human brain will be available in the next 50 years.[135] This includes a speed of 1 petaop (10^{15} operations per second) and storage of 10 terabytes (10^{13} characters). These capabilities will be on a computer that the user wears! It may be referred to as a body area network (BAN). They already have washable and wearable computers (<<http://www.media.mit.edu/~rehmi/cloth/>>). It will allow the storage and recall of everything a person reads, hears, and/or sees during their entire life. Furthermore, computers will be designed to calm the user rather than cause anxiety.

In the near future, limited advances are possible. It can be assumed that current software will have additional capabilities. For example, the next generation of web browsers will have better graphics, including three-dimensional capabilities.[136] Also, data will be presented in forms that make it easier to visualize and manipulate interactively, making it easier to understand.[137] Clinical decision support systems that physicians may use in diagnosis are expected to improve.[138] Different health professionals will be tied together by computers to improve patient care through such things as electronic drug utilization review.[139] In general, an increase in the amount of information and the way it is tied together will be seen.[82] More specifically for pharmacists, their practice sites will be redesigned to take advantage of automation of all dispensing functions, so that the pharmacists can spend more time on cognitive, business, and clinical functions—ensuring that patients have more information and better treatment and monitoring.[140] Those pharmacists who want to avoid cognitive functions will soon be out of a job if all they can do is count, pour, lick and stick; robotics are becoming increasingly common (one chain is already becoming fully automated[141]).

Of course, there will be other capabilities that pharmacists will find useful. For example, more capable intelligent agents will be available. These are small computer programs that can go out on the Internet and accomplish a task. An example is some of the software portals that extend search capabilities. Right now intelligent agents are seen, to a small extent, in programs that help to automatically set up meetings between numerous people through calendar and e-mail programs. Also, filters and portals will do a better job of allowing only the most relevant or desirable data to get through to the pharmacist. These things are currently available,[142] but have a long way to go.

Pharmacists will have to deal with digital identities, both their patients' and their own. In Germany, there are already identification cards for both patients and practitioners (<<http://www.abda.de/>>). The patient cards have encrypted medical information files on them and the practitioner cards have electronic authorization to review the medical information on the patient cards. Also, pharmacists may not know it, but some states make information about licensed practitioners available on the Internet. As might be expected, there may be information about such things as disciplinary action, but other items, such as the pharmacist's home address may come as a shock (e.g., <<http://www.hhs.state.ne.us/lis/lis.asp>>). Even further information may start appearing on the Internet, such as the American Medical Association's Accreditation Program (<<http://www.ama-assn.org/med-sci/amapsite/>>).

While much of the above deals with more clinical aspects of practice, the Internet may soon affect some of the most traditional aspects of pharmacy practice. The World Health Organization (WHO) is currently working toward recommendations on the international sale of prescriptions to patients via the Internet (e.g., your patients may already get their prescriptions filled from a third world country and have it expressed to them—check out <<http://www.prescriptionrx.com>>). Please note that President Clinton's call for establishment of an electronic free trade zone on Internet might have a large impact on this.[143]

Overall, it will be up to pharmacists to learn how to best use all of these capabilities to improve patient care and to obtain appropriate reimbursement for services. Others are selling drug information, medical books, and vitamins over the Internet to patients (Dr. Koop's Community Personal Drug Store [<<http://www.drkoop.com/hcrdrugstore/>>], and <<http://www.medixperts.com>>.[144] Also, a variety of well-known U.S. pharmacies are beginning to sell products, including prescription refills, via the Internet (see Appendix 5–12). It is predicted that on-line consumer health care will be up to 1.7 billion by 2003, including prescription drugs, over-the-counter products, nutraceuticals, and personal care products.[145] The National Association of Boards of Pharmacy have a process to approve Internet based pharmacies, called Verified Internet Pharmacy Practice Sites (VIPPS),[146] which is becoming very important as a number of less than reputable sites have been established to allow people to easily obtain prescription drugs, such as Viagra, with only electronic contact with a physician, if that much. It is expected that the amount of drugs sales via the Internet will increase 1000% between 1999 and 2002.[147] Also, physicians will be sending prescriptions over the web (see <<http://www.abaton.com>>). Other pharmacy services will have to follow for optimal economic survival of the profession. Pharmacists should try new technology and new ways to use that technology; it may seem crazy, but it may end up being a wonderful idea.[148]

To do all of this, pharmacists will have to learn how to use the technology, and they must be given continual training by their employers and through their own efforts. In addition to the technical aspects, pharmacists will also have to ensure that the quality of their information is good, which is not necessarily the case with Internet pharmacies.[149] Although pharmacy has long used computers for business type purposes, much of what this article discusses has not been covered in pharmacy training.[150] This will have to change. It will be up to pharmacists to embrace this powerful communication tool; to lead the way.

Acknowledgment

Portions of this chapter were reproduced, with permission, from Malone PM. Drug information technology and Internet resources. *J Pharm Pract* 1998;XI:196–218.

Study Questions

1. What search strategies can a pharmacist use in finding information on the Internet?

2. How can the quality of information be assessed for items located on the Internet?

3. How can a pharmacist use e-mail in practice situations (include distribution lists and listservers)?

4. What items can belong on a web site in your practice situation?

5. What Internet access does a practitioner need?

6. What are USENET news groups, how are patients using them, and what should a pharmacist know about them to discuss with the patients?

REFERENCES

1. Internet domain survey, January 2000. [cited 2000 Feb 16]:[1screen]. Available from: URL: http://www.isc.org/ds/WWW-200001/report.html.
2. Sandberg J. The next big blue thing. Newsweek 1999;CXXXIV(24):83.
3. Klein CN. Pharmacy and the Internet. Am J Health Syst Pharm 1995;52:2095.
4. Westberg EE, Miller RA. The basis for using the Internet to support the information needs of primary care. J Am Med Inform Assoc 1999;6:6–25.
5. Editors of ComputerTalk. The next generation: today's pharmacy students are wired to the future. A fascinating look at the innovative Shenandoah University School of Pharmacy. ComputerTalk 1998;18(6):14–23.
6. Ketchell DS, Freedman MM, Jordan WE, Lightfoot EM, Heyano S, Libbey PA. Willow: a uniform search interface. J Am Med Inform Assoc 1996;3:27–37.
7. Vecchione A. New data-collection tool speeds up reporting process. Hosp Pharmacist Report 1997;11(2):64.
8. Vine D, Corvalán E. 21st century physician's little black bag. Gratefully Yours 1997;Sept/Oct:1–3.
9. Rupley S. Calling the web. Smart phones get smarter. PC Magazine 1999;18(22):32.
10. Brown M, Brown B. Web phones. PC Magazine 2000;19(5):32–4, 36.
11. Currid C. Currid's ten commandments puts electronic mail use on top. InfoWorld 1992;14 (Sept 28):58.
12. Van Name ML, Catchings B. Quality Internet access is a business basic. PC Week 1999; 16(2):29.
13. Livingston B. Alexa provides additional ways to navigate the Web. InfoWorld 1998;20(8):44.
14. Ukens C, Vecchione A. How pharmacists are riding the technology tidal wave. Hospital Pharmacist Report 1997;[Technology and Pharmacy '97 Supplement]:22S–23S.

15. Ukens C. Technopharmacy. Drug Top 1998;142(21):56–67.

16. Jones MG. Telemedicine and the National Information Infrastructure: are the realities of health care being ignored? J Am Med Inform Assoc 1997;4:399–412.

17. Nicefaro ME. Internet use policies. Online 1998;23:31–3.

18. Modzelewski P. Internet connection alternatives. PC Magazine 1998;17(1):249–50.

19. Langa F. High speed surfing. Windows Magazine 1999 Feb;10(2):160–9.

20. Freed L, Derfler FJ, Jr. The faster web. PC Magazine 1999;18(8):158–62, 166, 168, 171, 174, 178.

21. Hafke D. Your own private Internet. Windows Magazine 1998;Feb:218–22, 226.

22. Scambray J, Broderick J. VPN growing pains. InfoWorld 1997;19(49):102–3, 106–8, 110, 112, 114, 116, 118, 120, 122.

23. Lapolla Stephanie. Saving time and lives over the Internet. Case study: hospital's VPN links doctors to confidential patient data. PC Week 1997;14(52):29, 37.

24. PC Week Labs Staff. IE 4 vs. Communicator: PC Week Labs sizes up the competition. PC Week 1997;14(43):69–80.

25. Johnson AH. Browser battle ends, but the war rages on. Windows Magazine 1998;9(1):90–2.

26. Clyman J. Face off. Internet Explorer 4.0 vs. Communicator. PC Magazine 1997;16(20):100–22.

27. Gardner D. Will Microsoft get the last laugh? InfoWorld 1997;19(47):65.

28. Bailes L. WinFAQ: PC viruses. Safe or sorry? Windows Magazine 1998;9(1):251–5.

29. Finnie S. Protection at the desktop. PC Magazine 1997;16(15):149–50.

30. Druffel L. Information warfare. In: Denning PJ, Metcalfe RM, editors. Beyond calculation. The next fifty years of computing. New York: Copernicus; 1997.

31. Livingston B. Drag and drop Net files with FTP tool. InfoWorld 1997;19(47):37.

32. The ABCs of FTP. Medicine on the Net 1997;3(12):24–7.

33. Ferguson T. Digital doctoring—opportunities and challenges in electronic patient-physician communication. JAMA 1998;280:1361–2.

34. Eng TR, Maxfield A, Patrick K, Deering MJ, Ratzan SC, Gustafson DH. Access to health information and support. A public highway or a private road? JAMA 1998;280:1371–5.

35. Ojala M. Beginning all over again: where to start a search. Online 1998;22(3):44–6.

36. Lindberg DAB, Humphreys BL. Medical informatics. JAMA 1997;277:1870–1.

37. Odlyzko AM. Will full online text have the last word? Medicine on the Net 1997;3(8):5–12.

38. McDonald CJ, Overhage JM, Dexter PR, Blevins L, Meeks-Johnson J, Suico JG, et al. Canopy computing. Using the web in clinical practice. JAMA 1998;280:1325–9.

39. Bourne DWA. Using the Internet as a pharmacokinetic resource. Clin Pharmacokinet 1997;33(3):153–60.

40. Rapoza J. HTML, XML get hitched. PC Week 1999;16(20):16.

41. Metcalfe B. Web father Berners-Lee shares next-generation vision of The Semantic Web. PC Week 1999;21(21):110.

42. Lidsky D. Home on the web. PC Magazine 1998;17(15):100–4, 108, 112, 116, 120, 124, 128, 131, 133, 135, 137, 139–41.

43. Engstrom P. To the online rescue: search engines designed with clinicians in mind. Medicine on the Net 1997;3(4):1–5.

44. Hersh WR, Brown KE, Donohoe LC, Campbell EM, Horacek AE. CliniWeb: managing clinical information on the World Wide Web. J Am Med Inform Assoc 1996;3:273–80.

45. The search is on for medical information. http://www.mwsearch.com/. Medicine on the Net 1997;3(10):18–19.
46. Morgan C. The search is on. Windows Magazine 1996;7(11):212–14, 216, 218, 220, 222, 224, 226, 230.
47. Lawrence S, Giles CL. Search the World Wide Web. Science 1998;280:98–100.
48. Search engines' tiny bite. PC Magazine 1999 Sept 1;18(15):9.
49. Sullivan D. Crawling under the hood. An update on search engine technology. Online 1998; 22(3):30–8.
50. Hock R. How to do field searching in web search engines. Online 1998;22(3):18–22.
51. Hock R. Web search engines features and commands. Online 1999;23(3):24–8.
52. Berinstein P. Turning visual: image search engines on the web. Online 1998;22(3):37–42.
53. Pemberton JK, Garman N, Ojala M. Head to head. Online 1998;22(3):24–8.
54. Livingston B. Finally, an effort is under way to make Net searches easier. InfoWorld 1999; 21(8):38.
55. Too much information. InfoWorld 1997;19(19):72–5, 78, 80, 82.
56. Notess GR. Toward more comprehensive web searching: single searching versus megasearching. Online 1998;March/April:73–6.
57. Lunt P. Search & retrieval—special agents find it for you. Imaging & Document Solutions 1999;8(4):46–54.
58. Feldman S. NLP meets the jabberwocky. Online 1999;23(3):62–72.
59. Sherman C. The future of web search. Online 1999;23(3):54–61.
60. Kurkul D. Free MEDLINE shakes up content providers: what it means for you. Medicine on the Net 1997;3(9):8–15.
61. Southwick K. Free MEDLINE ignites vendor wars. Medicine on the Net 1997;3(9):16–17.
62. Sikorski R, Peters R. Medical literature made easy. Querying databases on the Internet. JAMA 1997;277:959–60.
63. Detmer WM. Medline on the Web: ten questions to ask when evaluating a web based service. AMIA Internet Working Group Newsletter 1997;3(1):11–13.
64. Bailey WJ. Searching the Internet for drug information. Strategies for locating accurate and scientifically accepted information. [cited 1996 Jul 18]:[1 screen]. Available from: URL:http://www.drugs.indiana.edu/pubs/newsline/searching.html.
65. Talley CR. Trouble on the Internet. Am J Health-Syst Pharm 1997;54:757.
66. Rogers A. Good medicine on the web. The Internet is a powerful health resource, but watch where you surf. Newsweek 1998;CXXXII(8):60–1.
67. Bridges A, Thede LQ. Electronic education. Nursing education resources on the World Wide Web. Nurse Educator 1996;21(5):11–15.
68. Alexander J, Tate M. The web as a research tool: evaluation techniques. [cited 1997 April 14]: [1 screen]. Available from: URL: http://www.science.widener.edu/~withers/webeval.htm.
69. Jacobson T, Cohen L. Evaluating Internet resources. [cited 1997 April 14]:[1 screen]. Available from: URL: http://www.albany.edu/library/internet/evaluate.html.
70. Pines WL. The challenge of the Internet. Drug Info J 1998;32:277–81.
71. Health on the Net Foundation packs a punch with more than just quality. Medicine on the Net 1997;3(12):15–17.

72. Jadad AR, Gagliardi A. Rating health information on the Internet. Navigating to knowledge or to Babel? JAMA 1998;279:611–14.

73. Notess GR. Alexa: web archive, advisor, and statistician. Online 1998;22(3):29–30.

74. Silberg WM, Lundberg GD, Musacchio RA. Assessing, controlling, and assuring the quality of medical information on the Internet. JAMA 1997;277:1244–5.

75. Murray PJ. Click here—and be disappointed? Evaluating web sites. Computers in Nursing 1996;14(5):260–1.

76. Wu WK, Tucker T. Composing a pharmacy web page. US Pharmacist 1999;January:32, 34–6, 38, 40, 42–4.

77. Lowe HJ, Lomax EC, Polonkey SE. The World Wide Web: a review of an emerging Internet-based technology for the distribution of biomedical information. J Am Med Inform Assoc 1996;3:1–14.

78. Dalton M, Enos M, Halvachs F. Use of a private intranet system by a pharmacy and therapeutics committee. Hosp Pharm 1998;33:1365–71.

79. Mullich J. An obvious prescription. PC Week 1996;13(26):42, 46.

80. Reich P. Using Intranets in managed care. Medical Interface 1996;Nov:16.

81. Cox J. ELVIS lives at Eli Lilly. Network World 1996;13(52):72–3, 76, 78.

82. Gates B, Hemingway C. Business @ the speed of thought. Using a digital nervous system. New York: Warner Books; 1999.

83. Appleton EL. New recipes for learning. Inside Technology Training 1997;1(1):12–16, 18, 57.

84. Polyson S, Saltzberg S, Godwin-Jones R. A practical guide to teaching with the World Wide Web. Syllabus 1996;10(2):12, 14, 16.

85. Kaplan IP, Patton LR, Hamilton RA. Adaptation of different computerized methods of distance learning to an external Pharm.D. degree program. Am J Pharm Educ 1996;60:422–5.

86. Bell SJ. Mounting presentations on the web: presentation software, HTML or both? Online 1998;Sept/Oct:62–70.

87. Moore J. Stream your presentations from the web. Windows Sources 1998;Feb:108.

88. Hinman L. Streaming video: adding real multimedia to the web. Syllabus 1999;12(5):18–21.

89. Major MJ. Next generation Internet and video: emerging applications. Syllabus 1999;12(5):24, 26.

90. Alwang G. Meeting of the minds. PC Magazine 1998;17(4):179–82, 184, 186, 188, 190–2.

91. Levy L. Imaging takes publishing to new territories. Imaging Magazine 1998;7(3):16, 18, 20, 22.

92. Flahault A, Dias-Ferrao V, Chaberty P, Esteves K, Valleron A-J, Lavanchy D. FluNet as a tool for global monitoring of influenza on the web. JAMA 1998;280:1330–2.

93. Peters R, Sikorski R. Building your own. A physician's guide to creating a web site. JAMA 1998;280:1365–6.

94. Olsen G. 9 design and production stages for creating web presentations. Presentations 1997;11(4):31–3.

95. Schwartz M. Ways to doom your web site. Software Magazine 1998;18(4):26.

96. What makes a great web site? [cited 1999 May 13]:[1 screen]. Available from: URL: http://www.webreference.com/greatsite.html.

97. Giebel T. Make your site a success. PC Magazine 1999;18(16):36.

98. Hopp DI. Three topics integral to the use of the Internet for clinical trials: connectivity, communication, and security. Drug Info J 1998;32:933–9.

99. Guernsey L, Kiernan V. Journals differ on whether to publish articles that have appeared on the web. Chronicle Higher Educ 1998 July 17:Available from: URL: http://chronicle.com/free/v44/i45/45a02701.htm.

100. Machrone B. Perfect talk, perfect sense. PC Magazine 1998;17(3):85.

101. Kane B, Sands DZ, AMIA Internet Working Group. Guidelines for the clinical use of electronic mail with patients. J Am Med Inform Assoc 1998;5:104–11.

102. Stevens L. Communicating with your patients. The promises and pitfalls of e-mail. Medicine on the Net 1999;5(4):6–10.

103. Kuppersmith RB. Is e-mail an effective medium for physician-patient interactions? Arch Otolaryngol Head Neck Surg 1999;125(4):468–70.

104. Spielberg AR. On call and online. Sociohistorical, legal, and ethical implications of e-mail for the patient-physician relationship. JAMA 1998;280:1353–9.

105. Eysenbach G, Diepgen TL. Responses to unsolicited patient e-mail requests for medical advice on the World Wide Web. JAMA 1998;280:1333–5.

106. Borowitz SM, Wyatt JC. The origin, content, and workload of e-mail consultations. JAMA 1998;280:1321–4.

107. E-mail to eliminate drug confusion. Finger Lakes Times 1999;April 28:7.

108. Fitgerald WL Jr. Do you know where your e-mail messages are? Drug Top 1998;142(1):66.

109. Wolfe D. Avoiding e-mail litigation. Network Magazine 1999;14(1):25.

110. Steen M. Legal pitfalls of e-mail. Every company needs a clear policy, and IT needs to help draft it. InfoWorld 1999;21(27):65–6.

111. Mack J. Secrets of a successful e-mail discussion group moderator. Medicine on the Net 1999;5(4):12–13.

112. Peters R, Sikorski R. Digital dialogue. Sharing information and interests on the Internet. JAMA 1997;277:1258–60.

113. Faxless society. Newsweek 1999;CXXXIII(7):15.

114. Castagna R, Ginsburg L, Morgan C. Stop the e-mail madness! Windows Magazine 1997;8(10):243–51.

115. Howard B. Avoiding clueless e-mail. PC Magazine 1998;17(10):97.

116. Notess GR. Filtering the e-mail storm. Online 1998 Nov:[cited 1999 Nov]:[1 screen]. Available from: URL: http://www.onlineinc.com/onlinemag/OL1998/net11.html.

117. Brookshaw C. Web-based PIMS can help you stick to your schedule. InfoWorld 1999;21(19):57–8, 66.

118. Carre S. How to separate the Internet wheat from the chaff. Drug Top 1997;141(4):88, 90.

119. Seaboldt JA, Kuiper R. Comparison of information obtained from a Usenet newsgroup and from drug information centers. Am J Health-Syst Pharm 1997;54(1):1732–5.

120. Howe L. Patients on the Internet: a new force in healthcare community building. Medicine on the Net 1997;3(11):8–16.

121. Engstrom P. How a scientist tapped UseNet for clues to an inexplicable disease. Medicine on the Net 1997;3(3):1–4.

122. Trott B, Scannell E. Microsoft to open a new Office. InfoWorld 1998;20(7):35.

123. Verity J. IP shakes up long distance. Windows Sources 1998;Feb:58.

124. Keith MR. Televideo technology for patient couseling and education. Am J Health-Syst Pharm 1999;56(1):860–1.

125. Vecchione A. The net set. Hosp Pharm Rep 1999;April:38–40.

126. Melby MJ. Board of directors report on the Council on Professional Affairs. Am J Health-Syst Pharm 1999;56:664–7.

127. Angaran DM. Telemedicine and telepharmacy: current status and future implications. Am J Health-Syst Pharm 1999;56:1405–26.

128. Browserless news—free. PC Magazine 1999;18(17):66.

129. Rapoza J. The cost of free net tools. PC Week 1998;15(3):47.

130. Shankar G. PointCast adds broadcast tools. InfoWorld 1998;19(3):58C–58D.

131. Rapoza J. Personal feeds: all the news that's fit to push. PC Week 1998;15(3):47.

132. Dvorak JC. When push comes to shove. PC Magazine 1997;16(6):87.

133. Martin IG. Electronic labeling: a paperless future? Drug Info J 1998;32:917–19.

134. Collen MF. A vision of health care and informatics in 2008. J Am Med Inform Assoc 1999;6:1–5.

135. Bell G, Gray JN. The revolution yet to happen. In: Denning PJ, Metcalfe RM, editors. Beyond calculation. The next fifty years of computing. New York: Copernicus; 1997.

136. Trott B, Schwartz E. Explorer 5.0 takes on 3D. InfoWorld 1998;20(7):1, 24.

137. Hawkins DT. Information visualization: don't tell me, show me! Online 1999;23(1):88–90.

138. Hunt DL, Haynes RB, Hanna SE, Smith K. Effects of computer-based clinical decision support systems on physician performance and patient outcomes. A systematic review. JAMA 1998;280:1339–46.

139. Monane M. Matthias DM, Nagle BA, Kelly MA. Improving prescribing patterns for the elderly through an online drug utilization review intervention. A system linking the physician, pharmacist, and computer. JAMA 1998;280:1249–52.

140. Slezak M. Eckerd shoots for the moon. Am Druggist 1998;August:38–41.

141. ScriptPro sells Rite Aid on automation. Drug Top 1999;143(7):7.

142. Curle D. Filtered news services. Solutions in search of your problem. Online 1998 March/April:14–24.

143. Gebhart F. WHO to look at Internet prescription commerce. 1997;141(16):82.

144. Behan M. Selling from your website. Beyond Computing 1998;7(2):20–2, 24, 26, 30.

145. Internet Rx. PC Magazine 1999 July;18(3):10.

146. Breu J. NABP starts process of certifying sites as accepted pharmacies. Drug Topics 1999;143(19):19, 23.

147. Dear pharmacist. Pharmacists' Letter 1999;15(10):1.

148. If it sounds crazy, try it. Information Week 1994;Sept 5:32–7.

149. Gardner E. If this were a test, Drugstore.com would get a 'C'. Internet World 1999;5(14):1, 73.

150. Vecchione A. Pharmacy schools found wanting in their training on technology. Hosp Pharm Rep 1997 Sept;[Technology and Pharmacy '97 Supplement]:22S–23S.

151. Machrone B. It ain't worth a thing with no bandwidth swing. PC Week 1997;Aug 4:75.

152. Machrone B. Speed kills: the dial-up Internet. PC Magazine 1997;16(17):85.

153. Howard B. The cable modem guy. PC Magazine 1997;16(17):95.

154. Metcalfe B. Beep-beep! Road Runner's cable modem service offers really fast Internet access. InfoWorld 1998;20(8):115.

155. Nobel C, Berinato S. 1998 could be watershed year for DSL. PC Week 1997;14(51):1, 14.

156. Dodge J. Can DSL break the 'Year of' curse? PC Week 1997;14(51):2.

157. Riggs B. ADSL gets access call. LANTIMES 1998;15(4):1, 20.

158. Roberts-Witt SL. Highway in the sky. Internet World 1999;5(34):73–4, 76.

Chapter Six

Literature Evaluation I: Controlled Clinical Trials

Kristen W. Mosdell

Objectives

After completing this chapter, the reader will be able to:

- Explain the importance of literature evaluation to the practice of pharmacy.
- Describe why careful evaluation of medical literature is necessary before using study results for clinical decision making.
- Describe why poor quality biomedical literature is published.
- Define scientific fraud and explain how it may affect the biomedical literature.
- Describe the various venues where scientific literature is published and the peer-review process.
- Describe how experience of the investigator and resources available at the research site may influence quality of biomedical literature.
- Explain why the source of funding may bias study results.
- Describe the importance of abstracts in conveying study information and understand why structured abstracts are the preferred format.
- Explain the role of investigational review boards and informed consent.
- Describe why study objectives and hypotheses must be clearly defined.
- Differentiate between parallel and cross-over studies.
- Assess sample size of a study.
- Explain the concepts of controls, randomization, and blinding in clinical trials.
- Determine whether statistical tests used in a study are appropriate.
- Define intention-to-treat, subgroup, and interim analyses.
- Define the concepts of type I and type II errors.
- Interpret the meaning of *p* values, confidence intervals, and number needed to treat (NNT) and differentiate between clinical and statistical significance.

- Define internal and external validity of a study.
- Describe why study conclusions must be consistent with study results.
- Develop a strategy for routinely reviewing the biomedical literature.

Pharmacists in the new millennium face an explosion of biomedical information—currently over 20,000 biomedical journals are published annually.[1] It has been estimated that an individual would have to read 6000 journal articles each day just to keep ahead.[2] Continuing education programs and symposia help pharmacists keep up with this information; however, these resources may be subject to the bias of the author, sponsor of the program, or the literature used to prepare the programs or symposia. Pharmacists, therefore, must learn to systematically review and critique the biomedical literature. Skills in literature evaluation enable pharmacists to efficiently and effectively determine which treatment options represent therapeutic advances and which lack the potential to improve patient care and perhaps may even be harmful.

Literature evaluation skills are essential in many areas of pharmacy practice. Pharmacists are faced with an increasingly sophisticated patient population who educate themselves about drug therapy by consulting various individuals (e.g., health care professionals, purveyors of alternative medicine, family, and friends), searching the Internet, and reading both the medical literature and lay press. Such patients often seek the advice of a pharmacist to interpret information they have obtained. Likewise, physicians and other health care professionals often contact pharmacists for opinions regarding various aspects of therapy. Unbiased responses to these inquiries can only be provided after careful analysis of available studies. In addition, decisions on drug policy management, such as whether to add or delete a drug from the formulary, should be based on careful review of the literature.

Many assume that only high quality information meets the qualifications for publication and, therefore, the importance of developing skills in literature evaluation is questioned. Even if this were true, careful review of the literature would be necessary to determine whether the conditions of the study were similar to those routinely encountered in clinical practice. Additionally, even the most eloquent studies may show results that, though statistically significant, may be considered clinically irrelevant. The reality of the situation, however, is that much of the biomedical literature fails to meet standards for well-conducted studies. Various reviews have estimated that 40% to 50% of published articles in the medical and pharmacy literature have serious problems with design, statistical analysis, and conclusions.[3,4] Poorly conducted research is hazardous because it may result in substantial harm to patients and wastes resources, time, and money.[5]

How are studies fraught with flaws and bias ever published in reputable biomedical journals? This is a complex question. "Publish or perish," the situation where only those who publish in quantity become tenured academicians, forces many researchers to submit for publication studies that may be suboptimal in terms of quality or attempt to publish the same study or portions of the same study in multiple journals.[5-7]

Researchers may also lack appropriate knowledge in study design and statistical analysis to perform well-conducted investigations. Experts who critique manuscripts to determine their appropriateness for publication (i.e., peer reviewers) may also be deficient in such knowledge.[5] Even if peer reviewers recognize a study as flawed, they may consider it worthy of publication if the research is in an area of importance and its publication may stimulate further investigations. Readers must then recognize the results as preliminary with minimal potential to immediately influence patient care.

The most disturbing issue to consider, however, is the potential for scientific fraud. During 964 routine audits conducted by the Food and Drug Administration (FDA) from 1975 to 1983, fraudulent data were found to have been submitted by 59% (24/41) of investigators disciplined by the agency for scientific misconduct.[8] In another analysis of 235 articles retracted from journals, 86 (37%) were due to misconduct.[9] Alarmingly, these articles continued to be cited by other authors as valid work following publication of the retraction notice.[9]

Fabrication of data is difficult for anyone (including peer reviewers) to detect by simple review of manuscripts and requires that journals take further measures to ensure the validity of submitted data in the future.[6,7,10] Solutions that have been suggested by some experts include having all authors sign a statement confirming the validity of the data or having journals randomly audit raw data.[6,11] At a minimum, investigators should indicate in their manuscript that adequate trial records have been kept.[12]

This chapter explains basic concepts useful for evaluating controlled clinical trials. Chapter 7, Literature Evaluation II: Beyond the Basics, emphasizes skills for critically analyzing other types of research designs (e.g., case-control studies, follow-up studies, meta-analyses, etc.). Before beginning, one important caveat must be kept in mind. No study is perfect. Literature evaluation is the art of determining which flaws are acceptable and which strike a fatal blow to the study conclusions. Using the skills described in these two chapters, readers will be able to make these determinations.

Evaluating Clinical Trials (True Experiments)

In a clinical trial or true experiment, researchers administer a drug or treatment and follow the subjects forward in time (prospectively) to determine the effects of such treatment. Randomized controlled clinical trials, a type of true experiment, are the gold standard for determining cause and effect relationships.[13,14] The year 1998 marked the 50th anniversary of the first published, randomized clinical trial.[15] Over the years, much has been learned about proper conduct and reporting of randomized controlled clinical trials. The following section will review techniques for critically analyzing these studies.

JOURNAL, INVESTIGATORS, RESEARCH SITE, AND FUNDING

The literature evaluation process should begin by briefly scanning the article. The study should be published in a reputable journal where manuscripts undergo peer review before publication. During the peer-review process, study manuscripts that have been submitted for publication are critiqued by a panel of experts and then revised as suggested by these reviewers.[6] Studies that have been conducted appropriately and that are relevant to the journal's focus may subsequently be published.[6] Studies that fail the peer-review process may be submitted to alternate journals for consideration. If the research topic seems out of place for a particular journal, this may be an indication that the study was initially rejected for publication by peer reviewers from more pertinent journals. Highly competitive journals (e.g., *The New England Journal of Medicine*) accept fewer than one-third of submitted manuscripts for publication, whereas the publication rate is much higher for other journals.[6]

Clinical studies may also be published in other forums (Table 6–1). Before publication in peer-reviewed journals, studies may be published in the form of abstracts following presentation at scientific meetings. Such abstracts are meant to stimulate discussion among peers and allow results to be shared before publication in a peer-reviewed journal.[16] Abstracts are subject to a less stringent review process than articles published in peer-reviewed journals and are rarely detailed enough to allow clinical decisions to be based on their results.[16] In fact, many papers presented as abstracts at scientific meetings ultimately fail to meet the standards for publication when submitted to peer-reviewed journals.[16]

Results can be published as part of a symposium or journal supplement, a group of papers usually published as a separate issue or separate section of a journal, which are focused on a specific topic.[17] Such symposia, however, may be sponsored by the pharmaceutical industry for promotional purposes and may not undergo the same peer-review process as standard journal articles.[17,18] An evaluation of 242 articles found in

TABLE 6–1. HOW IS PRIMARY LITERATURE PUBLISHED?

- Article in peer-reviewed journal
- Abstract
- Component of symposium
- Letter to the editor

journals that routinely publish supplement issues found that quality scores were statistically lower for articles published in journal supplements compared to parent issues ($p = .01$).[18] In particular, discussion of issues such as compliance, baseline characteristics of subjects, major endpoints, study power, statistical analyses, and subject accountability were poorer in articles published in journal supplements compared to the parent journal.[18]

Reports of experience with a single patient or small group of patients with regard to drug efficacy or toxicity may be presented in the form of a letter to the editor, in which a description of the patient and results are briefly presented. Although these letters are reviewed by the editor before publication, they do not usually have to meet the rigorous standards necessary for publication as journal articles. They are meant to stimulate interest and conversation among readers of the journal.

Clinical studies are rarely, if ever, published in "throw-away" journals. Throw-away journals are characterized by being free to readers, having a high advertisement-to-text ratio, not being owned by professional societies, having a variable peer-review process, and not having a section for critical correspondence.[19] Articles published in such journals are of little benefit in clinical decision making.[19]

In addition to considerations regarding the journal, readers should assess whether the investigators have training and expertise in the area being studied and, preferably, a good track record of prior research.[20] A biostatistician should also have assisted in evaluation of data. Studies authored entirely by investigators working in the pharmaceutical industry are sometimes considered biased. Scientists from industry, however, often co-author articles with university and practice-based professionals in situations where a pharmaceutical manufacturer sponsors and coordinates a drug trial. Although such studies are less likely to be biased, readers need to carefully assess the methods, results, and conclusions. Most journals disclose affiliations of authors and sources of funding for studies, allowing potential conflicts of interest to be identified.[21]

To be listed as authors, individuals should contribute substantially to the research effort. The Uniform Requirements for Manuscripts Submitted to Biomedical Journals,[22] as well as many journals, provide guidelines for study authorship. Chapter 11, Professional Writing, addresses this topic in more detail. A recent proposal outlined a new system whereby all individuals who perform substantial work on a project are listed as contributors, along with a description of their various contributions.[23] One individual is also identified as guarantor for the integrity of the work.[23] These recommendations have been adopted by journals such as *The Lancet* and the *British Medical Journal*.[24] Contribution lists are more informative than order of authors in the byline. A recent review of contributions listed in the *British Medical Journal* found that author order in the byline did not correlate with contributions.[24] Political dynamics of research organizations may explain this discrepancy.[24] Interestingly, the same study also found that only 44% of authors met the criteria for authorship as defined by the International Committee of Medical Journal Editors.[24] Another analysis of 809 articles determined that 19% had evidence of honorary authors and 11% of ghost authors.[25] In the former case, authors who did not contribute substantially to the research effort received credit and in the latter, those who contributed substantially did not receive credit.

When reviewing biomedical literature, another important consideration is the research site. The research site should have appropriate resources and technology to effectively conduct the study and sufficient subjects who are similar to those routinely encountered in clinical practice to recruit for study entry.[20]

The reader should also note the source of study funding. Preferable sources of study funding include nonprofit organizations such as the National Institutes of Health (NIH) or the National Cancer Institute (NCI). Such organizations do not benefit financially from the study results. Funding by pharmaceutical manufacturers may indicate a possible bias because considerable financial gain may be accrued from a study demonstrating positive effects of a drug. This type of funding does not necessarily negate the study results, however. For example, studies conducted in support of a New Drug Application (NDA) often undergo extensive review by the FDA. In addition, most university- and practice-based investigators will report the results of a clinical study regardless of whether they are in favor of or reflect negatively against a product manufactured by the company who funded the project. Many pharmaceutical manufacturers provide study drugs and placebos for clinical trials. Unlike complete or partial financial support for a study, this practice usually does not indicate that a study is biased toward any particular therapy.

TITLE/ABSTRACT

The title of the article should be brief and catch the attention of readers interested in the topic.[5,20] The title should also be unbiased and should not indicate authors' preferences for any particular drug treatment. An example of a biased title would be, "The superiority of drug A versus drug B in the treatment of acute otitis media with effusion in children." More appropriately, such a study should be entitled, "A comparison of drug A versus drug B in the treatment of acute otitis media with effusion in children."

The abstract is the road map of a study, and briefly describes the purpose, methods, results, and conclusion of an investigation. By scanning the abstract, readers should be able to determine whether the study is of interest and deserves further review. Abstracts should be clearly written. Unfortunately, data are sometimes presented in the abstract that are not discussed in the body of the article, numerical values for data differ in these two sections, or important details of an investigation are not mentioned in the abstract.[5] Because abstracts only provide brief overviews of clinical studies, they cannot be used as substitutes for careful analysis of study methods, results, and conclusions. Although reading abstracts is less time consuming than critiquing an entire study, consideration of details contained in the body of articles (as will become obvious in the upcoming sections) is essential before applying study results to clinical practice.

Journals such as *The New England Journal of Medicine, Annals of Internal Medicine,* and the *British Medical Journal* have developed formats for structured abstracts.[26] Structured abstracts for clinical studies include the following sections: objective, research design, clinical setting, participants, interventions, main outcome measurements, results, and conclusions.[26] Structured abstracts were developed to improve the quality of abstracts in the medical literature and make them more informative. For further information related to abstracts, readers are referred to Appendix 11–2.

INTRODUCTION

The introduction section of a clinical study contains background information for the study, states study objectives and hypotheses, and indicates any planned subgroup or covariate analyses.[27] This section also addresses ethical issues related to conduct of the study.

Sufficient background information should be provided to demonstrate that the study is important and ethical.[5,13] Background information familiarizes readers with the research subject. Current treatment paradigms for the disease state being studied, limitations of these treatments, and reasons why the treatment under investigation may offer benefits should be discussed.[28] Data from completed preclinical and/or clinical studies should be summarized to justify that further study in the area is needed.[29] Background information should indicate that potential benefits outweigh risks to subjects entering the study. A study without potential to improve patient care wastes resources, time, and money and may harm the patient unnecessarily. When providing background information, authors should avoid citing only their own past research.

Study objectives or goals should be clearly stated by the investigators in the introduction of the article.[29] If they are not, the purpose of the investigation may not be clear and readers may come to erroneous conclusions regarding the study results. Poorly stated objectives make it difficult to read and evaluate clinical studies. If the investigators fail to state objectives, it may also be an indication that the study was not well planned and was haphazardly conducted. An example of a well-written objective is, "The study was designed to compare drug A 250 mg orally four times daily with drug B 200 mg orally once daily in the treatment of acute otitis media infection with effusion due to *Streptococcus pneumoniae, Moraxella catarrhalis,* or *Hemophilus influenzae* infections, as confirmed by tympanocentesis, in children aged 1 month to 6 years. A poorly written objective may state, "The goal of the study was to determine the effects of drug A and drug B in otitis media."

A research and null hypothesis must also be formulated for every study and should be stated in the introduction of an article. The research hypothesis or alternative hypothesis (H_A) tells readers what the investigators expected to find during the course of their study. For instance, the investigators may have believed that bacteriological cure for acute otitis media with effusion in children occurs more frequently with drug A than drug B and, therefore, designed their study to test this hypothesis. The null hypothesis (H_0), on the other hand, is the "no difference" hypothesis. It is the hypothesis that the investigators must reject to be able to accept the research hypothesis and the hypothesis upon which all statistical assumptions are based. In the previous example, the null hypothesis would be that frequency of bacteriological cure for acute otitis media with effusion in children is equal for both drug A and drug B. Unfortunately, authors rarely state both the null and research hypotheses in the study introduction. Although such information improves readers' understanding of the study methodology and statistical analyses, it is more common to find only the objective of the study noted in the introduction, and on occasion, the research hypothesis. Studies that fail to state both the null and research hypothesis may not automatically be classified as poor studies; however, they may be more difficult for readers to comprehend.

Ethical issues are usually addressed in the introduction of an article, but may sometimes be located in the methods section. Before initiation, study protocols involving human subjects should be reviewed by an investigational review board (IRB). An IRB consists of both health professionals and lay individuals who review study protocols and ensure that risk to subjects is minimal and that the consent form is written in such a way that subjects understand possible benefits and hazards associated with study entry. Subjects always have the right to refuse entry into a study, and the decision to participate must be made on a voluntary basis. Informed consent is mandatory for most studies except those in which routinely collected patient data (e.g., the medical record) are analyzed.[30] Readers should note whether the study protocol was reviewed by an IRB and that subjects signed informed consent forms. The role of IRBs is described in further detail in Chap. 17, Investigational Drugs.

METHODS

Study methodology is the most important section of a clinical study. The methods section contains information on the design, study population, instrumentation, and statistics used for the investigation. Results of studies with serious methodological flaws may be unreliable. The methods section should be sufficiently detailed to allow investigators to reproduce the study. Additionally, authors should state that the protocol is available upon request in case readers have additional questions regarding study methodology.[31]

Parallel Versus Cross-over Studies

During a parallel study, subjects receive only one treatment, while during a cross-over study, subjects receive all study drugs during the course of the study (Fig. 6–1).[13] Parallel studies are most appropriate when therapies are definitive or when disease states are self-limited (e.g., antimicrobials for infectious diseases). When disease states are chronic and/or highly variable (e.g., glaucoma, migraine headache), cross-over designs are more appropriate. Cross-over studies minimize error caused by variability among subjects because each subject serves as his or her own control. Cross-over studies also allow for efficient use of subjects. A smaller sample size is usually required in cross-over as compared to parallel studies.[32]

Several problems are unique to the use of cross-over designs and must be assessed when evaluating this type of study (Table 6–2).[32] If a subject is to receive both drug A and drug B during the cross-over study, sufficient time must elapse between treatments (washout period) so that the effects of the first treatment do not persist during the second treatment. When evaluating cross-over studies, a good rule of thumb to use is that washout periods should be equivalent to at least five half-lives of the study drug (the time for the drug to be eliminated totally from the body).

Another problem is the nature of chronic diseases.[32] Chronic diseases generally are not static, but have periods of remission and exacerbation. Response to study treatments may vary depending on severity of the disease state at the time the treatment is administered. If symptoms are more severe during treatment with drug A than drug B, drug B may erroneously be considered superior to drug A. Use of multiple cross-over periods helps to overcome this obstacle in assessing study results. In studies with multiple cross-over periods, the patient receives both drugs on more than one occasion

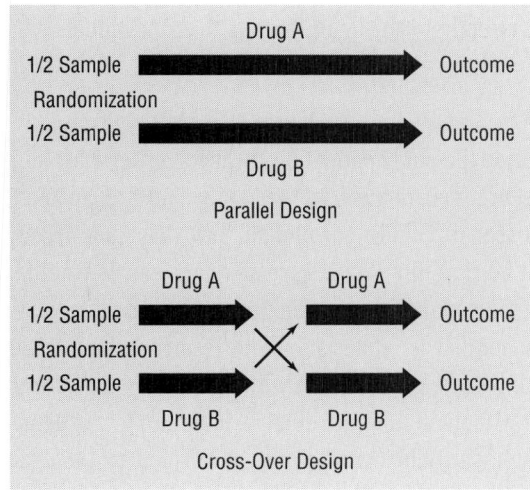

Figure 6–1. Parallel versus cross-over designs.

TABLE 6–2. IMPORTANT CONSIDERATIONS FOR CROSS-OVER STUDIES

- Washout period must be of sufficient duration to prevent carry-over effects.
- Multiple cross-over periods are useful when studying diseases with exacerbations and remissions.
- Subjects should be randomized to treatment order.
- Both investigators and subjects should be blinded to time when cross-over occurs.
- Subject drop-outs and deaths should be minimized.

allowing researchers to assess fluctuation in therapeutic response during the course of the study. Critical readers of cross-over studies need to consider whether variation in disease state severity may have influenced study results.

Another consideration relevant to cross-over studies is treatment order.[32] A subject may respond differently if drug A is given before drug B than if drug B is given before drug A. Consequently, it is essential that subjects are randomized to treatment order (randomization is discussed in detail in a subsequent section of this chapter). This technique assigns half of the subjects to initial treatment with drug A and half to drug B.

There are two other important points to evaluate when reading cross-over studies.[32] In cross-over studies, both subjects and investigators should be unaware of the point when cross-over occurs (i.e., they should be blinded to the cross-over period). This precaution is important because both physicians and patients may expect improvement in the condition during the second treatment phase if response was poor during the first treatment phase or vice versa if response was good initially. Blinding decreases the probability that patient or physician bias may influence study results. Drop-outs and deaths may also influence study results and should be minimized, if possible. In cross-over studies, each subject contributes at least two pieces of data for each measurement of outcome, and loss of patients during the course of the study results in substantial loss of data. In addition, it is impossible to determine whether patients who dropped out of a study would have responded differently to the drug therapy than individuals who completed the investigation.

Inclusion and Exclusion Criteria

Inclusion and exclusion criteria describe the study patients.[29] Inclusion criteria list subject characteristics that must be present for enrollment into the study and exclusion criteria list characteristics that, if present, preclude enrollment into the study. Study inclusion and exclusion criteria must be carefully stated so readers can assess whether the study sample is representative of the population to which the results are intended to be generalized.[13,29] Diagnostic criteria for disease states should be clearly defined.[33] It is inappropriate for investigators to simply state that children with acute otitis media with effusion were entered into the study without stating the clinical, laboratory, and demographic criteria that justified the diagnosis. Subjects who may be harmed by the drug therapy or who may confound the results of the study should be excluded from entry.

In the past, women of childbearing age were routinely excluded from clinical studies because of potential risks and liability concerns relative to fetal exposure to drug therapy, despite the fact that many women practice effective hormonal and barrier birth control methods.[34] Minorities have also been excluded due to concerns surrounding altered drug response or lack of availability of these patients for inclusion in drug trials.[34] Many pharmacokinetic and bioequivalence studies, for example, routinely use healthy male volunteers who may not be representative of patients in clinical practice. Safety, efficacy, and pharmacokinetics/pharmacodynamics, however, can differ substantially by gender and race. Therefore, authors should enroll subjects who are likely to receive the medication, including women and minorities, to better determine efficacy and to assess side effects that otherwise would remain unrecognized if these groups were excluded.[34] Additionally, the FDA expects safety and efficacy data to be analyzed by important demographic subgroups and can refuse to file an NDA that fails to analyze safety and efficacy information appropriately by gender.[35,36]

Readers must assess whether the study sample is representative of patients routinely encountered in clinical practice. For example, a study of acute otitis media with effusion done in an emergency room setting may not be representative of outpatient practice, because patients who seek medical attention in an emergency room may be more ill and of a lower socioeconomic status. Often, practitioners wish to apply study results to complicated patients with multiple disease states who differ substantially from the study sample. This practice must be done with caution because these patients may respond differently and experience more adverse events than the study patients.

Readers must also determine whether any patient groups permitted entry into the study may have confounded the study results. If in the example of acute otitis media with effusion, children with recurrent infections or those who had received antibiotics within the past 2 weeks were permitted entry into the study, response rates would be lower than would have been expected if this patient group had been excluded.

Sample Size

A sample is a subgroup from the entire population of patients with a particular disease state who would be eligible to enter the study. Samples are used because of logistic, financial, and resource constraints that prohibit studying an entire population.

One of the most important areas to critique when evaluating clinical studies is sample size. Investigators should state how sample size was determined for the study. There is no magic number that indicates an appropriate number of study subjects. Sample size varies from study to study based on the factors discussed below.

Readers can feel confident that sample size for a study was adequate if the number of patients who completed the study (not the number of patients who entered the study) equals the investigators' initial sample size calculations presented in the methods section of the article. Unfortunately, the issue of sample size is often overlooked in clinical studies and sample size calculations for the study are not stated. This omission is of particular concern when the results of a study indicate that study treatments are equal. When this scenario is encountered, readers must ask themselves, "Was the sample size large enough to detect a statistically significant difference between treatments" (see discussion of type II errors in a later section). When authors avoid a discussion of sample size in an article, quite often the sample was too small. Several nomograms and tables have been published to assist readers in determining whether an appropriate sample size was used in a clinical trial.[37,38] On the other hand, if a statistically significant difference in efficacy or safety is observed, then sample size was large enough to determine inequality between the groups; however, treatment effects may be overestimated if sample size is smaller than what would have been determined using sample size calculations due to the influence of outlier data (Fig 6–2).[14,30] Studies with inadequate samples sizes generally are not strong enough to directly influence patient care, but may be considered pilot studies capable of stimulating further research in an area. The fact that such studies are hypothesis forming should be clearly stated in the discussion section of the article.[39]

Sample size must be determined before initiation of an investigation. If sample size is considered while the study is ongoing, investigators may inappropriately decide to discontinue the study when results reflect their expectations or hypotheses.[30] If sample size is too small, probability of detecting a statistically significant difference between treatment groups may be low (see discussion of type II errors in a later section). There is also less likelihood that the sample is representative of the population when a small sample size is used (Fig 6–2).[14] On the other hand, an extremely large sample is probably more representative of the population, but may allow one to find statistically significant differences between treatment groups that are weak and lack clinical significance (Fig 6–2).[14,40]

Sample size should be based on four factors: alpha or level of significance (i.e., the probability of a false-positive result), beta (i.e., the probability of a false-negative result), delta (i.e., the amount of difference that one wants to detect between treatment groups), and variance or standard deviation (Table 6–3).[30,41] Investigators should determine what magnitude of response would be considered clinically important to avoid too small or too large a sample size and to increase the likelihood that statistically significant results

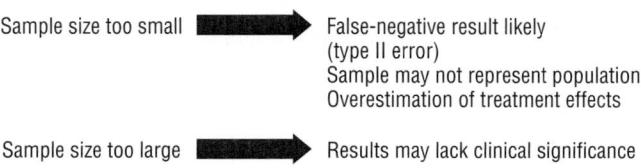

Figure 6–2. Inappropriate sample size risks.

TABLE 6–3. DETERMINANTS OF SAMPLE SIZE

- Alpha or level of significance (i.e., probability of false-positive result)
- Beta (i.e., probability of false-negative result)
- Delta (i.e., amount of difference to be detected)
- Standard deviation (i.e., variation)

will also be clinically relevant.[40,42] Sample size calculations should be based on the primary endpoint.[39,43] If there are multiple primary endpoints, the sample size needed to evaluate each of the endpoints should be calculated and the largest sample size required to evaluate all endpoints selected for the study.[39]

Readers do not need to understand how to calculate sample size because standard statistical texts can be consulted for this information. However, it is important to note whether the investigators discuss how sample size was calculated for the study and whether the final number of evaluable subjects equals this amount. Because drop-outs and deaths are likely during the course of a study, the final number of subjects may be smaller than initial sample size calculations and, therefore, the likelihood of a false-negative result may be increased. Many investigators will add an additional 10% or 20% to their initial calculations to ensure an adequate sample size at study completion.[43] The following excerpt from a study entitled "High-dose acyclovir compared with short-course preemptive ganciclovir therapy to prevent cytomegalovirus disease in liver transplant recipients. A randomized trial"[44] exemplifies how authors should justify sample size of a study: "We estimated that at least 20 patients in each group would be needed to detect a decrease in CMV disease from 35% with standard acyclovir prophylaxis to 5% with ganciclovir (alpha = .05, power = .80)."

Often, sample size needed to determine efficacy and safety of a treatment is large, and adequate subjects for the trial cannot be recruited from a single investigational site. In these situations, multicenter trials are conducted.[33] Such trials present unique challenges. Efforts to minimize the likelihood of obtaining different outcomes at different centers must be undertaken. For example, all centers must understand the protocol and receive adequate training on how to conduct the trial. Reports of multicenter trials should state whether differences in efficacy and safety were observed between sites. Sites that accrued patients should also be listed.[31]

Controls

A drug may exert psychological benefits even if it is pharmacologically inactive. Factors such as the natural history of the disease, extensive monitoring and ancillary care, chance, or bias can influence the efficacy and safety outcomes of clinical trials.[33] For example, studies on pain management have demonstrated that placebos are effective in providing pain relief in more than one-third of patients who receive them.[45] Because of this potential influence, controls are necessary in clinical studies to ascertain true physiological actions of drugs. Studies that are uncontrolled may exaggerate clinical benefits of drugs or show benefit where none exists. Results from uncontrolled trials are generally considered preliminary and rarely influence patient care unless the disease previously was uniformly fatal or if available treatments were ineffective or nonexistent.[33]

Two types of controls are typically encountered when reading the biomedical literature, placebo and active. In placebo-controlled trials, the control group receives a placebo that is identical to the study drug in terms of appearance, taste, smell, and other characteristics, but does not contain the active ingredient. The placebo should be described in detail in the methods section of the article.[46] Placebo-controlled studies are useful for determining whether a drug is effective. They also help to determine whether clinical effects are due to the treatment or another confounding variable.[47] Placebo controls are often used when efficacious treatments for a disease are unavailable.[33]

Active controls are used when efficacy and safety of two or more drugs need to be compared or when it would be unethical to administer a placebo. For example, a placebo-controlled study of a new antibiotic for acute otitis media would be unethical because appropriate antibiotic therapy is readily available. The current gold standard (i.e., the most effective and least harmful therapy available for treatment of the disease) should be used as the active control.[48] Appropriate dosage regimens for both the study drug and active control should be administered. When patient response to the drug therapy is variable, investigators should consider titrating dosage to therapeutic effect.[29] If the active control is given at a subtherapeutic dose, the investigation may be biased in favor of the study drug. Studies using active controls can be difficult to interpret if a gold standard is not available for comparison or if occurrence of the outcome parameter (e.g., migraine headaches, postoperative nausea and vomiting) is highly variable.[48] In the latter case, authors may have difficulty determining whether a decrease in event rates is due to efficacy of the study treatments or variability of the outcome parameters.[48] For example, consider an active-controlled study that concludes drugs A and B are equally efficacious in preventing postoperative nausea and vomiting. Because event rates without treatment are not generated, it is unknown whether both drugs decreased the incidence of postoperative nausea and vomiting or whether susceptibility of the study population to postoperative nausea and vomiting was low.[48]

Historical controls are also occasionally used. These studies use data from previously conducted trials or groups of previously treated patients for comparison with the current study population. Historical controls are useful in situations where new therapies offer such an advantage over previous options that it would no longer be ethical to subject patients either to placebo or active controls. For example, if a new drug was developed that reversed the pathology of Alzheimer's disease, comparison with active or placebo controls may not be ethical. In general, historical controls are only appropriate when the previous study conditions (e.g., inclusion and exclusion criteria, outcome variables) are identical to those in the current study.[49] However, because time of data collection affects patient response, historical controls are considered of limited value.

A final consideration that deserves mention is that all interventions other than the therapy being investigated should be identical in both the treatment and control groups.[50] Interventions such as physician care and counseling impact therapeutic outcome. If the treatment group receives more comprehensive care than the control group, the study becomes biased toward the new drug therapy whether or not the drug is pharmacologically superior.

Outcome Variables

Investigators should define variables to be measured and the amount of difference between treatment and control groups that the study is designed to detect (e.g., 10% difference in cure rate for children receiving drug A versus drug B for the treatment of acute otitis media with effusion).[27,30] Clinical outcomes should be relevant, clearly defined, objective, and clinically and biologically significant.[33,51] For example, it is more important to determine whether an antihypertensive agent decreases mortality from vascular complications than whether the drug lowers systolic and diastolic blood pressure.[51] The primary and secondary endpoints should be specified a priori (i.e., before the study is conducted) to avoid data dredging for statistically significant results at the conclusion of the study.[12,33] Clearly stated operational definitions are needed when outcome variables are vague (e.g., response, partial response, failure). If authors fail to describe variables in detail, readers may be unable to determine whether the outcome measurements appropriately meet the study objectives.[29] In addition, subsequent authors would have difficulty reproducing the study for future investigations.

Small studies are often adequate for assessing treatment effects when surrogate endpoints are used (e.g., blood pressure in hypertensive subjects, viral load in subjects infected with HIV), whereas large studies are often necessary for determining clinical outcomes (e.g., survival).[33] Although this represents a potential advantage, surrogate endpoints should only be used when they have been correlated with clinical endpoints and validated in previous clinical trials.[33]

Methodology used to measure outcome variables should be up to date and considered the current "gold standard."[28] Instruments used to measure variables should be justified.[29] For example, if serum drug concentrations are measured, authors should clearly explain the assay technique used in the study and its sensitivity and specificity. Studies focused on subjective parameters should provide literature demonstrating the validity of measurement tools such as questionnaires and visual analog scales. If errors in measurement are likely, or if the tools used for measurement have not been validated, data are questionable.

Variables should be measured at appropriate intervals and for an appropriate length of time to ensure that both positive and negative aspects of a therapy are adequately assessed.[28] Both the treatment and placebo groups should be followed with the same intensity.[12] For example, a study investigating a new cholesterol lowering agent should continue for a sufficient length of time to determine whether the agent prevents cardiovascular complications such as myocardial infarction, stroke, and death. Efficacy can also decrease over time if tolerance develops. Study duration should be of sufficient length to adequately assess the efficacy and safety profile of the treatment. Additionally, many adverse events only develop after prolonged treatment. Examples include pulmonary toxicity with amiodarone, cardiotoxicity with adriamycin, and cataracts with corticosteroids.

Randomization

Randomization is an important aspect of study design. When studies are randomized, subjects have an equal and independent chance of receiving any of the treatment modalities.[14] Randomization is equivalent to flipping a coin and helps ensure that treatment groups are similar in regard to clinical and socioeconomic factors that may affect treatment outcome.[51,52] Randomization helps diminish patient and investigator bias by prohibiting investigators from assigning drug treatments. In nonrandomized studies, physicians may be tempted to place patients who are more ill on the treatment they believe to be most efficacious, thereby biasing the study. Alternately, investigators may place healthier patients on the study drug in an attempt to demonstrate its superiority.[29] A recent analysis of published clinical studies concluded that, on average, nonrandomized trials tend to overestimate treatment outcomes; however, effects may also be underestimated, reversed in direction, masked, or similar to results from randomized trials.[53]

Randomization requires that an unpredictable treatment sequence be generated that remains concealed until subjects are allocated to treatment.[54] Proper methods of randomization include use of random number tables, computer-generated random numbers, or lotteries.[14] Assigning subjects to treatment groups via nonrandom techniques is inappropriate. Often authors state that patients were randomly allocated to treatment groups when in fact nonrandom techniques were used. Common nonrandom techniques that authors categorize as random include assignment of patients to treatments using phone numbers, days of the week, or hospital admission numbers or alternating treatments as patients are enrolled in the study.

Information on how the allocation schedule was concealed should also be provided.[27,54] Allocation schedules may be concealed through telephone assignment by pharmacy or clinical trial office personnel, numbered or coded bottles, or sequentially numbered opaque, sealed envelopes.[54] The latter method is considered the least desirable because envelopes can be manipulated by study personnel.[54] When questioned, investigators have admitted using various methods to determine randomization codes including opening unsealed envelopes, holding translucent envelopes up to light bulbs, deciphering randomization codes posted on bulletin boards, and searching for randomization codes in the principle investigator's files.[54]

Randomization can be simple (unrestricted) or balanced (restricted).[54] Simple randomization is accomplished by referring to a list of random numbers.[54] If sample size of the study is small, a risk of simple randomization is having uneven numbers of patients in each treatment group.[54] To overcome this problem, balanced randomization is sometimes used. For balanced randomization, blocks of patients (e.g., every 10 consecutively enrolled patients) are randomized to ensure that similar numbers of patients are allocated to each treatment group.[54] If the trial is unblinded, block size should be varied during the study to prevent individuals from deciphering the randomization code.[54] Restrictive randomization can also be used if certain factors are known to be prognostic (e.g., disease severity, age). In this situation, individuals can be stratified by presence or absence of the factor and randomized within each stratification group.[33,54] Alternately, subjects can be matched for prognostic factors and then one member of each pair randomized to receive treatment or control.[33]

Because individuals responsible for performing randomization have knowledge of treatment allocation, they should not determine subject eligibility, administer treatments, or assess outcomes to avoid introducing bias into the study.[12] Authors should state how individuals assigning treatments were separated from those conducting the clinical trial.[27] Furthermore, to minimize bias, investigators should not be aware of trends in data at the time of treatment allocation and data analysts should be unaware of randomization schema.[12]

It is difficult to be confident about the results of a nonrandomized trial, unless the treatment undergoing investigation decreases mortality and traditional strategies ultimately resulted in death.[51] When nonrandomized trials are encountered, readers must judge whether the magnitude of the treatment effects is so large that they could not be due to chance alone.[51] Of course the probability of error in this situation is large.

Statistically significant differences in patient characteristics may occur despite proper randomization, especially if sample size is small.[50] For example, consider a randomized study in which two drugs, A and B, are being compared for the treatment of severe infections. Morbidity and mortality are found to be lower in patients treated with drug A compared to drug B. However, upon close examination one notes that patients who received drug B had more severe infections than those treated with drug A. In this scenario, study outcome may be a function of disease severity and not drug therapy. Because of this problem, investigators should statistically compare demographic data of treatment and control groups. Readers should assess whether any statistically or clinically significant differences in demographic variables could potentially have biased the results.[50] If confounding variables are found to exist, authors should adjust data using statistical techniques such as analysis of covariance.[50] If after these statistical manipulations the original results do not differ substantially from the adjusted results, it is unlikely that the demographic differences in treatment and control groups affected the study outcome.[50]

Blinding

Both investigators and subjects involved in a clinical study usually have an opinion about the therapy undergoing investigation.[50] Subject response and researcher evaluation may be affected by these views. Blinding helps prevent these biases from influencing study results and ensures that monitoring and ancillary care are applied equally to both treatment and control groups.[33] Mechanisms for blinding the study and similarities between the treatment and control (e.g., appearance, taste, smell) should be described in clinical trial reports.[27] The location of the code and whether or not the blind was broken during the clinical trial should also be discussed.[27]

In a single-blind study, either patients or investigators are unable to identify the treatment (active or control) assigned; the alternate group (i.e., patient or investigator) is aware of therapy being administered (Table 6–4).[29] In a double-blind study, neither investigators nor patients are aware of treatment assignments.[29] Studies that involve interpretation of diagnostic tests such as electrocardiograms, computer tomography, electroencephalopathy, and so forth often blind the evaluators of the data (e.g., cardiologists, radiologists, neurologists), as well as the investigators and patients, a situation sometimes referred to as a triple-blind study. Data entry personnel should also be blinded to treatment allocation.[12] Additionally, study or pharmacy personnel that dispense the medication may be blinded to treatment allocation. For example, in a multicenter study, randomization and blinding may be done by the study sponsor in a centralized location and then forwarded to the sites for distribution to subjects.

Adequacy of blinding can be assessed by asking subjects, investigators, outcome evaluators, and data entry personnel which treatment they believe was received.[27,30] A 50% or lower guess rate indicates that blinding was successfully achieved.

TABLE 6–4. TYPES OF BLINDING

Type of Blinding	Definition
Single-blind	Either subjects or investigators are unaware of assignment of subjects to active or control groups
Double-blind	Both subjects and investigators are unaware of assignment of subjects to active or control groups
Triple-blind	Both subjects and investigators are unaware of assignment of subjects to active or control groups; another group involved with interpretation of data is also unaware of subject assignment

Sometimes multiple placebos are necessary to achieve blinding.[29] For example, a study comparing sedation using continuous intravenous infusion of a benzodiazepine versus continuous nasogastric administration would require use of two placebos—a double dummy study. In this situation, half of the patients would receive active intravenous infusion and placebo nasogastric infusion and half would receive placebo intravenous infusion and active nasogastric infusion.

Blinding improves the validity of all studies, but is most important when outcome variables are subjective rather than objective.[29,33] Blinding is difficult, if not impossible in some situations, such as when drug therapy is compared to surgical procedures or when certain drug characteristics (e.g., side effects, physicochemical properties, taste, smell) allow easy detection of active versus control drug. For example, studies involving drugs with anticholinergic actions are challenging because patients and investigators are aware that active drug is being administered when side effects such as dry mouth and constipation develop. If a study cannot be blinded, outside evaluators who are unaware of the treatments received should analyze the data, and the possibility of study bias should be discussed in the study report.[30,33]

Data Collection

Several points need consideration in regard to data collection. Accuracy of measurements taken at study initiation may differ from those obtained toward study conclusion.[14] As investigators become more familiar with study methodologies, data collection techniques may improve. To avoid this problem, careful instruction on study methodology and technology should be given to investigators before commencing a study in order to reduce variability and avoid inconsistent data.[13,14] Validation of data collection forms and instruments must also be undertaken.[13] In addition, reliability of repeated measures should be verified through use of correlation coefficients.[30] Accuracy of computer data entry should also be determined periodically by comparing a portion of patient records to computer printouts.[14]

Compliance

Subject compliance may also influence results and should be evaluated.[30] There are many disadvantages to commonly used methods of compliance monitoring such as pill counts and urine or serum drug concentrations, but more accurate methods such as use of computerized prescription vials often are not feasible because of their expense.[55] Monitoring of compliance is particularly important in studies where subjects receive medications on an outpatient basis and are responsible for self-administration of the study drugs. If study results indicate that a treatment is ineffective, but compliance for the study drug was low, lack of therapeutic benefit may be due to poor compliance of the study subjects rather than lack of efficacy of the drug therapy. Therapies with poor compliance during clinical trials may also be difficult to apply to clinical settings for reasons such as intolerance or inconvenience.

Investigators should also confirm that subjects did not take other prescription or over-the-counter medications and did not receive additional medical care during the course of the study.[13] Such factors may bias study results. Subject and investigator compliance with the study protocol should be addressed by the authors.[13] Information on compliance during clinical trials may help practitioners assess whether individuals in their practice setting will have difficulty complying with the therapy or may discontinue therapy due to adverse effects.[28,33]

Statistical Analyses

Errors in statistical analysis of data are commonly encountered and invalidate study conclusions. Therefore, readers should determine whether appropriate statistical methods were used for data analysis. Several guidelines for the use of statistics in medical journals have been published.[56,57] Chapter 10, Clinical Application of Statistical Analysis, discusses these concepts; however, several points deserve mention at this juncture.

Statistical tests are based on the study design and the type of data represented by outcome variables used for study endpoints.[58] There are four types of data—nominal, ordinal, interval, and ratio (Table 6–5). Nominal data are categorical (e.g., male/female, complete response/partial response/treatment failure). Ordinal data reflect a ranking (e.g., 1+/2+ edema, ⅙ to ⅚ heart murmurs). Interval data have measurable equal distance between data points, but no absolute zero (e.g., temperature in degrees Fahrenheit). Ratio data are similar to interval data except an absolute zero point is present (e.g., serum drug concentrations, temperature in degrees Kelvin).[59] Each type of data builds on the last, with nominal data being the weakest and interval/ratio data the strongest.[58] Categories for nominal data should be specified a priori to avoid data dredging for statistically significant results at the conclusion of the study.[12]

Statistics are either descriptive or inferential.[52] Descriptive statistics, as the name implies, describe the data and include medians, means, modes, and standard devia-

TABLE 6–5. TYPES OF DATA

Type of Data	Definition	Examples
Nominal	Categorical data	Yes/no; male/female; response/no response/partial response
Ordinal	Data reflects ranking	Visual analog scales; Likert scales
Interval	Data with measurable equal distances between points but no absolute zero	Temperature in degrees Fahrenheit
Ratio	Data with measurable equal distances between points and an absolute zero	Temperature in degrees Kelvin; serum drug concentrations

tions.[52] Readers should carefully assess the use of means in studies. Means provide little information if the data are extremely variable.[52] They also are of limited value if the data are ordinal in nature, because performing mathematical calculations on data that cannot be quantified is inappropriate.[58] In such cases, the median or mode should be used.

When variability of data is minimal, results are more reliable. Variability is assessed by examining the standard deviation (SD) of the data—the larger the standard deviation, the greater the variability. Sixty-eight percent of observations measured in a study will fall within 1 standard deviation, 95% within 2 standard deviations, and 99.73% within 3 standard deviations.[58] Many studies erroneously use standard error of the mean (SEM) rather than standard deviation to describe variability of data. Because standard error of the mean is equal to the standard deviation divided by the square root of the sample size, use of this statistic reduces the perceived variability of the data, especially with large sample sizes.[52] Rather than provide information on variability of data in the sample, standard error of the mean should be used as an estimate of the true mean of the population.[58] Ninety-five percent of the time, true mean of the population lies within two standard errors of the sample mean.[33,58]

Inferential statistical tests allow conclusions to be drawn from the data.[52,59] Parametric tests such as the t-test and analysis of variance (ANOVA) are used when distribution of the data is normal and symmetric, whereas nonparametric tests such as chi-square and the Kruskall-Wallis test are used when data do not have a bell-shaped distribution.[59] Parametric tests are generally used for interval or ratio data and nonparametric tests for nominal or ordinal data.[59] When a subject contributes more than one data point to an analysis, statistical tests appropriate for paired samples must be used.[59]

Statistical tests are either one-sided or two-sided (also referred to as one-tailed or two-tailed). A one-sided test is used when the direction of the relationship between outcome variables is known (i.e., the variables can only vary in one direction from their original value). For example, a one-tailed test is appropriate for diseases that are uniformly fatal where any improvement in survival would be considered a beneficial effect of the drug. A two-sided test is used when the direction is unknown. For example, consider a drug being investigated for the treatment of asthma. If it is known the drug will improve pulmonary function tests (PFTs), a one-sided test can be used; however, if the drug may either improve or worsen PFTs, a two-sided test would be used. A two-sided test requires a stronger relationship to achieve statistical significance than a one-sided test and is therefore often considered the preferred method.[14] Whether one-sided or two-sided tests are used for study analyses should be specified a priori.[12]

Readers should determine whether statistical tests used in the study were appropriate. Studies in which statistics were used incorrectly are unreliable and should not be used for making clinical decisions. Charts and guidelines for determining the most appropriate statistical test based on type of data and study design have been published in the literature.[58,60–69] Refer to Chap. 10 for more detailed information on specific statistical applications.

Inferential statistics generate p values.[52] The calculated p value is the probability of obtaining the result observed in the study if the result is entirely due to chance.[70] The data are considered statistically significant when the calculated p value is less than alpha or the level of significance. By convention, the level of significance is usually set at .05, meaning that the results have a less than a 5% probability of having occurred due to chance alone. Absolute values for calculated p values should be presented with the results of a study. For example, if the calculated p value for the study comparing drug A to drug B for the treatment of acute otitis media with effusion is .07 (i.e., a value greater than .05), the results would not be considered statistically significant, but if the p value was .001 (i.e., a value less than .05), the results would be statistically significant.

Although p values indicate whether a treatment has an effect, they do not indicate the magnitude of the effect.[42] Furthermore, statistical significance does not always equal clinical importance. For example, if sample size were large enough, a difference of 2% in bacteriological cures between drug A and drug B for acute otitis media with effusion may be found to be statistically significant, but of little clinical relevance. It is important to realize that the magnitude of the p value does not indicate the degree of clinical significance of the data.[52] A p value of <.05 indicates that there is a 95% chance that additional replications of this study would find the same amount of difference between groups, whereas a p value of <.0005 indicates a 99.95% probability.[52] The p value says nothing about whether the difference between groups would be considered clinically important.[52] For additional information on clinical significance, see "Application of Study Results to Clinical Practice" in a subsequent section.

There are several other points that must be considered when evaluating statistical analyses of studies. Investigators should avoid analyzing the data using multiple statistical tests because this action increases the likelihood of encountering a chance finding (i.e., increases the likelihood of obtaining a false-positive result).[14,70] One outcome variable should be designated as the primary endpoint for the study and one statistical test should be used to analyze this variable.[49] If the chosen statistical test for this primary endpoint does not indicate a statistically significant difference between treatment and control groups, investigators should resist examining multiple subgroups that initially were not designated for analysis in the study protocol.[49] Because an infinite number of factors may have influenced study outcome, the temptation to dredge data when results are not significant is great.[49] For example, suppose that no statistically significant differences are found when drug A is compared to drug B for the treatment of acute otitis media with effusion. In this scenario, the investigators may be tempted to reanalyze the data by dividing patients according to age or infecting organism. For instance, the investigators may decide to conduct further statistical analyses after the study is completed if they believe that statistically significant differences exist between drug A and drug B in patients aged 6 months to 1 year or patients infected with *Streptococcus pneumoniae*. Problems of subgroup analysis include insufficient subjects in the subgroups (i.e., small sample size) to allow differences between groups to be detected and the necessity to use multiple statistical tests to conduct the analyses, thus increasing the likelihood of a chance finding.[49] Subgroup analyses are only useful when the results show an extremely large difference between treatment and control groups that could not have occurred by chance alone, the decision to conduct subgroup analyses was determined before the study was initiated, only a few subgroups were analyzed, and previously conducted studies have shown similar results.[33,71] Otherwise, results of subgroup analyses should only be used for generation of future study ideas and should not be considered as evidence that a drug should be used in a particular patient population.[33,71]

A final consideration with regard to statistical analyses is the use of interim analyses. When interim analyses are performed, the data are examined at one or more points during the investigation before study termination is scheduled.[71,72] Journal articles may present the results of an interim analysis alone, or both the interim and final results for the study. Interim analyses are usually used to monitor the safety and efficacy of drug therapies at periodic intervals throughout the course of a study and help ensure that a study is ethical. Interim analyses may also be used to monitor progress of a study, adjust sample size, assist with dose finding, provide reassurance of drug activity, or aid decisions regarding manufacturing scale-up.[73,74] If interim analyses demonstrate unacceptable hazards or extreme efficacy of an agent before the study is scheduled for completion, the investigators may consider stopping the trial prematurely. Whenever subjects are evaluated for an extended period of time (e.g., months to years) during an investigation, authors should consider planning interim analyses at specified intervals.

The decision to conduct interim analyses, number and timing of interim analyses, parameters that will be assessed, statistical methods to be used, methods for blinding data during interim analyses, and criteria for discontinuing trials should always be determined a priori.[31,73,74] Interim analyses should be conducted by individuals who are not determining subject eligibility, administering treatments, or assessing outcomes.[73] To avoid introducing bias into a study, results of interim analyses should not be shared with individuals directly involved with conduct of the study.[73] Often, data monitoring committees (DMCs) are convened that oversee the scientific and ethical aspects of trials, provide unbiased evaluations of efficacy and safety, monitor the impact of safety and efficacy data from other clinical trials on the ongoing trial, and provide recommendations to the sponsor regarding study amendments or termination.[74]

A problem of interim analyses is that if the data are collected at a "random high," the safety or efficacy results tend to be exaggerated.[49] Because sample size increases as the study progresses, subsequent data analyses often show decreased differences between treatment and control groups and reduced statistical significance from those initially observed.[49] As stated, authors should avoid analyzing data using more than one statistical test; however, interim analyses entail multiple looks at the data and therefore require careful statistical planning including adjustment of p values required for significance.[72–74]

RESULTS

Data

Data should be presented in a clear and understandable format. Investigators who are skilled at writing manuscripts are able to explain even difficult concepts related to their results to the readers.[5] When results are presented in a confusing manner, it most likely reflects haphazard collection of data and lack of clearly defined study objectives rather than a deficiency in knowledge on the part of the reader.[5]

Authors should indicate in the article how original data can be obtained, if desired (e.g., investigator, National Auxiliary Publishing Service*).[31] Confidence intervals and/or p values should be provided for any statistical analyses performed on the data.[75] Efficacy results should be described in sufficient detail for readers to perform their own analyses of the data, if desired.[30,33] Information on adverse effects should include severity of the event, how it was managed, and whether it was believed to be drug related.[33] Variables that may have affected the prognosis in the control and treatment groups should be identified.[27] If conduct of the study deviated from the protocol, reasons for the discrepancy should be provided (i.e., investigator error, patient noncompliance, laboratory error).[31]

Data should be presented as actual numbers, rather than percentage changes alone.[31] Readers can use these numerical data to verify that all patients studied were represented in the calculations, the calculations were accurate, and the statistical analyses performed on the data were appropriate. Data presented in the abstract, charts, figures, and text should be identical and mathematical tabulations for charts and tables should be accurate.[75] Readers should check for errors in these data presentations. Graphs should also be carefully examined by readers. Visual presentation of the data can be varied by scales used for the x- and y-axes.[75] Narrowing the range of scale dramatizes the results, while increasing the range of scale minimizes the results.[75]

---

*National Auxiliary Publishing Service: ASIS/NAPS, c/o Microfiche Publications, PO Box 3513, Grand Central Station, New York, NY 10163-3513.

Authors should avoid artificially inflating data by presenting the number of observations rather than the number of subjects as sample size.[75] Observations for all subjects should be represented and presented in a manner that allows readers to conduct their own analyses, if desired.[52,75] If data for each of the measurements are not available for all subjects, reasons for the discrepancies should be carefully explained.[30]

Clinical trial reports should state the number of subjects screened, enrolled, treated, completing, and failing to complete the trial.[12] Reasons for study drop-outs should also be described.[28] A flowchart comparing flow of participants (e.g., screened, enrolled, dosed, withdrawn, completed) and timing of primary and secondary outcome measures for treatment and control groups is recommended.[27]

The average duration of the trial for each treatment group, and the study initiation and completion dates should be stated.[12] Explanations should be provided for why studies were terminated early (e.g., adverse events, superior clinical efficacy) or late (e.g., poor subject accrual).[12] Readers should take note of when the study was conducted compared to when it was published because several years may elapse between study completion and publication.[46] Justification for the relevance of data to clinical practice at the time of publication should be provided.[12] Data that are too old may no longer be clinically useful because standards of practice may have changed. A survey of 3394 life sciences faculty in 50 universities reported that their research results had been delayed by more than 6 months at least once in the last 3 years.[76] Reasons for these delays included allowing time for patent application or negotiation, protecting scientific leads, slowing dissemination of undesired results, or resolving disputes over ownership of intellectual property. Delays in publication were significantly associated with academic–industry research relationships and engagement in the commercialization of university research.

Two types of data analysis may be performed. Analyses of data from evaluable subjects assesses only subjects who complete the study, whereas an "intention-to-treat" analysis also evaluates data from subjects who die or drop out of the study.[30] Intention-to-treat analyses are important because subjects who fail to complete a trial may differ from those followed to study termination. Often, subjects who fail to complete a study are those with the worst outcomes.[28] Therefore, results of intention-to-treat analyses may differ dramatically from those obtained when only data from evaluable subjects are examined, especially when the drop-out rate is high.[30,50] For these reasons, intention-to-treat analyses are often considered stronger than those using only evaluable subjects and are preferred by the FDA. Intention-to-treat analyses use one of three methods for data manipulation—the subject's last score or measurement at the time of discontinuation, the average score or measurement for the entire group, or the worst score or measurement for the entire group.[28] Authors should specify which method was used in the intention-to-treat analysis.[28]

Type I and Type II Errors

A type I error occurs when the investigators accept the research hypothesis when it is incorrect (e.g., a false-positive result) (Table 6–6).[43] The probability of a type I error is equal to alpha or the level of significance and by convention is usually set at .05. When a statistically significant difference is found between treatment groups at a significance level of .05 (e.g., $p < .05$), there is a 1 in 20 probability that it was a chance finding and does not indicate a true difference between treatment and control groups.[14] For example, consider that the study comparing drug A and drug B in the treatment of acute otitis media with effusion showed that drug A was statistically better than drug B in achieving bacteriological cure at a significance level of .05%. For this study, there is a 95% probability that these results represent a "true" difference between efficacy for drugs A and B and a 5% probability that the results are a chance finding or false-positive result. Type I error is rarely discussed by the investigators, but should be considered by readers. Study results are never 100% accurate; there is always the possibility that the results are a chance finding that would not be replicated if the study were repeated.

On the other hand, type II errors (e.g., a false-negative result) can occur whenever investigators conclude that two treatments are equally efficacious or equally safe (see Table 6–6). Type II errors are usually the result of chance or inadequate sample size. A review of 383 randomized clinical trials having negative results found that sample sizes were large enough to detect a 25% or 50% difference in only 16% and 36% of articles, respectively, and only 32% of articles reported sample size calculations.[77]

The probability of making a type II error is equal to beta. Type II errors are related to the power of a study, which is defined as the ability to detect a difference if a difference actually exists and is calculated as 1-beta.[38] The greater the power of a study or ability to detect a difference, the less likely the possibility of a type II error or false-negative result. By convention, beta is usually set at 10% or 20% and a power of 80% or 90% (i.e., 1-beta) is considered acceptable.

The magnitude of beta and power depend on the amount of difference the treatment causes (it is easier to detect a large difference), the number of events in control

TABLE 6–6. TYPE I AND TYPE II ERRORS

	Reality in Population	
Statistical Results of Study	*No Difference*	*Difference*
Null hypothesis rejected	Type 1 error Probability = alpha False positive	Correct results
Null hypothesis accepted	Correct results	Type II error Probability = beta False negative

subjects (the more occurrences in control subjects, the easier it is to detect a beneficial effect of the drug under investigation on these occurrences), alpha, and sample size.[38]

Consider that the study comparing drug A and drug B for the treatment of acute otitis media with effusion demonstrated that bacteriological cure rates between the two drugs were not statistically significant. If the authors stated in the methodology that beta for the study was .10 or .20 (i.e., an 80% to 90% chance of detecting a difference if a difference actually exists), then a 10% to 20% probability of a false-negative result exists. This is an acceptable risk. However, if the investigators failed to state beta or power of their investigation, it may indicate an attempt to avoid the topic because power of their study was low. Alternately, investigators may not be knowledgeable about the concepts of beta and power. To put the importance of beta and power into perspective, if study power is 50%, flipping a coin to see which treatment is more efficacious would be as likely to produce a true result as conducting the actual clinical trial.

Remember, beta stated in the study reflects the original sample size calculation. If number of evaluable subjects at the conclusion of the study is smaller than the original sample size calculation, beta increases and power decreases.[14] Whenever researchers conclude that treatments are equally efficacious or safe, investigators should discuss the power of their study, including whether the number of subjects completing the study allowed sufficient power for a statistically significant difference to be detected.

If sample size was not determined a priori, a post hoc power calculation can be conducted[77]; however, some experts believe such analyses are inappropriate and recommend use of confidence intervals (see the section on "Application of Study Results to Clinical Practice").[39,42] These experts argue that power calculations ensure an adequately designed study by applying pre-experimental probabilities to hypothetical results. Once data are generated, these probabilities are no longer valid.[39] The situation has been likened to convincing a lottery winner (postexperimental condition) that buying a lottery ticket wastes money (pre-experimental condition).[39,78]

Study Validity

After reviewing a study, readers should consider whether the results are valid. Studies should be analyzed in terms of two types of validity—internal and external. Internal validity refers to the extent to which the study results reflect what actually happened in the study (e.g., Are the results consequent to the drug under investigation or are they the result of another confounding factor?). Such confounding factors can include events that develop between initial and final measurements, changes that occur in subjects during the course of the study, accuracy of instruments and the investigators taking measurements, selection of subjects in a nonrandomized manner, and drop-outs and deaths that occur during the study resulting in elimination of important data points.[79] Reasons for drop-outs and deaths should be carefully explained so readers may ascertain whether loss of these data points influenced study outcome.[30] Patients who drop out of a study because of uncontrollable circumstances such as accidents or personal situations unrelated to the study medication may be less of a concern than patients who drop out because of intolerable side effects related to the study medication. When drop-outs and deaths are not mentioned in a clinical trial or when they exceed 10% in a study lasting 3 months or less or 15% in a study of a duration exceeding 3 months, results may be significantly affected.[46] One method that has been suggested to ascertain whether drop-outs significantly affected study outcome is to assume that all drop-outs would have had a negative outcome to the drug therapy. If conclusions do not change after this maneuver, the probability of drop-outs biasing the study results are minimal, although such methodology may result in the risk of a type II error.[51]

External validity is the degree to which the study results can be applied to patients routinely encountered in clinical practice (e.g., Are the conditions of the study replicable or do factors such as concomitant medication use and presence of additional disease states in study subjects make it impossible to generalize results?).[79] If study conditions are not similar to those routinely encountered in clinical situations, the results may not be applicable to patient care.

CONCLUSIONS/DISCUSSION

The conclusions/discussion section allows authors to provide an interpretation of their data and how it relates to clinical practice. Study conclusions should be consistent with results and related to the initial study question. Results should be compared to a systematic review of all previously published data (see Chap. 7).[80] Both studies that are in agreement with and those whose results conflict with the investigators' results should be discussed.[75] Readers should be alerted to any potential study limitations that may have biased results. Any recommendations for use of a drug in clinical settings should be based on well-conducted research in which benefits of therapy outweigh potential risks, and preferably, where cost-effectiveness of therapy has been demonstrated.[30] Results should only be generalized to patient populations and conditions similar to those of the investigation.[30]

REFERENCES

The references used by authors for support of the study should be briefly scanned. Current literature on the topic from respected biomedical journals should be well represented. Authors should avoid citing only their own research efforts and publications.

ACKNOWLEDGMENTS

Sources of funding and other support (e.g., drug supply) should be acknowledged at the conclusion of the article.[31] Individuals who contributed to the research effort, but do not qualify for authorship, should also be listed.[31] In the case of multicenter trials, investigational sites participating in the study are often listed in this section.

APPLICATION OF STUDY RESULTS TO CLINICAL PRACTICE

Appendix 6–1 reviews questions that should be asked when evaluating clinical research studies. Several authors have also published checklists for assessing clinical studies.[28,81,82]

Recently, there has been a call for structured reporting of randomized controlled trials.[12,27,31] Structured reporting is defined as "providing sufficiently detailed information about the design, conduct, and analysis of the trial for the reader to have confidence that the report is an accurate reflection of what occurred during the various stages of the trial."[12] Proponents of this movement believe structured reporting will provide readers with uniform and standardized information for all randomized controlled trials and assist in determining the usefulness of treatments in clinical practice.[12]

Initially, guidelines were developed independently by two separate groups, the Standards of Reporting Trials (SORT) group[12] and the Asilomar Working Group on Recommendations for Reporting of Clinical Trials in the Biomedical Literature.[31] Later, representatives from both groups met to develop a single set of recommendations, the Consolidated Standards of Reporting Trials (CONSORT) statement.[27] The CONSORT statement provides a checklist of information that should be included in clinical trial reports, recommends use of a diagram to illustrate flow of participates during the study, and proposes using five new subheadings—protocol, assignment and masking in the methods section, and subject flow/follow-up and analysis in the results section.[27] Several journals have adopted the CONSORT guidelines including *Annals of Internal Medicine,* the *British Medical Journal, JAMA,* and *The Lancet.*[54,80]

In addition to published checklists, a stepwise process can also be used to determine the usefulness of an article to clinical practice (Fig. 6–3).[13,33,71] First, read the title and abstract. If they appear interesting and relevant to your clinical practice, continue. Next, scan the figures and tables in the article to determine whether the data are adequately reported, a control group is used, and outcomes are clinically relevant. The results should then be reviewed for adequacy of data reporting (e.g., compliance, adverse events, reasons for study drop-outs) and appropriateness of statistical analyses. If the results are important to clinical practice, the study methods should be critiqued. Determine whether study subjects are similar to patients routinely seen in clinical practice. Readers should also consider whether the requirements for use of a therapeutic

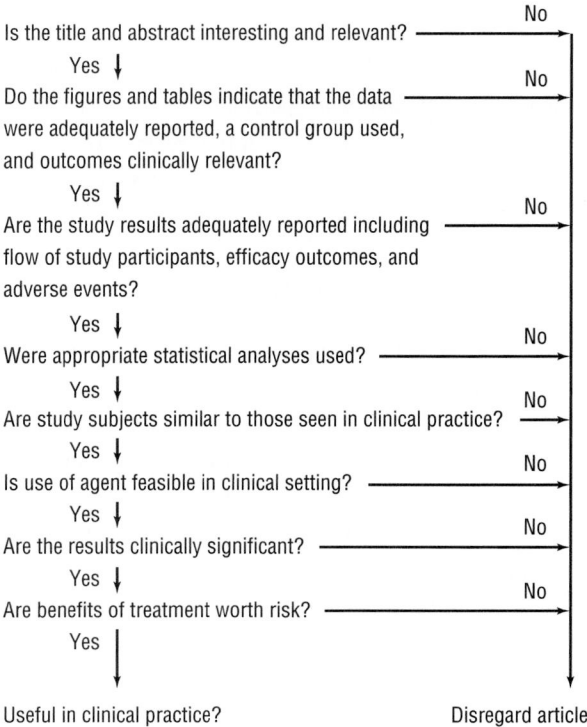

Figure 6–3. Step-wise approach to evaluating the literature.

agent are feasible in their practice settings.[51] For example, certain pharmacotherapeutic agents require close monitoring of laboratory parameters, which may not be possible in all clinical settings. Readers should next ascertain the clinical importance of the study data (e.g., Is the magnitude of the treatment response large enough to be clinically relevant?). Readers should establish whether the benefits of the treatment are worth the associated risks and cost. If the outcome of the above review is positive, the article can be filed for future reference. If time permits, the discussion and introduction can be perused.

Traditionally, health care professionals have relied heavily on the *p* value to determine whether the study results prove or disprove the research hypothesis. However, as stated, statistically significant results (e.g., $p < .05$) mean that there is less than a 5% probability of observing data of the magnitude obtained in the study because of chance alone.[40] Statistically insignificant results (e.g., $p \geq .05$) only demonstrate that the study was inconclusive, but do not prove the null hypothesis.[40] Future studies using more sensitive methods of measurement and/or a greater number of subjects may show a positive effect of the drug therapy.[40] Therefore, tests for statistical significance do not indicate the degree of clinical importance of the study data.[40] Regardless of statistical significance, studies may be either clinically important or clinically irrelevant.[71]

Confidence intervals may assist in making decisions concerning the clinical relevance of study data.[49] Currently, confidence intervals are underreported in the literature of pharmacy and medicine, but have gained more attention in recent years and may soon become the norm, rather than the exception. Confidence intervals represent the variability of the study data and are usually smaller when sample size is large.[71] From 95% confidence intervals, readers are able to determine the range that includes the true value for the population 95% of the time.[71] This concept is illustrated in the example below.

Consider the scenario in which a new antihypertensive agent is studied to determine whether it decreases the rate of myocardial infarction. The results indicate that the antihypertensive decreases myocardial infarction by 11% with a 95% confidence interval of –2% to 25%. This confidence interval indicates that the antihypertensive may actually be of no benefit (e.g., low range of the confidence interval is a negative value) and the study is inconclusive. Confidence intervals are useful regardless of whether the results were determined to be statistically significant or insignificant. If the investigators conclude that the treatment is beneficial because a statistically significant result was found (i.e., $p < .05$), look at the low range of the confidence interval (e.g., –2%). Is this value clinically important? If the investigators conclude that a treatment is not beneficial because results were statistically insignificant (i.e., $p > .05$), look at the upper range of the confidence interval (e.g., 25%). Is this value clinically important? If the low end of the confidence interval in a statistically significant study is not clinically significant, the study results may not be useful for patient care.[71] If the high end of the confidence interval in a statistically insignificant study is clinically important, further studies with the drug therapy may prove that the agent has therapeutic benefit and the results may be considered clinically important.[71]

Another useful parameter for assessing clinical importance of study data is the number needed to treat (NNT). NNT indicates the number of patients who need to be treated for every one patient who will benefit from the therapy and is a measure of clinical significance.[83] NNT is calculated as the reciprocal of the absolute risk reduction as illustrated in the following example.[83,84] Consider again a study designed to determine whether a new antihypertensive agent reduces acute myocardial infarction. Of subjects receiving the new drug, 3% have an acute myocardial infarction, compared to 6% in the placebo group. The absolute risk reduction is 0.06 – 0.03 = 0.03 and the NNT is 1/0.03 or 33. In this scenario, 33 patients would have to be treated for every one acute myocardial infarction prevented. NNT is rarely, if ever, discussed in an article, but may be calculated by readers. Readers must determine if the number represented by the NNT is a reasonable use of resources for the benefit produced.[83] The higher the NNT, the less beneficial the treatment to society in general.

FROM CONCEPT TO PRACTICE

To become proficient in literature evaluation, readers must routinely critique the biomedical literature. Deciding where to begin can be a formidable task. Because the amount of published literature is vast, one can easily become lost in an information jungle. Therefore, it is important to develop a strategy for periodically reviewing the biomedical literature.[85,86] Articles that are pertinent to your practice focus and likely to change standard of practice and/or directly impact patient care are worth investing time for critical analysis and review.[85,86]

Articles can be identified by routinely scanning the tables of contents of journals that publish research relevant to your practice area.[85,86] For a broader scope, *Current Contents,* a weekly journal that lists the tables of contents for over 1250 journals, or *Inpharma,* a newsletter that abstracts significant articles from about 1800 journals, can be browsed.[86] Journals that critique articles for research quality prior to publication, such as *ACP Journal Club,* are useful for identifying well conducted and clinically relevant research.[86] Search strategies for bibliographic databases (e.g., Medline) that identify articles in your focus area can be developed.[86] For a fee, some bibliographic databases and on-line vendors will automatically perform searches using predefined terms and forward citations via e-mail. A commitment to improving literature evaluation skills and keeping abreast of the medical literature can easily be made by allotting time each week to visit the local medical library. Journal clubs, where members share critiques of pertinent articles, are another excellent means for developing literature evaluation skills while benefiting from the expertise of colleagues.[86,87]

CONCLUSION

Literature evaluation is a skill that requires understanding of the basic concepts of research methods and statistics. It is important to remember that flaws can be found in all studies. Readers must ask themselves whether the study flaw could have affected study results to the point that they are invalid. Once the principles of literature evaluation are mastered, the pharmacist is able to make unbiased clinical judgments regarding drug therapy based on results of clinical studies, thereby improving the level of pharmaceutical care. Although thousands of articles are published yearly, only a select few will meet the standards presented in this chapter.

Acknowledgment

The author would like to thank Dr. James Visconti, PhD, Professor of Pharmacy Practice, and Director, Drug Information, University Hospitals and the Arthur G. James Cancer Hospital & Research Institute and College of Pharmacy, The Ohio State University, for his insight and assistance in preparing this chapter. Dr. Visconti was Dr. Mosdell's preceptor during her drug information fellowship at The Ohio State University and taught her most of the concepts presented in this chapter.

Study Questions

1. Provide examples of how literature evaluation skills can be used in the practice of pharmacy.

2. An article is published about the beneficial effects of a new treatment option for the prevention of cerebrovascular accidents. The article is published in a well-respected, peer-reviewed medical journal. The article is later retracted from the journal after it is discovered that the data were fraudulent.
   a. Describe the peer-review process.
   b. Why is it difficult to identify fraudulent data through the peer-review process?
   c. What solutions have been suggested to avoid publication of fraudulent data?

3. During clinical rounds, a pharmacist is asked whether inhaled corticosteroids are effective for the management of chronic obstructive pulmonary disease. The pharmacist conducts a literature search to identify relevant articles on the subject.
   a. The pharmacist locates several articles published in peer-reviewed journals or journal supplements. Case reports and meeting abstracts are also identified. What issues should the pharmacist consider regarding the forum for publication of these data?
   b. The research was conducted by investigators practicing in urban teaching hospitals, community settings, or managed care facilities. How may the training of the investigators or resources at the research site influence the study results?
   c. The research has been funded through various mechanisms including pharmaceutical manufacturers, the American Lung Association, and the National Heart, Lung, and Blood Institute. Can source of funding potentially bias results?
   d. The pharmacist reviews the abstracts for each of the articles identified. What are the components of a structured abstract? Why is it inappropriate to rely entirely on study abstracts when making clinical decisions?

5. An investigator identifies a new therapy for the treatment of osteoarthritis. He plans to conduct a randomized, controlled clinical trial to evaluate the safety and efficacy of this treatment.
   a. Why is it necessary for the investigator to obtain approval of an investigational review board (IRB) before initiation of the study?
   b. The subjects will be required to sign an informed consent before entrance into the study. What is informed consent?
   c. What would be an appropriate objective, research hypothesis, and null hypothesis for this study?
   d. What factors would the investigator consider for determination of sample size?
   e. Which is more appropriate for this study—a parallel or cross-over design?

6. A new antimicrobial, drug A, was compared to standard therapy, drug B, for the treatment of acute otitis media. Patients aged 2 to 5 years who did not receive other antimicrobials within 30 days of study initiation were enrolled into the study. Subjects were recruited from the emergency room population of an urban teaching hospital. The results indicate that drug A was statistically better than drug B in eradication of microorganisms associated with acute otitis media. While working at a managed care facility, a physician asked you whether drug A would be an appropriate therapy for an 18-month-old child with recurrent otitis media who has failed to respond to standard treatments. Based on results of this study, how would you respond?

7. A study is conducted to compare a new antihypertensive agent to standard therapy for prevention of cardiovascular events (e.g., cerebrovascular accidents, myocardial infarction). One hundred patients with stage 1 hypertension (systolic: 140 to 149 mmHg, diastolic: 90 to 99 mmHg) are enrolled in the study. After 1 year, no statistically significant differences ($p = .14$) are observed between the new therapy and standard treatment in rate of cardiovascular events.
   a. Could duration of treatment have influenced results?
   b. Is there a possibility of a type I or type II error? Why?

8. Compare and contrast placebo, active, and historical controls. Under what circumstances would each be used? Why is it important to use controls in clinical trials?

9. Addition of a therapeutic vaccine to highly effective antiretroviral therapy (HEART), a cocktail usually consisting of two reverse transcriptase inhibitors and a protease inhibitor, is evaluated for the treatment of human immunodeficiency virus (HIV) infection. Patients are randomized to receive HEART therapy alone or in combination with the vaccine. The endpoints of the study include $CD4^+$ cell counts and viral

load. Secondary endpoints include Karnofsky performance status (scale from 0 to 100) and quality of life.

a. Are study endpoints appropriate? Why?

b. What methods could be used to randomize patients to study treatments? Differentiate between unrestricted and restricted randomization.

c. Who should be blinded to study treatment and how could blinding of these individuals be accomplished?

d. What type of data are being measured (i.e., nominal, ordinal, interval, or ratio) and what types of statistical analyses would be appropriate for this study?

10. A new agent is compared to placebo for treatment of osteoporosis. Females aged 65 years or older were enrolled in the study. Forty-eight percent of the subjects received estrogen therapy concomitantly during the study. One hundred fifty patients were enrolled and 120 completed the study. The power of the study was 80% and the level of significance was set at .05. At the conclusion of the study, an intent-to-treat analysis was conducted and bone mass was found to be significantly better in the treatment versus the control group ($p = .014$). The primary reason for study withdrawal was intolerable side effects (lower calf pain, dizziness).

a. Why is it important to conduct intent-to-treat analyses?

b. Is there a possibility of a type I or type II error in this study? What is the probability of such an error?

c. Consider potential problems of internal and external validity that may have occurred in this study.

d. The investigators wanted to know whether efficacy differed between those receiving and not receiving concomitant estrogen therapy. A subgroup analysis to investigate this question was conducted. When is it appropriate to conduct subgroup analyses and what problems are associated with subgroup analyses?

11. Two chemotherapeutic regimens, A and B, are compared for the treatment of non-Hodgkins lymphoma. Complete responses are noted in 60% of patients treated with regimen A and 80% with regimen B (difference: 20%, 95% confidence interval, 5% to 35%).

a. Do the confidence intervals indicate that the results are clinically significant?

b. Calculate the NNT for this study? Are the results clinically significant?

12. Two cholesterol-lowering agents are being compared. The endpoint of the study is number of myocardial infarctions and cerebrovascular accidents. The study will be conducted over a 5-year period with interim analyses at 1 and 3 years. What is an interim analysis and what benefit would it play in this study scenario?

13. Outline a plan for keeping up with the medical literature in your clinical practice setting.

REFERENCES

1. Lowe HJ, Barnett GO. Understanding and using the medical subject headings (MeSH) vocabulary to perform literature searches. JAMA 1994;271:1103–8.
2. Slawson DC, Shaughnessy AF, Bennett JH. Becoming a medical information master: feeling good about not knowing everything. J Fam Pract 1994;38:505–13.
3. Glantz SA. Biostatistics: how to detect, correct and prevent errors in the medical literature. Circulation 1980;61:1–7.
4. Thorn MD, Pulliam CC, Symons MJ, Eckel FM. Statistical and research quality of the medical and pharmacy literature. Am J Hosp Pharm 1985;42:1077–82.
5. Bulman JS. A critical approach to the reading of analytical reports. Br Dent J 1988;165:180–2.
6. Relman AS. Publishing biomedical research: roles and responsibilities. Hastings Cent Rep 1990 May/June:23–7.
7. Berk RN. Threats to the quality of peer-reviewed radiology journals: identification of the problem and possible solutions. Am J Radiol 1988;150:19–21.
8. Shapiro MF, Charrow RP. Scientific misconduct in investigational drug trials. N Engl J Med 1985;312:731–6.
9. Budd JM, Sievert M, Schultz TR. Phenomena of retraction. Reasons for retraction and citations to the publications. JAMA 1998;280:296–7.
10. MacDermott RP. Fraudulent research in science: the responsibility of the peer reviewer. Cancer Invest 1991;9:703–5.
11. Sun M. Peer review comes under peer review. Science 1989;244:910–12.
12. The Standards of Reporting Trials Group. A proposal for structured reporting of randomized controlled trials. JAMA 1994;272:1926–31.
13. Weintraub M. How to evaluate reports of clinical trials. P & T 1990 Dec:1463–76.
14. Niemcryk SJ, Kraus TJ, Mallory TH. Empirical considerations in orthopaedic research design and data analysis. Part I: strategies in research design. J Arthroplasty 1990;5:97–103.
15. Doll R. Controlled trials: the 1948 watershed. Br Med J 1998;317:1217–20.
16. Gorman RL, Oderda GM. Publication of presented abstracts at annual scientific meetings: A measure of quality? Vet Hum Toxicol 1990;32:470–2.
17. Bero LA, Galbraith A, Rennie D. The publication of sponsored symposiums in medical journals. N Engl J Med 1992;327:1135–40.
18. Rochon PA, Gurwitz JH, Cheung CM, Hayes JA, Chalmers TC. Evaluating the quality of articles published in journal supplements compared with the quality of those published in the parent journal. JAMA 1994;272:108–13.
19. Rennie D, Bero LA. Throw it away, Sam. The controlled circulation journals. CBE Views 1990;13:31–5.

20. Department of Clinical Epidemiology and Biostatistics, McMaster University Health Sciences Centre. How to read clinical journals: I. Why to read them and how to start reading them critically. CMAJ 1981;124:555–8.

21. International Committee of Medical Journal Editors. Conflict of interest. Ann Intern Med 1993;118:646–7.

22. International Committee of Medical Journal Editors. Uniform requirements for manuscripts submitted to biomedical journals. JAMA 1997;277:927–34.

23. Rennie D, Yank V, Emanuel L. When authorship fails. A proposal to make contributors accountable. JAMA 1997;278:579–85.

24. Yank V, Rennie D. Disclosure of researcher contributions: A study of original research articles in The Lancet. Ann Intern Med 1999;130:661–70.

25. Flanagin A, Carey LA, Fontanarosa PB, Phillips SG, Pace BP, Lundberg GD, et al. Prevalence of articles with honorary authors and ghost authors in peer-reviewed medical journals. JAMA 1998;280:222–4.

26. Haynes RB, Mulrow CD, Huth EJ, Altman DG, Gardner MJ. More informative abstracts revisited. Ann Intern Med 1990;113:69–76.

27. Begg C, Cho M, Eastwood S, Horton R, Moher D, Olkin I, et al. Improving the quality of reporting of randomized controlled trials. The CONSORT statement. JAMA 1996;276:637–9.

28. Basskin L. How to evaluate the validity and usefulness of published randomized clinical trials. Formulary 1997;32:279–86.

29. Cuddy PG, Elenbaas RM, Elenbaas JK. Evaluating the medical literature. Part I: Abstract, introduction, methods. Ann Emerg Med 1983;12:549–55.

30. Reisch JS, Tyson JE, Mize SG. Aid to the evaluation of therapeutic studies. Pediatrics 1989;84:815–27.

31. The Asilomar Working Group on Recommendations for Reporting of Clinical Trials in the Biomedical Literature. Checklist of information for inclusion in reports of clinical trials. Ann Intern Med 1996;124:741–3.

32. Louis TA, Lavori PW, Bailar JC, Polansky M. Crossover and self-controlled designs in clinical research. N Engl J Med 1984;310:24–31.

33. Bigby M, Gadenne AS. Understanding and evaluating clinical trials. J Am Acad Dermatol 1996;34:555–90.

34. Wermeling DP, Selwitz AS. Current issues surrounding women and minorities in drug trials. Ann Pharmacother 1993;27:904–11.

35. CDER. Food and Drug Administration. Guideline for the study and evaluation of gender differences in clinical evaluation of drugs. Washington, D.C.: U.S. Government Printing Office; July 22, 1993.

36. CDER. Food and Drug Administration. Guideline for the format and content of the clinical and statistical section of new drug applications. Washington, D.C.: U.S. Government Printing Office; July, 1988.

37. Young MJ, Bresnitz EA, Strom BL. Sample size nomograms for interpreting negative clinical studies. Ann Intern Med 1983;99:248–51.

38. Detsky AS, Sackett DL. When was a "negative" clinical trial big enough? How many patients you needed depends on what you found. Arch Intern Med 1985;145:709–12.

39. Fayers PM, Machin D. Sample size: how many patients are necessary? Br J Cancer 1995; 72:1–9.

40. Sheehan TJ. The medical literature. Let the reader beware. Arch Intern Med 1980;140:472–4.

41. McLarty JW. How many subjects are required for a study? Clin Pharm 1988;7:694–6.

42. Borenstein M. Hypothesis testing and effect size estimation in clinical trials. Ann Allergy Asthma Immunol 1997;78:5–11.

43. Hogan JW, Peipert JF. Power and sample size. Clin Obstet Gynecol 1998;41:257–66.

44. Singh N, Yu VL, Mieles L, Wagener MM, Miner RC, Gayowski T. High-dose acyclovir compared with short-course preemptive ganciclovir therapy to prevent cytomegalovirus disease in liver transplant recipients. A randomized trial. Ann Intern Med 1994;120:375–81.

45. Turner JA, Deyo RA, Loeser JD, Von Korff M, Fordyce WE. The importance of placebo effects in pain treatment and research. JAMA 1994;271:1609–14.

46. Chalmers TC, Smith H, Blackburn B, Silverman B, Schroeder B, Reitman D, et al. A method for assessing the quality of a randomized control trial. Control Clin Trials 1981;2:31–49.

47. Lyons DJ. Use and abuse of placebo in clinical trials. Drug Info J 1999;33:261–4.

48. Tramer MR, Reynolds DJM, Moore RA, McQuay HJ. When placebo controlled trials are essential and equivalence trials are inadequate. Br Med J 1998;317:875–80.

49. Pocock SJ. Current issues in the design and interpretation of clinical trials. Br Med J 1985;290:39–42.

50. Guyatt GH, Sackett DL, Cook DJ. Users' guides to the medical literature. II. How to use an article about therapy or prevention. A. Are the results of the study valid? JAMA 1993;270:2598–601.

51. Department of Clinical Epidemiology and Biostatistics, McMaster University Health Sciences Centre. How to read clinical journals: V: To distinguish useful from useless or even harmful therapy. CMAJ 1981;124:1156–62.

52. Yancey JM. Ten rules for reading clinical research reports. Am J Surg 1990;159:533–9.

53. Kunz R, Oxman AD. The unpredictability paradox: review of empirical comparisons of randomised and non-randomised clinical trials. Br Med J 1998;317:1185–90.

54. Schulz KF. Randomized controlled trials. Clin Obstet Gynecol 1998;41:245–56.

55. Stichele RV. Measurement of patient compliance and the interpretation of randomized clinical trials. Eur J Clin Pharmacol 1991;41:27–35.

56. Bailar JC, Mosteller F. Guidelines for statistical reporting of articles for medical journals. Amplifications and explanations. Ann Intern Med 1988;108:266–73.

57. Altman DG, Gore SM, Gardner MJ, Pocock SJ. Statistical guidelines for contributors to medical journals. Br Med J 1983;286:1489–93.

58. Elenbaas RM, Elenbaas JK, Cuddy PG. Evaluating the medical literature. Part II: Statistical analysis. Ann Emerg Med 1983;12:610–20.

59. Niemcryk SJ, Kraus TJ, Mallory TH. Empirical considerations in orthopaedic research design and data analysis. II: the application of data analytic techniques. J Arthroplasty 1990;5:105–10.

60. Gaddis ML, Gaddis GM. Introduction to biostatistics: Part 1, Basic concepts. Ann Emerg Med 1990;19:86–9.

61. Gaddis GM, Gaddis ML. Introduction to biostatistics: Part 2, Descriptive statistics. Ann Emerg Med 1990;19:309–15.
62. Gaddis GM, Gaddis ML. Introduction to biostatistics: Part 3, Sensitivity, specificity, predictive value, and hypothesis testing. Ann Emerg Med 1990;19:591–7.
63. Gaddis GM, Gaddis ML. Introduction to biostatistics: Part 4, Statistical inference techniques in hypothesis testing. Ann Emerg Med 1990;19:820–5.
64. Gaddis GM, Gaddis ML. Introduction to biostatistics: Part 5, Statistical inference techniques in hypothesis testing with nonparametric data. Ann Emerg Med 1990;19:1054–9.
65. Gaddis ML, Gaddis GM. Introduction to biostatistics: Part 6, Correlation and regression. Ann Emerg Med 1990;19:1462–8.
66. Guyatt G, Jaeschke R, Heddle N, Cook D, Shannon H, Walter S. Basic statistics for clinicians: 1. Hypothesis testing. CMAJ 1995;152:27–32.
67. Guyatt G, Jaeschke R, Heddle N, Cook D, Shannon H, Walter S. Basic statistics for clinicians: 2. Interpreting study results: Confidence intervals. CMAJ 1995;152:169–73.
68. Jaeschke R, Guyatt G, Shannon H, Walter S, Cook D, Heddle N. Basic statistics for clinicians: 3. Assessing the effects of treatment: Measures of association. CMAJ 1995;152:351–7.
69. Guyatt G, Walter S, Shannon H, Cook D, Jaeschke R, Heddle N. Basic statistics for clinicians: 4. Correlation and regression. CMAJ 1995;152:497–504.
70. Brown GW. P values. Am J Dis Child 1990;144:493–5.
71. Guyatt GH, Sackett DL, Cook DJ. Users' guides to the medical literature. II. How to use an article about therapy or prevention. B. What were the results and will they help me in caring for my patients? JAMA 1994;271:59–63.
72. Lewis RJ. An introduction to the use of interim data analyses in clinical trials. Ann Emerg Med 1993;22:1463–9.
73. Sankoh AJ. Interim analyses: An update of an FDA reviewer's experience and perspective. Drug Information Journal 1999;33:165–76.
74. Facey KM, Lewis JA. The management of interim analyses in drug development. Stat Med 1998;17:1801–9.
75. Elenbaas JK, Cuddy PG, Elenbaas RM. Evaluating the medical literature, Part III: Results and discussion. Ann Emerg Med 1983;12:679–86.
76. Blumenthal D, Campbell EG, Anderson MS, Causino N, Louis KS. Withholding research results in academic life science. Evidence from a national survey of faculty. JAMA 1997;277:1224–8.
77. Moher D, Dulberg CS, Wells GA. Statistical power, sample size, and their reporting in randomized controlled trials. JAMA 1994;272:122–4.
78. Goodman SN, Berlin JA. The use of predicted confidence intervals when planning experiments and the misuse of power when interpreting results. Ann Intern Med 1994;121:200–6.
79. Campbell DT, Stanley JC. Experimental and quasi-experimental designs for research. Chicago: Rand McNally; 1963. pp. 5–6.
80. Clarke M, Chalmers I. Discussion sections in reports of controlled trials published in general medical journals. Islands in search of continents? JAMA 1998;280:280–2.
81. Cho MK, Bero LA. Instruments for assessing the quality of drug studies published in the medical literature. JAMA 1994;272:101–4.

82. Verhagen AP, de Vet HCW, de Bie RA, Kessels AGH, Boers M, Bouter LM, et al. The Delphi list: A criteria list for quality assessment of randomized clinical trials for conducting systematic reviews developed by Delphi consensus. J Clin Epidemiol 1998;51:1235–41.

83. Wiffen PJ, Moore RA. Demonstrating effectiveness—the concept of numbers-needed-to-treat. J Clin Pharm Ther 1996;21:23–7.

84. Cook D, Sackett DL. On the clinically important difference. ACP J Club 1992 September/October:A16–7. Editorial.

85. Shaughnessy AF, Bucci KK, Slawson DC. How to be selective in reading the biomedical literature. Am J Health-Syst Pharm 1995;52:1116–8.

86. Cook DJ, Meade MO, Fink MP. How to keep up with the critical care literature and avoid being buried alive. Crit Care Med 1996;24:1757–68.

87. Linzer M, Brown JT, Frazier LM, DeLong ER, Siegel WC. Impact of a medical journal club on house-staff reading habits, knowledge, and critical appraisal skills. A randomized control trial. JAMA 1988;260:2537–41.

Chapter Seven

Literature Evaluation II: Beyond the Basics

Carrie J. Johnson • Kristen W. Mosdell • Linda R. Young

Objectives

After completing this chapter, the reader will be able to:

- Describe the types of study designs published in the biomedical literature.
- Compare the differences between a case study and an *n*-of-1 trial.
- Discuss the potential utility, important features, and questions to ask when evaluating an *n*-of-1 trial.
- Describe guidelines for the conduct of stability studies.
- State the methods used in bioequivalence trials, criteria for establishing bioequivalence, and potential sources of error in bioequivalence trials.
- Describe situations where cohort, case-control, and cross-sectional study designs are most useful and disadvantages of these designs.
- Define relative risk as it relates to cohort studies and odds ratios as they relate to case-control studies.
- Describe limitations of data provided in case studies.
- Describe types of bias that may enter into the results of a survey and what investigators might do to help control these types of bias.
- Differentiate between a narrative review, systematic review, and meta-analysis.
- Distinguish between a quantitative and a qualitative systematic review, and list key questions to ask when evaluating a systematic review.
- Identify potential sources of error and bias in a meta-analysis.
- Discuss the use and evaluation of practice guidelines.
- Describe potential errors in the interpretation of data from postmarketing adverse event surveillance studies.
- Discuss the use and analysis of programmatic research.

The randomized, controlled clinical trial is often the focus of drug information responses and therapeutic decision making; however, there are situations where other types of research designs are more effective in answering specific questions or are the only data available to answer the questions. For example, only a handful of small controlled trials may be available to address a particular clinical situation. This is apparent in the many small trials of streptokinase, tissue plasminogen activator (tpa), and aspirin in the treatment of stroke. In this case, a meta-analysis may be more effective at answering the question because data from these small trials could be pooled to achieve the statistical power needed to answer the question. As another example, it may not be feasible to study the toxicity of certain agents in controlled clinical trials, and epidemiological research such as case-control or cohort studies must be employed to answer a question. Many types of research studies are published in the biomedical literature, and are discussed in this chapter.

Evaluation of controlled clinical trials (true experiments) was discussed in Chap. 6, Literature Evaluation I: Controlled Clinical Trials. The principles discussed in that chapter also apply to other types of study designs; however, literature evaluation skills unique to these designs must also be mastered to use these studies effectively. The goal of this chapter is to introduce readers to other types of literature frequently encountered and to describe techniques for evaluating this literature beyond what was discussed in the previous chapter. True experiments (*n*-of-1 trials, survey research, stability and bioequivalence studies), observational studies (cohort, case-control, cross-sectional, case studies or case series, survey research, and postmarketing surveillance studies), systematic reviews (qualitative, quantitative, and meta-analyses), and outcomes research (quality of life and pharmacoeconomics) will be addressed. Study design, utility, and evaluation techniques specific to each type of literature are discussed (Table 7–1).

True Experiments

Techniques for evaluating clinical trials, a type of true experiment, were reviewed in Chap. 6. *N*-of-1 trials, analytical research such as stability studies, and pharmacokinetic research such as bioequivalency studies are also classified as true experiments and will be discussed in the following sections. An overview of programmatic research, another type of true experiment important to pharmacy practice, also will be provided in this section. Techniques beyond those described in Chap. 6 are necessary for evaluating these designs and, following an initial description of the purpose of the study design, are described in detail below.

TABLE 7–1. STUDY DESIGNS COMMONLY ENCOUNTERED IN THE BIOMEDICAL LITERATURE

Study Design	Study Purpose
Clinical study (true experiment)	Determine cause and effect relationships
N-of-1 study	Compare effects of drug to control during multiple observation periods in a single patient
Stability study	Evaluate stability of drugs in various preparations (e.g., ophthalmologic, intravenous, topical, oral)
Bioequivalence study	Assess the bioequivalency of two or more products
Programmatic research	Determine impact and/or economic value of services
Follow-up (cohort) study	Determine association between various factors and disease state development
Case-control (trohoc) study	Determine association between disease states and exposure to various risk factors
Cross-sectional study	Identify prevalence of characteristics of diseases in populations
Case study or series	Report observations in a single patient or series of patients
Survey research	Study the incidence, distribution, and relationships of sociological and psychological variables through use of questionnaires applied to various populations
Postmarketing surveillance study	Evaluate use and adverse effects associated with newly approved drug therapies
Narrative review	Nonsystematic, subjective summary of data from multiple studies
Systematic review	Systematic, qualitative, and objective summary of data from multiple studies
Meta-analysis	Combine, statistically evaluate, and summarize data from multiple studies
Outcomes studies (pharmacoeconomic and QOL measures)	Compare outcomes (quality of life) and costs (pharmacoeconomics) of drugs therapies or services

N-OF-1 TRIALS

Randomized, controlled trials are not feasible for many diseases and therapies. Furthermore, if results from controlled trials are available, restrictive inclusion criteria of the trial may make it difficult to apply results from the trial to individual patients routinely encountered in clinical practice.[1] N-of-1 trials are useful when the beneficial effects of a particular treatment in an individual patient are in doubt. It is advantageous if the treatment has a short half-life (allowing multiple cross-over periods without carry-over effects) and is being used for symptomatic relief of a chronic condition.[1,2] An n-of-1 trial can be used to determine whether a drug is effective in an individual patient.[2] Taken as a whole, a group of n-of-1 trials can help to identify characteristics that differentiate responders from nonresponders.[2] Trials of multiple doses can identify the most effective dose and the clinical endpoints most influenced by the drug.[2]

N-of-1 trials attempt to apply the principles of clinical trials such as randomization and blinding to individual patients.[1] An n-of-1 trial can be likened to a cross-over study conducted in a single subject in that a patient receives treatments in pairs (one period of the experimental therapy and one period of either alternative treatment or placebo) in random order.[2] As described below, the study usually consists of several treatment periods that are continued until effectiveness is proven or refuted.[2] Randomization to active drug or placebo and blinding of the physician and patient to the treatment being administered helps to reduce treatment order effects, placebo effects, and observer bias. Desired outcomes are identified prior to initiation of the study to ensure that objective criteria that are meaningful to both the physician and patient are used to assess treatment efficacy.[1]

N-of-1 trials may improve appropriate prescribing of drugs in individual patients. For example, carbamazepine may be an option for relief of pain in a patient with diabetic neuropathy, but definitive information on the efficacy of such treatment is limited. Therefore, the investigators may conduct an n-of-1 trial to determine whether such therapy is useful in this patient. N-of-1 trials are especially useful when long-term treatment with a particular drug may result in toxicity and the physician wishes to determine whether benefits outweigh potential risks.[1]

The effectiveness of n-of-1 trials has been evaluated.[3,4] Of 57 n-of-1 trials completed, 50 (88%) provided a definite clinical or statistical answer to a clinical question leading to the conclusion by the authors that n-of-1 trials were useful and feasible in clinical practice.[3] Of 34 completed n-of-1 trials evaluated over a 2-year period, 17 (50%) were judged to provide definitive results.[4] Overall, physician confidence in the therapy was found to increase or decrease depending on the direction of trial results.[4]

When encountering a published n-of-1 trial, several considerations must be made. General requirements have been recommended for n-of-1 trials.[5] Readers should determine whether the treatment target (or measure of effectiveness) was evaluated during each treatment period.[5] The measure of effectiveness can be a symptom or diagnostic test result, but must be directly relevant to the patient's well-being (e.g., the Visual Analog Scale for pain in the example of carbamazepine). Two other critical characteristics of an n-of-1 study are that there is rapid improvement when effective treatment is begun and that there is rapid regression of this improvement upon discontinuation of treatment.[5]

Cook and associates have identified other questions to ask when evaluating n-of-1 trials.[2] These include: (1) Was the treatment period long enough to include an exacerbation of the condition? (A general rule is that if an event occurs an average of once every x days, then a clinician needs to observe $3x$ days to be 95% confident of observing at least one event.) (2) Can a clinically relevant treatment target be measured? (It is advisable to measure symptoms or the patient's quality of life directly, with patients rating each symptom at least twice during each study period.) (3) Can sensible criteria for stopping the trial be established? (Specification of the number of treatment pairs in advance strengthens the statistical analysis of the results and it has been advised that at

TABLE 7–2. COMPARISON OF *N*-OF-1 TRIALS AND CASE STUDIES

	Case Study	*N*-of-1 Trial
Design	Retrospective (most often)	Prospective
Predefined methods	No	Yes
Clearly defined outcome measures	No	Yes
Randomization	No	Yes
Blinding	No	Yes
Multiple treatment periods	Not usually	Yes

Source: *Adapted from Spilker.[21]*

least two pairs of treatment periods are conducted before unblinding.)[2] Questions to ask when evaluating *n*-of-1 trials are provided in Appendix 7–1.

N-of-1 trials provide more objective information than case reports (as will be described in a later section) (Table 7–2) and are useful for providing definitive information for drug prescribing in individual patients. This is reflected in the fact that publication of such studies has increased in recent years.

STABILITY STUDIES/IN VITRO STUDIES

Stability studies determine the stability of drugs in various preparations (e.g., ophthalmologic, intravenous, topical, oral) under various conditions (e.g., heat, freezing, refrigeration, room temperature). Stability studies are extremely important to the practice of pharmacy. For example, pharmacists who prepare intravenous solutions for use by patients at home often want to know how long a drug admixed in a particular solution is stable or if freezing increases the length of time an admixture is stable in order to determine how many intravenous admixtures may be dispensed at a time. It is also important for pharmacists involved with extemporaneous compounding to know the length of time a particular preparation is stable.

Unfortunately, the quality of stability studies conducted in the past has been poor, which prompted Trissel and Flora[6] to prepare guidelines for stability studies. These guidelines state that investigators conducting stability studies should provide a complete description of study methodology and test conditions. Appropriate, validated assays should be used. Samples should include a baseline "time zero" measurement and an appropriate number of samples to assess stability over the time period. For example, if the goal of the study is to determine the stability of an antibiotic at room temperature then taking measurements at, for example, time zero and 30 days may not be adequate. Planning the study so that testing is done at multiple time points (i.e., time zero, 6 hours, 12 hours, 18 hours, 24 hours, etc.) would yield more information about the degradation timeline of the product. As with all studies, conclusions should be consistent with the results. Questions to ask when evaluating stability studies are provided in Appendix 7–1.

BIOEQUIVALENCE STUDIES

An ever-increasing number of generic products are becoming available in the marketplace and there is a need to establish that the quality, safety, and efficacy of these generic drugs are the same as the brand name product.[7] The health care practitioner is often placed in the position of having to select one from among several apparently equivalent products for individual patients or for use on formularies of health care organizations. The more skilled the health care practitioner is at interpreting the data, the more comfortable he or she will be in selecting the appropriate product for the specific patient or organization.

Bioequivalence trials are often conducted under standardized conditions in a small number of normal, healthy adult volunteers because of availability and lack of confounding factors in this population.[8] Data from healthy volunteers, however, may not reflect the population for whom the medication is prescribed. Single doses of the test and reference drugs are administered and blood or plasma levels of the drug are measured over time. Multidose studies are also conducted on occasion to establish bioequivalence at steady state. A cross-over study design is used so that the subject serves as his own control, thus improving the precision of the results.[9]

Bioequivalent products are products that are equivalent in rate and extent of absorption (by definition, the rate and extent of absorption differ by $-20\%/+25\%$ or less).[8] The area under the blood concentration time curve (AUC), the peak height concentration (C_{max}), and the time of the peak concentration (T_{max}) are the primary phamacokinetic parameters used to assess the rate and extent of drug absorption. Two formulations that differ by $-20\%/+25\%$ or less in rate and extent of absorption are considered bioequivalent. These criteria are based on an arbitrary medical decision that, for most products, a $-20\%/+25\%$ difference in the concentration of the active ingredient in blood will not be clinically significant.[8] Additionally, for approval of a generic product, a manufacturer must show that a 90% confidence interval for the ratio of the mean response of its product compared to that of the innovator product is within the limits of 0.8 to 1.25 (80% to 125%).[8]

When evaluating bioequivalence studies, readers should note whether the acceptable age and weight range for the subjects is defined in the methods and clinical parameters used to characterize a normal, healthy adult (e.g., physical examination observations, hematologic evaluations) are described.[10] Subjects should be free of all drugs, including caffeine, nicotine, and other recreational drugs, for at least 2 weeks prior to testing and usually fast overnight prior to dosing.[10] Subjects are usually nonsmokers and may also have limitations placed on their caffeine intake because both factors may affect blood levels of the product in question. Bioequivalency testing may be performed in the fasting and fed states to assess the impact of food on bioavailability; however, the intake of food should be closely monitored and controlled. Food can impact the rate and absorption of some products. For example, a high-fat meal may affect absorption of highly lipophilic products. Additionally, the methods should define sample collection times, which should be based on the half-life of the drug.[10]

When examining the results of bioequivalence studies, lack of statistical significance does not equate with bioequivalence.[10] The rate and extent of absorption for products must be compared. This is a commonly encountered problem. Tests for statistical significance are generally based on the premise that two products are assumed to be the same until proven otherwise. DiSanto[10] provides the example that "if the data presented are highly variable (wide range of values identified by a large standard deviation), it would be possible to show that there was no statistically significant difference between an AUC of 100 units versus an AUC of 40 units." In this example, the test for statistical significance does not demonstrate that the AUCs are truly similar; it actually shows that the data were too variable from patient to patient to be able to detect a 60 unit (%) difference in areas, even if it existed.[10]

One of the most common errors in the use of bioavailability data is comparing two products based on data obtained from separate studies.[10] Different subject populations, study conditions, and assay methodologies are reasons why comparisons of data from different studies are dangerous and can lead to false conclusions.[10] For example, a formulary committee may locate two generic products that each individually have shown equivalence to the brand product in two separate studies. The false conclusion can be made that both generic products are bioequivalent to each other. As another example, for some products, multiple assays are available for measuring serum levels. Using the same assay, the results for the two drugs may demonstrate equivalence; however, if one assay type is used for the reference drug and another assay type is used for the test drug, the results may not demonstrate equivalence because the sensitivity and specificity of assays may be different.

It is very important, therefore, that a thorough investigation of the methods of the bioequivalence study be made. All subjects should receive the drug under the same conditions, and all blood levels should be taken at the same time. The reader must be assured that confounding factors (e.g., increased weight, increased alcohol intake, initiation of smoking) were minimized between treatment periods (cross-over periods). For example, if a patient started to smoke during the cross-over period, the serum levels of the drug may be affected on the next assay because smoking may alter the pharmacokinetics of the drug.

Current Food and Drug Administration (FDA) regulations require bioequivalence between the generic product and the brand name product be demonstrated, but do not require that bioequivalence among generic copies of the same brand name drug be demonstrated. As a result, it is a concern whether these generic drugs can be used interchangeably. To address this issue, the FDA has developed a revised guideline that is available in draft form (<<http://www.fda.gov/cder/guidance/index.htm>>), which proposes population bioequivalence for drug prescribability (prescription of a drug product to a patient for the first time) and individual bioequivalence for drug switchability (transfer of the patient from one drug to another).[9] This change will better meet the needs of patients and health care practitioners both in initiating therapy (prescribability) and in changing therapy (switchability).

As a guide to health care practitioners in evaluating the bioequivalence of prescription drug products, the scientific and medical evaluations by the FDA are published in the USPDI Volume III. Approved Drug Products and Legal Requirements ("Orange Book") and are also available on the FDA web site at <<http://www.fda.gov/cder/orange/adp.htm>>.[8] A coding system is used for efficient determination of the equivalence status of a particular product (first letter) and to provide additional information based on the FDA's evaluations (second letter). This coding system is described in the initial pages of the USPDI. Products rated A are considered therapeutically equivalent to their pharmaceutical equivalents. Products rated B may have documented bioequivalence problems, or there may be a significant potential for such problems and no adequate studies demonstrating bioequivalence. A rating of B may also indicate that the quality standards are inadequate or the FDA has insufficient data to determine equivalence. For example, multisource products having the same strength, same ingredients, same dosage form, and same route(s) of administration will usually be coded AB if there is a study submitted demonstrating bioequivalence.[8] A product coded BX is one for which the data is not sufficient to determine therapeutic equivalence and the product is assumed to be therapeutically inequivalent.

Bioequivalence studies represent an increasingly important part of the medical literature. When evaluating such trials for application in clinical practice, it is important to focus on the methods of the study. Specifically, the reader must determine if a crossover study design was used, if the assay was validated, and if consistent conditions were maintained to minimize subject variability (i.e., food intake, timing of blood levels, and nicotine use). Questions to ask when evaluating bioequivalence studies are provided in Appendix 7–1.

PROGRAMMATIC RESEARCH

Another type of true experiment important to the practice of pharmacy is research focused on the impact and economic value of programs and services provided by pharmacists in community and institutional settings. Programmatic research is particularly important because limited resources and budget constraints demand that only those services that improve patient care in a cost-effective manner be implemented. The economic value of many widely available pharmacy services, including drug information, CPR team involvement, and discharge patient counseling, has not been adequately studied.[11]

The methodology of studies evaluating pharmacy programs and services should be carefully analyzed.[11] Patients using the program or service should be compared to a control group of patients who do not use the program or service. Alternatively, periods before and after implementation of the program or service may be compared. The program or service under investigation should be clearly defined. Studies may be conducted from various perspectives—patient, provider, third-party payer, society—and, therefore, the focus of the investigation should be specified. Costs, if measured, should include all economic costs related to providing the program or service (see Chap. 8, Pharmacoeconomics). Finally, outcome parameters that are relevant and meaningful should be used to determine effectiveness of the program or service.

Observational Study Designs

True experiments provide the highest level of evidence for establishing cause-and-effect relationships. Under certain circumstances, however, it is impossible or unethical to perform such a trial. For instance, if an agent is particularly toxic and of no therapeutic value, it would be unethical to ask subjects to voluntarily expose themselves to the agent and impossible to recruit patients for such a study.[12] An example of this type of situation is in the evaluation of risk factors for diseases such as cancer. An investigator wishing to evaluate the toxicity of environmental or industrial hazards or the teratogenicity of drugs administered during pregnancy would have to employ epidemiologic research techniques such as follow-up (cohort) or case-control studies to study these problems. These research techniques allow associations rather than cause-and-effect relationships to be determined and are discussed in the following sections. Two other observational research designs, cross-sectional and case studies or case series, will also be discussed.

In evaluating the overall results of any observational study (case-control, cohort, cross-sectional, or case studies), it is important to remember that an association between exposure and outcome does not necessarily prove causation.[13] The reader of such studies must consider other factors not addressed by the investigators that are possibly related to both the exposure and outcome.[13]

FOLLOW-UP (COHORT) STUDIES

In a follow-up study, a group of subjects exposed to the factor of interest are compared to an unexposed group of subjects and followed prospectively. Development of a disease state of interest is observed during the study period.[12] For example, consider the hypothetical situation where drug A has become available for the prevention of myocardial infarction in patients with coronary artery disease; however, there is some concern that drug A actually increases death through proarrythmic effects. A follow-up study could compare subjects exposed to drug A and those not exposed to drug A with the primary endpoint being the incidence of sudden death.

Cohort studies are most useful for examining relatively common diseases with shorter biological intervals for the development of disease.[13] This is because of the cost to maintain follow-up, which is one of the primary disadvantages of cohort studies. For example, performing a cohort study analyzing the effect of increased fiber on cholesterol levels would be less costly than looking for the development of colon cancer in the sample population.

When evaluating cohort studies, the research question must be stated clearly and unambiguously with relevant inclusion and exclusion criteria described in detail.[14] It is imperative that exposed and unexposed individuals be similar in terms of demographic characteristics so that susceptibility to the disease state is equal except for the presence of the risk factor under investigation.[15] This is best achieved if subjects are randomized to exposure or nonexposure; however, in the case of questions of toxicity, randomization is not feasible.[15] Selection bias can occur if exposed and unexposed subjects do not have an equal chance of developing the outcome due to differential exposure to an important causative agent.[14] For example, if a trial was assessing the impact of asbestos exposure on lung cancer and more patients in the nonexposed group were smokers, then there is selection bias. Bias can also occur if the outcome is not similarly assessed in both the exposed and unexposed groups.[13] Furthermore, information bias can occur if the same efforts to measure outcomes are not made for both groups.[14] Bias may further be introduced if there are different follow-up rates for the two groups. In this case, the outcome incidences would reflect follow-up rates rather than exposure to the risk factor.[14] To accurately assess the results of a cohort study, the reader must thoroughly examine the methods of the study for evidence of any of these types of bias.

Attributable risk and/or relative risk is calculated from the data and provides information about the incidence of outcomes.[12] For example, consider the hypothetical situation presented in Table 7–3 in which the effects of industrial formaldehyde exposure on the development of chronic respiratory illness (i.e., chronic obstructive pulmonary disease and emphysema) were assessed. Risk for the development of respiratory illness is 200/2000 or 0.10 for those exposed to formaldehyde and 30/2000 or 0.01 for unexposed subjects. Attributable risk is the difference of these two values or (0.10 – 0.01) or 0.09, which translates to 90 per 1000 exposures. Relative risk is equal to the ratio of these two numbers (0.10/0.01) or 10. In this case, risk of respiratory illness is 10 times greater in individuals exposed to formaldehyde. If relative risk is equal to 1, the risk is the same

TABLE 7–3. EFFECT OF INDUSTRIAL FORMALDEHYDE EXPOSURE ON THE DEVELOPMENT OF RESPIRATORY ILLNESS—FOLLOW-UP STUDY

Risk Factor	Respiratory Illness	No Respiratory Illness	Total
Formaldehyde exposure	200	1800	2000
No industrial exposure to formaldehyde	30	1970	2000
Total	230	3770	4000

for both exposed and unexposed subjects and if it is less than 1, the risk is less for individuals exposed to the factor.[12,15] Attributable risk can also be used to demonstrate a protective effect (e.g., folic acid has been shown to decrease the risk of colon cancer).

It is important to remember that relative risk gives an idea of the size of the effect, but does not provide information about precision or statistical significance of the result.[14] Calculation of 95% confidence intervals are necessary for evaluation of the statistical significance of the results. Because a relative risk of 1 indicates no difference between groups, if the confidence interval includes 1, the results are not statistically significant. The wider the confidence interval, the less precise the result. In the situation described above, the relative risk is 10. If the 95% confidence interval is 7 to 14, then the risk of formaldehyde contributing to respiratory illness is at least 7 times and up to 14 times greater in individuals exposed to formaldehyde. The confidence interval provides an idea of the clinical significance of the results by providing a range of results in which the true value for the population lies.

One of the primary disadvantages of cohort studies is the cost of follow-up. For example, if the outcome is rare, it takes many years for adequate assessment of disease development or to establish disease-free status.[13] Studies where loss to follow-up exceeds 20% in either the exposed or nonexposed cohort should be interpreted with caution.[13] For these reasons, alternate designs such as case-control studies are often undertaken. Questions to ask when evaluating cohort studies are provided in Appendix 7–1.

CASE-CONTROL STUDIES

Case-control studies are a type of observational study that offer an epidemiologic research alternative to cohort studies, which require a large number of participants, and are often expensive and time-consuming.[12] In a case-control study, participants (i.e., cases) with a particular characteristic (e.g., disease) are compared to a similar group of participants without the characteristic (i.e., controls) to determine risk factors associated with development of the characteristic.[12,16,17] Those factors that occur more frequently in cases than controls may be associated with development of the characteristic.

For our hypothetical product, drug A, a case-control study design would be useful in determining if more deaths from arrhythmia occurred in groups treated with drug A than those who did not receive this agent.

Case-control studies are commonly conducted because they are relatively inexpensive and simple to perform. Case-control studies are more useful than follow-up studies when diseases occur infrequently or many years after exposure.[16] This type of study design is considered the most efficient design for studying rare diseases.[13] Because case-control studies are conducted in the opposite direction of randomized clinical trials and follow-up studies, and are designed to determine cause rather than effect, they are sometimes called "trohoc" studies (i.e., "cohort" spelled backward).[16] Figure 7–1 compares the design of case-control studies to that of follow-up studies.

Readers should understand that there are several limitations inherent to case-control studies, most of which are due to their retrospective design.[17] A prominent disadvantage of the case-control study design is that information about the exposure and outcome are collected simultaneously, so it is difficult to sort out the temporal relationship of the two.[14] Predisposition to disease should be similar in both cases and controls, except for exposure to the risk factor under investigation.[17,18] Many different factors or the interaction of many different factors may influence development of disease. It is extremely difficult to ensure that both cases and controls have equal exposure to all factors, other than the variable under investigation, which may contribute to disease.

Furthermore, it is often difficult to determine if the exposure preceded the outcome, a situation termed protopathic bias, where the disease may lead to exposure to the risk factor rather than vice versa.[14,18] For example, abnormal vaginal bleeding may be an early sign of uterine cancer. Vaginal bleeding, however, may lead to prescribing of hormonal therapies such as progesterone. An investigator may later erroneously conclude that use of progesterone was associated with development of uterine cancer when in fact the cancer preceded use of progesterone.[18]

Matching is often used to ensure that cases and controls are similar. With matching, each case has a control that is comparable in terms of demographic and exposure characteristics. It is often difficult to determine which variables should be used for matching cases to controls (e.g., sex, age, date of admission, etc.) and such matching allows assessment of only the risk factor under investigation and no other variables that may have contributed to disease.[16,17,19] Matching, however, may have a negative impact on the interpretation of study results if cases and controls are matched on a factor that is itself related to exposure.[13]

Some experts have suggested use of several control groups selected on the basis of different criteria in an attempt to reduce some of the biases discussed.[16] If results of comparing the cases to the various control groups are in agreement, bias in the control

Follow-Up Study (Cohort)

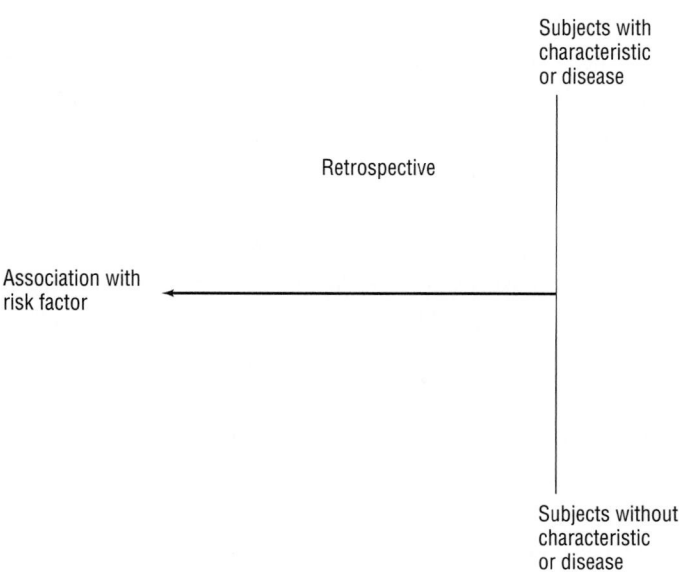

Subjects exposed to
risk factor

Prospective

Development of disease
or characteristic

Subjects unexposed to
risk factor

Case-Control Study

Subjects with
characteristic
or disease

Retrospective

Association with
risk factor

Subjects without
characteristic
or disease

Figure 7–1. Follow-up and case-control study questions.

groups is unlikely to be present.[16] Overall, due to the retrospective nature of case-control studies, the two major methodological issues include the appropriate selection of the control group and the accurate determination of the level of exposure.[14]

Exposure of study subjects to the risk factor should reflect what occurs in the general population. If subjects with higher or lower rates of exposure to the risk factor are excluded from the study, determination of possible associations between the exposure and a particular disease may be biased and inaccurate.[16,18] Case-control studies often use subjects drawn from hospitalized populations, whose exposure to the risk factor may differ from individuals in the community, a problem termed "Berkson's bias."[16]

Cases and controls should undergo the same criteria for evaluation, because presence of disease is more likely to be found in individuals who undergo extensive diagnostic testing.[18] Diagnostic tests used to determine the presence or absence of the disease under investigation (e.g., endoscopy for ulcer disease) should be performed in both the cases and controls. In addition, individuals performing the tests should be blinded to the presence or absence of the risk factor to eliminate "diagnostic-review bias."[16,18] A problem is that many diagnostic tests can only be performed in individuals suspected of having a particular disease state due to the considerable risks associated with their use.

Also of note is that historical data used in case-control studies may be inaccurate or incomplete.[16,17] When patients are interviewed regarding historical events, anamnestic equivalence may not be ensured.[18] For example, patients with the disease state may be more likely to recall events preceding development of the disease than patients who are healthy, because patients with disease are more likely to have contemplated factors that may have contributed to disease development (recall bias). There should be some explanation in the study addressing the issue of recall bias. Investigators who collect data also may question individuals exposed to the disease more intensely than control subjects. To reduce variation in data obtained for cases and controls, data collectors should be blinded to the status of the participants as cases or controls.[16]

During case-control studies, odds ratios are calculated. Consider the situation presented in Table 7–4 where industrial exposure to formaldehyde in patients with and without respiratory illness is assessed. Odds of exposure to formaldehyde is 20/180 or 0.11 in the cases with respiratory illness and 2/197 or 0.01 in the controls and the odds ratio is calculated as 0.11/0.01 or 11, which approximates the risk ratio determined in the follow-up study example. Odds ratio is an estimate of risk ratio.[12] The interpretation is the same: greater than one, increased risk; equal to one, no effect; less than one, protective effect. As with cohort studies, 95% confidence intervals should be calculated.[15] Questions to ask when evaluating case-control studies are provided in Appendix 7–1.

CROSS-SECTIONAL STUDIES

Cross-sectional or "prevalence" studies can be thought of as a "snapshot" because data are collected and evaluated at a single point in time.[14,20] Cross-sectional studies are most ideally suited for generating, as opposed to testing, hypotheses.[14] Typical examples of cross-sectional studies are surveys that evaluate opinions or situations at a fixed point in time and studies focused on description, diagnosis, and mechanisms of disease states.[20] For our hypothetical situation concerning drug A, a cross-sectional study design could be developed to look into a large insurance database and determine how many people died suddenly within 5 years of receiving drug A. Cross-sectional studies are relatively quick and easy to perform and may be useful for measuring current health status or setting priorities for disease control.[14]

A study is classified as cross-sectional because measurements are taken at a single point in time, even though the observations may cover a period of several months or years.[20] For example, a survey of drug abusers is cross-sectional when the questionnaire is administered once; however, the questions contained in the survey may focus on drug habits over the past 10 years.

As in other observational trial designs, the research question and the relevant inclusion and exclusion criteria must be clearly and unambiguously stated.[14] Also, selection of cases must be clearly described because the starting point for the study is the disease status of the patient.[13]

Problems that may occur during cross-sectional studies include errors in data collection and transient effects that may influence observations.[20] Because measurements occur at only one point in time, inaccuracies in data collection may go unnoticed because there is no prior data for comparison. In studies where multiple observations occur, outlier data, which may represent data collection errors, are more easily recognized. Transient effects are temporary occurrences that are found at the time the cross-sectional study is conducted, but would not be identified if the study were repeated. A good example of transient effects are student evaluations of university professors. If a professor chooses to have students evaluate a course after a particularly grueling exam-

TABLE 7–4. INDUSTRIAL FORMALDEHYDE EXPOSURE IN PATIENTS WITH RESPIRATORY ILLNESS—CASE-CONTROL STUDY

Risk Factor	Respiratory Illness	No Respiratory Illness	Total
Formaldehyde exposure	20	2	22
No industrial exposure to formaldehyde	180	195	375
Total	200	197	397

ination, chances are the evaluations would be poor based on students' response to the examination just taken. However, if the evaluations were administered after a curve had been applied for final grades, students may reflect on the course positively based on overall knowledge they received from the instructor, rather than a single negative experience. Transient effects are difficult to identify by the evaluator of the study. They may only be uncovered through retrospective evaluation of the study by the investigator. The investigator must perform a thorough assessment of all factors that may have impacted the results of the trial. Questions to ask when evaluating cross-sectional studies are provided in Appendix 7–1.

CASE STUDIES AND CASE SERIES

In contrast to *n*-of-1 trials, a case study (a type of observational study) does not apply principles of clinical trials such as randomization and blinding to individual patients and simply reports on the clinical course of a particular patient. The case study is usually retrospective and does not involve multiple treatment periods, whereas an *n*-of-1 trial is prospective and includes multiple treatment periods. Comparisons of single patient clinical trials (*n*-of-1) and case-studies are presented in Table 7–2.[21]

In a case study or case series, observations related to a drug or technology being applied to a single patient or group of patients are described.[22] The results are either not compared to a control group or may be compared to a group of previously treated patients (historical controls).

The interpretation of case studies can be difficult.[23] The design of and methods for conducting a case study are not well defined or agreed upon.[23] For example, beneficial effects attributed to the drug or treatment under investigation may actually be a function of spontaneous regression of the signs and symptoms of the disease, a placebo effect, and/or physicians' attitudes that may influence patient outcome.[22]

Case studies, however, are an integral part of the biomedical literature. They have played an important role in identifying treatments for rare disorders where large subject pools cannot be identified.[23] Case studies or case series may also be useful for early recognition of drug toxicities and teratogenicity.[20] When possible, results should be confirmed with randomized clinical trials. Case studies and case series serve as an important initial step in the formulation of hypotheses.[22] Only when case studies or case series show a beneficial effect of a drug or treatment in diseases whose outcomes are consistently grim or when all other treatments have failed can the results be applied to patients in clinical practice.[20,22] Questions to ask when evaluating case studies or case series are provided in Appendix 7–1.

Survey Research

Survey research is used to study the incidence, distribution, and relationships of sociological and psychological variables.[24] This type of research gathers information from a sample to generalize findings to a larger, "target" population.[25] Data obtained from survey re-search have been used for many purposes, including helping investigators to identify, assess, and compare respondents' ideas, feelings, plans, beliefs, and demographics.[25] In pharmacy, surveys may be used to determine how programs should be implemented by utilizing the opinions of experts with experience in a particular area, to study the effectiveness of a program by questioning individuals who have used its services, or to understand the attitudes and behaviors of patients or members of the profession. For example, directors of pharmacy may survey other hospitals to determine salary ranges to decide whether salary increases are needed to remain competitive in the job market. The ability to critically evaluate such literature has become a necessity for the practicing pharmacist due to an increased emphasis on this type of research in the medical literature.[25]

There are two basic types of surveys published in the biomedical literature. Descriptive surveys attempt to identify psychosocial variables such as attitudes, opinions, knowledge, and behaviors in a population, while explanatory surveys attempt to explain causal relationships between variables.[26] These dependent variables such as knowledge and behavior are often compared to independent variables such as age, sex, or education.[27]

Several types of data are collected in survey research and include incidence, attitudinal, knowledge, and behavior measurements. Incidence data try to determine the occurrence of events without drawing any relationships between variables.[27] An example of incidence data is the morbidity or mortality data reported weekly in the Centers for Disease Control's *Morbidity and Mortality Weekly Report* (<<http://www2.cdc.gov/mmwr>>). Manpower data are also incidence data frequently reported in pharmacy literature.[27] The number of residency-trained specialists in drug information centers is an example of data that might be collected in a nationwide manpower survey. Attitudinal data such as job satisfaction surveys often try to compare this dependent variable with independent variables such as age, education, or salary. Knowledge data attempt to document a person's knowledge or level of understanding about a specific topic. Examples include surveys asking physicians' knowledge of retail prices of medications or pharmacists' knowledge of state pharmacy laws.[27] Behavior data document what a person actually does in a particular situation rather than what he or she says he does on a mail survey. Observing the number of specific points that a pharmacist addresses during patient education sessions is an example of behavior data.[27]

Data collection for surveys may involve questionnaires, examination of historical records, telephone interviews, face-to-face interviews, or panel interviews.[28] Well-conducted surveys have several important characteristics—they are objective and carefully planned, data are quantifiable, and subjects surveyed are representative of the target population.[28] In evaluating survey research, just like any other research, one must ask if the results are reliable and valid and if they can be generalized.[25]

Four sources of error have been described that can threaten the precision and accuracy (i.e., reliability) of mail survey results and must be evaluated by readers.[25] The first type of error, coverage error (sampling bias), occurs when there is a discrepancy between the target population and the population from which the sample was derived.[25] This type of error can compromise the ability to generalize the results of the study.[25] For example, people without telephones or unlisted numbers would be excluded from a sample frame of names from a telephone directory.

Sampling error (or random error) occurs when the researcher surveys only a subset (sample) of all possible subjects within the population of interest.[25] The use of random sampling procedures and larger sample sizes can be used to minimize sampling error. Sampling error is a statistical term that describes the rate of random error in sample selection. It describes the variation around the true value of the population mean seen when multiple samples are pulled from the same population.[29] Sample error is reported usually as the mean ± 1 standard error from the mean.

Measurement error (response bias) occurs when the collection of data is influenced by the interviewer or when the survey item itself is unclear from the respondent's point of view.[25] When measurement error occurs, a subjects' response cannot be compared to other responses.[25] The survey method used to collect the data may be one source of measurement error.[25] Face-to-face interviewers may influence the responses of the person being surveyed.[25] The survey instrument itself may be ambiguous and open to interpretation.[25] Bias can be introduced into a survey by the cover letter or sponsoring body; either may lead the respondent to one desired response rather than measuring the true response.[25] A fourth type of measurement error occurs when a respondent replies with a preferred or more socially acceptable answer rather than the real answer. A well-designed survey takes into account the abilities and motivation of the respondent to respond correctly (i.e., written at the appropriate educational level). To increase the reliability and minimize the impact of measurement errors, parallel forms (usually consisting of alternatively worded items placed throughout the survey) can be used. Correlation coefficients between the parallel items or survey instruments must be calculated in order to compare responses.[25]

It may be difficult to assess measurement because, oftentimes, the original questionnaire used as the survey instrument is not published.

The fourth source of error described by Harrison and Draugalis is nonresponse error (nonresponse bias), which occurs when "a significant number of subjects in the sample do not respond to the survey and when responders differ from nonresponders in a way that influences, or could influence, the results."[25] Generally, researchers strive for response rates in the 80% to 90% range so that nonresponders will not alter the author's conclusions.[27] Other authors argue that response rates of 80% for face-to-face interviews, 70% for telephone interviews, and 50% for mailed questionnaires are acceptable.[26] Additionally, evaluating the responses of early versus late responders presumes that the late responders are more like the nonresponders, which may not hold true.

To accurately assess the survey's validity (robustness) and evaluate these potential sources of error and bias, the methods section, which must be explicit, should be heavily scrutinized. Foremost, a description of study methodology with enough detail to replicate the study should be provided. Additionally, the methods section should relate each type of error associated with survey research and state how the investigators attempted to control for those errors.[29]

Attempts to assess validity of the survey and efforts made to validate factual data should be described. For example, demographics of individual hospitals can be verified through the use of American Hospital Association data. Additionally, asking more than one question, through the use of parallel forms as described above, about a concept can increase the internal validity of a survey.[25] For example, a respondent who answers yes to a positively worded statement would be expected to answer no to the same concept when worded in a negative fashion. A coefficient alpha that measures correlation between items should be calculated and reported in the article if this technique is used.[25] The coefficient alpha is interpreted in the same fashion that coefficients of reliability are interpreted; that is, 0 indicates no consistency between responses and 1 indicates complete consistency.

The methods section should report the sample size, along with a description of how it was determined. The validity of both survey research and clinical trials relies on sample size. To have sufficient statistical power to demonstrate a difference between two groups, studies must have an adequate sample size. In designing survey research, the population of interest is first determined then subdivided into smaller groups around a variable of interest. For example, the population of interest may be all patients who attend a pharmacist-managed asthma clinic. This population could be subdivided into smaller groups based on the severity of their asthma and then surveyed as to their level of customer satisfaction. In establishing the sample size for survey research, investigators must then determine the minimum number of subjects that must be sampled for the sample to be representative of the entire population.[29] This determination is made by consulting references that describe variability in sampling.[29]

Additionally, the reader should evaluate the comprehensiveness, probability of selection, and efficiency of the sample frame. A sample is comprehensive if all members of the population had a chance to be chosen and no one was systematically excluded.[29] Determining the efficiency of a sample relates to how well the sample frame excluded individuals who are not the subject of the survey. For example, to survey elderly people, it is appropriate to survey all households to determine if elderly individuals live there.[29] In addition to providing information about the sampling frame, the methods section should provide a description of the interviewers (age, sex, ethnicity, etc.) and the effect that interviewers may have had on the data.

Sampling strategy and response rates should also be stated. The methods section should supply the reader with enough information to assure that nonresponse error was assessed and measures were taken to control it.[25] Higher response rates resulting in more accurate results can be attained through repeated attempts at follow up with initial nonrespondents.[36] For example, phone surveys should be attempted at varying times of the day and a second reminder postcard should be sent for mailed surveys. Additionally, one way to minimize the problem of poor response rates is to sample (by phone) a small group of nonresponders to determine if their responses differ substantially from responders, although this may not be possible.[28] If the results do not differ, the survey remains valid. Furthermore, the authors should relate as much information about the nonrespondents as is possible. Although survey result information has not been gathered, the authors may have demographic and geographic data based on addresses and other information originally obtained.

The methods section should also describe techniques used to assess the reliability (i.e., can the results of the survey be repeated by another investigator) of the survey instrument and present the results of reliability estimates.[25] In general, the higher the reliability estimate, the more confidence the reader may place in the results published.[25] Chapter 10, Clinical Application of Statistical Analysis, provides a more complete review of reliability coefficients. Additionally, any relevant elements of the survey research administration process (i.e., whether a pretest or pilot test was used) should be described. A pretest or pilot test is "an assessment of a questionnaire made before full-scale implementation to identify and correct problems such as faulty questions, flawed response options, or interviewer training deficiencies."[30] Subjects administered the pretest not only answer the survey questions, but also answer questions about the clarity, length, and ease of understanding of the actual instrument and may contribute other questions they think should be included.[26]

Of note, informed consent is generally not required in survey research because the risk is minimal and the respondent has the opportunity to withdraw from participating every time a new question is asked.[29] If the respondent does withdraw part way through the survey or interview, the data should not be included in the final analysis. In situations where sensitive information might potentially harm the subject, asking for an informed consent document to be signed allows the researchers the opportunity to reassure their commitment to confidentiality and reinforce the limits of how the data can be used.

Surveys are a commonly used research tool and are capable of providing a wealth of information on many aspects of a given target population. Ensuring the validity of information gained through survey research, however, relies on critical evaluation of the results through a thorough assessment of the study's methods.[25] A guide for the critique of mail survey research has been published[25] and questions to ask when evaluating survey research are available in Appendix 7–1.

Postmarketing Surveillance Studies

Prior to approval by the FDA, drugs undergo testing in a limited number of patients. Once approved, experience in patients escalates and previously unrecognized, rare adverse events may be identified. The drug also may be found to be useful for conditions not described in the product labeling.

Postmarketing surveillance studies are phase IV studies that follow drug use after market approval and are sometimes referred to as pharmacoepidemiologic studies. They are useful in identifying new, potentially serious effects of drugs. Several drugs have been discontinued from the market after approval following identification of such problems (e.g., flosequinan, felbamate, zomepirac). Postmarketing surveillance studies also allow assessment of drug use outside of product labeling and may identify areas for further research.

Many types of study designs are used in phase IV studies including cross-sectional, case-control, cohort, and even experimental designs (randomized controlled clinical trials). These studies can answer questions about drug interactions, identify potential new indications for the product, and gather information about the consequences of overdose and efficacy in a larger and broader population (patients with different disease states and demographics that may not have been fully evaluated in the original clinical trials).[31] The principles of literature evaluation described in previous sections are also applicable to these studies.

Perhaps one of the most important functions of postmarketing surveillance is in the area of adverse event reporting. Currently, most of the information on postmarketing safety of the product comes from spontaneous adverse reaction reports. Reporting of events associated with a product by the health care practitioner to a regulatory agency or the pharmaceutical company that markets the product are the primary means for gathering this information. Each pharmaceutical company is required to maintain a database of these spontaneous reports. This database is monitored for increases in frequency of certain events or the appearance of serious unexpected events. If it is determined that there is a causal relationship between the drug and the event, the product labeling may be changed to reflect either new events or events with increasing frequency.

There are several limitations to this type of data collection. The information is taken from the reporter who must make a diagnosis and assessment of causality, data may be underreported because it is a voluntary system and this may bias the estimation of incidence, reports may vary in quality and thoroughness, and the database may not be suitable for detecting adverse reactions with high background rates in the population.[31] See Chap. 16, Adverse Drug Reactions and Medication Misadventures, for additional information. Questions to ask when evaluating postmarketing surveillance studies are provided in Appendix 7–1.

Overviews

Review articles that discuss treatment of disease states or clinical aspects of drug therapy are considered tertiary literature (although they can be used like secondary sources because they will lead the reader to primary literature references). Review articles consist of an analysis and interpretation of previously conducted research studies. Review articles enable pharmacists to gain insight into a topic or question of interest and may provide more current information than textbooks; however, they may be subject to the biases of the authors and inaccuracies in the literature search.[32] Standard (narrative) reviews of the literature, which do not apply systematic methods and answer broad rather than focused clinical questions, have largely been replaced by systematic reviews (including meta-analyses). Because of their increased visibility in the medical literature, it is important to be able to distinguish attributes of meta-analyses compared to qualitative systematic reviews of the literature. It is of parallel importance for the practitioner to be able to evaluate both primary and tertiary literature. For this reason, this section comparing narrative (nonsystematic) reviews and qualitative and quantitative (meta-analyses) systematic reviews follows.

Overviews are becoming more prevalent in the literature and are being relied on as an efficient method for keeping up with the large amount of information presented to the health care professional each day. The term "overview" encompasses three very different entities—the nonsystematic (narrative) review, the systematic review (qualitative review), and the meta-analysis (quantitative review).

Table 7–5 compares the characteristics of nonsystematic reviews, systematic (qualitative) reviews, and meta-analyses.

It is important to note that it is not uncommon to find that the conclusions of general overviews, systematic reviews, or meta-analyses conflict with one another.[33,34] Differences in research methodology may explain conflicting conclusions noted in selected published studies. Other explanations for discordant conclusions include differences in study populations, type of intervention, or study endpoint, as well as chance.[34] The purpose of review articles is to determine the "truth" among conflicting and variable primary literature; however, this may not be accomplished or may conflict with results from other reviews and readers need to determine whether studies included in the review apply to their situation.

NONSYSTEMATIC REVIEWS

A narrative review (or nonsystematic review) is a summary of research that lacks a description of systematic methods. Narrative reviews are generally considered tertiary (general) literature because they provide much the same information as found in textbooks, but are sometimes used like secondary references because they also contain

TABLE 7–5. COMPARISON OF NONSYSTEMATIC REVIEWS, QUALITATIVE SYSTEMATIC REVIEWS, AND QUANTITATIVE SYSTEMATIC REVIEWS (META-ANALYSES)

Characteristic	Nonsystematic Review	Qualitative Systematic Review	Quantitative Systematic Review
Clinical question	Generally described	Specifically defined	Clearly defined and focused
Literature search	Methods of literature search usually not explicitly described	Explicit description of pre-defined and comprehensive search strategy	Explicit description of pre-defined and comprehensive search strategy
Studies included	Rarely described	Predefined inclusion and exclusion criteria	Predefined inclusion and exclusion criteria
Includes unpublished literature	Not usually	Possibly	Possibly
Blinding of reviewers	No	Yes	Yes
Analysis of data	Subjective	Objective	Objective
Results statistically evaluated	No	No	Yes

Source: Adapted from Cook, Mulrow, and Haynes.[37]

extensive bibliographies. Narrative reviews may pertain to clinical information or to topics related to pharmacy administration (e.g., Pharmacy and Therapeutics Committees). Techniques can be applied to evaluate the quality of narrative reviews (Appendix 7–1). Such skills are necessary considering the poor quality of many published narrative reviews.[32] As a specific example of the shortcomings of narrative reviews, Joyce, Rabe-Hesketh, and Wessely[35] found that citation of the literature is influenced by the review authors' discipline and nationality. This study also found that, of 89 reviews, only 3 (3.4%) described the methods used in the literature search.

QUALITATIVE SYSTEMATIC REVIEWS

If the purpose of nonsystematic reviews is to find the truth, then "the purpose of the systematic review is finding the whole truth."[36] Cook and associates describe systematic reviews as scientific investigations with predefined methods and original studies as their "subjects."[37] Two general types of systematic reviews exist. The term "qualitative systematic review" has been applied to a summary of results of primary studies where the results are not statistically combined.[37] In contrast, a quantitative systematic review, or meta-analysis, has been described as a systematic review that uses statistical methods to combine the results of two or more studies.[37] Perhaps, more appropriately, meta-analyses can be thought of as a specific methodological and statistical technique (or tool) for combining quantitative data. Table 7–5 illustrates the primary differences between qualitative and quantitative systematic reviews.[37]

Systematic overviews of the medical literature that summarize scientific evidence (in contrast to unsystematic narrative reviews that mix together opinions and evidence) are becoming increasingly prevalent. These overviews address questions of treatment, causation, diagnosis, or prognosis.[33] Because a systematic, qualitative approach is used in identifying and analyzing primary literature, systematic reviews are often considered superior to nonsystematic (narrative) reviews of any given topic.

Qualitative systematic reviews should concentrate on a clearly defined issue that is of importance to practice.[33,34] Specific criteria should be used to select articles from the primary literature to be included in the review.[33] For valid conclusions to be derived from qualitative systematic reviews, the authors must define the study population or topic of interest and include only those studies that used valid research methods.[33] For example, authors would have the choice of assessing patients who are either pre- or postmenopausal in a qualitative systematic review focused on the utility of chemotherapy in improving survival following mastectomy in breast cancer patients. The conclusions of the qualitative systematic review are likely to be very different depending on the patient population selected. In addition, authors would probably find a collection of studies that used a variety of research techniques. Poorly controlled, nonrandomized, unblinded studies should be excluded from the analysis. Only those studies that meet strict criteria for validity as discussed in Chap. 6, Literature Evaluation I, Controlled Clinical Trials, should be included in the review.

Authors should use a variety of resources to identify studies for the qualitative systematic review. Use of a single database is not likely to capture all relevant studies; a combination of databases, study bibliographies, and experts in the field should be used to identify studies for evaluation.[33,34]

Consideration should be given to inclusion of unpublished (e.g., data on file at the manufacturer or personal communication with investigators) and published studies, because it has been determined that published studies are more often of a positive nature than unpublished studies, a situation termed publication bias.[33] Because assessment of studies may be subjective and biased, two or more authors should critique the studies and all should concur on which studies will be included in the qualitative systematic review.[33]

Data should be summarized in table format.[33] Outcomes described in the qualitative systematic review article should be meaningful, and, if the trial is a clinical trial, clinically important.[33] For example, improved survival is a more important endpoint than reduction in tumor size in breast cancer patients. Authors should also assess benefits versus risks associated with the therapy under review, if possible.[33]

"All reviews, narrative and systematic alike, are retrospective, observational research studies and are therefore subject to systematic and random error."[37] Just as for nonsystematic reviews, techniques can be applied to evaluate the quality of systematic reviews.[38] Questions to ask when critiquing systematic reviews are provided in Appendix 7–1.

QUANTITATIVE SYSTEMATIC REVIEWS (META-ANALYSES)

Meta-analyses are now widely used to provide supporting evidence for clinical decision making. Meta-analysis is a technique that has been developed to provide a quantitative and objective assessment.[40] In a meta-analysis, results of previously conducted clinical trials are combined and statistically evaluated.[40,41] Meta-analyses are designed to provide greater insight into clinical dilemmas than individual clinical trials. They are especially useful when previous studies have been inconclusive or contradictory, or in situations where sample size may have been too small to detect a statistically significant difference between treatment and control groups (i.e., low power). Sacks and colleagues[41] have described the following purposes for performing a meta-analysis: "(1) to increase the statistical power for primary endpoint and for subgroups, (2) to resolve uncertainty when reports disagree, (3) to improve estimates of size of effect, (4) to answer new questions not posed at the start of individual trials, and (5) to bring about improvements in the quality of the primary research."

Meta-analysis has been used to address important clinical questions such as whether aspirin reduces the risk of pregnancy-induced hypertension, cholesterol decreases mortality, fluoxetine increases suicidal ideations, or estrogen replacement therapy increases the risk of breast cancer.[40] Meta-analysis can be used to look at both clinical trials and epidemiologic research, such as follow-up and case-control studies, and is particularly useful when definitive trials cannot be conducted, results of available trials are inconclusive, or while awaiting the results of definitive trials.[40-42] For the hypothetical situation regarding drug A used for the treatment of myocardial infarction, suppose that there are a number of small clinical trials suggesting that the product increases sudden death through proarrythmic effects. A meta-analysis could be performed to statistically combine the results of these small trials and increase the power of the finding (association or lack of association of drug A with increased sudden death).

Methodological problems with meta-analyses have lead to controversy surrounding their use in clinical decision making. When results from multiple trials are combined, the biases of the individual studies are incorporated and new sources of bias arise. The quality of the meta-analysis depends on the quality of the individual studies used to develop the meta-analysis.[39] Indeed, LeLorier and co-workers[39] have compared the results of a series of large, randomized controlled trials with those of previously published meta-analyses examining the same questions. They found that the outcomes of the 12 large, randomized, controlled trials studied were not predicted accurately by the meta-analyses published previously on the same topics 35% of the time.[39] The randomized, controlled clinical trials corresponded to meta-analyses in terms of population studied, therapeutic intervention, and at least one outcome. In this study, 46% of divergences in results involved a positive meta-analysis being followed by a negative randomized, controlled trial while the remaining 54% of identified divergences involved a negative meta-analysis followed by a positive randomized, controlled trial. Reasons for divergences as cited by the authors included the heterogenicity of the trials included in the meta-analyses and publication bias (tendency of investigators to preferentially submit studies with positive results for publication).[39]

Several points should be considered when evaluating meta-analyses. A quality meta-analysis must clearly define the clinical question to be addressed by the analysis.[41,42] As with qualitative systematic reviews, details of literature searches that were conducted to locate primary research articles must be given and criteria for inclusion of studies in the meta-analysis must be determined prior to conducting the analysis.[40-42] Because computerized searches may not locate all of the relevant articles, other resources such as textbooks, experts in the field, and reference lists from clinical studies should also be consulted.[41]

Trials included in and excluded from the meta-analysis should be listed. Strict standards should be established prior to the initiation of the meta-analysis to ensure that the criteria used for the inclusion of participants, the administration of the principle treatment, and the measurement of outcome events are similar in all trials studied.[39] Types of patients, their diagnosis, treatments, and therapeutic endpoints used in the original clinical studies should be given. The source of financial support for the original articles (because this may represent study bias) should also be addressed.[41,42] Interpretation of results of meta-analyses are limited by what studies were (or were not) included, how well the studies were (or were not) done, and how homogenous (or heterogenous) the studies were.[13]

A major problem of meta-analyses is the issue of publication bias found by LeLorier and associates[39] described above.[40,41] It has been documented that investigators are more likely to publish studies that demonstrate positive effects of drugs. Therefore, studies that show lack of efficacy are less likely to be located than those that demonstrate beneficial effects of a drug. Additionally, as discussed, controversy exists over whether data from unpublished studies should be included in the meta-analysis, because such studies have not been scrutinized through the peer-review process.[43]

Authors need to address the validity of articles used in the meta-analysis (see Chap. 6) such as randomization techniques, compliance, blinding and intention-to-treat analyses.[40,41] Some experts believe that studies should be weighted based on quality, but this practice is controversial because such assessments are subjective.[40]

The studies should be similar enough to allow pooling of data.[41,42] Statistical tests that evaluate homogenicity should be used to assess similarity of studies.[42] The more statistically significant the results of these tests, the more likely differences in study results are due to chance alone. If results of tests of homogenicity are not significant, the studies are heterogenous and differences in study results may be due to research design, rather than chance alone. Caution should be used when pooling results of heterogenous studies.

To reduce bias in the meta-analysis, only the methods section of the individual studies should be used to determine which studies are appropriate for inclusion. Investigators collecting data should be blinded to the names of the original articles' authors, place of publication of the article, and final results.[41,42]

Appropriate statistical analyses should be undertaken (usually the Mantel-Haenzel test), probability of false-positive (e.g., type I error) and false-negative (e.g., type II error) results should be discussed, and 95% confidence intervals, which provide the range of values where the true value lies 95% of the time, should be calculated.[41]

Finally, sensitivity analyses should be conducted to determine how the results of the meta-analysis vary depending on use of different assumptions, tests, and criteria and the economic implications of the meta-analysis should be considered.[41,42] Use of the above criteria when conducting meta-analyses has improved in recent years.[41] However, recently the usefulness of meta-analysis has been questioned when the results of subsequent randomized, controlled trials did not support previously published meta-analyses on the same subject as described above.[39] Questions for readers to consider when evaluating the quality of published meta-analyses have been published and are provided in Appendix 7–1.[44]

Overall, meta-analyses should be interpreted with caution, remembering that conclusions depend on the quality of the studies included and findings of subsequent randomized, controlled trials may differ from those of the meta-analysis.[13] Meta-analyses, on the surface, appear to be an extremely valuable tool allowing the practitioner to efficiently stay abreast of new information; however, oversimplification may lead to inappropriate conclusions.[39] Like all types of research evidence meta-analyses require careful analysis to determine their validity and their applicability in practice.[43]

Of note, an important source of systematic reviews (both qualitative and meta-analyses) is the *Cochrane Handbook* (published by the COCHRANE Collaboration), which is available in paper, CD-ROM, and Internet format (<<http://hiru.mcmaster.ca/COCHRANE/DEFAULT.htm>>). Recently, 36 reviews published in the COCHRANE Database of Systematic Reviews were compared to a randomly selected sample of 39 meta-analyses or systematic reviews published in journals indexed by MEDLINE in 1995.[46] Cochrane reviews were more likely to include a description of the inclusion and exclusion criteria (35/36 vs. 18/39; $p < .001$) and an assessment of trial quality (36/36 vs. 12/39; $p < .001$). By June 1997, 18 of 36 Cochrane reviews had been updated as compared to 1 of 39 reviews listed in MEDLINE. Overall, the authors concluded that "Cochrane reviews appeared to have greater methodological rigor and were more frequently updated than systematic reviews or meta-analyses published in paper-based journals."[46]

Practice Guidelines

Evidence-based practice guidelines are developed through systematic reviews of the literature appropriately adapted to local circumstances and values. According to Zinberg, practice guides are created primarily for the purpose of "improving the quality of health care, decreasing costs, diminishing professional liability, and improving consistency of practice."[47] Key questions to consider when reviewing a practice guideline have been proposed.[48] These questions primarily rely on how accurately the guideline reflects the research used to produce it and are summarized in Appendix 7–1.

A useful guideline allows the reader to examine the range of therapeutic options for a given disease and the most appropriate choice for a specific patient.[49] Although the publication of practice guidelines has been increasing in the biomedical literature, well-developed guidelines are still uncommon.[49]

Some key issues to consider when evaluating a practice guideline include questions about validity (are the recommendations strong) and reliability (would the same conclusion be reached if another group of investigators attempted to develop the guideline), generalizability of the results to a wide population, and methods used to identify, select, rate, and combine the evidence.[48] Other issues important to the evaluation of practice guidelines include whether or not the guideline is regularly updated to incorporate new evidence as it is made available and peer reviewed.

Practice guidelines are becoming an increasingly important part of the biomedical literature and are further discussed in Chap. 9, Evidence-Based Clinical Guidelines.

Health Outcomes Research

Health outcomes research encompasses the areas of pharmacoeconomics and quality of life assessments. Evaluation of these types of studies will be discussed in this section.

PHARMACOECONOMIC STUDIES

Readers are referred to Chap. 8 for information on evaluating these types of trials.

QUALITY OF LIFE MEASURES

Health-related quality of life (HR-QOL) includes many dimensions or domains of health status such as physical, social and cognitive functioning, mental health, symptom tolerance, and overall well-being.[50] Each dimension of health may be reported as a composite score or as a subscore for each specific dimension. For example, the Short-Form 36 (SF-36), a generic quality of life (QOL) instrument, measures eight health concepts (pain, vitality, social functioning, etc.), which can be scored individually or grouped to provide summary scores (overall physical health and overall mental health).[51] The addition of HR-QOL measures to clinical and economic trials of medical interventions allows the evaluator to assess the impact at the level of the individual. QOL reporting has been increasing in the last decade (from 1% in 1980 to about 4% in 1997); however, Sanders and colleagues[52] reported that only 5% of all randomized controlled trials and 10% of cancer studies reported HR-QOL measures. QOL is a relatively new concept and these findings may reflect confusion about the term "quality of life" and the resultant lack of a conceptual basis for HR-QOL measures.[53]

Generic instruments are available for general use in different populations for measuring changes in HR-QOL across a broad spectrum of diseases and treatments. They are composed of a standard set of health dimensions. One of the most commonly used generic instruments is the SF-36. Because this type of instrument can be used for different diseases and patient populations, the results derived from generic instruments can be used to compare impact of different treatments in the same disease, or impact of treatments across diseases. They many not, however, be able to detect QOL differences within a specific disease state. Specific instruments, such as the Health Assessment Questionnaire (HAQ), are required to obtain disease-specific or population-specific QOL information. These types of instruments are not suited for cross-condition comparison.

When evaluating studies that report HR-QOL measures, there are several issues the reader must keep in mind. For most HR-QOL instruments, changes in score that constitute clinically important differences are not known.[54] This makes interpretation of HR-QOL results from clinical trials difficult. The availability of a benchmarking process for determining clinically important differences would improve interpretation of HR-QOL results from clinical trials.[54] For example, the Expanded Disability Status Scale is used for grading levels of disability in multiple sclerosis and ranges from 0 to 10. Varying levels of disability are broken down by 0.5 unit increments (i.e., "no disability" falls into the 1 to 1.5 range and "minimal disability" falls into the 2 to 2.5 range). If a new agent for the treatment of multiple sclerosis demonstrates an improvement of 0.25 (i.e., causes that patient's score to decrease from 1.5 to 1.25) on this scale, it is difficult to determine whether or not this is a clinically important difference.

Gill and Feinstein[55] evaluated how well HR-QOL is being measured in the medical literature. Seventy-five articles were randomly selected for inclusion in the analysis. Investigators conceptually defined HR-QOL in only 11 (15%) of the 75 articles, identified target domains in only 35 (47%), gave reasons for selecting the HR-QOL instrument in 27 (36%), and aggregated results into a composite "HR-QOL score in only 13 articles (17%). The authors concluded that HR-QOL is a uniquely personal perception, denoting the way individual patients feel about their health status and/or nonmedical aspects of their lives, and that most measurements of HR-QOL in the medical literature do not capture this important concept."[55]

The consistency and availability of standards for measuring HR-QOL are lacking. Of the 67 studies sampled in a bibliographic study by Sanders and associates,[52] 48 used 62 different pre-existing instruments and a further 15 studies reported new measures.[52] Additionally, culturally defined factors may impact patient HR-QOL and its assessment. Validity of HR-QOL measures across different cultures or subcultures is rarely reported.[56] Accurate measurement of HR-QOL is very difficult without extensive validation efforts in every cultural population of interest. As more experience is gained with QOL studies, the issues of clinical significance and validated instruments may be resolved. Readers must understand that this field is growing rapidly and being perfected.

When reviewing QOL studies, response rates are critical for reporting HR-QOL as nonresponse can introduce serious bias. The fact that response rates were unreported in almost a half of the trials analyzed by Sanders and co-workers[52] was a matter of concern. The authors also found that selective reporting of favorable or statistically significant results was a problem.[52]

Important aspects of trials reporting on HR-QOL data have been identified and questions to ask when reviewing trials that report on HR-QOL have been proposed and are reviewed in Appendix 7–1.[57,58] Foremost, the validity and the applicability of the HR-QOL instrument to the disease state or treatment under investigation should be documented.[57] The HR-QOL instrument should be sensitive to changes in the patients' status throughout the clinical trial and should measure aspects of the patient's lives that the patients consider to be important.[57,58] Additionally, if the HR-QOL instrument is used multiple times, a training effect may occur by which the performance of either the patient or assessor or both improves or is modified simply through the multiple use of the instrument.[57] The reviewer of such a trial needs to ask if this type of effect was present and how it may have influenced the results. A final question in reviewing trials that present HR-QOL data is whether all sites in a multicenter trial performed the HR-QOL analyses.[57]

Conclusion

Many types of study designs are published in the biomedical literature. Each type of design is appropriately geared to answer specific clinical questions and each has a unique set of problems. Careful evaluation using the techniques outlined in this chapter is necessary for appropriate application of the results from these studies to clinical practice.

Study Questions

1. Describe the differences between odds ratio and relative risk as they pertain to cohort and case-control studies. Why is it important to use confidence intervals when describing these parameters?

2. Describe how the validity of results obtained through survey research is assessed.

3. For each of the following scenarios, identify the type, advantages and disadvantages, and important points to consider when critiquing each study design.
   a. A physician designs a cross-over study to prospectively evaluate the use of ibuprofen for chronic fatigue syndrome in an individual patient.

b. Leucovorin calcium and fluorouracil often have been combined in the same solution and infused over multiple days by using a portable infusion pump. However, precipitation and clogging of the portable pump lines and catheters have been reported. A study was conducted to further evaluate the compatibility of this combination.

c. An investigator evaluates the question of whether or not different levothyroxine products can be use interchangeably.

d. It is hypothesized that hormone replacement therapy (HRT) in postmenopausal women may play a beneficial role in preventing osteoporosis. A group of patients receiving HRT and a group of patients not receiving HRT are followed over a 20-year period. The development of osteoporosis as assessed by bone mineral density in each group is compared and the relative risk associated with the use of HRT and the development of osteoporosis is calculated.

e. There is a concern that the use of HRT in postmenopausal women may cause an increased risk of breast cancer. A study is conducted to test this hypothesis. A group of patients admitted to the hospital with the diagnosis of breast cancer is compared to a group of patients admitted to the hospital without breast cancer. The groups are matched by age, sex, date of admission, and other confounding factors such as alcohol use. Use of HRT in each group is assessed and compared. An odds ratio for the risk of breast cancer related to the use of HRT is calculated.

f. An investigator identifies a study sample of women aged 20 to 45 years. During a single office visit, the investigator measures bone mass in the women. He also questions them about their past and present exercise habits. The investigator determines that women involved with rigorous exercise before the onset of menses have a greater bone mass.

g. A pharmacist notes that a patient develops erythema multiforme after administration of phenytoin. The pharmacist reports her observations regarding this patient.

h. A smoking cessation clinic has been developed and implemented at a community pharmacy. A questionnaire is mailed to all patients using the clinic within the past month to assess patient satisfaction.

i. A new antipsychotic agent is approved by the FDA. Following approval, the manufacturer of the antipsychotic agent creates a registry with several major hospitals and health maintenance organizations to monitor how the drug is used and the adverse effects associated with the use of the drug.

j. A pharmacist publishes an educational summary describing the types, use, side effect profile, and cost of available oral contraceptives.

k. A pharmacist systematically gathers and analyzes the evidence for efficacy and cost effectiveness of topical treatments of superficial fungal infections of the skin and nails of the feet. An explicit description of methods used in selecting and analyzing the data is provided. Statistical analysis is not used in combining the results of individual trials.

l. Conflicting reports exist about the effect of combining heparin with thrombolytic therapy on mortality in acute myocardial infarction. An investigator systematically identifies both published and unpublished studies in this area, combines the results, and statistically evaluates the data.

m. Guidelines for the use of thrombolytics are developed and published to aid in appropriate prescribing of these agents.

n. An investigation of the impact of intensive therapy (drug therapy, blood glucose monitoring, exercise, and diet) on the quality of life for diabetic patients is conducted and published.

REFERENCES

1. Larson EB, Ellsworth AJ. N-of-1 trials: increasing precision in therapeutics. ACP J Club 1993 July/August:A16–A17. Editorial.

2. Cook DJ. Randomized trials in single subjects: the N of 1 study. Psychopharmacol Bull 1996;32:363–7.

3. Guyatt GH, Keller JL, Jaeschke R, Rosenbloom D, Adachi JD, Newhouse MT. The *n*-of-1 randomized controlled trial: clinical usefulness. Our three year experience. Ann Intern Med 1990;112:293–9.

4. Larson EB, Ellsworth AJ, Oas J. Randomized clinical trials in single patients during a 2-year period. JAMA 1993;270:2708–12.

5. Guyatt G, Sackett D, Taylor DW, Chong J, Roberts R, Puosley S. Determining optimal therapy-randomized trials in individual patients. N Engl J Med 1986;314:889–92.

6. Trissel LA, Flora KP. Stability studies: five years later. Am J Hosp Pharm 1988;45:1569–71.

7. Chow SC. Individual bioequivalence—a review of the FDA draft guidance. Drug Info J 1999;33:435–44.

8. The United States Pharmacopeial Convention, Inc. Food and Drug Administration center for drug evaluation and research approved drug products with therapeutic equivalence evaluations. USPDI 19th ed., Volume III: Approved drug products and legal requirements. Massachusetts; 1999. pp. I/5–I/17.

9. FDA. Guidance for industry. In vivo bioequivalence studies based on population and individual bioequivalence approaches. Draft Guidance. Rockville (MD): U.S. Department of Health and Human Services, Food and Drug Administration, Center for Drug Evaluation and Research (CDER); 1997.

10. DiSanto AR. Bioavailability and bioequivalency testing. In: Gennaro AR, Chase GD, Marderostan AD, Harvey SC, Hussar DA, Medwick T, et al, editors. Remington's Pharmaceutical sciences. 18th Edition. Pennsylvania: Mack Publishing Company; 1990. pp. 1451–8.

11. Willett MS, Bertch KE, Rich DS, Eveshehefsky L. Prospectus on the economic value of clinical pharmacy services. A position statement of the American College of Clinical Pharmacy. Pharmacotherapy 1989;9:45–56.

12. Feinstein AR, Horwitz RI. Double standards, scientific methods, and epidemiologic research. N Engl J Med 1982;307:1611–7.

13. Dolan MS. Interpretation of the literature. Clin Obstet Gynecol 1998;41:307–14.

14. Peipert JF, Glennon Phipps M. Observational studies. Clin Obstet Gynecol 1998;41:235–44.

15. Hartzema AG. Guide to interpreting and evaluating the pharmacoepidemiologic literature. Ann Pharmacother 1992;26:96–8.

16. Hayden GF, Kramer MS, Horwitz RI. The case-control study. A practical review for the clinician. JAMA 1982;247:326–31.

17. Niemcryk SJ, Kraus TJ, Mallory TH. Empirical considerations in orthopaedic research design and data analysis. Part I: Strategies in research design. J Arthroplasty 1990;5:97–103.

18. Horwitz RI, Feinstein AR. Methodologic standards and contradictory results in case-control research. Am J Med 1979;66:556–64.

19. Gullen WH. A danger in matched-control studies. JAMA 1980;244:2279–80.

20. Bailar JC, Louis TA, Lavori PW, Polansky M. A classification of biomedical research reports. In: Bailar JC, Mostellar F, editors. Medical Uses of Statistics. 2nd ed. Boston: NEJM Books, 1992. pp. 141–56.

21. Spilker B. Single Patient Clinical Trials. Guide to Clinical Trials. New York: Lippincott-Raven; 1996. pp. 277–82.

22. Jaeschke R, Sackett DL. Research methods for obtaining primary evidence. Int J Technol Assess Health Care 1989;5:503–19.

23. Lukoff D, Edwards D, Miller M. The case study as a scientific method for researching alternative therapies. Altern Ther Health Med 1998;4:44–52.

24. Kerlinger FN. Foundations of behavioral research. 2nd ed. New York: Holt, Rinehart & Winston; 1973. p. 401.

25. Harrison DL, Draugalis JR. Evaluating the results of mail survey research. J Am Pharm Assoc 1997;NS37:662–6.

26. Shi L. Health services research methods. In: Williams S, editor. Delmar series in health services administration. Albany: International Thomson Publishing; 1997.

27. Manasse H, Lambert R. Types of research: a synopsis of the major categories and data collection methods. Am J Hosp Pharm 1980;37:694–701.

28. Segal R. Designing a pharmacy survey. Top Hosp Pharm Manage 1985 May:37–45.

29. Fowler F. Survey research methods. In: Bickman L, Rog D, editors. Applied Social Research Methods Series. Vol. 1, Newbury Park (CA): Sage; 1993.

30. Fairman K. Going to the source: a guide to using surveys in health care research. J Manag Care Pharm 1999;5:150–9.

31. Spilker B. Classification and description of phase IV postmarketing study designs. Guide to clinical trials. New York: Lippincott-Raven; 1996. pp. 44–58.

32. Mulrow CD. The medical review article. State of the science. Ann Intern Med 1987;106:485–88.

33. Oxman AD, Cook DJ, Guyatt GH. Users' guides to the medical literature. VI. How to use an overview. JAMA 1994;272:1367–71.

34. Oxman AD, Guyatt GH. Guidelines for reading literature reviews. CMAJ 1988;138:697–703.

35. Joyce J, Rabe-Hesketh S, Wessely S. Reviewing the reviews. The example of chronic fatigue syndrome. JAMA 1998;280:264–6.

36. Mulrow CD, Cook DJ, Davidoff F. Systematic reviews: critical links in the great chain of evidence. Ann Intern Med 1997;126:389–91. Editorial.

37. Cook DJ, Mulrow CD, Haynes RB. Systematic reviews: synthesis of best evidence for clinical decisions. Ann Intern Med 1997;126:376–80.
38. Greenhalgh T. Papers that summarize other papers (systematic reviews and meta-analyses). Br Med J 1997;315:672–5.
39. LeLorier J, Gregoire G, Benhaddad A, Lapierre J, Derderian F. Discrepancies between meta-analyses and subsequent large randomized, controlled trials. N Engl J Med 1997;337:536–42.
40. Gibaldi M. Meta-analysis. A review of its place in therapeutic decision making. Drugs 1993; 46:805–18.
41. Sacks HS, Berrier J, Reitman D, Pagano D, Chalmers TC. Meta-analyses of randomized control trials. An update of the quality and methodology. In: Bailar JC, Mosteller F, editors. Medical uses of statistics. 2nd ed. Boston: NEJM Books; 1992. pp. 427–42.
42. Einarson TR, Leeder JS, Koren G. A method for meta-analysis of epidemiological studies. Drug Intell Clin Pharm 1988;22:813–24.
43. Cook DJ, Guyatt GH, Ryan G, Clifton J, Buckinham L, William A, et al. Should unpublished data be included in meta-analyses? Current conviction and controversies. JAMA 1993;269:2749–53.
44. Thacker SB, Stroup DF, Peterson HB. Meta-analysis for the practicing obstetrician-gynecologist. Clin Obstet Gynecol 1998;41:275–81.
45. Hunt DL, McKibbon KA. Locating and appraising systematic reviews. Ann Intern Med 1997;126:532–8.
46. Jadad AR, Cook DJ, Jones A, Klassen TP, Tugwell P, Moher M, Moher D. Methodology and reports of systematic reviews and meta-analyses. JAMA 1998;280:278–80.
47. Zinberg S. Practice guidelines—a continuing debate. Clin Obstet Gynecol 1998;41:343–7.
48. Hayward RS, Wilson MC, Tunis SR, Bass EB, Guyatt G. Users' guide to the medical literature. VIII. How to use clinical practice guidelines. A. Are the recommendations valid? JAMA 1995;274:570–4.
49. Wilson MC, Hayward RS, Tunis SR, Bass EB, Guyatt G. Users' guide to the medical literature. VIII. How to use clinical practice guidelines. B. What are the recommendations and will they help you in caring for your patients? JAMA 1995;274:1630–2.
50. Rizzo JD, Powe NR. Methodological hurdles in conducting pharmacoeconomic analyses. Pharmacoeconomics 1999;15:339–55.
51. Guyatt GH, Jaeschke R, Feeny DH, Patrick DL. Measurements in clinical trials: choosing the right approach. In: Spilker B, editor. Quality of Life and Pharmacoeconomics in Clinical Trials. 2nd ed. Philadelphia: Lippincott-Raven; 1996. pp. 41–58.
52. Sanders C, Egger M, Donovan J, Tallon D, Frankel S. Reporting on quality of life in randomised controlled trials: bibliographic study. Br Med J 1998;317:1191–4.
53. Leplege A, Hunt S. The problem of quality of life in medicine. JAMA 1997;278:47–50.
54. Samsa G, Edelman D, Rothman ML, Williams GR, Lipscomb J, Matchar D. Determining clinically important differences in health status measures. A general approach with illustration to the Health Utilities Index Mark II. Pharmacoeconomics 1999;15:141–55.
55. Gill TM, Feinstein AR. A critical appraisal of the quality of quality-of-life measurements. JAMA 1994;272:619–26.
56. Yabroff KR, Linas BP, Schulman K. Evaluation of quality of life for diverse patient populations. Breast Cancer Res Treat 1996;40:87–104.

57. Spilker B. Quality of life trials. Guide to clinical trials. New York: Lippincott-Raven; 1996. pp. 370–8.

58. Guyatt GH, Naylor CD, Juniper E, Heyland DK, Jaeschke R, Cook DJ. Users' guides to the medical literature. XII. How to use articles about health-related quality of life. JAMA 1997; 277:1232–7.

Chapter Eight

Pharmacoeconomics

James P. Wilson • Karen L. Rascati

Objectives

After completing this chapter, the reader will be able to:

- List the advantages and disadvantages of the different types of pharmacoeconomic analyses.
- List and explain 10 steps that should be found in a well-conducted pharmacoeconomic study.
- List the six steps in a decision analysis.
- Apply the use of pharmacoeconomic evaluation techniques to the formulary decision process, including decision analysis.
- Apply a systematic approach to evaluation of the pharmacoeconomic literature.
- List at least four applications specific to pharmacy, where pharmacoeconomic methodology is commonly employed.

Many changes have taken place in health care recently. The introduction of new technologies, including many new drugs, has been among these changes. In 1999, the Federal Food and Drug Administration's (FDA) Center for Drug Evaluation and Research (CDER) approved 90 new drugs compared to 62 in 1994.[1] As the number of new drugs continues to increase, so does their cost, rising 2.7% between January and June of 1997.[2] The increase in the number of new drugs combined with the increased cost of these drugs provides a great challenge for managed care organizations as they struggle to deliver quality care while minimizing costs.

Pharmacy and Therapeutics (P&T) Committees are responsible for evaluating these new drugs and determining their potential value to organizations. Evaluating drugs for formulary inclusion can often be an overwhelming task. The application of pharmaco-economic methods to the evaluation process may help streamline formulary decisions.

This chapter presents an overview of the practical application of pharmaco-economic principles as they apply to the formulary decision process. For a more in-depth review of the principles and concepts of pharmacoeconomics, please refer to the references at the end of the chapter.

Pharmacoeconomics—What Is It and Why Do It?

Pharmacoeconomics has been defined as the description and analysis of the costs of drug therapy to health care systems and society—it identifies, measures, and compares the costs and consequences of pharmaceutical products and services.[3] Decision makers can use these methods to evaluate and compare the total costs of treatment options and the outcomes associated with these options. To show this graphically, think of two sides of an equation—the inputs (costs), used to obtain and use the drug, are used to produce health-related outcomes (Fig. 8-1).

The center of the equation, the drug product, is symbolized by the symbol ℞. If just the left-hand side of the equation is measured without regard for outcomes, this is a cost analysis (or a partial economic analysis). If just the right-hand side of the equation is measured without regard to costs, this is a clinical or outcome study (not an economic analysis). To be a true pharmacoeconomic analysis, both sides of the equation must be considered and compared.

Models of Pharmacoeconomic Analysis

The four types of pharmacoeconomic analyses all follow the diagram shown in Fig. 8-1—they measure costs or inputs in dollars and assess the outcomes associated with these costs. Pharmacoeconomic analyses are categorized by the method used to assess outcomes. If the outcomes are assumed to be equivalent, the study is called a cost-minimization analysis; if the outcomes are measured in dollars, the study is called a

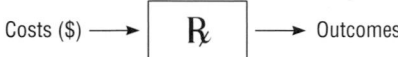

Figure 8–1. The pharmacoeconomic equation.

TABLE 8–1. THE FOUR TYPES OF PHARMACOECONOMIC ANALYSIS

Methodology	Cost Measurement Unit	Outcome Measurement Unit
Cost-minimization analysis (CMA)	Dollars	Assumed to be equivalent in comparable groups
Cost-benefit analysis (CBA)	Dollars	Dollars
Cost-effectiveness analysis (CEA)	Dollars	Natural units (life-years gained, mm Hg blood pressure, mMol/L blood glucose)
Cost-utility analysis (CUA)	Dollars	Quality-adjusted life-year (QALY) or other utilities

cost-benefit analysis; if the costs are measured in natural units (cures, years of life, blood pressure), the study is called a cost-effectiveness analysis; if the outcomes take into account patient preferences (or utilities), the study is called a cost-utility analysis (Table 8–1). Each type of analysis includes a measurement of costs in dollars. Measurement of these costs is discussed first, followed by further examples of how outcomes are measured for these four types of studies.

Assessment of Costs

First, the assessment of costs (the left-hand side of the equation) will be discussed. A discussion of the four types of costs and adjustments for the timing of costs follow.

TYPES OF COSTS

"Costs" are calculated to estimate the resources (or inputs) that are used to produce an outcome. Pharmacoeconomic studies categorize "costs" into four types. "Direct medical costs" are the most obvious costs to measure. These are the medically related inputs used directly to provide the treatment. Examples of direct medical costs include those associated with pharmaceutical products, physician visits, emergency room visits, and hospitalizations. "Direct nonmedical costs" are costs directly associated with treatment, but are not medical in nature. Examples include the cost of traveling to and from the physician's office or hospital, babysitting for the children of a patient, and food and lodging required for the patient and their family during out-of-town treatment. "Indirect costs" involve costs that result from the loss of productivity due to illness or death. Please note that the accounting term "indirect costs," which is used to assign overhead, is different from the economic term, which refers to a loss of productivity of the patient or the patient's family due to illness. "Intangible costs" include the costs of pain, suffering, anxiety, or fatigue that occur because of an illness or the treatment of an illness. It is difficult to measure or assign values to intangible costs.

Treatment of an illness may include all four types of costs. For example, the cost of surgery would include the direct medical costs of the surgery (medication, room charges, laboratory tests, physician services), direct nonmedical costs (travel and lodging for the preoperative day), indirect costs (due to the patient missing work during the surgery and recuperative period), and intangible costs (due to pain and anxiety). Most studies only report the direct medical costs. This may be appropriate, depending on the objective or perspective of the study. For example, if the objective is to measure the costs to the hospital for two surgical procedures that differ in direct medical costs (for example, using high-dose versus low-dose aprotinin in cardiac bypass surgery), but that are expected to have similar nonmedical, indirect, and intangible costs, measuring all four types of costs may not be warranted.

To determine what costs are important to measure, the perspective of the study must be determined. "Perspective" is a pharmacoeconomic term that describes whose costs are relevant based on the purpose of the study. Economic theory suggests that the most appropriate perspective is that of society. Societal costs include costs to the insurance company, costs to the patient, and indirect costs due to the loss of productivity. Although this may be the most appropriate perspective according to economic theory, it is rarely seen in the pharmacoeconomic literature. The most common perspectives used in pharmacoeconomic studies are the perspective of the institution (hospital or clinic) or the perspective of the payer. The payer perspective may include the costs to the third-party plan or the patient or a combination of the patient co-pay and the third-party plan costs.

TIMING ADJUSTMENTS FOR COSTS

When costs are estimated from information collected for more than a year before the study or for more than a year into the future, adjustment of costs is needed. If retrospective data are used to assess resources used over a number of years, these costs should be adjusted to the present year. For example, if the objective of the study is to estimate the difference in the costs of antibiotic A versus B in the treatment of a specific type of infection, information on the past utilization of these two antibiotics might be collected from a review of medical records. If the retrospective review of these medical records dates back for more than a year, it may be necessary to adjust the cost of both medications by calculating the number of units (doses) used per case and multiplying this number by the current unit cost for each medication.

If costs are estimated based on dollars spent or saved in future years, another type of adjustment, called discounting, is needed. There is a time-value associated with money. Most people (and businesses) prefer to receive money today, rather than at a later time. Therefore a dollar received today is worth more than a dollar received next year—the time-value of money. "Discount rate," a term from finance, approximates the cost of capital by taking into account the projected inflation rate and the interest rates of borrowed money and estimates the time-value of money. From this parameter, the present value (PV) of future expenditures and savings can be calculated. The discount factor is equal to $1/(1 + r)^n$, where r is the discount rate and n is the year the cost or savings occur. For example, if the costs of a new pharmaceutical care program are $5000 per year for the next 3 years, and the discount rate is 5%, the PV of these costs is $14,297 [$5000 year 1 + $5000/1.05 year 2 + $5000/(1.05)^2$ year 3]. The most common discount rate currently seen in the literature is 5%, the approximate cost of borrowing money today.

Assessment of Outcomes

The methods associated with measuring outcomes (the right-hand side of the equation) will be discussed in this section. As shown in Table 8–1, there are four ways to measure outcomes, and each type of outcome measurement is associated with a different type of pharmacoeconomic analysis. The advantages and disadvantages of each type of analysis will be discussed in this section.

COST-MINIMIZATION ANALYSIS

For a cost-minimization analysis (CMA), costs are measured in dollars, and outcomes are assumed to be equivalent. One example of a CMA is the measurement and comparison of costs for two therapeutically equivalent products, like glipizide and glyburide.[4] Another example is the measurement and comparison of using prostaglandin E_2 on an inpatient versus an outpatient basis.[5] In both cases, all the outcomes (e.g., efficiency, incidence of adverse drug interactions) are expected to be equal, but the costs are not. Some researchers contend that a CMA is not a true pharmacoeconomic study, because although costs are measured, outcomes are not. Others say that the strength of a CMA depends on the evidence that the outcomes are the same. This evidence can be based on previous studies, publications, FDA data, or expert opinion. The advantage of this type of study is that it is relatively simple compared to the other types of analyses because outcomes need not be measured. The disadvantage of this type of analysis is that it can only be used where outcomes are assumed to be identical.

Examples

A hospital needs to decide if it should add a new intravenous antibiotic to the formulary, which is therapeutically equivalent to the current antibiotic used in the institution and has the same side effect profile. The advantage of the new antibiotic is that it only

TABLE 8–2. EXAMPLE OF COST MINIMIZATION

Type of Cost	Every 8 Hours	Once Daily
Drug acquisition cost	$43.70	$55.39
Minibag cost	$29.32	$10.90
Preparation cost	$13.81	$6.20
Administration costs	$67.63	$25.13
Total cost	$154.46	$97.62

NOTE: Costs are presented in Canadian dollars.

has to be administered once per day (versus three times a day for the comparison anti-biotic). Because the outcomes are expected to be nearly identical, and the objective is to assess the costs to the hospital (e.g., the hospital perspective), only direct medical costs need to be estimated and compared. The direct medical costs include the daily costs of each medication, the pharmacy personnel time used in the preparation of each dose, and the nursing personnel time used in the administration of each dose. Even if the cost of the new medication is a little higher than the cost of the current antibiotic, the lower cost of preparing and administering the new drug (once a day versus three times per day) may offset this difference. Direct nonmedical, indirect, and intangible costs are not expected to differ between these two alternatives and they need not be included if the perspective is that of the hospital, so these costs are not included in the comparison.

Mithani and Brown[6] examined once daily intravenous administration of aminogly-coside versus the conventional every 8 hour administration (Table 8–2). The drug acquisition cost was $Can 43.70 under every 8 hours dosing, and $Can 55.39 for the single dose administration. Not including laboratory drug level measurements, the costs of minibags ($29.32), preparation ($13.81), and administration ($67.63) were $Can 110.76 for the three times daily administration, versus $Can 42.23 (minibags $10.90, preparation $6.20, and administration $25.13) for the single daily dose. With essentially equivalent clinical outcomes, the once daily administration of the aminoglycoside minimized hospital costs ($97.63 versus $154.46).

COST-BENEFIT ANALYSIS

A cost-benefit analysis (CBA) measures both inputs and outcomes in monetary terms. One advantage to using a CBA is that alternatives with different outcomes can be compared, because each outcome is converted to the same unit (dollars). For example, the costs (inputs) of providing a pharmacokinetics service versus a diabetes clinic can be compared with the cost savings (outcomes) associated with each service, even though different types of outcomes are expected for each alternative. Many CBAs are performed to determine how institutions can best spend their resources to produce monetary benefits. For example, a study conducted at Walter Reed Army Medical Center looked at costs and savings associated with the addition of a pharmacist to its medical teams.[7] Discounting of both the costs of the treatment or services and the benefits or cost savings are needed if they extend for more than a year. Comparing costs and benefits (outcomes in monetary terms) is accomplished by either of two methods. One method divides the estimated benefits by the estimated costs to produce a benefit-to-cost ratio. If this ratio is more than 1.0, the choice is cost beneficial. The other method is to subtract the costs from the benefits to produce a net benefit calculation. If this difference is positive, the choice is cost beneficial. The example at the end of this section will use both methods for illustrative purposes.

Another, more complex, use of CBA consists of measuring clinical outcomes (for example, avoidance of death, reduction of blood pressure, reduction of pain) and placing a dollar value on these clinical outcomes. This type of CBA is not seen often in the pharmacy literature, but will be discussed here briefly. This use of the method still offers the advantage that alternatives with different types of outcomes can be assessed, but a disadvantage is that it is difficult (and some argue distasteful) to put a monetary value on pain, suffering, and human life. There are two common methods that economists use to estimate a value for these types of consequences—the human capital approach and the willingness-to-pay approach. The human capital approach assumes that the values of health benefits are equal to the economic productivity that they permit. The cost of disease is the cost of the lost productivity due to the disease. A person's expected income before taxes and/or an inputed value for nonmarket activities (e.g., housework and childcare) is used as an estimate of the value of any health benefits for that person. The human capital approach was used when calculating the costs and benefits of administering a meningococcal vaccine to college students. The value of the future productivity of a college student was estimated at $1 million in this study.[8] There are disadvantages to using this method. A person's earnings may not reflect their true value to society, and this method lacks a solid literature of research to back this notion. The willingness-to-pay method estimates the value of health benefits by estimating how much people would pay to reduce their chance of an adverse health outcome. For example, if a group of people is willing to pay, on average, $100 to reduce their chance of dying from 1:1000 to 1:2000, theoretically a life would be worth $200,000 [$100/(.001 − .0005)]. Problems with this method include that what people say they are willing to pay may not correspond to what they actually would do, and it is debatable if people can meaningfully answer questions about a .0005 reduction in outcomes.

Example

An independent pharmacy owner is considering the provision of a new clinical pharmacy service. The objective of the analysis is to estimate the costs and monetary bene-

TABLE 8–3. CBA EXAMPLE CALCULATIONS

	Year 1 Dollars [No Discounting in Year 1]	Year 2 Dollars [Discounted Dollars]	Year 3 Dollars [Discounted Dollars]	Total Dollars [Discounted Dollars]	Benefit-to-Cost Ratio Dollars [Discounted Dollars]	Net Benefit Dollars [Discounted Dollars]
Costs of A	$50,000 [$50,000]	$20,000 [$19,048]	$20,000 [$18,140]	$90,000 [$87,188]	$120,000/90,000 = 1.33:1 [$114,376/87,188 = 1.31:1]	$120,000 − 90,000 = 30,000 [$114,376 − 87,188 = 27,188]
Benefits of A	$40,000 [$40,000]	$40,000 [$38,095]	$40,000 [$36,281]	$120,000 [$114,376]		
Costs of B	$40,000 [$40,000]	$30,000 [$28,571]	$30,000 [$27,211]	$100,000 [$95,782]	$135,000/100,000 = 1.35:1 [$128,673/95,782 = 1.34:1]	$135,000 − 100,000 = 35,000 [$128,673 − 95,782 = 32,891]
Benefits of B	$45,000 [$45,000]	$45,000 [$42,857]	$45,000 [$40,816]	$135,000 [$128,673]		

fits of two possible services over the next 3 years (Table 8–3). Clinical service A would cost $50,000 in start-up and operating costs during the first year, and $20,000 in year 2 and year 3. Clinical service A would provide an added revenue of $40,000 each of the 3 years. Clinical service B would cost $40,000 in start-up and operating costs the first year and $30,000 for year 2 and year 3. Clinical service B would provide an added revenue of $45,000 for each of the 3 years. Table 8–3 illustrates the comparison of both options using the perspective of the independent pharmacy with no discounting and when a discount rate of 5% is used. Although both services are estimated to be cost beneficial, clinical service B has both a higher benefit-to-cost ratio and a higher net benefit when compared to clinical service A.

COST-EFFECTIVENESS ANALYSIS

A cost-effectiveness analysis (CEA) measures costs in dollars and outcomes in natural health units such as cures, lives saved, or blood pressure. This is the most common type of pharmacoeconomic analysis found in the pharmacy literature. An advantage of using a CEA is that health units are common outcomes practitioners can readily understand and these outcomes do not need to be converted to monetary values. On the other hand, the alternatives used in the comparison must have outcomes that are measured in the same units. If more than one natural unit outcome is important when conducting the comparison, a cost-effectiveness ratio should be calculated for each type of outcome. Outcomes cannot be collapsed into one unit measure in CEAs as they can with CBAs (outcome = dollars) or CUAs (outcome = quality-adjusted life-years [QALY]). Because CEA is the most common type of pharmacoeconomic study in the pharmacy literature, many examples are available. Bloom and colleagues[9] compared two medical treatments for gastroesophageal reflux disease (GERD), using both "healed ulcers confirmed by endoscopy" and "symptom-free days" as the outcomes measured. Law and associates[10] assessed two anti-diabetic medications by comparing the "percentage of patients who achieved good glycemic control" as the outcome measure.

A cost-effectiveness grid can be used to illustrate the definition of "cost effectiveness." In Table 8–4, cells D, G, and H (lightly shaded cells) are cost-effective choices,

TABLE 8–4. COST-EFFECTIVENESS GRID

Cost Effectiveness	Lower Cost	Same Cost	Higher Cost
Lower effectiveness	A	B	C
Same effectiveness	D	E	F
Higher effectiveness	G	H	I

TABLE 8–5. LISTING OF COSTS AND OUTCOMES

Alternative	Costs for 12 Months of Medication	Lowering of LDL in 12 Months
Current preferred medication	$1,000	25 mg/dL
New medication	$1,500	30 mg/dL

while cells B, C, and F (darker shaded cells) are not cost effective, and the remaining cells might be cost-effective if the added benefits are determined to be worth the added costs. The unshaded cells, A, E, and I are situations when a more subjective, complex judgment is needed.

Example

A managed care organization (MCO) is trying to decide whether to add a new cholesterol-lowering agent to its preferred formulary. The new product has a greater effect on lowering cholesterol than the current preferred agent, but a daily dose of the new medication is also more expensive. Using the perspective of the MCO (e.g., direct medical costs of the product to the MCO), the results will be presented three ways. Table 8–5 presents the simple listing of the costs and benefits of the two alternatives. Table 8–6 shows the cost-effectiveness ratio for each alternative. Table 8–7 shows the marginal (or incremental) cost effectiveness (the extra cost of producing one extra unit) of the new medication compared to the current medication. A marginal cost-effectiveness ratio is calculated by determining the added cost divided by the added benefit. Most economists agree that a marginal cost-effectiveness ratio is the more appropriate way to present CEA results. Because the costs and benefits of the medications are estimated for only 1 year, discounting is not needed.

Clinicians must then wrestle with this information—it becomes a "clinical call." Many economists will argue that this uncertainty is why cost effectiveness may not be the preferred method of pharmacoeconomic analysis.

COST-UTILITY ANALYSIS

A cost-utility analysis (CUA) takes patient preferences, also referred to as "utilities," into account when measuring health consequences. The most common unit used in con-

TABLE 8–6. COST-EFFECTIVENESS RATIOS

Alternative	Costs for 12 Months of Medication	Lowering of LDL in 12 Months	Average Cost per Reduction in LDL
Current preferred medication	$1,000	25 mg/dL	$40 per mg/dL
New medication	$1,500	30 mg/dL	$50 per mg/dL

TABLE 8–7. MARGINAL COST-EFFECTIVENESS RATIO

Alternative	Costs for 12 Months of Medication	Lowering of LDL in 12 Months	Marginal Cost per Marginal Reduction in LDL
Current preferred medication	$1,000	25 mg/dL	
New medication	$1,500	30 mg/dL	$\dfrac{\$1,500 - \$1,000}{30 \text{ mg/DL} - 25 \text{ mg/dL}} = \$100$ per mg/dL

ducting CUAs is QALYs, which incorporates both the quality and quantity of life. The advantage of using this method is that different types of health outcomes can be compared using one common unit (QALYs) without placing a monetary value on these health outcomes (like CBA). The disadvantage of this method is that it is difficult to determine an accurate QALY value. This is a relatively new type of outcome measure and is not understood or embraced by many providers or decision makers. Therefore, this method is rarely seen in the pharmacy literature. One reason researchers are working to establish methods for measuring QALYs is the belief that 1 year of life (a natural unit outcome that can be used in CEAs) in one health state should not be given the same weight as 1 year of life in another health state. For example, if two treatments both add 10 years of life, but one provides an added 10 years of being in a healthy state and the other adds 10 years of being in a disabled health state, the outcomes of the two treatments should not be considered equal. Adjusting for the quality of those extra years is warranted. When calculating QALYs, 1 year of life in perfect health has a score of 1.0 QALY. If health-related quality of life (HR-QOL) is diminished by disease or treatment, 1 year of life in this state is less than 1.0 QALY. This unit allows comparisons of morbidity and mortality. By convention perfect health is assigned 1.0 per year and death is assigned 0.0 per year, but how are scores between these two determined? Different techniques for determing scales of measurement for QALY are discussed below.

There are three common methods for determining these scores: rating scales, standard gamble, and time trade-off. A rating scale consists of a line on a page, somewhat like a thermometer, with perfect health at the top (100) and death at bottom (0). Different disease states are described to subjects and they are asked to place the different disease states somewhere on the scale indicating preferences relative to all diseases described. As an example if they place a disease state at 70 on the scale, the disease state is given a score of 0.7 QALYs.

The second method for determining patient preference (or utility) scores is the standard gamble method. For this method, each subject is offered two alternatives. Alternative one is treatment with two possible outcomes: either the return to normal health or immediate death. Alternative two is the certain outcome of a chronic disease state for life. The probability (p) of dying is varied until the subject is indifferent be-

TABLE 8–8. SELECTED QALY ESTIMATES

Disease State	QALY Estimate
Complete health	1.00
Moderate angina	0.83
Breast cancer: removed breast, unconcerned	0.80
Severe angina	0.53
Cancer spread; constant pain; tired; not expected to live long	0.16
Death	0.00

SOURCE: *From Kaplan.[11]*

tween alternative one and alternative two. As an example, a person considers two options: a kidney transplant with a 20% probability of dying during the operation (alternative one) or dialysis for the rest of his life (alternative two). If this percent is his point of indifference (he would not have the operation if the chances of dying during the operation were any higher than 20%), the QALY is calculated as $1 - p$ or 0.8 QALY.

The third technique for measuring health preferences is the time trade-off method. Again the subject is offered two alternatives. Alternative one is a certain disease state for a specific length of time t, the life expectancy for a person with the disease, then death. Alternative two is being healthy for time x, which is less than t. Time x is varied until the respondent is indifferent between the two alternatives. The proportion of the number of years of life a person is willing to give up $(t - x)$ to have her remaining years (x) of life in a healthy state is used to assess her QALY estimate. For example, a person with a life expectancy of 50 years is given two options: being blind for 50 years or being completely healthy (including being able to see) for 25 years. If the person is indifferent between these two options (she would rather be blind than give up any more years of life), the QALY for this disease state (blindness) would be 0.5. Table 8–8 contains examples of disease states and QALY estimates for each disease state listed.

As one might surmise, QALY measurement is not regarded as being as precise or "scientific" as natural health unit measurements (like blood pressure and cholesterol levels) used in CEAs. Some issues in the measurement of QALYs are debated in the literature. One issue concerns whose viewpoint is the most valid. An advantage of having patients with the disease of interest determine health state scores is that these patients may understand the effects of the disease better than the general population, whereas some believe these patients would provide a biased view of their disease compared with other diseases. Some contend that health care professionals could provide good estimates because they understand various diseases, and others argue that these professionals may not rate discomfort and disability as seriously as patients or the general population.

Another issue that has been addressed regarding patient preference or utility score measures is the debate over which is the "best" measure. Utility scores calculated using one method may differ from those using another. Finally, utility measures have been criticized for not being sensitive to small, but clinically meaningful, changes in health status.

Example

An article by Kennedy and co-workers[12] assessed the costs and utilities associated with two common chemotherapy regimens (vindesine and cisplatin [VP], and cyclophosphamide, doxorubicin, and cisplatin [CAP]) and compared the results with the costs and utilities of using best supportive care (BSC) in patients with non–small cell lung cancer. The perspective was that of the health care system, or the payer. Using the time-trade off (TTO) method, treatment utility scores were estimated by members of the oncology ward. Although the chemotherapy regimens provide a longer survival (VP = 214 days, CAP = 165 days) than BSC (112 days), the quality of life TTO score was higher for BSC (0.61) compared with the chemotherapy regimens (0.34). When survival time is multiplied by the TTO scores, the use of BSC results in an estimated 0.19 QALYs, which is similar to VP (0.19 QALYs), but higher than CAP (0.15 QALY). The costs to the health care system for the three options are about $5,000 for BSC, $10,000 for VP, and $7,000 for CAP.* Cost-utility ratios are calculated similarly to cost-effectiveness ratios, except that the outcome unit is QALYs. Therefore the cost-utility ratio is about $26,000/QALY for BSC and about $44,000 to $52,000/QALY for the chemotherapy regimens. Because BSC is at least as effective, as measured by QALYs, and is less expensive than the other two options, a marginal cost-utility ratio does not need to be calculated. Marginal cost utility ratios only need to be calculated to estimate the added cost for an added benefit, not when the added benefit comes at a lower cost.

Performing an Economic Analysis

Conducting a pharmacoeconomic analysis can be challenging. Resources (time, expertise, data, money) are limited. Data used to construct a model may be impossible to obtain due to lack of computer automation. Comparative studies of drug treatments may not be available or poorly designed. Results of clinical trials may not apply at the institution performing the analysis due to lack of resources.

---

*The authors reported median costs instead of average costs due to the non-normality of the cost data.

Methods for conducting a pharmacoeconomic analysis have been described. All four types of analyses described (CMA, CBA, CEA, and CUA) should follow 10 general steps. A modified practical approach to these steps based on the work developed by Jolicoeur and colleagues[13] will be reviewed.

STEP 1: DEFINE THE PROBLEM

This step is self-explanatory. What is the question or objective that is the focus of the analysis? An example might be, "The objective of the analysis is to determine what medications for the treatment of urinary tract infections (UTIs) should be included on our formulary." Perhaps one of the drugs being evaluated is a new drug recently approved by the FDA. Should the new drug be added to the drug formulary? The important thing to remember in this step is to be specific.

STEP 2: DETERMINE THE STUDY'S PERSPECTIVE

It is important to identify from whose perspective the analysis will be conducted. As mentioned in the Assessment of Costs section, this will determine the costs to be evaluated. Is the analysis being conducted from the perspective of the patient or from that of the hospital, clinic, insurance company, or society? Depending on the perspective assigned to the analysis, different results and recommendations based on those results may be identified. If you are deciding on whether to add a new antibiotic to your formulary for treating UTIs, the perspective of the institution or payer would probably be used.

STEP 3: DETERMINE SPECIFIC TREATMENT ALTERNATIVES AND OUTCOMES

In this step, all treatment alternatives to be compared in the analysis should be identified. This selection should include the best clinical options and/or the options that are used most often in that setting at the time of the study. If a new treatment option is being considered, comparing it with an outdated treatment or a treatment with low efficacy rates is a waste of time and money. This new treatment should be compared with the next best alternative or the alternative it may replace. Keep in mind that alternatives may include drug treatments and nondrug treatments. For the UTI example, a new antibiotic would probably be compared with nitrofurantoin or sulfa drugs, or even the use of cranberry juice—"old" or "gold standard" therapy—but still the usual and most commonly used therapy. Today's expensive new chemical entities are very unlikely to cost less than the standard therapy, so they are often compared to the most recent, most expensive drug used as alternative therapy.

The outcomes of those alternatives should include all anticipated positive and negative consequences or events that can be measured. Remember, outcomes may be measured in a variety of ways—lives saved, emergency room visits, hospitalizations, adverse drug reactions, dollars saved, QALYs, and so forth. For the UTI example, cure rates would be the most important outcome.

STEP 4: SELECT THE APPROPRIATE PHARMACOECONOMIC METHOD OR MODEL

The pharmacoeconomic method selected will depend on how the outcomes are measured (see Table 8–1). Costs (inputs) for all four types of analyses are measured in dollars. When all outcomes for each alternative are expected to be the same, a CMA is used. If all outcomes for each alternative considered are measured in monetary units, a CBA is used. When outcomes of each treatment alternative are measured in the same nonmonetary units, a CEA is used. When patient preferences for alternative treatments are being considered, a CUA is used. For the UTI example, cure rates are a natural clinical unit measure, so a CEA would be conducted.

STEP 5: MEASURE INPUTS AND OUTCOMES

All resources consumed by each alternative should be identified and measured in monetary value. The cost for each alternative should be listed and estimated (see Assessment of Costs section). The types of costs that will be measured will depend on the perspective chosen in step 2. When evaluating alternatives over a long period of time (e.g., greater than 1 year), the concept of discounting should be applied. For the UTI example, if the perspective is an acute-care hospital, only inpatient costs of treatment are measured. If the perspective is that of the third-party payer, all direct medical costs for the treatment are included whether they are provided on an inpatient or outpatient basis.

Measuring outcomes can be relatively simple (e.g., cure rates) or relatively difficult (e.g., QALYs). Outcomes may be measured prospectively or retrospectively. Prospective measurements tend to be more accurate and complete, but may take considerably more time and resources than retrospective data retrieval. For the UTI example, cure rates attributed to the new product may be estimated from previous clinical trials, expert opinion, or measured prospectively in the population of interest.

STEP 6: IDENTIFY THE RESOURCES NECESSARY TO CONDUCT THE ANALYSIS

The availability of resources to conduct the study is an important consideration. Lack of access to important data can severely limit the validity of an analysis, as can the accuracy of the data itself. Data may be obtained from a variety of sources, including clinical trials, medical literature, medical records, prescription profiles, or computer databases. Before proceeding with the project, evaluate whether reliable sources of data are accessible or the data can be collected within the timeframe and budget allocated for the project.

STEP 7: ESTABLISH THE PROBABILITIES FOR THE OUTCOMES OF THE TREATMENT ALTERNATIVES

Probabilities for the outcomes identified in step 3 should be determined. This may include the probability of treatment failures or success or adverse reactions to a given treatment or alternative. Data for these can be obtained from the medical literature, clinical trials, medical records, expert opinion, prescription databases, as well as institutional databases. For the UTI example, probabilities of a cure rate for the new medication can be found in clinical trials or obtained from the FDA approved labeling information. Probabilities of cure rates for the previous treatments (e.g., sulfas) can also be found in clinical trials or by accessing medical records. If prospective data collection is conducted, the probabilities of all alternatives will be directly measured instead of estimated.

STEP 8: CONSTRUCT A DECISION TREE

Decision analysis can be a very useful tool when conducting a pharmacoeconomic analysis (see the section on Decision Analysis for a step-by-step review). Constructing a decision tree creates a graphic display of the outcomes of each treatment alternative and the probability of their occurrence. Costs associated with each treatment alternative can be determined and the respective cost ratios derived. An example using a decision tree will be provided in the Decision Tree Analysis section.

STEP 9: CONDUCT A SENSITIVITY ANALYSIS

Whenever estimates are used, there is a possibility that these estimates are not precise. These estimates may be referred to as "assumptions." For example, if the researcher assumes the discount rate is 5%, or assumes the efficacy rate found in clinical trials will be the same as the effectiveness rate in the general population, this is a "best guess" used to conduct the calculations. A sensitivity analysis allows one to determine how the results of an analysis would change when these "best guesses" or assumptions are varied over a relevant range of values. For example, if the researcher makes the assumption that the appropriate discount rate is 5%, this estimate should be varied from 0% to 10% to determine if the same alternative would still be chosen within this range.

This method will help determine the "robustness" of the analysis. Do small changes in probabilities produce significant differences in the outcomes of the treatment alternatives? Another example of a sensitivity analysis will be provided in the Decision Analysis section.

STEP 10: PRESENT THE RESULTS

The results of the analysis should be presented to the appropriate audience, such as P&T committees, medical staff, or third-party payers. The steps outlined in this section should be employed when presenting the results. State the problem, identify the perspective, and so on. It is imperative to acknowledge or clarify any assumptions.

Although none of the above models are perfect, their utility may lead to better decision making when faced with the often difficult task of evaluating new drugs or technology for health care systems.

What Is Decision Analysis?

Decision analysis is a tool that can help visualize a pharmacoeconomic analysis. Decision analysis is the application of an analytical method for systematically comparing different decision options. A key word (decision analysis) search in MEDLINE and International Pharmaceutical Abstracts (IPA) revealed that approximately one-half of the over 1000 citations and almost all of the 134 decision analysis citations, respectively, were published in the 1990s. Decision analysis graphically displays choices and performs the calculations needed to compare these options. It assists with selecting the best or most cost-effective alternative. Decision analysis is a tool that has been utilized for years in many fields, but has been applied to medical decision making more frequently in the last 10 years. This method of analysis assists in making decisions when the decision is complex and there is uncertainty about some of the information.

Discussions of the medical uses of decision analysis have been included in collections of pharmacoeconomic bibliographies,[14-18] and in such specific topic areas as cost-effectiveness studies,[19] CUAs,[20] CBAs,[21] CMAs,[22] policies,[23] formulary processes,[24] pharmacy practices,[25] and drug product development.[26]

STEPS IN DECISION ANALYSIS

The steps in the decision process are enumerated in greater detail in several articles[27-30] and are relatively straightforward, especially with the availability of computer programs that greatly simplify the calculations.[31] Articles reporting a decision analysis should include a picture of the decision tree, including the costs and probabilities utilized. The steps in a decision analysis will be outlined using the UTI example. The steps involved in performing a decision analysis include the following.

Step One: Identify the Specific Decision (a Therapeutic or Medical Problem)

Clearly define the specific decision to be evaluated (what is the objective of the study?). Over what period of time will the analysis be conducted (the episode of care, a year, etc.)? Will the perspective be that of the ill patient, the medical care plan, an institution/organization, or society? Specifying who will be responsible for the costs of the treatment will determine how costs are measured. For the UTI example, the decision was whether to add a new antibiotic to the formulary to treat UTIs. The perspective was that of the institution and the time period is 2 weeks.

Step Two: Specify Alternatives (in the Simplest Form, Two Different Drugs or Treatments, A or B)

Ideally, the two most effective treatments or alternatives should be compared. In pharmacotherapy evaluations, makers of innovative new products may compare or measure themselves against a standard (read as older, more well-established) therapy. This is most often the case with new chemical entities. For pharmaceutical products, dosage and duration of therapy should be included. When analyzing costs and outcomes of pharmaceutical services, these services should be described in detail. For the UTI example, the use of the new medication (drug A) will be compared with that of a sulfa drug (drug B).

Step Three: Specify Possible Outcomes and Probabilities

Consequences and outcomes calculated in dollars yield a CBA; in natural medical units, such as mg/dL, a CEA. For each potential outcome, an estimated probability must be determined (e.g., 95% probability of a cure, or a 7% incidence of side effects). Table 8–9 shows the outcomes and probabilities for the UTI example.

TABLE 8–9. OUTCOMES AND PROBABILITIES, UTI EXAMPLE

	Drug A	Drug B
Effectiveness probability	.95	.85
Side effect probability	.05	.15
Cost of medication	$120	$100
Cost of side effects	$50	$50

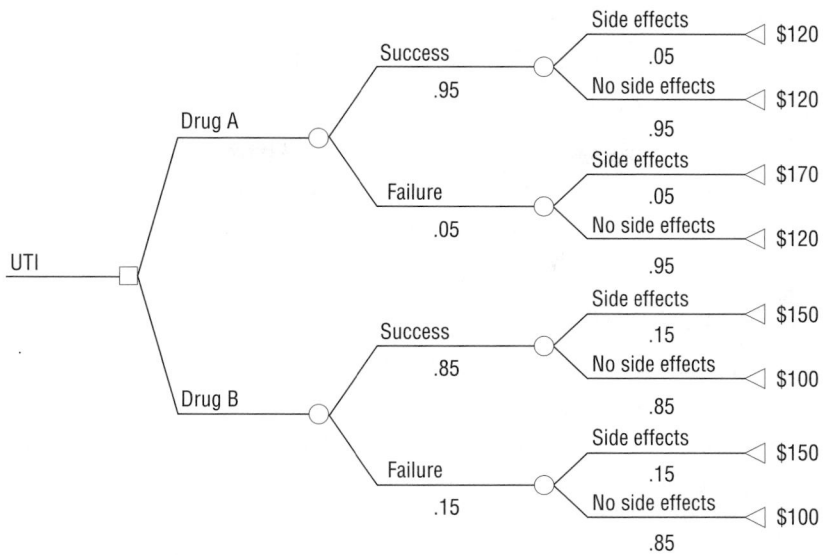

Figure 8–2. Decision tree for UTI example.

Step Four: Draw the Decision Analysis Structure

Lines are drawn to joint decision points (branches or arms of a decision tree), represented either as choice nodes, chance nodes, or final outcomes. Nodes are places in the decision tree where decisions are allowed; a branching becomes possible at this point. There are three types of nodes: (1) a choice node is where a choice is allowed (as between two drugs or two treatments), (2) a chance node is a place where chance (natural occurrence) may influence the decision or outcome expressed as a probability, and (3) a terminal node is the final outcome of interest for that decision. Probabilities are assigned for each possible outcome and the sum of the probabilities must add up to one. Most computer-aided software programs utilize a square box to represent a choice node, a circle to represent a chance node, and a triangle for a terminal branch or final outcome. Figure 8–2 illustrates the decision tree for the UTI example.

TABLE 8–10. CALCULATIONS EXAMPLE: DECISION ANALYSIS CALCULATIONS FOR DRUG A

Drug A	Cost	Probability	Probability × Cost
Outcome 1	$120 + $50 = $170	0.95 × 0.05 = 0.0475	$8.08
Outcome 2	$120	0.95 × 0.95 = 0.9025	$108.30
Outcome 3	$120 + 50 = $170	0.05 × 0.05 = 0.0025	$0.42
Outcome 4	$120	0.05 × 0.95 = 0.0475	$5.70
Total		1	$122.50

TABLE 8–11. CALCULATIONS EXAMPLE: DECISION ANALYSIS CALCULATIONS FOR DRUG B

Drug B	Cost	Probability	Probability × Cost
Outcome 1	$100 + $50 = $150	0.85 × 0.15 = 0.1275	$19.12
Outcome 2	$100	0.85 × 0.85 = 0.7225	$72.25
Outcome 3	$100 + $50 = $150	0.15 × 0.15 = 0.0225	$3.38
Outcome 4	$100	0.15 × 0.85 = 0.1275	$12.75
Total		1	$107.50

Step Five: Perform Calculations

The first consideration should be the present value, or cost, of money. If the study is over a period of less than 1 year, actual costs are utilized in the calculations. If the study period is greater than 1 year, then costs should be discounted (converted to present value). For each branch of the tree, costs are totaled and multiplied by the probability of that arm of the tree. These numbers (costs × probabilities) calculated for each arm of the option are added for each alternative. Example calculations are given in Tables 8–10, 8–11, and 8–12. The UTI example would be a cost-effectiveness type of study, so the difference in the cost for each arm would be divided by the difference in effectiveness for each arm to produce a marginal cost-effectiveness ratio (see Table 8–12).

Step Six: Conduct a Sensitivity Analysis (Vary Cost Estimates)

Because these models are constructed with our best guesses, a sensitivity analysis is conducted. The highest and lowest estimates of costs and probabilities are inserted into the equations, to determine the best case and worse case answers. These estimates should be sufficiently varied to reflect all possible true variations in values. For the UTI example, the new drug (drug A) would be added to the formulary if the committee thought the added cost ($150) was worth the added benefit (one more successful treatment) (see Table 8–12). Some might not agree with the probability of the side effects of drug A; however, because the therapy is new, they may believe 5% may be an underestimate. If we increase this estimate to a 10% side effect rate for the new drug and recalculate the marginal cost-effectiveness ratio, the recalculated ratio would be $175 per added treatment success. Again the committee would have to decide if the added cost is worth the added benefit.

TABLE 8–12. MARGINAL COST-EFFECTIVENESS RATIO FOR EXAMPLE

	Alternative Costs of Drug and Treating Side Effects	Effectiveness in Treating UTI	Marginal Cost per Treatment Success
Drug A	$122.50	95%	$\dfrac{\$122.50 - 107.50}{0.95 - 0.85} = \$150$
Drug B	$107.50	85%	

Decision analysis is being used more commonly in pharmacoeconomic evaluations. The use and availability of computer programs[32] to assist with the multiple calculations makes it fairly easy for someone to automate their evaluations.[33]

Steps in Reviewing Published Literature

It is more likely, as a practicing pharmacist, that you will be asked to evaluate published literature on the topic of pharmacoeconomics, rather than actually conduct a study. When evaluating the pharmacoeconomics literature for making a formulary decision, or selecting a "best" product for your institution, a systematic approach to evaluating the pharmacoeconomics literature can make your task easier.

Several authors[13,33–37] cite methodology to assist in systematically reviewing the pharmacoeconomic literature. If a study is carefully reviewed to ensure the author(s) included all meaningful components of an economic evaluation, the likelihood of finding valid and useful results is high. The steps for evaluating studies are similar to the steps for conducting studies, because the readers are determining if the proper steps were followed when the researcher conducted the study. When evaluating a pharmacoeconomic study, at least the following 10 questions should be considered.

1. Was a well-defined question posed in an answerable form? The specific questions and hypotheses should be clearly stated at the beginning of the article.
2. Is the perspective of the study addressed? The perspective should be explicitly stated, not implied.
3. Were the appropriate alternatives considered? Head-to-head comparisons of the best alternatives provide more information than comparing a new product or service with an outdated or ineffective alternative.
4. Was a comprehensive description of the competing alternatives given? If products are compared, dosage and length of therapy should be included. If services are compared, explicit details of the services make the paper more useful. Could another researcher replicate the study based on the information given?
5. What type of analysis was conducted? The paper should address if a CMA, CEA, CBA, or CUA was conducted. Some studies may conduct more than one type of analysis (i.e., a combination of a CEA and a CUA). Some studies, especially older published studies, incorrectly placed in the title of the article a reference to a benefit or effectiveness analysis, when many were actually CMA studies.
6. Were all the important and relevant costs and outcomes included? Check to see that all pertinent costs and consequences were mentioned. Compare their list to your practice situation.

7. Was there justification for any important costs or consequences that were not included? Sometimes, the authors will admit that although certain costs or consequences are important, they were impractical (or impossible) to measure in their study. It is better that the authors state these limitations, than to ignore them.

8. Was discounting appropriate? If so, was it conducted? If the treatment cost or outcomes are extrapolated for more than 1 year, the time-value of money must be incorporated into the cost estimates.

9. Are all assumptions stated? Were sensitivity analyses conducted for these assumptions? Many of the values used in pharmacoeconomic studies are based on assumptions. For example, authors may assume the side effect rate is 5%, or that compliance with a regimen will be 80%. These types of assumptions should be stated explicitly. For important assumptions, was the estimate varied within a reasonable range of values?

10. Was an unbiased summary of the results presented? Sometimes, the conclusions seem to overstate or overextrapolate the data presented in the results section. Did the authors use unbiased reasonable estimates when determining the results? In general, do you believe the results of the study?

Many articles, several journals, and numerous texts have been devoted to pharmacoeconomics. Research and further development and refinement of the analysis tools are ongoing. We can expect the literature on pharmacoeconomics to continue to expand rapidly, not only for use in proving the value of new therapies, but invalidating the worth of standard therapies. Draugalis,[33] Baskin,[34] and Greenhalgh[35] among others, cite references to assist readers in understanding and assessing economic analyses of health care, as well as providing checklists (with examples and explanations) to evaluate published articles.

Selected Pharmacoeconomics Web Sites

Articles that provide an overview of the field of pharmacoeconomics, its changing methodologies, and recent advances can often be found at Internet sites devoted to this area of specialization. These sites usually highlight articles that may not be drug or therapy specific, but many present an overview or validation of methodologies. Several pharmacoeconomic web sites are included as references. They were selected because they include multiple links to other pharmacoeconomic related sites.

- Canadian Coordinating Office of Health Technology Assessment <<http://www.ccohta.ca>>
- Cochrane Collaboration Home Page <<http://hiru.mcmaster.ca/cochrane>>
- Department of Defense Pharmacoeconomic Center <<http://www.pec.ha.osd.mil>>
- HealthEconomics.Com <<http://www.healtheconomics.com>>
- Institute of Health Economics <<http://www.ipe.ab.ca>>
- International Society for Pharmacoeconomics and Outcomes Research <<http://www.ispor.org/links.html>>
- Pharmaceutical Economics and Policy (University of Southern California) <<http://www.usc.edu/go/pharmecon>>

Conclusion

Many pharmacy and therapeutics committees continue to be challenged with managing costs of pharmacotherapy. Pharmacoeconomic models can be useful tools for evaluating the costs of pharmaceuticals. The ability to objectively measure and compare costs may also produce better decisions about the choice of pharmaceuticals for a formulary. Decision analysis is one of the many tools finding increased utilization in the field of medicine, and pharmacoeconomics specifically. As the science of pharmacoeconomics becomes more standardized, rigorous comparisons among several papers on the same topic will be possible (and necessary).

Study Questions

1. Describe the differences in CEA, CBA, CMA, and CUA.

2. What are the steps in the decision analysis process?

3. Why is a sensitivity analysis performed as part of the decision analysis?

4. Will all articles presenting pharmacoeconomic studies contain essentially the same "parts" of a study? Why?

REFERENCES

1. U.S. Department of Health and Human Services. CDER 1998 report to the nation. January 1998.

2. Mehl B, Santell JP. Projecting future drug expenditures—1998. Am J Health-Syst Pharm 1998; 55:127–36.

3. Bootman JL, Townsend RJ, McGhan WF. Introduction to pharmacoeconomics. In: Bootman JL, Townsend RJ, McGhan WF, editors. Principles of pharmacoeconomics. 2nd ed. Cincinnati (OH): Harvey Whitney Books; 1996. p. 5–11.

4. Nadel HL. Formulary conversion from glipizide to glyburide: A cost-minimization analysis. Hosp Pharm 1995;30(6):467–9, 472–4.

5. Farmer KC, Schwartz WJ, Rayburn WF, Turnball G. A cost-minimization analysis of intracervical Prostaglandin E_2 for cervical ripening in an outpatient versus inpatient setting. Clin Ther 1996;18(4):747–56.

6. Mithani H, Brown G. The economic impact of once-daily versus conventional administration of gentamicin and tobramycin. PharmacoEconomics 1996;10(5):494–503.

7. Bjornson DC, Hiner WO, Potyk RP, Nelson BA, Lombardo FA, Morton TA, et al. Effects of pharmacists on health care outcomes in hospitalized patients. Am J Hosp Pharm 1993;50: 1875–84.

8. Jackson LA, Schuchat A, Gorsky RD, Wenger JD. Should college students be vaccinated against meningococcal disease? A cost-benefit analysis. Am J Public Health 1995;85(6):843–5.

9. Bloom BS, Hillman AL, LaMont B, Liss C, Schwartz JS, Stever GJ. Omeprazole or ranitidine plus metoclopramide for patients with severe erosive oesophagitis. PharmacoEconomics 1995;8(4): 343–9.

10. Law AV, Pathak DS, Segraves AM, Weinstein CR, Arneson WH. Cost-effectiveness analysis of the conversion of patients with non-insulin-dependent diabetes mellitus from glipizide to glyburide and of the accompanying pharmacy follow-up clinic. Clin Ther 1995;17(5):977–87.

11. Kaplan RM. Utility assessment for estimating quality-adjusted life years. In: Sloan FA, editor. Valuing health care: costs, benefits, and effectiveness of pharmaceuticals and other medical technologies. Cambridge (NY): Cambridge University Press; 1995.

12. Kennedy W, Reinharz D, Tessier G, Contandriopoulos AP, Trabut I, Champagne F, et al. Cost-utility analysis of chemotherapy and best supportive care in non-small cell lung cancer. PharmacoEconomics 1995;8(4):316–23.

13. Jolicoeur LM, Jones-Grizzle AJ, Boyer JG. Guidelines for performing a pharmacoeconomic analysis. Am J Hosp Pharm 1992;49:1741–7.

14. McGhan WF, Lewis NJW. Basic bibliographies: pharmacoeconomics. Hosp Pharm 1992; 27:547–8.

15. Wanke LA, Huber SL. Basic bibliographies: cancer therapy pharmacoeconomics. Hosp Pharm 1994;29:402.

16. Skaer TL, Williams LM. Basic bibliographies: biotechnology pharmacoeconomics I. Hosp Pharm 1994;29:1053–4.

17. Skaer TL, Williams LM. Basic bibliographies: biotechnology pharmacoeconomics II. Hosp Pharm 1994;29:1136.

18. McGhan WF. Basic bibliographies: pharmacoeconomics. Hosp Pharm 1998;33:1270, 1273.

19. Duggan AE, Tolley K, Hawkey CJ, Logan RF. Varying efficacy of *Helicobacter pylori* eradication regimens: cost effectiveness study using a decision analysis model. Br Med J 1998;316:1648–54.

20. Messori A, Trippoli S, Becagli P, Cincotta M, Labbate MG, Zaccara G. Adjunctive lamotrigine therapy in patients with refractory seizures: a lifetime cost-utility analysis. Eur J Clin Pharmacol 1998;53(6):421–7.

21. Ginsberg G, Shani S, Lev B. Cost benefit analysis of risperidone and clozapine in the treatment of schizophrenia in Israel. PharmacoEconomics 1998:Feb 13;231–41.

22. Sesti AM, Armitstead JA, Hall KN, Jang R, Milne S. Cost-minimization analysis of hand held nebulizer vs metered dose inhaler protocol for management of acute asthma exacerbations in the emergency department. ASHP Midyear Clinical Meeting; 32: MCS-7: 1997: New Oreleans, December 8–12, 1996.

23. Hinman AR, Koplan JP, Orenstein WA, Brink EW. Decision analysis and polio immunization policy. Am J Public Health 1988;78:301–3.

24. Kessler JM. Decision analysis in the formulary process. Am J Health-Syst Pharm 1997;54:S5–S8.

25. Einarson TR, McGhan WF, Bootman JL. Decision analysis applied to pharmacy practice. Am J Hosp Pharm 1985;42:364–71.

26. Walking D, Appino JP. Decision analysis in drug product development. Drug Cosmet Ind 1973; 112:39–41.

27. Rascati KL. Decision analysis techniques practical aspects of using personal computers for decision analytic modeling. Drug Benefit Trends 1998;July:33–6.

28. Richardson WS, Detsky AS. Users' guides to the medical literature. Part 7. How to use a clinical decision analysis. Part A. Are the results of the study valid? JAMA 1995;273:1292–5.

29. Richardson WS, Detsky AS. Users' guides to the medical literature. Part 7. How to use a clinical decision analysis. Part B. What are the results and will they help me in caring for my patients? JAMA 1995;273:1610–3.

30. Baskin LE. Practical pharmacoeconomics. Cleveland (OH): Advanstar Communications; 1998.

31. Decision tree and influence diagram software [cited 1999 Sept 21]: Available from: URL: http://faculty.fuqua.duke.edu/daweb/dasw6.htm.

32. Sacristán JA, Soto J, Galende I. Evaluation of pharmacoeconomic studies: utilization of a checklist. Ann Pharmacother 1993;27:1126–32.

33. Draugalis JR. Assessing pharmacoeconomic studies. In: Bootman JL, Townsend RJ, McGhan WF, editors. Principles of pharmacoeconomics. Cincinnati: Harvey Whitney Books; 1996. pp. 278–89.

34. Baskin LE. How to evaluate the validity and usefulness of pharmacoeconomic literature. In: Practical pharmacoeconomics. Cleveland: Advanstar Communications; 1998. pp. 95–102.

35. Greenhalgh T. How to read a paper: Papers that tell you what things cost (economic analyses). Br Med J 1997;315:596–9.

36. Drummond MF, Richardson WS, O'Brien BJ, Levine M, Heyland D. Users' guides to the medical literature. XIII. How to use an article on economic analysis of clinical practice. A. Are the results of the study valid? Evidence-Based Medicine Working Group. JAMA 1997;277(19): 1552–7.

37. O'Brien BJ, Heyland D, Richardson WS, Levine M, Drummond MF. Users' guides to the medical literature. XIII. How to use an article on economic analysis of clinical practice. B. What are the results and will they help me in caring for my patients? Evidence-Based Medicine Working Group [published erratum appears in JAMA 1997; Oct 1:278(13):1064]. JAMA 1997:277(22); 1802–6.

9

Chapter Nine

Evidence-Based Clinical Practice Guidelines

Kevin G. Moores

Objectives

After completing this chapter, the reader will be able to:

- Define clinical practice guidelines.
- Describe the role of clinical practice guidelines in pharmacy practice and the pharmacist's role in development and use of these guidelines.
- Identify various sources of published guidelines and organizations currently involved in guideline activities.
- Describe various intended purposes for the development and implementation of clinical practice guidelines.
- Explain the methodology for development of clinical practice guidelines.
- Describe the critical process of the systematic review of scientific evidence to assess clinical benefits and harms of therapeutic interventions in the early steps for drafting clinical practice guidelines.
- Apply structured criteria to evaluate the validity of clinical practice guidelines.
- Identify the key issues in interpreting clinical practice guidelines and issues involved in their implementation.
- Explain the interdependent relationship between clinical practice guidelines and outcomes research.
- Describe how clinical practice guidelines are used in a continuous quality improvement process.
- Describe the use of practice guidelines to strengthen the dialogue between patients and health care providers with the goal of empowering the patient to participate in a shared decision making process.

Evidence-based clinical practice guidelines are "systematically developed statements to assist practitioner and patient decisions about health care for specific circumstances."[1] Clinical practice guidelines are developed by a variety of groups and organizations including federal and state government, professional societies and associations, managed care organizations, third-party payers, quality assurance organizations, and utilization review groups. The purpose of the guidelines, development methods used, format of the documents, and the strategies for dissemination or implementation vary widely. Considering the potential for clinical practice guidelines to influence thousands to millions of decisions on medical interventions, it is incumbent upon all health care practitioners to be thoroughly familiar with criteria to judge the validity of guidelines, and be skilled in determining their appropriate application.

Development and implementation of clinical practice guidelines has many characteristics in common with traditional activities performed by drug information practitioners, such as evaluation of new drugs for formulary consideration, medication use evaluation, and quality improvement. Many of the skills required for guideline development are required of drug information practitioners, including literature search and evaluation, epidemiology, biostatistics, clinical expertise, writing, editing, formatting, and education. Drug information practitioners benefit from the use of clinical practice guidelines as information resources for their work, and are logical professionals to participate in guideline development and implementation.

The primary attraction for health care practitioners in properly developed, valid practice guidelines is that they provide a concise summary of current best evidence on what works and what does not in consideration of specific health care interventions. New information and technology in health care are developed at a rapid pace. It is very difficult for individual practitioners to systematically evaluate the benefits and risks of all new technology, including drugs. By presenting a summary of best evidence, guidelines assist the practitioner in decision making for specific patients and also facilitate discussion of care options most consistent with individual patient needs and preferences. Guidelines may also enhance provider communication and continuity of care, especially when decisions are made by multiple providers in different care settings.[2]

There is a growing awareness in health care that a significant time lag occurs in getting research information into practice. There are several examples of treatments that have been well studied and proven effective that are substantially underutilized, and interventions that have been proven ineffective or harmful that continue to be provided.[3] One of the goals of development and implementation of evidence-based clinical practice guidelines is to help speed up the process of "getting evidence into practice."

Clinical practice guidelines to assist with health care decision making and identify indicators for monitoring quality of care are frequently mentioned in connection with efforts to improve quality and efficiency of services. The key issues in reorganizing the

U.S. health care system are access to care, cost, and quality. Quality currently is a major focus as evidenced by recent legislative proposals for specific requirements of health insurance coverage, patients' bill of rights, as well as the critical recommendations in the report from the President's Advisory Commission on Consumer Protection and Quality in the Health Care Industry[3]; and the conclusions of The Institute of Medicine National Roundtable on Health Care Quality.[4]

Methods currently recommended as the most valid for development of clinical practice guidelines emphasize an evidence-based approach, formal quantitative techniques to calculate risks and benefits, and incorporation of the patient's preference. The concepts of an evidence-based approach and use of the rules of evidence are critical elements that will be reviewed in detail in this chapter in the section on methodology for clinical practice guideline development. The "evidence-based health care" movement, and the implementation of continuous quality improvement programs have stimulated growth in guideline development. There have also been advancements in methods of evaluating and summarizing the best available evidence, for example, systematic reviews, meta-analyses, and decision analyses. Development of new information databases of systematic reviews, and new informatics resources facilitate the production of clinical practice guidelines and improve access to this information.

This chapter presents a review of the background for why clinical practice guidelines have become a common element in health care; describes the activities of selected major organizations involved with guidelines; reviews evidence-based methods for guideline development, evaluation, and implementation; discusses the role of practice guidelines in quality improvement efforts; and provides directions to locate sources of guidelines and further information.

Historical Background and Review of Key Issues and Publications

Although practice guidelines have been in existence for a long time, the past decade has seen significant changes in emphasis, use, and methods for development. Clinical practice guidelines are being developed throughout the health care industry and have been in most proposals for health care reform including legislation proposed by the Clinton Administration in 1992.[5] A survey of physician medical groups and independent practice associations in 1996 found that 87% were developing or implementing guidelines to accomplish either cost containment or quality improvement goals.[6]

Regardless of the fact that national legislation failed to be enacted, the issues are being addressed at the state level and by business, various third-party payers, and health care providers. The clinically oriented goals of practice guidelines include improving the frequency of appropriate care, reducing unnecessary or inappropriate care, and ultimately improving patient outcomes. The success of clinical practice guidelines in reaching these goals depends on many factors such as appropriate selection of topics, methods of guideline development, implementation strategies, mechanisms of feedback, and incentives to providers.

In the remaining paragraphs of this section, background information on significant issues and key papers published in the last several years that outline the framework for current activities in the development of clinical practice guidelines will be provided. This background information will increase understanding of some of the reasons for the prominent role of clinical practice guidelines in health care reform proposals, and why many health care organizations and providers have become active in this area. This information is in this text for several reasons. (1) A significant percentage of clinical practice guidelines relate to provisions of medications; pharmacists must be prepared to evaluate guidelines and know when and how to use them when making therapeutic decisions. (2) Until recently the literature on this topic included very little participation by pharmacists. (3) It is important for pharmacists to be aware of the momentum that has been generated in this area. (4) It is essential that pharmacists become more actively involved to ensure that all appropriate considerations are given to pharmaceutical care issues in the development and implementation of clinical practice guidelines.

Without question, one of the key factors leading to the call for increased use of practice guidelines is the rate of growth of health care costs in the United States. Strategies that have been implemented to reduce expenditure growth include new approaches to utilization review, reimbursement via diagnosis-related groups (DRG), encouragement of health maintenance organization enrollments (HMOs), capitation, and a multitude of other measures. However, these strategies have not been sufficient.

According to the Health Care Financing Administration (HCFA) total health care expenses in the United States in 1997 were $1.092 trillion, representing 13.5% of gross domestic product (GDP).[7] Even though health care expenses have stabilized at approximately 13½% of GDP for the past 5 years and the rate of growth in spending has been modest at 5% per year in this period, HCFA analysts projected that beginning in 1998, national health spending would again begin to grow faster than the rest of the economy. By 2002, the agency projected that national health expenditures would total $2.1 trillion, an estimated 16.6% of GDP.[8,9]

As costs for health care have escalated and consequently the cost for health care insurance and employee benefits, many employers have changed from passive payers to aggressive purchasers. As aggressive purchasers, they are exerting more influence over payment rates, where patients receive care, and even the content of care.[9] One way this influence is executed is the encouragement or requirement for providers to use protocols or guidelines for some services. If these protocols or guidelines are developed properly, they have the potential to reduce unnecessary care and unwarranted practice variation. However, there is also the potential to simply restrict access to care.

It is theorized that appropriate use of practice guidelines will result in reduction of unnecessary procedures or treatments, thus resulting in "painless" cost control. For example, it is estimated that the high rates of cesarean section in the United States add more than $1 billion to costs without improving overall neonatal or maternal birth outcomes.[10] Implementation of guidelines could perhaps cut those costs.

An additional factor stimulating interest in guidelines has been the studies showing large variations in the rate with which specific procedures are performed in different geographic areas. Several studies conducted by researchers at Dartmouth, the Rand Corporation, and others have demonstrated significant variation in hospitalization rates, rates of surgery for prostatic hyperplasia, endarterectomy, coronary angiography, and other health care utilization in both inpatient and outpatient settings.[11] The differences in patterns of care could not be explained by case mix, inadequacies in data or methods of analysis, or any other confounding factors. These variations in provision of care were not accompanied by evidence of differences in outcome. The fact that apparently similar patients are treated in such widely different ways casts doubt on the knowledge base, the decision making process, or both. Clinician uncertainty about the relevant risks and benefits for various treatments is thought to be part of the reason for these variations. Providing guidelines that summarize the available evidence and expert opinion would be useful in reducing the magnitude of practice variation and inappropriate care.

Geographic variations in health care continue to be an active area in research. The current medical literature contains several recent studies of practice variation. The President's Advisory Commission report on quality in health care (explained in more detail below) also provides several references related to variations in discharge rates, hysterectomy, cesarean delivery, care for patients with myocardial infarction, diabetes, asthma, hypertension, and many others.[3]

The third key factor proposed to have stimulated growing interest in practice guidelines is research indicating considerable inappropriate use of many services including laboratory tests, diagnostic and surgical procedures, prescription medications, and hospital admissions or length of stay.[1] One example study involved the review of more than 4500 hospital records of Medicare patients. This study found that one-sixth of those undergoing coronary angiography and upper gastrointestinal endoscopy, and one-third of those undergoing carotid endarterectomy, had procedures that a consensus panel considered inappropriate.[12] Another study reported a significant frequency of inappropriate medication prescribing for the elderly.[13] Using data from the 1987 National Medicaid Expenditure Survey, Wilcox and colleagues[13] reviewed data for 6171 people more than 65 years of age for the incidence of prescribing of 20 drugs judged to be inappropriate for use in the elderly. A total of 23.5% of these people received at least one of the contraindicated drugs. A separate study of 1100 California nursing home residents revealed that 21% received inappropriate medications during a 1-month period.[14] When dosage or length of use were considered, inappropriate medication use rose to 40%. Additional examples of more recent studies of failure to achieve targets for accepted care are provided in the section on quality improvement in this chapter. The President's Advisory Commission report states that "there is ample empirical evidence to substantiate the existence of significant overutilization of services, which some have estimated to be as high as 30 percent of total health care delivered in the United States."[15]

A fourth factor that is well recognized by practitioners is that much of health care is characterized by considerable uncertainty about the health outcomes expected from the use or nonuse of various services or treatments. Clinical research documenting the effectiveness of many services does not exist, particularly at the level of very specific patient circumstances.

Whether based on the issue of rising costs, unexplained variations, inappropriate care, or uncertain outcomes, similar conclusions are being reached by many. More research is needed on outcomes and effectiveness of health care services, and the results of this research should be combined with other empirical data to formulate specific, evidence-based clinical practice guidelines.

Three key articles outlining these issues were published in 1988. One was an editorial published in the *New England Journal of Medicine* by Relman[16] stating that the third revolution in medical care was beginning. He called this the "Era of Assessment and Accountability." Relman reviews the issues of the rising costs of health care, which he believes are caused primarily by increasing volume and intensity of medical services. He spoke of the growing concern about the unknown quality and outcomes of many medical services and evidence of the large geographic variations in use of certain services, unaccompanied by difference in outcome. He states that to control costs without arbitrarily reducing access to care or lowering quality, more must be known about the safety, appropriateness, and effectiveness of drugs, tests, and procedures, and the way care is provided. Relman also refers to two other key papers published in 1988: one, by Ellwood, which calls for a major national program of "outcomes management"[17]; and one by Roper and colleagues with HCFA,[18] which describes the federal government's interest in the improvement of clinical practice and assessment of medical effectiveness. Familiarity with the content of the arguments in these papers provides improved understanding of the current "outcomes movement" and the call for greater emphasis on development and use of clinical practice guidelines.

Ellwood[17] states in his article that "the healthcare system has become an organism guided by misguided choices; it is unstable, confused, and desperately in need of a central nervous system that can help it cope with the complexity of modern medicine." He continues by explaining that the problem is the system's inability to measure and understand the effects on the patient's quality of life caused by the choices made by patients, payers, and physicians. "The result is that we have uninformed patients, skeptical payers, frustrated physicians, and besieged healthcare executives."[17]

To react to these problems Ellwood suggests that the system adopt a technology for collaborative action that he labeled "outcomes management." He describes this as a technology of patient experience designed to help patients, payers, and providers make rational medical care–related choices based on better insight into the effect of these choices on the patient's health and quality of life. Ellwood states that outcomes management will draw on four maturing techniques. The first one he mentions is greater reliance on standards and guidelines that can be used in selecting appropriate interventions. Second, Ellwood discusses the techniques for routinely and systematically measuring the functioning and well-being of patients, along with disease-specific clinical outcomes at appropriate time intervals. Third, he mentions the pooling of clinical and outcome data on a massive scale. Powerful information systems, standardized data collection methods, and the ability to integrate data from various sources will be critical to achieving this step. Fourth is analysis and dissemination of results from the database most appropriate to the concerns of each decision maker (providers, patients, policymakers, payers). Through this methodology, outcomes research and clinical practice guidelines work interdependently, with the guidelines delineating the usual care practices and types of data to be collected, and the results of outcomes data being used to update (i.e., improve) practice guidelines. In this way, outcomes management fits the model of continuous quality improvement.

Ellwood also compares outcomes management to the clinical trial in that it consists of the same basic steps: a carefully designed and followed protocol, measurements of results, data pooling, analysis, and dissemination. Outcomes management lacks the purposeful randomization of a clinical trial, but has the advantage of providing information about the results of the natural variations that occur in routine medical practice and would help by providing data on outcomes of patients who would be ineligible for typical clinical trials due to extremes of age, concomitant therapies, or other comorbidities.

Roper and colleagues at HCFA discuss an initiative to evaluate and improve medical practice.[18] They report the decision of the Department of Health and Human Services, through HCFA and the Public Health Services (PHS), to begin an active role in improving the quality of the information that guides medical practice. They state that HCFA sees the assessment of medical effectiveness and the improvement of clinical practice as a process involving the following four steps: (1) monitoring via an ongoing universal database to characterize the health status of the population involved (Medicare beneficiaries), monitoring the outcomes of interventions, and screen for emerging trends; (2) analyzing variations in medical care in terms of both practice patterns and outcomes and conducting more detailed investigation of the causes of outcomes variations; (3) assessing the outcomes of interventions by retrospective or prospective study with observational analysis or randomized controlled trials; and (4) offering feedback and education for practitioners via the peer-review organization (PRO) system, professional societies, journals, medical schools, and the PHS. These initiatives are also designed to link the Department of Health and Human Services with health care providers, researchers, medical educators, private purchasers, and consumer groups in a continuous, long-term, cooperative effort. Roper concludes that these efforts hold valuable possibilities, including better information for practitioners and patients for use in making decisions, improved guidelines for medical practice, greater protection from malpractice suits when guidelines are followed, and improved information for patients to address their expectations.

By 1989, a future role for the federal government in developing practice guidelines received broad-based support. In a January 1989 report to the Bush administration, the National Leadership Commission on Health Care (a blue-ribbon panel, co-chaired by former Presidents Carter, Ford, and Nixon, that included prominent health leaders) recommended expanded federal support for effectiveness research and development of national practice guidelines.[19] In the spring of 1989, Congress introduced a series of bills calling for expanded federal funding for effectiveness research and the creation of a formal Public Health Services agency with responsibility for the development and dissemination of practice guidelines. The practice guideline legislation was strongly supported by organized medicine including the American Medical Association (AMA). This support was provided in part to promote the use of guidelines as an alternative to expenditure targets.

In November 1989, Congress amended the Public Health Service Act to create the Agency for Health Care Policy and Research (AHCPR). Under the terms of Public Law 101-239 (also known as Omnibus Budget Reconciliation Act of 1989 [OBRA '89]) this agency was given responsibility for supporting research, data development, and other activities to "enhance the quality, appropriateness and effectiveness of health care services." The AHCPR was also charged with the responsibility to "arrange for" the development and periodic review and updating of (1) clinically relevant guidelines that may be used by physicians, educators, and health care practitioners to assist in determining how diseases, disorders, and other health conditions can most effectively and appropriately be prevented, diagnosed, treated, and managed clinically; and (2) standards of quality, performance measures, and medical review criteria through which health care providers and other appropriate entities may assess or review the provision of health care and assure the quality of such care.[20] This legislation reflects the increased importance of this issue in national health policy and elevated the activities of the AHCPR to the level of a full PHS agency, on the same level as the Centers for Disease Control, the National Institutes of Health, and the Food and Drug Administration (FDA).

The mission of the AHCPR continues to be to support, conduct, and disseminate research that improves access to care and the outcomes, quality, cost, and utilization of health care services.[21] The specific methods and activities of the Agency have changed. More information about the Agency's current activities is provided in the section on methodology for clinical practice guideline development below.

By the early 1990s, it was clear that analysis of practice variation, outcomes research, and the development of clinical practice guidelines was becoming a major activity within the health care industry. Therefore, to ensure that appropriate considerations are given to pharmaceutical care issues, it is critical that pharmacists be actively involved in the development and implementation of clinical practice guidelines. Pharmacists previously had assumed the health care leadership role in the areas of drug utilization review, drug usage evaluation, drug regimen review, and medication use evaluation. Pharmacists have also been actively and significantly involved in the development and implementation of prescribing guidelines or protocols for restricted use drugs through the Pharmacy and Therapeutics committee process in hospitals, health maintenance organizations, state Medicaid programs and other practice settings (see Chap. 14 for additional information). These activities are similar in nature to clinical practice guideline development and demonstrate that pharmacists have the skills and experience required to be key participants in this process.

Clinical Practice Guidelines and Quality Improvement in Health Care

Quality in health care has emerged as one of the major issues in the U.S. health care system. The national media have focused attention on high profile individual cases of error in health care such as a fatal overdose of cancer chemotherapy, surgery on the wrong limb, and similar incidents. An Associated Press poll conducted in February 1999 found that when asked "What is your biggest concern about health care?" the top two responses were the ability to pick their doctor of choice (28%), followed closely by the quality of care (23%).

There have been exposés on television "news" programs and in popular magazines about pharmacists who did not catch potentially serious drug interactions. The national news also broadcast the results of a meta-analysis of prospective studies which estimated that 2.2 million hospitalized patients experienced a serious adverse drug reaction in 1994, and that there were 106,000 fatal adverse drug reactions (ADRs), which would make this the fourth to sixth leading cause of death.[22] Another study reported that fatal medication errors more than doubled for inpatients from 1983 to 1993, and increased more than eightfold for outpatients.[23]

Donald Berwick from the Institute for Healthcare Improvement recently stated that it is usually easier to defend the status quo than to change it. However, he continued, evidence is mounting that the excellence of the status quo is a sentimental illusion. Berwick advocates using modern systems theory and the "plan-do-study-act" model for continuous quality improvement to redesign the health care system, increase the frequency of appropriate care and improve the health outcomes of patients.[24]

In an editorial published in the New England Journal of Medicine, Marcia Angell, MD, stated "the American health care system is at once the most expensive and the most inadequate system in the developed world, and it is uniquely complicated."[25] In support of this statement she continued, "In 1997 we spent about $4,000 per person on health care, as compared with the next most expensive country, Switzerland, which spent $2,500. Yet 16 percent of our population has no health insurance at all, and many of the rest have only very limited coverage."[25]

Fred Brown, American Hospital Association chairman, speaking at the Association's annual meeting in 1999, emphasized that "as the new millennium approaches, health care providers must work to restore public trust and confidence."[26] It is clear that quality improvement, measurement of quality, and reporting of quality measures are critical components of the health care system.

Evidence-based clinical practice guidelines are an important tool in clinical health care continuous quality improvement programs. Both processes require an analysis of the best available evidence to develop a recommended course of action. Continuous quality improvement has been used in industry for many years and has been slowly implemented in health care over the past decade. Two key national reports related to quality in health care were recently produced, one from the Institute of Medicine (IOM), the other from a Presidential Advisory Commission. Certain aspects of these reports on health care quality have particular importance to clinical practice guidelines and are presented below. Activities of the major organizations in health care quality (e.g., Joint Commission on the Accreditation of Healthcare Organizations [JCAHO], National Committee for Quality Assurance [NCQA], Foundation for Accountability [FACCT], Institute for Healthcare Improvement [IHI], and the American Medical Accreditation Program [AMAP]) also have relevance to clinical practice guidelines.[27-29]

The IOM National Roundtable on Health Care Quality, addressed quality of care problems in the United States.[4] The roundtable identified important issues related to measurement, assessment, and improvement of quality of care and concluded that a national focus on improving health care quality is imperative. The reasons supporting this conclusion included: (1) the quality of health care can be defined and measured, (2) problems in health care quality are serious and extensive, (3) although a number of successes have been achieved in improving quality there is still no clear role model of exemplary delivery systems, and (4) taken together these circumstances require a major effort to rethink and reengineer how we deliver, assess and try to improve the quality of health care services.[4]

For the measurement of health care quality, the IOM roundtable stated that both process and outcome measures were required. They noted that attention must be directed to both populations and individuals and that measurements must be able to assess the quality of the systems of care, not just the performance of individuals. Health care professionals practice within groups and systems of care. The functioning of those systems in preventing errors, coordinating care among settings and various practitioners, and ensuring that relevant and accurate health care information is available when needed, are critical factors in ensuring high-quality care. They emphasized that health care professionals must stay abreast of the dynamic knowledge base in medicine and use that knowledge appropriately.[4] Guidelines are especially intended to support these last two functions.

The roundtable described quality problems as occurring in three categories: (1) underuse—the failure to provide a service when it would have produced a favorable outcome, (2) overuse—a service is provided when its potential for harm exceeds possible benefit, and (3) misuse—an appropriate service has been selected but a preventable complication occurs. The literature over the last few years contains many studies that have documented underuse of effective services. Example of underuse referenced by the roundtable included undetected and untreated hypertension or depression, failure to immunize children, prenatal care begun too late, and failure to use thrombolytics, beta-blockers, aspirin, and angiotensin-converting enzyme (ACE) inhibitors for myocardial infarction. Properly developed and implemented guidelines can help to correct these underuse quality problems. Overuse of health care services is also common in the U.S. system. The roundtable reviewed several studies that documented overuse of antibiotics and a number of different surgical procedures performed for inappropriate indications. The roundtable also reviewed several studies related to misuse and errors in health care.[4]

The IOM roundtable recommended several approaches to quality improvement. Those that have common elements with clinical practice guidelines include improvement in training health care practitioners in the use of the avalanche of rigorous data on efficacy, improvement in the information infrastructure, implementation of continuous quality improvement as an integral part of a scientific (evidence-based) approach to improving clinical practice, and providing patients the opportunity and information needed to participate in decision making about their care. The IOM roundtable provided a great deal of information that is useful for health care practitioners involved in quality improvement activities including development of guidelines. Additional information about the roundtable's work is available at <<http://www.iom.edu/>>.

On March 26, 1997, President Clinton appointed an Advisory Commission to "address changes occurring in the health care system and recommend such measures as may be necessary to promote and assure health care quality and value, and protect consumers and workers in the health care system."[30] Secretary of Health and Human Services, Donna E. Shalala, and the Secretary of Labor, Alexis M. Herman co-chaired this commission. The final report from the Commission was approved on March 12, 1998. The Commission recommended the following statement: "The purpose of the health care system must be to continuously reduce the impact and burden of illness, injury, and disability and to improve the health and functioning of the people of the United States."[30]

The report from the Commission included more than 50 recommendations to advance the effort to improve the quality of health care in the United States. The basic philosophy of the recommendations center on continuous quality improvement. The core aims for improvement set by the commission are to (1) reduce the underlying causes of illness, injury, and disability; (2) expand research on new treatments and evidence of effectiveness; (3) ensure the appropriate use of health care services; (4) reduce health care errors; (5) increase patients' participation in their care; and (6) address oversupply and undersupply of health care resources.

The Commission specifically recommended that the expanded research include basic, clinical, preventive, and health services research. They stated that the continued development and dissemination of evidence-based information can help to guide practitioners' actions and the development and implementation of management policies that can influence practice to improve quality. In an effort for more complete and rapid dissemination of quality of care information, the Commission recommended public and private collaboration to synthesize evidence on effective health care practices, develop practice protocols, and provide technical assistance to practitioners to access and incorporate these guidelines into practice. "Synthesizing the existing clinical literature and developing clinical practice guidelines are essential steps in support of evidence-based health care practices." The Commission also addressed the need to invest in health care information systems to collect, analyze, and provide access to the information for practitioners, patients, and policy decision makers required to support the quality improvement effort and to get evidence into practice.

To focus the health care industry on these goals the Commission recommended creation of two complementary organizations, one public and one private. The public organization, The Advisory Council for Health Care Quality, is charged with identifying national goals and specific objectives for improvement and track progress in meeting those goals and objectives. The Advisory Council also should establish goals and objectives for quality measurement and reporting by health care organizations and providers, and track compliance with the Consumer Bill of Rights and Responsibilities. The Council should report annually to the President and Congress on the Nation's progress in improving health care quality. The private organization, The Forum for Health Care Quality Measurement and Reporting should identify core quality measures for standardized reporting, and promote the focused development of enhanced core measures for the future. The Forum should create and implement a plan for measuring health care quality and reporting the results to the public. The Forum should also coordinate its activity with the Advisory Council. The Commission emphasized that both organizations would include public and private sector representation, and that the public–private coordination and communication were key to the effectiveness of the effort.

On March 13, 1998, President Clinton directed the Secretary of Health and Human Services to establish a Quality Interagency Coordination task force to meet the recommendations of the Quality Commission report, and stated that a permanent Health Care Quality Council should be established by any new health care quality legislation. On June 17, 1998, Vice President Gore launched the planning committee that will create the Forum for Health Care Quality Measurement and Reporting. The Forum will be composed of representatives from provider, purchasing, insurance, accreditation, government, labor unions, and patient communities. In addition to achieving the goals noted above, the Forum is intended to eliminate duplicative and overlapping demands for information from health care providers and plans, which occur because of variable requirements for Medicaid, Medicare, different States, and commercial requests.[31] James R. Tallon Jr., President of the United Hospital Fund of New York, is the executive director of the planning committee for the Forum, and Gail L. Warden, CEO of the Henry Ford Health System, is the committee Chair. More details of the planning committee activities and membership are available at <<http://www.qualityforum.org/>>.

Three major health care accrediting/quality assurance organizations have gotten a jump on the Forum to devise a systematic approach to setting measurement priorities, identifying common criteria to be used in performance measurement, and adopting a standard framework for evaluating new measures. The JCAHO, the NCQA, and the AMAP have established a coordinating body, the Performance Measurement Coordinating Council (PMCC).[32] It is hoped that the PMCC will help to lower costs of performance measurement by reducing redundant or overlapping measurement activities, and make the data more useful by standardizing data requirements among different systems.[33] These organizations are also participating in the planning activities of the Forum.

These efforts to improve coordination, gain efficiency, and improve the value of the results are in essence continuous quality improvement (CQI) efforts in themselves. The data resulting from accreditation and quality assurance programs will be available for use in further improving quality of services. Many of the results will also be useful in the process of producing practice guidelines.

Another responsibility of the President's Commission was to produce a proposed Consumer Bill of Rights and Responsibilities. The proposed bill of rights, released November 20, 1997, addressed issues related to information disclosure, choice of providers and plans, access to emergency care, participation in treatment decisions, respect and nondiscrimination, confidentiality of information, complaints and appeals, and consumer responsibilities for their health and care. The requirement for consumers to have the right and responsibility to fully participate in all decisions related to their health care is particularly related to clinical practice guidelines. The proposal stated that physicians and other health professionals should provide patients with sufficient information and opportunity to decide among treatment options consistent with the informed consent process including all risks, benefits, and consequences to treatment or nontreatment. Clinical practice guidelines serve as a resource to assist in this process. The patient responsibilities included maximizing healthy habits (e.g., diet, exercise, not smoking), working collaboratively with health care providers, and participating in prevention activities. These responsibilities are also consistent with the philosophy of clinical practice guidelines. The full Consumer Bill of Rights and Responsibilities is available at <<http://www.hcqualitycommission.gov/final/append_a.html>>.

Examples of continuous quality improvement programs, that have utilized practice guidelines in the process of improving care, have been published. Since 1992, HCFA has been implementing a CQI approach to ensuring quality of care for its Medicare beneficiaries. The first project of this program is the Cooperative Cardiovascular Project (CCP), which focuses on treatment of patients with acute myocardial infarction (AMI). The CCP began with the development of quality indicators for the treatment of AMI based heavily on clinical practice guidelines from the American College of Cardiology and the American Heart Association.[34] The PROs in Alabama, Connecticut, Iowa, and Wisconsin measured performance on indicators of appropriate use of reperfusion, aspirin, beta-blockers, ACE inhibitors, smoking cessation counseling, and avoidance of calcium channel blockers. The PROs provided the results of compliance rates with the indicators to participating hospitals in their state in 1994, and encouraged implementation of CQI programs for the treatment of AMI. Results of monitoring in 1996 demonstrated improvement on all indicators in the four states, and a reduction in 30-day and 1-year mortality as well. Also in comparison with states not in the project, the performance on the indicators was better and was associated with reduced mortality.

Investigators working with the Minnesota Clinical Comparison and Assessment Program conducted a randomized controlled trial in 37 community hospitals in Minnesota.[35] They studied the use of education provided by opinion leaders and performance feedback to implement clinical practice guidelines to improve quality of care for AMI. The intervention hospitals increased the appropriate use of aspirin from 77% to 90% of patients, and the appropriate use of beta-blockers from 49% to 80%. Both of these changes were significantly better than the control hospitals. The AHCPR was one of the funding agencies in this study.

The AHCPR report "The Challenge and Potential for Assuring Quality Health Care for the 21st Century" references numerous other examples of successful projects in various settings using similar methods to improve quality for coronary artery bypass surgery and angioplasty, reduce unnecessary cesarean delivery, reduce asthma deaths and emergency department visits, increase influenza vaccination rates, reduce pressure ulcers, and prevent adverse drug reactions.[36]

The U.S. Department of Health and Human Services, through many of its operating divisions, has identified improvement in quality of health care and efficiency of health care services as a priority of their activities in 1999 and beyond. The divisions primarily included in this effort are the National Institutes of Health (NIH), the FDA, the Centers for Disease Control and Prevention (CDC), the AHCPR, and HCFA. Some of the specific programs for health care quality improvement (e.g., building the evidence base for health care, putting prevention into practice, and getting evidence into practice) are especially the focus of the AHCPR.

Practice guidelines highlight key clinical information needed at the major decision points in management of a disease, and therefore define the core content of the medical record. Explicit standardized definitions characteristic of good guidelines assist consistent entry of this information into the medical record, and also facilitate the development of objective criteria or indicators for evaluation of care. The purpose of both clinical practice guidelines and evaluation instruments is to increase the quality and value of care. The guideline explores the rationale and evidence behind recommendations for care and the evaluation instruments turn the guideline recommendations into quantifiable measures of care actually provided. A rational approach to the evaluation instrument would be to emphasize the major recommendations of guidelines, especially those well supported by the highest level of scientific evidence to identify aspects of care most likely to relate to overall quality.

Quality of care is a critical emphasis in health care today and clinical practice guidelines are one of the tools that are used in quality improvement efforts. Clinical practice guidelines by themselves are not the solution to quality of care problems, but used within a systems approach and when directed at providing needed valid information to the right people at the right time in the right format, they can improve decision making, reduce errors of omission, and help to correct overuse, underuse, and errors, as called for by the Institute of Medicine National Roundtable and the President's Advisory Commission.

Evidence-Based Practice and Clinical Practice Guidelines

Evidence-based medicine (EBM) is a philosophy of practice and an approach to decision making in the clinical care of patients. Sackett and colleagues[37] have defined EBM as the "conscientious, explicit and judicious use of current best evidence in making decisions about the care of individual patients." The practice of EBM refers to integrating individual clinical expertise with the best available external clinical evidence from systematic research. EBM is often mistaken for or reduced to just one of its several components, critical appraisal of the literature. However, EBM requires both clinical expertise and an intimate knowledge of the individual patient's situation, beliefs, priorities, and values to be useful. External evidence must be used to inform but not replace individual clinical expertise. It is clinical expertise that determines if the external evidence may be applied to the individual patient, and if so, how it should be used in decision making by the patient and the health care provider. The development and application of clinical practice guidelines is one of the tools used in EBM. An understanding of EBM is necessary to understand recommended methods for production and implementation of guidelines.

Physicians working at McMaster University in Hamilton, Ontario, first used the terminology "evidence-based medicine." This group, called "The Evidence-Based Medicine Working Group," published a description of what they considered a new paradigm for medical practice and teaching.[38] In this article they present their views on changes that are occurring in medical practice relating to the use of medical literature to more effectively guide decision making. They state that the foundation for the paradigm shift rests in the significant developments in clinical research over the past 30 years, particularly the randomized controlled trial. Also considered important is meta-analysis as a method of summarizing the results of a number of randomized trials that may have profound effects on setting treatment policy.

The Evidence-Based Medicine Working Group cites the following changes that document the development of the new philosophy: (1) proposals to apply the principles of clinical epidemiology to day-to-day clinical practice; (2) numerous articles published instructing clinicians on how to access, evaluate, and interpret the medical literature; (3) growing demand for courses that instruct physicians on how to use the medical literature; (4) improvements in the format of journal articles; (5) textbooks with more rigorous review of available evidence; (6) new information resources like the American College of Physicians (ACP) Journal Club; and (7) the development of practice guidelines based on rigorous methodological review.

The practice of EBM focuses on five linked activities[39]: (1) convert information needs into a clearly defined answerable clinical question, (2) conduct a systematic search for the best available evidence for the problem, (3) evaluate the validity and applicability of the evidence, (4) prepare a synthesis or summary of the evidence for decision making and implement the decision in practice, and (5) evaluate performance and follow-up on any areas for improvement. Those that are familiar with the literature in drug information practice will recognize that these activities are remarkably similar to the systematic approach to drug information requests as outlined by Watanabe and colleagues over 20 years ago.[40] This process is very similar to the approach to drug information questions today (see Chap. 2).

Recent advances in information technology have made it much easier to search the medical literature. Access (via the Internet, on-line, or CD-ROM) to electronic databases such as MEDLINE, International Pharmaceutical Abstracts (IPA), the Iowa Drug Information Service (IDIS), and others provide the tools to rapidly sort thousands and even millions of published articles. These databases allow one to find articles that address the specific subject of the clinical problem or question that is of interest. Availability of these systems on local area networks, wide area networks, and the Internet have made them accessible virtually everywhere (see Chap. 5).

With the announcement on June 26, 1997, that MEDLINE was available free on the World Wide Web, use by the general public has greatly increased. In March 1998, 7.6 million searches were done on PubMed and Internet Grateful Med; more than the 7.4 million done for the entire year of 1996. The general public now does almost one-third of these searches.[41] The National Library of Medicine (NLM) has now expanded the resources available with "Medline*plus*." This new site includes not only MEDLINE, but also other search databases from NLM, NIH, National Cancer Institute (NCI), HCFA, AHCPR, Healthfinder, and other government resources. This site provides links to medical dictionaries, major associations and clearinghouses, publications and news items, directories of health professionals and health facilities, and libraries that provide health information services for the public.[42]

Consumer access to databases like MEDLINE, and the wide range of information available on the Internet from major health care professional organizations, pharmaceutical manufactures, and government sites, has the potential to support a much more sophisticated and informed population. The public is taking more interest in their own health and in seeking information about prevention and treatment of specific illnesses. Some of the information available via the rapidly expanding technology is very good, accurate, and helpful information; however, much of it is misleading or false and potentially dangerous. In any case, the expanded interest in health care information, and availability of information to the public, will continue to place increasing pressure on health care providers to stay current with valid scientific information, develop the skills to evaluate the evidence, and assist their patients in understanding the difference between reliable and suspect information.

Some general practitioners have identified a potential advantage of the evidence-based philosophy for health care to be empowerment of the general practitioner as (1) a knowledgeable and enthusiastic professional, (2) an advocate for their patients, and (3) a resource manager and commissioner of services. They note that not only do the skills required for evidence-based practice provide the patient's personal doctor with a strategy for keeping up to date on caring and curing, but they also enable the doctor to educate, defend, and negotiate on behalf of patients in a true primary care-led health care system.[43]

In a survey of general practitioners in the United Kingdom the respondents thought the best way to move from opinion-based medicine to evidence-based medicine is by using evidence-based guidelines developed by their colleagues.[44] Health care professionals face the complicated reality of constantly changing and increasing medical knowledge. What is required to practice effective, high-quality medicine is not an encyclopedic memory but the skills to acquire and critically assess the specific information that is necessary to make clinical decisions.

The educational model in health care must recognize that the knowledge base required to practice high-quality medicine is growing at unprecedented speed. A rough index of the rapidity with which medical knowledge about efficacy has accumulated can be obtained by examining the number of randomized controlled trials that have been published in peer-reviewed literature. In 1966 there were just over 100 articles per year compared to 10,000 in 1995. The first 5 years of this 30-year period account for only 1% of the articles; the last 5 years account for half.

Most (if not all) colleges of medicine and pharmacy have incorporated some component of problem-based learning in their curriculum within the last several years. This learner-centered approach to teaching is in many ways parallel to the philosophy of EBM. In essence, the equivalent steps involve identifying information needs or questions, conducting a search for the best evidence to address the question, conducting an evaluation of that evidence, preparing a synthesis and conclusion for action, and evaluating performance.

Michael Green, MD, and Peter Ellis, MD, recently described the EBM curriculum implemented in the Yale Primary Care Residency.[45] They also explained the reasoning for implementing this new method of training. They noted that

> with the proliferation of clinical trials and observational studies, the usefulness of an increasing amount of clinical maneuvers can be confirmed. However, many physicians on the front lines of patient care do not apply this growing evidence base, perhaps owing to lack of access, skills, or acceptance. In response to these needs, medical educators, as well as advisory groups such as the Accreditation Council for Graduate Medical Education, and the Association of American Medical Colleges, have called for the introduction

of clinical epidemiology, biostatistics, critical appraisal, and medical informatics into medical school and graduate medical education curricula.

The objectives of their curriculum were that the participants would demonstrate (1) the ability to pose a focused answerable question when faced with an uncertain scenario, (2) the ability to conduct an efficient search on MEDLINE, (3) the ability to critically appraise the published report of a clinical study, (4) the ability to incorporate their evaluation of the evidence into their decision making for individual patients, (5) an increase in their use of evidence from clinical research to help solve the clinical problems they encounter, (6) an appreciation of the advantages of practicing EBM, and (7) an opinion that the EBM curriculum is a valuable educational experience.

Shin and associates[46] conducted a study of the effect of problem-based, self-directed undergraduate education on life-long learning. They compared the up-to-date knowledge for the treatment of hypertension (as an example topic to test continued learning 5 to 15 years after graduation) between graduates of a medical school curriculum using problem-based, self-directed learning and a traditional curriculum. They found that the graduates of the problem-based curriculum demonstrated significantly higher current knowledge for appropriate management of hypertension.

Several other articles have been published recently that describe the implementation of learner-centered and evidence-based strategies for medical education. Curry and colleagues (from Northwestern University Medical School, Boston University School of Medicine, and the University of Oklahoma College of Medicine at Tulsa) describe learner-centered strategies in clerkship education.[47] Bordley and colleagues (from University of Rochester School of Medicine, Brown University School of Medicine, and the University of North Dakota School of Medicine and Health Sciences) describe "evidence-based medicine: a powerful tool for clerkship education."[48] Reilly and Lemon describe "evidence-based morning report: a popular new format in a large teaching hospital" at Cook County Hospital and Rush Medical College Internal Medicine Residency.[49] Numerous other programs are teaching and practicing EBM; the ones mentioned are only a small sample. EBM is clearly gaining many supporters.[50-52]

The *British Medical Journal* recently published a series of seven articles looking at international trends in continuing medical education.[53-59] Major themes of these articles include individual responsibility for health professionals to direct their own learning; self-assessment and specific needs directed education; wider aspects of continuing professional development including computer literacy, literature appraisal, information management, problem solving skills, and EBM; improved working and collaboration among different health professionals to achieve gains in quality and savings in cost; innovative portfolio-based programs to capture learning issues and achievements that occur in everyday practice; programs for better communications with patients and other health care providers; programs based on skill development rather than the traditional lecture format, distance learning, and use of technology to support learning; focus on education that will affect behaviors and improve outcomes of care; problem-based learning and small group activities; quality improvement tools; and programs based on the theories of adult learning.

The philosophy of EBM is consistent with the philosophy of clinical practice guidelines. The decision making process of EBM is supported by access and use of clinical practice guidelines. Health and Human Services Secretary Donna Shalala, PhD, who co-chaired the President's Advisory Commission (as described in the quality improvement section) said that the final report of the Commission provides a "fundamentally different vision of where we're going in the healthcare system, moving us toward a quality based, evidence-based system, it reinvents health care in this country."[60]

Methodology for Clinical Practice Guideline Development

A thorough understanding of the methodology used for clinical practice guideline development is critical for pharmacists (considering the rapidly increasing demand for participation in the process). This understanding will prepare pharmacists for involvement in appropriate evaluation and implementation of these guidelines. A lack of understanding of the requirements for guideline development could lead to inappropriate interpretation, acceptance of inappropriate levels of enforcement or implementation of the guideline, and consequent provision of ineffective or adverse therapy.

Several methods for developing practice guidelines have been described including informal consensus development, formal consensus development, evidence-based guideline development, and explicit guideline development.[61] For decades developers have used informal consensus as the basis of guideline development. These guidelines were produced following a meeting of an expert panel in which agreement was reached through open discussion, sometimes producing recommendations in a single meeting. The actual guideline document would often provide only the recommendation, with little background on the evidence that was used or information on the methodology of the group. This practice made it difficult or impossible for readers to verify the accuracy of the recommendation or to determine that bias did not significantly influence the results. Informal consensus development remains a common approach to developing practice guidelines because it is a relatively fast, easy, and inexpensive process. However, this approach generally results in guidelines of questionable quality. The fact that explicit methods for how the decisions were made are often not provided leaves doubt about how consensus was reached. Treatment recommendations are notoriously fallible when they are the result of efficacy evaluations based primarily on opinion. In addition, the ability to implement such "black box" guidelines will be seriously hampered based on the inability of the user to verify the accuracy and a resultant lack of confidence.[61]

The formal consensus development process is used by the NIH Consensus Development Program.[62] The NIH uses a structured 2.5-day conference in which guidelines are developed in closed session after a plenary session and open discussion, and are presented to an audience and press conference on the third day.[61] In some instances the usual 2.5-day format of the conference is not sufficient and alternative formats are used.[63] It should also be noted that substantial advanced planning occurs for presentations of up-to-date reviews of available evidence by experts. This process provides more structure than informal consensus; however, it has been criticized for its requirement to produce recommendations in a relatively short period, the absence of explicit criteria, the variability in the type and degree of referencing of the recommendations to the literature, and the inconsistent degree of labeling recommendations as to the level of certainty provided by empirical evidence.

The method that was used by the AHCPR is the evidence-based model or a variation of the evidence-based model that has been referred to as the "explicit approach."[64] This method is currently believed to provide the most scientific rigor for practice guideline development. It also emphasizes extensive documentation and communication of the methods and evidence used to make recommendations. This method will be described in detail in this text and is based on the writing of Eddy[64–67] and the Manual for Clinical Practice Guideline Development prepared by Woolf, which was supported by the AHCPR.[68]

Even though the AHCPR no longer produces guidelines directly, the methodology developed has been adopted, and in some cases slightly modified, by other groups. The AHCPR evidence-based guideline methodology is still recognized as a rigorous and valid method. Additional information about activities of the AHCPR is provided below. This information is valuable for anyone involved in producing or implementing clinical practice guidelines considering that the AHCPR is the lead agency within the U.S. Department of Health and Human Services, which sponsors and conducts research with a goal to increase the evidence base for health care, to assist with getting evidence in to practice, and to improve quality of care.

Between 1990 and 1996, AHCPR-supported panels produced 19 clinical practice guidelines. The Agency discontinued the guideline development program in the fall of 1996 after recognizing that convening separate national panels to develop each guideline was expensive and time consuming. The demand for evidence-based information far exceeded the resources that could be devoted to the guideline development program. Furthermore, the Agency recognized that many professional organizations, health plans, and commercial firms were producing thousands of guidelines. Therefore the

Agency initiated the "Evidence-Based Practice Program," and now serves as a science partner with private- and public-sector organizations to develop "evidence reports." Evidence reports are based on comprehensive reviews and rigorous analysis of relevant scientific evidence. These reports are intended for use as the scientific foundation for public and private organizations to develop tools (including guidelines, technology assessments, and quality indicators) for improving quality of care.

The AHCPR currently is composed of 13 major functional components, one of which is the Center for Practice and Technology Assessment. This center directs the "evidence-based practice program," which consists of (1) evidence-based practice centers developing evidence reports and technology assessments, (2) the Internet-based national guideline clearinghouse, (3) the U.S. Preventive Services Task Force, and (4) research and evaluation on translating evidence-based findings into clinical practice.[69] On June 25, 1997, the AHCPR announced the awarding of 5-year contracts to 12 institutions in the United States and Canada to serve as Evidence-Based Practice Centers.[70] A list of these centers is available on the AHCPR web site. These centers, which are consortia of methodologists and clinical experts, work with public- and private-sector organizations to produce the synthesis of the best available evidence, and ensure that products are useful and improve care. Professional organizations and associations, health care provider groups, health plans, public and private purchasers, states, and others use this evidence-based foundation to implement their own practice guidelines, clinical pathways, review criteria, performance measures, and other tools to improve the quality of care.

Other centers in the AHCPR that are closely related to the Center for Practice and Technology Assessment include the Center for Outcomes and Effectiveness Research, which conducts and supports studies on the outcomes of diagnostic, therapeutic, and preventive health care services and procedures; the Center for Primary Care Research, which conducts and supports studies of primary care, and clinical, preventive, and public health policies and systems; the Center for Quality Measurement and Improvement, which conducts and supports research on the measurement and improvement of the quality of health care, including consumer surveys that measure satisfaction with health care services and systems; and the Center for Information Technology, which conducts and supports studies of health information systems, computerized patient record systems, and medical decision analysis, including data standards, automated medical records, and decision support systems.[69]

The AHCPR also conducts research for developing and improving information technology. Informatics is an area of research that is critical to translating research evidence into practice. Information technology is vital for health care delivery systems to efficiently measure and improve the quality of care. Seamless information systems linking administrative, financial, and clinical data that can follow patients no matter where or from whom they receive care are needed. Outcomes studies that assess what works best in clinical practice rely on information technology to provide accurate data and analysis. Informatics studies currently being conducted by the AHCPR are evaluating computerized decision support systems, automating access to relevant guidelines in the practice setting at the point of care, computerized drug monitoring systems for dosage checking and alerts to possible adverse drug events, and others.[71]

It must be recognized that the detailed approach described by the AHCPR is time consuming, technically demanding, and costly. In the experience of the AHCPR, exclusive of staff time, the cost for developing their clinical practice guidelines was estimated to range from $350,000 to $1 million each.[1] The main variable was the number of questions the expert panel addressed that required preparation of literature reviews. It should be noted that this involves a 12-month process that produces a science-based, pilot-tested, peer-reviewed guideline document. Another point of perspective in terms of the cost of developing guidelines is that this cost is not unlike that of conducting a single controlled trial, which may have comparatively limited effects on clinical decisions. The American Heart Association reported that many professional societies have developed guidelines using member volunteers supported by a small staff at a cost ranging from $10,000 to $200,000.[2]

It is not practical to expect that all clinical practice guidelines will be developed using all of the detailed methodology described in this chapter. In making the decision to use this methodology, consideration must be given to the target audience for the guideline, the condition or treatment that will be the subject of the guideline, what type of evidence is available on the subject, the anticipated benefits from preparing the guideline, what methods will be used to implement and/or enforce the guideline, and what financial, technical, and personnel resources are available. Based on limitations that may exist in any of these factors it may not be possible to achieve the goals of this methodology. This fact should also be kept in mind when evaluating available practice guidelines.

Eddy describes five objectives for guideline development: (1) the method should produce guidelines that are accurate (i.e., the outcomes that will occur if the guideline is followed should be as predicted); (2) the method should be accountable, enabling readers to review the data and reasoning behind the recommendations; (3) it should anticipate the health and financial consequences of applying the guideline (both to the individual and to a population); (4) it should facilitate resolution of conflicts with other guidelines; and (5) it should facilitate application of the policy.

In preparation of the manual for the AHCPR, Woolf describes in detail four analytic steps in guideline development methodology: (1) definition of the process, (2) assessment of the clinical benefits and harms, (3) assessment of health policy issues, and (4) preparation of the practice guideline document. Some of the details of these four steps will be provided, but it is impractical to cover all of the details within this chapter. Sufficient information will be provided to allow the reader to understand the process and to be able to evaluate guidelines. For pharmacists who will participate in guideline development, it is recommended that further preparation be undertaken. A vast amount of information is available from the resources described in the section of this chapter on sources of clinical practice guidelines. The Internet sites from McMaster University and Oxford, and the Cochrane Handbook (available for download at <<http://hiru.mcmaster.ca/cochrane/cochrane/resource.htm>>) are highly recommended. In addition the American College of Cardiology and the American Heart Association have published a detailed description of their guideline development methodology.[72] The American College of Chest Physicians Fifth ACCP Consensus Conference on Antithrombotic Therapy provides excellent descriptions of many of the critical issues of guideline development, and serves as a current example of valid guidelines.[73]

The clinical practice guideline "Heart Failure: Evaluation and Care of Patients with Left-Ventricular Systolic Dysfunction,"[74] released June 1994 by the AHCPR, will be used as a case example to illustrate specific points in the review of guideline development. This guideline is now in need of updating, but is a good example to illustrate the development process. Additional guidelines on the treatment of heart failure have been published by the American College of Cardiology/American Heart Association, and would also require updating with recent primary literature on the use of beta-blockers, among other things.

The first two events, which occur before the formal clinical practice guideline development process is undertaken, are (1) selection of a topic and (2) appointing an expert panel. The topic of heart failure was chosen by the AHCPR for several reasons including[74]:

- More than 2 million Americans have heart failure and 400,000 new cases are diagnosed each year.
- The 5-year mortality for congestive heart failure (CHF) is approximately 50%.
- Total treatment costs for CHF were more than $10 billion in 1990 (only $230 million of that total were for medication).
- Proper management can reduce morbidity and mortality of CHF.
- Data indicate that deficiencies exist in the level of care currently provided to patients.
- Studies have shown wide practice variations in terms of resource use and costs.

Therefore, this condition meets many priorities for guideline development, including high prevalence, high morbidity and mortality, availability of effective treatments, demonstrable evidence of opportunity to improve the quality of and cost effectiveness of care, and significant practice variation. For producing the heart failure guideline, AHCPR contracted with the Rand Corporation and an expert panel was appointed including five cardiologists, two cardiac surgeons, one internist-geriatrician, one general internist, one family physician, one pulmonologist, one clinical pharmacist, two nurses, and two consumer representatives.

The first analytic step for the panel is to define the goals and clarify the topic. It is important to specifically define the target condition and types of patients for which the guideline is intended to apply, the clinical interventions that will and will not be considered, and the type of provider and practice setting in which the guideline will be applicable. The panel should specify the outcomes that it would like to see changed as a result of implementing the guideline. It is also important for the panel to give consideration to the information needs of the intended users of the guideline. Appropriate consideration for target user needs and interests should be included throughout guideline preparation to maximize the acceptability and usability of the final product and ensure that goal outcomes are achieved. A topic that is defined on too broad of a scope will be unrealistic in terms of the review of scientific evidence and providing usable recommendations that may be applied to individual patients. Clearly identifying the outcomes that the guideline is intended to improve will provide a rational basis for the analytic process that follows and help to keep the topic focused. It is also important that a record-keeping system be established so that the rationale for each decision made by the panel is traceable. Example worksheets that may facilitate this process are provided in Woolf's manual.[68]

The next critical step in the clarification process is the development of the "evidence model." The panel prepares a graphical flowchart describing expectations of how clinical outcomes will be influenced by the guideline and the type of evidence that must be gathered. This exercise is intended to help the panel think through the natural history of the disease process, the sequence of intermediate effects of an intervention to reach the desired outcome, and potential adverse effects that may be encountered. Figures 9-1 and 9-2 (from the AHCPR guideline[74]) represent two portions of the analytic model prepared for the heart failure guideline. Figure 9-1 represents the overview of evaluation and care of patients with heart failure, and Fig. 9-2 represents the subcomponent dealing with pharmacologic management.

This framework is used by the panel to help clearly define questions the guideline will address and, therefore, what literature must be included in the next step. The importance of this phase cannot be overemphasized. Just as in the systematic approach to a drug information question, it is critical to first clearly define the question to be successful in searching for the necessary evidence and subsequently be able to provide useful, valid conclusions.

To define the goals for the heart failure guideline,[74] the panel identified several aspects of care for heart failure patients that the guideline was intended to improve including the following items.

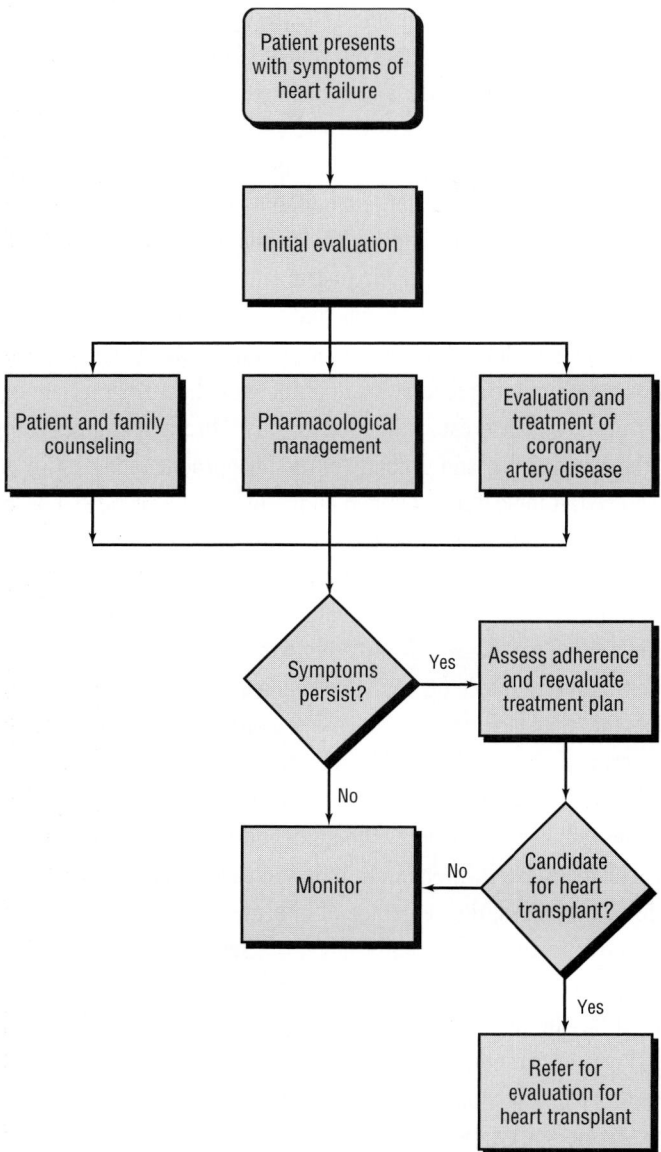

Figure 9–1. Overview of evaluation and care of patients with heart failure. *(SOURCE: From AHCPR Guidelines.[74])*

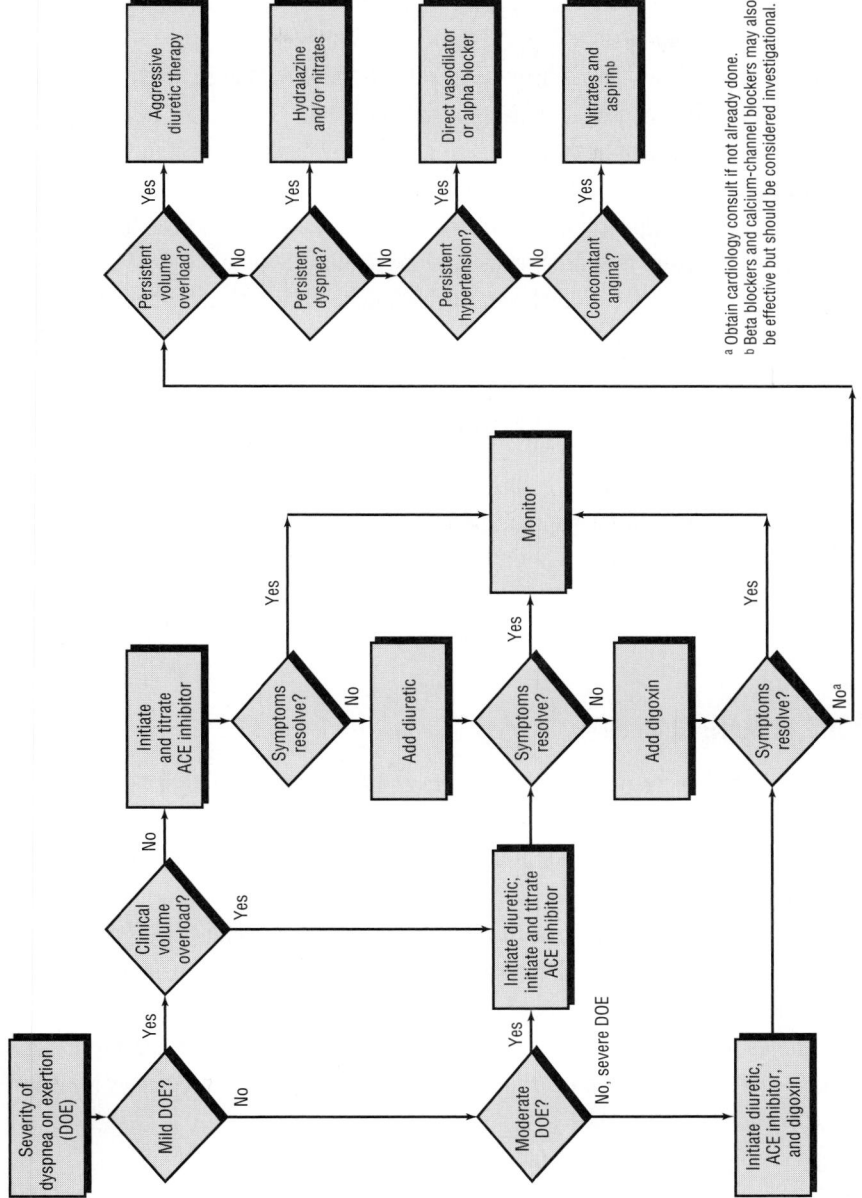

Figure 9–2. Pharmacologic management of patients with heart failure. *(SOURCE: From AHCPR Guidelines.)*

[a] Obtain cardiology consult if not already done.
[b] Beta blockers and calcium-channel blockers may also be effective but should be considered investigational.

ERRORS IN DIAGNOSIS

- Patients with symptoms suggestive of heart failure are often not thoroughly evaluated to rule out noncardiac causes before treatment for heart failure is instituted.
- Symptoms of heart failure may be attributed to chronic obstructive pulmonary disease (COPD) and treated inappropriately.
- Reversible causes of heart failure are not always identified, or if identified, they may be undertreated.
- Patients with peripheral edema may be inappropriately labeled as having heart failure when there is another cause for the edema.
- An initial measurement of left-ventricular function is not always obtained.
- Concurrent angina or other evidence of ischemia is not always properly evaluated.

ERRORS IN EVALUATION AND TESTING

- Chest x-ray, electrocardiography, echocardiography, and radionuclide studies are commonly used for monitoring patients' progress, rather than symptom- or activity-based measures.
- Holter monitoring is overutilized, leading to unjustified treatment of asymptomatic ventricular arrhythmias.

ERRORS IN MANAGEMENT

- Coexistent hypertension is often not treated aggressively enough.
- Patient, family, and caregiver education is often inadequate.
- Patients with heart failure that is not due to systolic dysfunction may be treated inappropriately.
- Practitioners may not instruct patients to monitor their weight closely.
- The possibility of revascularization is often not considered in patients who have severe coronary artery disease with left-ventricular systolic dysfunction.
- Patients with severe heart failure are often referred too late for heart transplantation, after severe decompensation and the development of secondary multisystem organ failure.
- Exercise prescriptions are underutilized.
- ACE inhibitors are often not initiated or are prescribed at suboptimal doses because of clinicians' concerns about possible side effects.
- Physicians frequently prescribe inadequate doses of diuretics in patients who continue to have overt volume overload despite modest doses of diuretics.

- Practitioners may fail to appreciate the potentially deleterious effects of certain pharmacological agents in heart failure (e.g., calcium blockers, nonsteroidal anti-inflammatory agents, beta-agonist inhalers).

To define the scope of the guideline, the panel elected to focus on the practical aspects of management of patients with heart failure caused by reduced left-ventricle systolic function (ejection fraction less than 35% to 40%). The panel elected *not* to address detailed management of diastolic dysfunction. Also, the guideline does not address medical management strategies specific to the in-hospital setting (e.g., pulmonary artery catheters, intra-aortic balloon pumps) or heart failure caused by surgically correctable valvular disease, aneurysm, or identifiable myocardial disease (e.g., amyloidosis, sarcoidosis).

By defining goals, limiting the scope, and constructing the evidence model, it is possible to see from the heart failure guideline example how this analytic step is performed. At this time it is also necessary to define the admissible evidence—the types of published or unpublished research to be considered so that an appropriate literature search may be performed to conduct the next step, the assessment of clinical benefits and harms.

Assessment of clinical benefits and harms is a process similar to preparing a drug evaluation monograph (see Chap. 14). The purpose of this process is to bring together all relevant empirical data regarding each of the "questions" identified in step 1 of the guideline development process. A thorough literature search must be conducted and the literature must be evaluated for the quality of the data. The literature retrieval process should include a search of the available bibliographic resources such as MEDLINE, *Current Contents, Excerpta Medica, Science Citation Index,* citations listed in published bibliographies, textbooks, and any literature that may be identified by researchers and other individuals on the "expert" list that the panel may create. Specific keywords and other search constraints, for example, Medical Subject Headings from MEDLINE (MeSH) terms, limits by publication year, language, randomized controlled trials, and so forth should be recorded to allow verification of the process. Each retrieved article should then be judged for its relevance and compliance to criteria for inclusion as predetermined by the panel. When possible, it is helpful to have more than one reviewer judge the inclusion of studies. A log should be kept of excluded studies and the rationale for their rejection.

There are a variety of methods for evaluating individual studies, many of which are discussed in other sections of this text (see Chaps 6 and 7). The purpose of this process is to identify issues with trial design or any biases that would affect internal or external validity. Issues to consider include the trial design (i.e., clinical trial, cohort study, case-control study, indirect evidence), sample size, statistical power, selection bias, inclusion/exclusion criteria, selection of control group, randomization methods, comparability of groups, definition of exposure or intervention, definition of outcome measures, accuracy and appropriateness of outcome measures, attrition rates, data collection methods, methods of statistical analysis, confounding variables, unique characteristics of the study population, and adequacy of blinding. Formal methods may also be used to assign a quality score to each trial.

A draft summary report of the evidence for each decision point (question) should be prepared for review by the panel. Example formats and sample tables are provided in Woolf's manual.[68] Table 9–1 is an example of an evidence table from the heart failure guideline.[74] A formal narrative summary should also be provided with the draft evidence table and include the following information: (1) specific information about the direction (positive or negative) and magnitude of the effect of an intervention, (2) a range of uncertainty of the estimate (e.g., a 95% confidence interval), (3) the ability to generalize the results to clinical practice, (4) gaps in the evidence, and recommendations for future study. In preparation of the heart failure guideline, the project staff with the AHCPR examined more than 1000 articles, 237 of which were specifically used to develop the recommendations.

Panel members are then asked to provide review comments on the report to address flaws in the literature review process, specific studies or data that were overlooked, errors in interpretation of studies, errors in the assessment of individual decision points, or errors in the overall assessment of benefits and harms. Panel members may also be asked to comment on the need to reconsider any of the "questions" that the guideline is intended to address or whether any time-consuming, optional techniques not done need to be performed to make decisions (e.g., meta-analysis, decision analysis, or focus groups) to assess patient preference or values for certain procedures or outcomes. At this point the AHCPR might also have the document distributed to outside reviewers to obtain their feedback on the same issues as requested in the review by the panel members.

The panel then reviews the revised evidence table of the benefits and harms for the various interventions and may elect to fill in gaps with expert opinion through the formal or informal consensus process. The panel discusses the strengths and weaknesses of the data and subsequently reaches conclusions on the benefits and harms of specific procedures or treatment. These conclusions are clearly stated to be based on high-quality data or consensus and explicitly document the rationale for the decisions and how they were reached. Once the panel has reached agreement on the quantitative description of the risks and benefits of various treatments, the next step is to begin to draft the practice guideline by constructing the "appropriateness profile." In this early step, each treatment or intervention may be classified as (1) appropriate (should definitely be performed in the specified case), (2) inappropriate (should definitely *not* be performed, or (3) in the "gray zone" (uncertain if should be performed).

TABLE 9-1. EFFECTS OF TREATMENT ON MORTALITY IN PATIENTS WITH LEFT-VENTRICULAR DYSFUNCTION OR CLINICAL HEART FAILURE

Study Author, Year	Study Population	N	Duration of Followup (years)	Treatment	Mortality Rate (percent)	Absolute Mortality Difference[a] (percent)	Symptomatic Hypotension[b] (percent)
Surgical Management of Heart Failure or Left-Ventricular Dysfunction							
Bounous et al., 1988[9]	First cardiac catheterization; EF ≤40%	710	3.0	CABG Medical	14[c] 32[c]	18 (Operative mortality NR)	— —
Medical Management of Left-Ventricular Dysfunction							
Pfeffer et al. (SAVE), 1992[15]	3–16 days after MI; EF ≤40%; no current heart failure	2,231	3.5[d]	Captopril Placebo	20.4 24.6	4.2	0.7
SOLVD Investigators (SOLVD Prevention Trial), 1992[16]	EF ≤35%; no heart failure	4,228	3.1[d]	Enalapril Placebo	14.8 15.8	NS	NR
Medical Management of Heart Failure							
Cohn et al. (VHeFT I), 1986[17]	Chronic heart failure, cardiac enlargement or EF <45%, and MVO₂ <25 mL/kg/min	642	3.0	HYD/ISDN Placebo	36.2 46.9	10.7	NR
CONSENSUS Trial Study Group, 1987[10]	New York Heart Association Class IV heart failure	253	1.0	Enalapril Placebo	36.2 52.4	16.2	5.5
SOLVD Investigators (SOLVD Treatment Trial), 1991[18]	Chronic heart failure; EF ≤35%	2,569	3.5[d]	Enalapril Placebo	35.2 39.7	4.5	2
Cohn et al. (VHeFT II), 1991[19]	Same as VHeFT I	804	2.5[d]	Enalapril HYD/ISDN	32.8 38.2	5.4	4.5

[a] All mortality differences are significant at $p < 0.05$ except where indicated (NS).
[b] Symptomatic hypotension requiring termination of the study drug.
[c] Adjusted for baseline prognostic factors.
[d] Mean duration of followup.

Notes: NR = not reported, NS = not significant, HYD/ISDN = hydralazine and isosorbide dinitrate, CABG = coronary artery bypass graft, EF = ejection fraction, MI = myocardial infarction, MVO₂ = maximum oxygen uptake, SAVE = Survival and Ventricular Enlargement, SOLVD = Studies of Left-Ventricular Dysfunction, VHeFT = Veterans Affairs Vasodilator Heart Failure Trial.
SOURCE: *From AHCPR Guidelines.*[74]

Reaching clear decisions on recommendations for clinical practices is often difficult because the data are not adequate to clearly label the practice appropriate or inappropriate. Unfortunately, many practices fall into this "gray zone" category because of uncertainties about the benefits and harms, variability in patients and in their responses to treatment, and differences in patient preferences about the desirability of outcomes and aversion to risk. The use of rigid language in an effort to produce clear-cut recommendations can be dangerous, particularly when presented as simplistic algorithms that fail to recognize the complexity of medical decision making and the need for individual clinical judgment. This danger can be avoided by describing uncertainty and providing broad boundaries for appropriate practice that allow for legitimate differences of opinion. Attempts to develop rigid guidelines when the data are not conclusive is clearly worse than having no written guidelines.

To this point, decisions regarding appropriate recommendations for patient management are based only on consideration of clinical benefits and risks. In consideration of the potential effects on the quality of health care and the acceptability of the guidelines to practitioners, it is critical that these decisions be based on what is best for the patient's well-being. Any contamination of the process by cost issues or "policy" issues at this stage will ultimately produce an unsatisfactory guideline. This is not to say that cost issues and feasibility issues are not important to consider—they clearly are if the guideline is to be applicable in the real world—but this must be done in a distinctly separate step of the process. Any final recommendations that are modified for reasons other than clinical benefit must include explicit documentation of the rationale. It is appropriate and responsible to base recommendations for preferred therapies on the results of cost-effectiveness or cost-utility analyses, but the panel should apply the same degree of scientific rigor as with the clinical issues. Also, the panel should document the degree of influence the cost issues had on the recommendations.

In an environment in which resources are unlimited, it would not be necessary to consider cost and feasibility issues. However, to produce a practice guideline that is usable, feasibility issues should be addressed. To the extent that data are available, cost estimates should be included. In the guideline development process used by the AHCPR, a report on health policy issues is prepared for use by the expert panel for making final recommendations. The review of health policy issues should follow a comprehensive approach similar to that used in reviewing evidence for clinical benefits and harms. Relevant literature should be collected, evaluated, and summarized using explicit criteria. The expertise of a health economist may be required to assist in examining some of the issues. The specific health policy issues recommended for review in the AHCPR manual[68] include effect of the guideline on limited resources (costs and cost effectiveness, availability of qualified providers, equipment, ancillary services); medical ethics; concerns of patients and caretakers; concerns of practitioners (interference with autonomy, time pressures, need for decision support to have information available at the right time, need for specific skills, special characteristics of local patient population, local guidelines, reimbursement, medicolegal issues); and concerns of payers (provider accountability, precertification, utilization review and quality assurance, cost effectiveness). The AHCPR also holds an open forum to allow groups or individuals that have an interest or expertise in these topics to provide oral and written testimony.

The use of information regarding feasibility issues such as equipment and personnel availability are relatively straightforward. The use of cost information in the decision making process for practice guidelines remains controversial and requires development and research to determine the most efficient and effective methods. The panel may elect not to use cost information in the decision making process for guideline recommendations. However, it would still be useful for cost information to be summarized and provided as an overlay or an appendix to help both the developers and users of guidelines understand the financial implications of following or not following the guidelines.

When consensus is reached within the panel on the estimates of benefits and risks of each treatment, the appropriateness profile has been prepared, and the health policy issues have been considered, the first draft of the clinical practice guideline may be prepared. The entire process has focused on explicit methodology, the requirement for decisions to be made on the basis of the best available evidence, and clear and thorough documentation of the decision making rationale. This explicit process must now be carried through in the preparation of the guideline document. Specific criteria have been recommended for this purpose.[1,61,64,68] For example, the AHCPR has detailed eight desirable attributes of clinical practice guidelines[1] that are provided in this chapter in the section on evaluation of clinical practice guidelines. Knowledge of these criteria is needed in order to be prepared to write practice guidelines, as well as judge the validity of guidelines currently available.

It is important to consider the information needs of the guideline's user. Practitioners will want specific, qualitative estimates of the relevant health outcomes, a statement of the strength of the evidence and expert judgment supporting the guidelines, information on patient preferences, projections of cost, details of the reasoning behind the recommendations, and the ability to review the data independently if they so choose. Guidelines should be written such that they may be perceived as an explanation of the thinking process that is used in evaluating and applying the information. If guidelines are perceived as information only, they may be rejected as the "cookbooks" that practitioners fear guidelines will become. Such guidelines would also not achieve the educational goals to focus further research efforts (outcomes research or other) on gaps in the current evidence.

Eddy has published the most succinct description of the recommended content of a "policy statement."[64] A clinical practice guideline, such as the AHCPR guideline on heart failure, may contain several policy statements. Eddy recommends a content and format that is similar to a research article and includes 13 main sections (this material is condensed and slightly modified).

1. *Summary of the Policy*—This is a one- to three-line statement that should be clear, concise, specific and as operational as possible. An example statement from the AHCPR guideline[74] is "Asymptomatic patients who are found to have moderately or severely reduced left-ventricular systolic function (ejection fraction <35–40 percent) should be treated with an ACE inhibitor to reduce the chance of developing clinical heart failure. (Strength of Evidence = A)." Note that the patient description (reduced left-ventricular ejection fraction) is defined with specific criteria (EF <35% to 40%). This is important to make the statement clear and specific. Also, note that the statement is accompanied by a grade designation of the strength of evidence (A); this grading system will be explained in more detail in a later section. A complete clinical practice guideline may include numerous policy statements regarding a variety of treatment issues, prevention, education, diagnosis, or other aspects involving the particular disease or condition.

2. *Background*—The background should answer the broad question, "Why is this policy being written?" It might describe basic information regarding the prevalence of the condition, a known problem in quality of care for the condition, or a recent change in the recommended treatment.

3. *Health Problem*—This section should clearly delineate the health problem addressed in the guideline, the interventions that are compared, specific details of patients to whom the policy may apply (similar to inclusion/exclusion criteria for a clinical trial), any restrictions on practitioners who should provide the treatment, or the setting (e.g., specialty certification or training, facilities, equipment).

4. *Health and Economic Outcomes*—This section should identify the health outcomes (e.g., 5-year survival, rate of hospitalization, incidence of MI) and economic costs (e.g., costs for hospitalization, medication costs, procedure costs, laboratory costs) that were considered in the design of the policy.

5. *Evidence*—A detailed description of the evidence is a critical element in assessing the validity of a guideline. The methods used to locate evidence about the effect of the treatment on the outcome of the disease should be clear, and specify which evidence was accepted or excluded and why, how the evidence was interpreted, and what subjective judgments were used to supplement the evidence from controlled trials.

6. *Effect on Health and Economic Outcomes*—This is the core information desired by practitioners. It should provide the quantitative estimates of the benefits and risks of the intervention, the economic outcomes when possible and appropriate,

and should express a range of uncertainty. The question of health and economic effects of providing or not providing the interventions should be answered. This information is key to allow patient participation in shared decision making.

7. *Methods Used to Derive Estimates of Outcomes*—This section should describe how estimates were made for the information in section 6 including whether models were used such as decision analysis, sensitivity analysis, or meta-analysis. Decision analysis is an objective method that identifies the relationship between various decision options and possible consequences, assigns a value and probability to each of the consequences, and calculates which decision pathway leads to the maximum value. Sensitivity analysis mathematically determines the effect on the conclusion if the value of one of the variables (which may have been assigned an estimated value) is changed. For example, if the estimated efficacy or toxicity rate of one of the treatments is doubled, would that change which treatment is recommended? Meta-analysis involves critical review of the quality of individual studies, and statistically combines the results of the studies when appropriate in order to more precisely calculate the magnitude (or direction) of a treatment effect.

8. *Preference Judgment*—This section describes the judgments made about the desirability of the health outcomes and the source of the preference judgments (e.g., survey of patients, consensus process of expert panel).

9. *Instruction for Tailoring Guidelines*—Factors that should be considered when applying the guideline (e.g., patient variables, setting, provider) and estimates of how the effects of these factors will alter the estimated outcomes are helpful for users to apply the guidelines locally.

10. *Conflicts with Other Policies*—If other organizations have issued a different recommendation for the same health problem, the variation should be addressed, and an explanation for the difference should be provided. If the authors of the conflicting statement did not describe their rationale and the evidence base for their recommendation, it may not be possible to reconcile the conflict.

11. *Comparisons with Other Interventions*—Within the guideline, comparisons are made with other interventions for the same condition. In this section, however, Eddy recommends that the interventions in the guideline be put in context with other interventions in health care in a more global sense including other conditions, perhaps in terms of a cost-benefit, cost-effectiveness, or cost-utility analysis. For example, the cost effectiveness of the treatments or interventions for heart failure may be compared with cost effectiveness for treatments for hypertension or hyperlipidemia.

12. *Caveats*—This section may describe any expected developments or new information that could modify the recommendations and a suggested date for review.

For example, although not specifically identified in the AHCPR guideline, Parmley noted in an editorial[75] that there were two studies in progress: "one may provide new information on the effects of calcium channel blockers on patients with heart failure and the other is a large trial organized by the NIH to compare digoxin and placebo on mortality in patients with heart failure." The results of these studies will need to be considered so that guideline recommendations may be altered, if necessary.

13. *Authors of the Policy*—The guideline document should include the authors of the policy and their expertise, along with statements of any conflicts of interest. Phillips recently expressed the importance of making conflicts of interest explicit in any guideline.[76] These conflicts, as noted by Phillips, may involve financial interests such as those of pharmaceutical companies or professional organizations that may try to protect their interests.

Depending on the subject of the clinical practice guideline, more or less emphasis may be placed on the various sections of the guideline document. In addition, recommendations for future research may be included with the document. The process of developing practice guidelines often calls attention to the gaps in scientific information. The direction provided for future research may be one of the most important results of the practice guideline development process. Practice guidelines that fail to address research priorities may discourage innovation and negatively influence funding decisions for needed research in the involved area. For the few examples that exist in which clear answers are already provided by high-quality scientific evidence, waste of research resources may be avoided by stopping generation of data that would not increase understanding of a disease process or its treatment. The AHCPR heart failure guideline identifies 15 main areas for future research that were inadequately studied in available literature.

Extensive detail on the issues of formatting practice guidelines and "wordsmithing" are beyond the scope of this chapter; however, a few points are worth noting. Essentially, effective formatting means presenting guidelines in physical arrangement or media that can be readily accessed, understood, and applied by the intended users. The major "formats" are freetext, algorithms, flowcharts, and decision trees. Significant work is being done in some institutions to structure guidelines in computerized decision support programs.

For example, the Department of Clinical Epidemiology, LDS Hospital, Salt Lake City has developed a computer decision support program to aid in empiric antibiotic selection.[77] An evaluation of this program demonstrated that it provided recommendations for an antibiotic regimen that improved care compared to regimens selected by physicians not using the program. Key features of this program are that it provides information that is readily available at the time decisions need to be made, it is based on extensively evaluated evidence, it is convenient to use, and the rationale for the recommendations is available on command for the user by "windowing" back to whatever level of detail he or she wishes. The evaluation of this program also demonstrated that 88% of physicians stated they would recommend the program to other physicians, 85% said the program improved antibiotic selection, and 81% said they believed the program improved patient care.

Further evaluation of this computer-aided decision support program for anti-infective selection has shown improved clinical outcomes of care as well as significant cost savings and reduced length of stay.[78] The information technology incorporated patient care protocols, expert-derived logic, hospital-specific epidemiological data, and patient-specific data. The logic of all of the recommendations was available in the system for review by the clinician, who also could override the protocol if needed. This allowed for further quality assurance of the system and of the care provided in a CQI process. The use of best available evidence in evaluation of antibiotic selection for development of patient care protocols combined with local practitioner involvement, local patient data, immediate availability of recommendations with clear logic, and CQI concepts are key features of this system.

The AHCPR publishes its guidelines in three formats, the *Clinical Practice Guideline, Quick Reference Guide for Clinicians,* and a *Consumer Version.* The *Clinical Practice Guideline on Heart Failure* is a 121-page book providing significant detail for the majority of items described. The *Quick Reference Guide for Clinicians* is a 20-page booklet that presents the clinical algorithms, tables of information, brief explanations, and pertinent references. It is a "distilled" version of the *Clinical Practice Guideline* intended as a ready reference for daily use. The consumer version is a small booklet for the general public to increase patient knowledge and involvement in health care decision making; it is available in English and sometimes Spanish versions. These guidelines are also available in the CD-ROM format and via on-line access (further detail is provided in this chapter in the section on sources of guidelines).

The language of the recommendations in clinical practice guidelines may have significant influence on the interpretation and impact of the guideline. The words *must, should,* or *may* must be selected carefully and applied appropriately.

The authors of practice guidelines must be careful not to overstate the confidence with which they define proper care. In discussion of the impact of practice guidelines on patient care, Woolf recommends a three-tiered model for guideline enforcement based on the level of scientific evidence and clinical quality of the guideline.[5] High-quality guidelines that define optimal care with certainty should have a relatively high level of enforcement. At the other end of the spectrum, guidelines with weak scientific evidence would be suitable for education, but it would be inappropriate to require that patients and practitioners follow them or that they be used for reimbursement decisions or provider credentialling.

Eddy suggests that the terms *standards, guidelines,* and *options* be used to provide flexibility in practice policy.[67] He suggests that *standards* must be applied rigidly when the health and economic consequences of an intervention are sufficiently well known and there is virtual unanimity (>95%) among patients about the desirability of the outcome. A *guideline* should be followed in most cases, but deviations could be justified based on patient factors, the setting, or other reasons. In this case, evidence is adequate to identify at least some of the important outcomes, and a majority (60% to 95%) of individuals would favor the practice (use or nonuse of the intervention). *Options* are neutral with respect to recommending the use of an intervention, and practitioners and patients should be given sufficient freedom to make an individual choice.

For purposes of qualifying its recommendations, the AHCPR uses a literature quality rating system. Seven levels of evidence have been defined for the panel's use. The levels depend on the study design, the quality of the studies, sample size, and the consistency of results across centers. The seven levels are:

I. Evidence from large, well-conducted, randomized, controlled trials.
II. Evidence from small, well-conducted, randomized, controlled trials.
III. Evidence from well-conducted cohort studies.
IV. Evidence from well-conducted case-control studies.
V. Evidence from uncontrolled or poorly controlled studies.
VI. Conflicting evidence but tending to favor the recommendation.
VII. Expert opinion.

The panel will then grade each recommendation in the clinical practice guideline based on the quality of the evidence on a three-level system:

A. *Good evidence*—Evidence from well-conducted, randomized, controlled trials or cohort studies (Levels I through III)
B. *Fair evidence*—Evidence from other types of studies (Levels IV through VI)
C. *Expert opinion* (Level VII)

This grading level for each recommendation is helpful for guideline users to realize the level of evidence supporting the recommendation. This is also important in determining how a guideline is implemented and enforced. It is clearly inappropriate to attempt to rigidly enforce a grade-C recommendation, whereas compliance may usually be expected with grade-A recommendations.

For further information regarding the rules of evidence and clinical recommendations, the reader may also wish to review the work of Guyatt and co-workers, who have previously described the philosophy of the "rules of evidence and clinical recommendations," used by the American College of Chest Physicians in their consensus Conference on Antithrombotic Therapy.[79] The more recent level of evidence rating and grade of recommendation includes consideration for meta-analysis, the consistency of results across the studies, the bounds of the confidence interval, and a balance of the benefits versus the risks of therapy.

To complete the formal development process (as recommended by the AHCPR), following the first draft of the clinical practice guideline, the expert panel members complete a review of the document and make recommendations for revision. The second draft is then sent for peer review to members of the "expert list," which includes individuals or organizations that participated in the open forum, and other organizations that will later have an important role in implementing or promoting the guideline. There were 40 professional organizations and individuals involved in this process for the Heart Failure Guideline. The next step is pretesting the guideline in practice settings. The pretesting panel is given clear instructions on the observations that are considered most useful and are asked to keep written notes of their experiences, observations, and suggestions. A summary report of these observations is provided to the development panel. In the final revision steps, the panel should examine all review comments and pretesting results in an unbiased fashion. A disposition record that documents how each recommendation was handled and the rationale for inclusion or exclusion in the final document should be kept.

The guideline development process may be viewed in the philosophy of continuous quality improvement from several aspects. The methodology emphasizes building quality in the production process, use of scientific principles and data, and plans to conduct follow-up studies on the outcomes of the use of the guideline, which are then used to update and improve the guideline.

Evaluation of Clinical Practice Guidelines

Many guidelines have been developed based on weak methods, incomplete literature reviews, and an overreliance on opinion. Such guidelines may be influenced by bias, conflicts of interest, and political motives. It is the responsibility of practitioners to evaluate the quality of guidelines, reject poor quality guidelines, and provide objective reasons why such guidelines should not be used. To a certain extent, knowledge of who developed a guideline is helpful in evaluating its quality. Guidelines prepared under the direction of the AHCPR can be expected to follow the detailed methodology described in the previous section of this chapter. In addition, the AMA, the ACP, the American Heart Association (AHA), the American College of Cardiology (ACC), the RAND Corporation, and others have all endorsed similar methodologies that emphasize the evidence-based approach, appropriate use of consensus, and thorough documentation of procedures and decision making rationale. Even though the development and review procedures used by these professional organizations provide some assurance, the quality and validity of a guideline cannot be discerned solely by knowing who developed it. The use of objective evaluation criteria is important. Although not yet systematically studied for validity, suggested evaluation criteria are available from AHCPR, AMA, ACP, and Canadian Medical Association (CMA). The criteria from the AHCPR will be emphasized in the following material.

When evaluating a clinical practice guideline, one could review its documentation of methods and decision making rationale and compare it with the recommendations from AHCPR presented in the previous section on guideline development. One could also review the guideline and judge its consistency with the eight desirable attributes of clinical practice guidelines that have been delineated for the AHCPR by the IOM of the National Academy of Sciences. These eight attributes are as follows.

1. *Validity*—Practice guidelines are valid if, when followed, they lead to the health and cost outcomes projected for them. A prospective assessment of validity will consider the substance and quality of the evidence cited, the means used to evaluate the evidence, and the relationship between the evidence and recommendations.
   * *Strength of evidence*—Practice guidelines should be accompanied by descriptions of the strength of the evidence and the expert judgment behind them.
   * *Estimated outcomes*—Practice guidelines should be accompanied by estimates of the health and cost outcomes expected from the interventions in question compared with alternate practices. Assessments of relevant health outcomes will consider patient perceptions and preferences.
2. *Reliability/reproducibility*—Practice guidelines are reproducible and reliable if (a) given the same evidence and methods for guideline development, another set of experts produces essentially the same statements, and (b) given the same clinical circumstances, the guidelines are interpreted and applied consistently by practitioners.
3. *Clinical applicability*—Practice guidelines should be as inclusive of appropriately defined patient populations as evidence and expert judgment permit and explicitly state the population(s) to which statements apply.
4. *Clinical flexibility*—Practice guidelines should identify the specifically known or generally expected exceptions to their recommendations and discuss how patient preferences are to be identified and considered.
5. *Clarity*—Practice guidelines must use unambiguous language, define terms precisely, and use logical and easy-to-follow modes of presentation.

6. *Multidisciplinary process*—Practice guidelines must be developed by a process that includes participation by representatives of key affected groups. Participation may include serving on panels that develop guidelines, providing evidence and viewpoints to the panels, and reviewing draft guidelines.

7. *Scheduled review*—Practice guidelines must include statements about when they should be reviewed to determine whether revisions are warranted given new clinical evidence or professional consensus (or lack of it).

8. *Documentation*—The procedures followed in developing guidelines, the participants involved, the evidence used, the assumptions and rationales accepted, and the analytic methods employed must be meticulously documented and described.

In addition, the IOM has developed a more formal evaluation instrument to assess clinical practice guidelines. This instrument uses the eight attributes as a starting point but expands these attributes to a series of 46 questions with as many as 10 subquestions on some points, creating a 40-page evaluation document. Individual clinicians are not the intended users of this assessment instrument; however, a group or panel involved in development or implementation of clinical practice guidelines may wish to consider its use. The full instrument is available as Appendix B of Field and Lohr's *Guidelines for Clinical Practice: From Development to Use.*[1]

The CMA in collaboration with five other professional medical associations in Canada developed 14 guiding principles for the clinical practice guidelines process.[80] Comparison of a clinical practice guideline against these principles is another useful method for evaluation of the guideline by the practitioner. The CMA stated that the need for these guiding principles was a result of the more than 40 organizations that were actively involved in guideline development and more than 400 clinical practice guidelines in use in Canada. The Association also has stated that the rapidly increasing volume and complexity of medical research makes it difficult for physicians to incorporate research data into daily practice. The Association believes that guidelines assist physicians in the clinical decision making process and improve quality of care and outcomes, minimize risk, and enhance efficiency. They note that the guideline process is complex and includes needs assessment, development, implementation, evaluation, and revision; therefore, it requires expertise and experience to ensure effectiveness. These 14 guiding principles are intended to foster quality in the guideline process. These principles, divided into three categories, are as follows.

PHILOSOPHY AND ETHICS

1. The goal of clinical practice guidelines should be to improve quality of health care.
2. Clinical practice guidelines should be sufficiently flexible to allow patients and physicians to exercise judgment when choosing among available options.

3. Clinical practice guidelines should enable informed decision making by patients and physicians by enhancing professional learning, patient education, and patient–physician communication.

4. Clinical practice guidelines should recognize that the physician's primary responsibility is to his or her own patient, although it may have to be balanced against the needs of other people and society in general.

5. Ethical issues should be considered in all phases of the clinical practice guideline process.

METHODS

6. Organizations with clinical practice guideline programs should articulate clear goals and explicitly document processes for setting priorities and assigning resources to the development, implementation, evaluation, and revision of guidelines.

7. Clinical practice guidelines should be developed by physicians in collaboration with representatives of those who will be affected by the specific intervention(s) in question, including relevant physician groups, patients, and other health care providers as appropriate.

8. Developers of clinical practice guidelines should state the objectives and methods, and identify the intended users before the guideline is developed.

9. Clinical practice guidelines should (a) cite the specific evidence bearing on the conclusion, (b) indicate the strength of the evidence, and (c) specify the date of the most recent evidence considered.

10. Before implementation, clinical practice guidelines should be reviewed by expert and user groups and, if possible, tested through such mechanisms as field trials.

11. When appropriate, the developers of a clinical practice guideline should use a standardized summary to report the development process and key conclusions.

IMPLEMENTATION AND EVALUATION

12. The clinical practice guideline process should include specifically tailored, effective, and coordinated strategies for voluntary implementation that emphasize patient, physician, and other health care provider involvement.

13. The effectiveness of the clinical practice guideline process should be assessed with a well-designed program evaluation that incorporates user feedback.

14. Clinical practice guidelines should be reviewed and revised as advances in medical knowledge occur.

The Evidence-Based Medicine Working Group at McMaster University, Hamilton, Ontario, chaired by Guyatt, has had a significant influence on the development of the recommended methods for clinical practice guidelines. This group has also published an excellent series of articles[81-86] on various aspects of clinical practice guidelines and a "user's guide" to evaluation and use of guidelines[87,88] (also available at <<http://hiru. hirunet.mcmaster.ca/ebm>> or <<http://www.cche.net/>>).

Shaneyfelt and colleagues[89] conducted an evaluation of 279 guidelines published in peer-reviewed literature from 1985 to June of 1997. Using the principles of guideline development and reporting formulated by major medical organizations (essentially those described in this chapter) these researchers identified 25 key elements or criteria for guideline evaluation. These elements were reviewed and pilot tested by guideline developers, evaluators, implementers, and groups of practicing clinicians. Feedback was also solicited at three national workshops about practice guidelines. Overall, the mean number of standards satisfied by the guidelines out of 25 was 10.77 (SD 3.71) with a range of 2 to 24. Guidelines did show improvement from 1985 (mean 9.2 elements met) to 1997 (mean 12.6 elements met). Remarkably, of the guidelines reviewed, only 10.8% reported an expiration date or date of scheduled review, only 12.9% graded recommendations according to the strength of evidence, and only 14.3% quantified an estimated effect on health care costs. The guidelines reviewed in this study were produced by 69 different groups; 45% were produced by subspecialty medical societies, 33% by general medical societies, 16% by governmental agencies, and 6% by miscellaneous groups. The results of this study demonstrate that many published guidelines fail to follow recommended standards and underline the importance of guideline evaluation by practitioners and organizations.

The gold standard for guideline evaluation may ultimately be validation via controlled trials or other forms of scientific research.[90] Examples that have undergone this form of evaluation were mentioned in the section on quality improvement. Also with the efforts of AHCPR and others, research continues on validation of guidelines and methods to most effectively communicate and implement the guideline.

Implementation of Clinical Practice Guidelines

The most effective methods for implementing guidelines to achieve the desired effects of improved quality of care have not been determined. It appears that implementation strategies that use multiple methods and consider local practice and political characteristics will be the most likely to succeed. In a systematic review of adoption of clinical practice guidelines, variables that affected the success of implementation included qualities specific to the guidelines, characteristics of the health professional, characteristics of the practice setting, incentives, regulation, and patient factors.[91] The methods shown to be weak were traditional Continuing Medical Education (CME) and mailings. Moderately effective were audit and feedback, especially those that were concurrent, targeted to specific providers, and delivered by peers or opinion leaders. Strong methods were reminder systems, academic detailing, and multiple intervention systems.[91]

Cabana and colleagues[92] conducted a systematic review of the literature to review barriers to physician adherence to clinical practice guidelines. For this review the authors conducted a search for articles published between January 1966 and January 1998 that focused on clinical practice guidelines, practice parameters, clinical policies, national recommendations or consensus statements, and that examined at least one barrier to adherence. A barrier was defined as any factor that limits or restricts complete physician adherence to a guideline. The full text of 423 articles was examined and 76 met the criteria for inclusion in the review. After classifying possible barriers into common themes the authors identified seven general categories or barriers. Table 9–2 lists the seven categories of barriers and provides examples or a description of each barrier. The relative importance of different barriers will vary depending on the characteristics of the specific guideline, and on many local health care system characteristics. However, this review provides a "differential diagnosis for why physicians do not follow practice guidelines." Appropriate attention to these potential barriers in the planning and development of guidelines will facilitate successful implementation.

Computer-based clinical decision support is one method thought to facilitate guideline implementation. A systematic review of controlled trials assessing the effects of computer-based clinical decision support systems indicated that they can enhance clinical performance for drug dosing, preventive care, and other aspects of medical care, but were not convincing for effects on diagnosis.[93]

A randomized controlled trial of continuous quality improvement and academic detailing to implement clinical guidelines for the primary care of hypertension and depression produced mixed results.[94] The authors concluded that both academic detailing and CQI interventions involve complex social interactions that produce varied implementation across the different organizations.

An observational study of general practice in the Netherlands identified the following characteristics that influenced the use of guidelines: (1) specific attributes of the guidelines determine whether they are used in practice; (2) evidence-based recommendations are better followed in practice than those not based on scientific evidence; (3) precise definitions of recommended performance improve use; (4) testing the feasibility and acceptance of clinical guidelines among target groups is important; and (5) the people setting the guidelines need to understand the attributes of effective evidence-based guidelines.[95]

TABLE 9–2. BARRIERS TO PHYSICIAN ADHERENCE TO CLINICAL PRACTICE GUIDELINES

Barrier Category	Examples of Barriers Identified or Description of Barrier
Lack of awareness	• Did not know the guideline existed
Lack of familiarity	• Could not correctly answer questions about guideline content or self-reported lack of familiarity
Lack of agreement	• Difference in interpretation of the evidence • Benefits not worth patient risk, discomfort, or cost • Not applicable to patient population in their practice • Credibility of authors questioned • Oversimplified cookbook • Reduces autonomy • Decreases flexibility • Decreases physician self-respect • Not practical • Makes patient–physician relationship impersonal
Lack of self-efficacy	• Did not believe that they could actually perform the behavior or activity recommended by the guideline, e.g., nutrition or exercise counseling
Lack of outcome expectancy	• Did not believe intended outcome would occur even if the practice was followed, e.g., counseling to stop smoking
Inertia of previous practice	• This barrier relates primarily to motivation to change practice, whether the motivation is professional, personal, or social. It was also noted that guidelines that recommend eliminating a behavior are more difficult to implement than guidelines that recommend adding a new behavior
External barriers	• Patient resistance/nonadherence • Patient does not perceive need • Perceived to be offensive to patient • Causes patient embarrassment • Lack of reminder system • Not easy to use, not convenient, cumbersome, confusing • Lack of educational materials • Cost to patient • Insufficient staff or consultant support or other resources • Lack of time • Lack of reimbursement • Increased malpractice liability • Not compatible with practice setting

A systematic literature review and evaluation of 59 studies of guidelines was published in 1993.[96] The authors conducted an extensive literature search and identified 59 studies that they considered to have appropriate methods to evaluate the effect of guidelines on either physician behavior or patient outcomes. All but four of the studies showed some benefit from the guidelines; however, the magnitude of the benefit and the patient care significance was not impressive in all cases.

Several articles have also been published describing how medical informatics can be used to help clinicians find, use, and create practice guidelines.[97–100]

Eddy stated in a lecture to the IOM, "All the science in the world has no effect until it is implemented properly, and measuring performance is one of the most powerful tools for implementation."[101] Guidelines represent one beginning application of decision support systems to facilitate providing quality clinical care. When written well, practice guidelines should contain all the necessary elements of routine care for most individuals with a specific condition. They should prompt consideration of what specific characteristics of an individual patient might warrant departures from the guideline. Effectively implemented, such systems save clinicians time. They should be assisted by computerized systems that, among other functions, can catalogue past histories, check orders for medications against measures of hepatic and renal function, and schedule reminders for screening tests or preventive services. They should be part of the continuous improvement of systems of care. Guidelines will not be perfect at the outset, systems that use them must be constructed so that experience can be applied to improve the guidelines, just as the guidelines indicate where care delivery can be improved.[102]

Sources of Clinical Practice Guidelines

There are several mechanisms to locate completed clinical practice guidelines or systematic reviews. A web-based national guideline clearing house (NGC) <<http://www.guideline.gov>> has been created by the AHCPR, in cooperation with the AMA and the American Association of Health Plans. The mission of the NGC is to provide an accessible mechanism for obtaining objective, detailed information on clinical practice guidelines and to further their dissemination, implementation and use. Components of the NGC include structured abstracts about the guideline and its development; a utility for comparing attributes of two or more guidelines in a side-by-side comparison; synthesis of guidelines covering similar topics, highlighting areas of similarity and difference; links to full-text guidelines where available and/or ordering information for print copies; an electronic forum for exchanging information on clinical practice guidelines and their development, implementation, and use; and annotated bibliographies on guideline development methodology implementation and use. To be included in the NGC the following criteria must be met.

1. The clinical practice guideline contains systematically developed statements that include recommendations, strategies, or information that assists physicians and/or other health care practitioners and patients make decisions about appropriate health care for specific clinical circumstances.

2. The clinical practice guideline was produced under the auspices of medical specialty associations; relevant professional societies, public or private organizations, government agencies at the Federal, State, or local level; or health care organizations or plans. A clinical practice guideline developed and issued by an individual not officially sponsored or supported by one of the above types of organizations does not meet the inclusion criteria for NGC.

3. Corroborating documentation can be produced and verified that a systematic literature search and review of existing scientific evidence published in peer-reviewed journals was performed during the guideline development. A guideline is not excluded from NGC if corroborating documentation can be produced and verified detailing specific gaps in scientific evidence for some of the guideline's recommendations.

4. The guideline is in English, current, and the most recent version produced. Documented evidence can be produced or verified that the guideline was developed, reviewed, or revised within the last 5 years.

The NGC provides a search function for identifying guidelines by disease, producer, bibliographic source, characteristics of the guideline, date, clinical specialty, objective, target population, and many other factors. The search engine allows the use of Boolean operators, truncation, automatic concept mapping, textword searching, and multiple sort and display options. The NGC premiered in January 1999 with 286 guidelines and is expected to include an estimated 3500 within 3 years.

Many guidelines have been published in the peer-reviewed medical literature and can therefore be located in MEDLINE. A variety of search techniques may be used, but the most efficient may be to search for "practice guideline" in the publication type field of the record, or use the MeSH term "practice guidelines" in conjunction with other terms for the specific disease or therapy of interest. Additional publication types in the NLM record that may be searched include "consensus development conference," "consensus development conference, NIH," "guideline," "meta-analysis," and "review, academic." Systematic review articles are also useful in preparation of clinical practice guidelines. The key differences with systematic reviews compared to the old forms of narrative review articles are that the systematic review begins with a focused clinical question, involves a comprehensive search for evidence, uses criteria-based selection that are uniformly applied to include evidence in the review, performs rigorous critical appraisal of the studies chosen, and provides a quantitative summary of the evidence.[103] Literature search strategies have been published for locating systematic reviews.[104]

Internet access to the full text AHCPR guidelines is available at <<http://www.ahcpr.gov>>. The NIH Consensus Statements, NIH Technology Assessments, the U.S. Preventive Services Task Force Guide to Clinical Preventive Services, HIV/AIDS Treatment Information Service, Substance Abuse and Mental Health Services Administration, Center for Substance Abuse Treatment improvement protocols, and links to the CDC Guidelines Database are available on Health Services Technology Assessment Texts (HSTAT). HSTAT was developed by the NLM Information Technology Branch and can be accessed at <<http://text.nlm.nih.gov>>. The Combined Health Information Database at <<http://chid.nih.gov>> provides access to information from the NIH, CDC, and complementary and alternative medicine.

As mentioned, multiple professional organizations, academic centers, independent research centers, and government agencies are involved in development of clinical practice guideline activities. Updated information may be obtained by contacting these organizations directly and many have provided access to their guidelines on the Internet.

Two new databases are also available, which are useful for obtaining information to support an evidence-based practice—*Best Evidence* and the *Cochrane Library. Best Evidence* is the electronic presentation of all issues of *ACP Journal Club* (1991 to present) and *Evidence-Based Medicine* (1995 to present). It contains more than 1300 articles carefully selected for their scientific merit and clinical relevance. The articles present enhanced structured abstracts of original research and are accompanied by expert commentaries. *ACP Journal Club* and *Evidence-Based Medicine* are published bimonthly and include articles from approximately 85 journals. *Best Evidence* is available on CD-ROM and is distributed by the American College of Physicians, the BMJ Publishing Group, and the CMA. More information may be obtained about *Best Evidence* at <<http://www.acponline.org/catalog/electronic/best_evidence.htm>>.

The Cochrane Library is based on the work of an international collaboration of health care providers and scientists who engage in preparing, maintaining, and disseminating systematic reviews of relevant randomized controlled trials of health care.[105] This collaboration is named in honor of Archie Cochrane, who in 1979 wrote "it is surely a great criticism of our profession that we have not organized a critical summary, by specialty, adapted periodically, of all relevant randomized controlled trials." The Cochrane Library provides a collection of four databases on one CD-ROM—*The Cochrane Database of Systematic Reviews, The York Database of Abstracts of Reviews of Effectiveness, The Cochrane Controlled Trials Register,* and *The Cochrane Review Methodology Database.*

The *Cochrane Database of Systematic Reviews* is a collection of highly structured and systematic reviews of research evidence in specific areas of health care. Data are often combined statistically (with meta-analysis) to increase the power of the findings from multiple studies. This database includes over 326 complete reviews and is growing. This database also includes another 342 protocols, which are reviews that are in process.

The *York Database of Abstracts of Reviews of Effectiveness* includes structured abstracts of good quality systematic reviews from around the world that have been critically appraised by reviewers at the National Health Service Centre for Reviews and Dissemination at the University of York, England. This database also provides brief records of reviews that may be useful for background information, as well as the abstracts of reports produced by technology assessment agencies worldwide, and abstracts of reviews from the *ACP Journal Club.*

The *Cochrane Controlled Trials Register* is a bibliography of controlled trials identified by contributors to the Cochrane Collaboration as part of an international effort to create an unbiased source of data for systematic reviews of the medical literature. There are currently over 158,000 articles referenced in this bibliography.

The *Cochrane Review Methodology Database* is a bibliography of articles and books on the science of research evaluation and synthesis. It also contains an extensive handbook on conducting critical literature appraisal, and developing systematic reviews of the best available evidence on health care topics. More information is available about the Cochrane Collaboration and the Cochrane Library from the McMaster University evidence-based medicine web site at <<http://hiru.mcmaster.ca/cochrane/default.htm>>.

The Internet has rapidly become a useful tool for access to health care–related information. Many sites are potentially useful. Three excellent sites that are specifically designed to support EBM are the AHCPR web site listed above, the Health Information Research Unit at McMaster University (<<http://hiru.mcmaster.ca/>>), and the Centre for Evidence-Based Medicine at Oxford (<<http://cebm.jr2.ox.ac.uk/>>). These sites contain extensive information about systematic appraisal and use of evidence, worldwide projects for development of EBM, including clinical practice guidelines and links to many other quality sites.

Many activities conducted by professional organizations in pharmacy have principles in common with EBM and clinical practice guidelines. The following paragraphs briefly describe a few of these prominent activities.

The American Society of Health-System Pharmacists (ASHP) in 1990 created a policy-recommending body called the Commission on Therapeutics. This commission develops therapeutic guidelines defined as "systematically developed documents that assist health-care professionals on appropriate use of drugs for specific clinical circumstances."[106] With the publication of the ASHP Therapeutic Guidelines on Angiotensin-Converting-Enzyme Inhibitors in Patients with Left Ventricular Dysfunction,[107] the ASHP initiated an evidence-based style for its therapeutic guidelines.[108] The ASHP uses a process for preparation of the therapeutic guidelines similar to the one developed by the AHCPR.

The most recent therapeutic guideline from ASHP is on stress ulcer prophylaxis.[109] This extensive review coordinated by Brian L. Erstad, PharmD, and Kathryn L. Grant, PharmD, used the most current methods for guideline preparation including decision algorithms and a decision tree for pharmacoeconomic analysis. They employed methods for assessing the literature by using evidence tables, and categorized the recommendations according to the strength of evidence using a system based on recommendations from the Evidence-Based Working Group at McMaster. This system for defining levels of evidence takes into consideration the information provided in meta-analysis, the consistency of results across trials, and the bounds of the 95% confidence interval compared to the numerical threshold for clinically important benefit.

The American Pharmaceutical Association (APhA) has published the *APhA Guide to Drug Treatment Protocols: A Resource for Creating & Using Disease-Specific Pathways*.[110] This resource includes specific drug treatment protocols and an extensive handbook on the guideline development process and many issues surrounding the use of evidence-based guidelines. This resource was developed by the APhA to assist health professionals with their efforts to develop, use, and measure patient outcomes with disease-specific drug treatment protocols. The APhA uses a multidisciplinary process to develop the guidelines based on scientific evidence published in the peer-reviewed literature. New protocols are being produced and released on a continuing basis. Other Internet sources of clinical guidelines are listed in the appendices of Chap. 5.

Conclusion

Clinical practice guidelines have become a significant tool in health care with the focus on evidence-based practice. These guidelines fit well with the emphasis of continuous quality improvement techniques. Guidelines have the potential to assist medical decision making and ultimately improve the quality of care, improve patient outcomes, and make more efficient use of resources. Significant advances have been made in the methodology to produce valid guidelines. Information technology, and greater understanding of optimal methods for implementation of guidelines, will maximize their effect to improve quality of care. Pharmacists' active involvement in preparation of evidence-based clinical practice guidelines is vital to ensure that pharmaceutical care issues are addressed. A thorough understanding of evidence-based methodology will prepare the pharmacist to participate in this process.

Study Questions

The Agency for Health Care Research and Quality (formerly AHCPR) has set criteria for choosing a topic for development of evidence reports and systematic reviews. These criteria are very similar to those that have been recommended for professional organizations, integrated health systems, individual hospitals, or practitioners who plan to develop disease management programs.

1. Which of the following would *not* be consistent with the recommended criteria?
   a. Evidence of suboptimal treatment exists.
   b. The condition has a high prevalence in the general populations or in subgroups.
   c. There is little controversy or uncertainly about the effectiveness of management strategies.
   d. There is potential to influence patient decision making.
   e. Data are available to construct guidelines for best practices.

2. Which of the following is *not* considered to be part of the philosophy of the evidence-based practice of medicine?
   a. Life-long self-directed learning.
   b. Explicit use of best evidence in making decisions.
   c. Information management is critical.
   d. Evidence is restricted to randomized controlled trial or meta-analysis.
   e. Full informed participation by patients in decision making is encouraged.

3. Which of the following is considered to be a strong argument for implementation of evidence-based care?
   a. It eliminates reliance on clinical expertise, which is known to be invalid for clinical decision.
   b. It will reduce costs for providing health care.
   c. It supports self-directed continuing education, which has been shown to be more effective in maintaining current knowledge.
   d. It restricts decision making to evidence from randomized controlled trials so reliability of decisions is improved.
   e. Most practitioners already have the skills and are following this philosophy so it is a natural step to implement.

4. Which of the following is an important outcome from the development of clinical practice guidelines?
   a. The standardized practices will ensure cost savings in health care.
   b. More authority for decision making is given to administrators.
   c. The use of clinical practice guidelines reduces the reliance on clinical judgment.
   d. Gaps in the evidence are identified so that research funding can be focused on the area with the greatest potential to provide answers to important questions.
   e. Unemployment among drug information pharmacists is reduced.

5. Which of the following would be the best indicator to evaluate the validity of a clinical practice guideline?

a. Clear documentation of the criteria used to select evidence for guideline development.
b. The guideline was produced by a specialty organization.
c. The guideline was published in a peer-reviewed journal.
d. The guideline incorporated consensus development to provide treatment recommendations.
e. The guideline includes a decision tree.

6. *True or false?* Clinical practice guidelines have many elements in common with a continuous quality improvement (CQI) process.

7. Which of the following is *not* one of the most likely reasons that practice guidelines are inconsistently followed in clinical practice?
a. Practitioners lack awareness of the existence of the guideline.
b. Patients do not want to participate in decision making.
c. Practitioners do not have convenient access to the guideline at the time decisions are made.
d. Practitioners do not agree that the guideline will achieve the benefits intended.
e. Lack of motivation to change current practice.

8. Which of the following would be the strongest predictor of success in implementing a clinical practice guideline within a health care system?
a. National specialist experts recommend that the practices be implemented.
b. A multifaceted strategy with local input is used.
c. The guidelines are very rigid.
d. The guidelines cover areas where level I evidence is not available.
e. The chief of the service wants it to be done.

9. Which of the following groups have *not* been involved in developing clinical practice guidelines?
a. Subspecialty medical societies.
b. General medical societies.
c. Governmental agencies.
d. Pharmacy professional societies.
e. All of the above have been involved in guideline development.

10. Which of the following methodological standards for guideline development has been the least frequently followed?
a. Purpose of the guideline is specified.
b. The role of value judgments used by the developers is discussed.
c. The targeted health problem or technology is clearly defined.

d. Flexibility in the recommendations is specified.

e. Benefits and harms of specific health practices are quantified.

REFERENCES

1. Field JM, Lohr KN, editors. Guidelines for clinical practice: from development to use. Washington (DC): National Academy Press, 1992.

2. Jones RH, Ritchie JL, Fleming BB, Hammermeister KE, Leape LL. 28th Bethesda Conference. Task force 1: Clinical practice guideline development, dissemination and computerization. J Am Coll Cardiol 1997;29:1133–41.

3. President's Advisory Commission on Consumer Protection and Quality in the Health Care Industry. Quality first better health care for all Americans. 1998 June 15 [cited 1999 Jan 18]:[1 screen]. Available from: URL: http://www.hcqualitycommission.gov/final/execsum.html.

4. Chassin MR, Galvin RW. The urgent need to improve health care quality. Institute of Medicine National Roundtable on Health Care Quality. JAMA 1998;280:1000–5.

5. Woolf SH. Practice guidelines: a new reality in medicine. III. Impact on patient care. Arch Intern Med 1993;153:2646–55.

6. Fang E, Mittman BS, Weingarten S. Use of clinical practice guidelines in managed care physician groups. Arch Fam Med 1996;5:528–31.

7. Highlights of national health expenditures, 1997. [cited 1999 Feb 15]:[1 screen]. Available from: URL: http://www.hcfa.gov/stats/nhe-oact/hilites.htm.

8. National health care expenditure projections [cited 1999 Feb 15]:[1 screen]. Available from: URL: http://www.hcfa.gov/stats/nhe-proj/hilites.htm.

9. Inglehart JK. The American health care system: expenditures. N Engl J Med 1999;340:70–6.

10. Grumbach K, Bodenheimer T. Painful vs. painless cost control. JAMA 1994;272:1458–64.

11. Blumenthal D. The variation phenomenon in 1994 [editorial]. N Engl J Med 1994;331:1017–18.

12. Epstein AM. The outcomes movement—will it get us where we want to go? N Engl J Med 1990;323:266–70.

13. Willcox SM, Himmelstein DU, Woolhandler S. Inappropriate drug prescribing for the community-dwelling elderly. JAMA 1994;272:292–6.

14. Beers MH, Ouslander JG, Fingold SF, Morgenstern H, Reuben DB, Rogers W, et al. Inappropriate medication prescribing in skilled nursing facilities. Ann Intern Med 1992;117:684–9.

15. President's Advisory Commission on Consumer Protection and Quality in the Health Care Industry. Strengthening the market to improve quality. Chapter ten. Reducing errors and increasing safety in health care. 1998 July 19 [cited 1999 Jan 18]:[1 screen]. Available from: URL: http://www.hcqualitycommission.gov/final/chap10.html.

16. Relman AS. Assessment and accountability: the third revolution in medical care. N Engl J Med 1988;319:1220–2.

17. Ellwood PM. Shattuck lecture—outcomes management: a technology of patient experience [report]. N Engl J Med 1988;318:1549–56.

18. Roper WL, Winkenwerder W, Hackbarth GM, Krakauer H. Effectiveness in healthcare. An initiative to evaluate and improve medical practice. N Engl J Med 1988;319:1197–202.

19. Woolf SH. Practice guidelines: a new reality in medicine. I. Recent developments. Arch Intern Med 1990;150:1811–18.

20. Field JM, Lohr KN, editors. Clinical practice guidelines: directions for a new program. Washington (DC): National Academy Press, 1990.

21. AHCPR Strategic Plan. 1998 December 15 [cited 1999 Feb 9]:[1 screen]. Available from: URL: http://www.ahcpr.gov/about/stratpln.htm.

22. Lazarou J, Pomeranz BH, Corey PN. Incidence of adverse drug reactions in hospitalized patients: a meta-analysis of prospective studies. JAMA 1998;279:1200–5.

23. Phillips DP, Christenfeld N, Glynn LM. Increase in US medication-error deaths between 1983 and 1993. Lancet 1998;351:643–4.

24. Berwick DM, Nolan TW. Physicians as leaders in improving health care: a new series in Annals of Internal Medicine. Ann Intern Med 1998;128:289–92.

25. Angell M. The American health care system revisited—a new series. N Engl J Med 1999; 340:48.

26. Quality and accreditation initiatives update. 1999 February [cited 1999 Feb 9]:[1 screen]. Available from: URL: http://www.aha.org/quality/QualityUpdate5-98.html.

27. Bodenheimer T. The American health care system—the movement for improved quality in health care. N Engl J Med 1999;340:488–92.

28. Blumenthal D, Kilo CM. A report card on continuous quality improvement. Milbank Q 1998; 76:625–48.

29. Shortell SM, Bennett CL, Byck GR. Assessing the impact of continuous quality improvement on clinical practice: What it will take to accelerate progress. Milbank Q 1998;76:593–624, 510.

30. Presidents' Advisory Commission on Consumer Protection and Quality in the Health Care Industry. Message from the Commission. 1998 July 19 [cited 1999 Jan 18]:[1 screen]. Available from: URL: http://www.hcqualitycommission.gov/.

31. Mitka M. Renewed efforts to improve the quality of health care. JAMA 1999;281:404.

32. Friedrich MJ. Quality groups coordinate. JAMA 1999;281:599

33. Skolnick AA. JCAHO, NCQA, and AMAP establish council to coordinate health care performance measurement. Joint Commission on Accreditation of Healthcare Organizations, National Committee for Quality Assurance, American Medical Accreditation Program. JAMA 1998;279: 1769–70

34. Marciniak TA, Ellerbeck EF, Radford MJ, Kresowik TF, Gold JA, Krumholz HM, et al. Improving the quality of care for Medicare patients with acute myocardial infarction: results from the Cooperative Cardiovascular Project. JAMA 1998;279:1351–7.

35. Soumerai SB, McLaughlin TJ, Gurwitz JH, Guadagnoli E, Hauptman PJ, Borbas C, et al. Effect of local medical opinion leaders on quality of care for acute myocardial infarction: a randomized controlled trial. JAMA 1998;279:1358–63.

36. The Challenge and Potential for Assuring Quality Health Care for the 21st Century. From quality measures to quality care: Examples of quality improvement at work. [cited 1999 Feb 9]: [2 screens]. Available from: URL: http://www.ahcpr.gov/qual/21stcenb.htm.

37. Sackett DL, Rosenberg WM, Gray JA, Haynes RB, Richardson WS. Evidence-based medicine: what it is and what it isn't. Br Med J 1996;312:71–2.

38. Evidence-Based Medicine Working Group. Evidence based medicine. A new approach to teaching the practice of medicine. JAMA 1992;268:2420–5.

39. Sackett DL, Richardson WS, Rosenberg W, Haynes RB. Evidence-based medicine: how to practice & teach EBM. New York: Churchill Livingstone; 1997.

40. Watanabe AS, McCart G, Shimomura S, Kayser S. Systematic approach to drug information requests. Am J Hosp Pharm 1975;32:1282–5.

41. Lauer B, Kuller A, Wessel C. MEDLINE and the new health care consumer. J Am Pharm Assoc 1999;39:92.

42. Medlineplus. [cited 1999 Feb 17]:[1 screen]. Available from: URL: http://www.nlm.nih.gov/medlineplus.

43. Rogers S. Evidence-based learning for general practice. Br J Gen Pract 1997;47:52–3.

44. McColl A, Smith H, White P, Field J. General practitioner's perceptions of the route to evidence based medicine: a questionnaire survey. Br Med J 1998;316:361–5.

45. Green ML, Ellis PJ. Impact of an evidence-based medicine curriculum based on adult learning theory. J Gen Intern Med 1997;12:742–50.

46. Shin JH, Haynes RB, Johnston ME. Effect of problem-based, self directed undergraduate education on life-long learning. CMAJ 1993;148:969–76.

47. Curry RH, Hershman WY, Saizow RB. Learner-centered strategies in clerkship education. Am J Med 1996;100:589–95.

48. Bordley DR, Fagan M, Theige D. Evidence-based medicine: a powerful educational tool for clerkship education. Am J Med 1997;102:427–32.

49. Reilly B, Lemon M. Evidence-based morning report: a popular new format in a large teaching hospital. Am J Med 1997;103:419–26.

50. Levin A. Evidence-based medicine gaining supporters. Ann Intern Med 1998;128:334–6.

51. Bryan CS, Evidence-based medicine: try it, you'll like it. J S C Med Assoc 1997;93:352–4.

52. Waeckerle JF, Cordell WH, Wyer P, Osborn HH. Evidence-based emergency medicine: integrating research into practice. Ann Emerg Med 1997;30:626–8.

53. Towle A. Changes in health care and continuing medical education for the 21st century. Br Med J 1998;316:301–4.

54. Davis D. Continuing Medical Education. Global health, global learning. Br Med J 1998;316:385–9.

55. Fox RD, Bennett NL. Learning and change: implications for continuing medical education. Br Med J 1998;316:466–8.

56. Bashook PG, Parboosingh J. Recertification and the maintenance of competence. Br Med J 1998;316:545–8.

57. Holm HA. Quality issues in continuing medical education. Br Med J 1998;316:621–4.

58. Southgate L, Dauphinee D. Maintaining standards in British and Canadian medicine: the developing role of the regulatory body. Br Med J 1998;316:697–700.

59. Headrick LA, Wilcock PM, Batalden PB. Interprofessional working and continuing medical education. Br Med J 1998;316:771–4.

60. Prager LO. Report sets health care improvement goals, stops short of urging mandates. American Medical News 1998; April 6 41:3, 21–2.

61. Woolf SH. Practice guidelines: a new reality in medicine. II. Methods of developing guidelines. Arch Intern Med 1992;152:946–52.

62. Perry S. The NIH consensus development program. A decade later. N Engl J Med 1987;317: 485–8.

63. Guidelines for the planning and management of NIH consensus development conferences 1995 March [cited 1999 Feb 22]:[1 screen]. Available from: URL: http://odp.od.nih.gov/consensus/about/process.htm.

64. Eddy DM. Clinical decision making: from theory to practice. Guidelines for policy statements: the explicit approach. JAMA 1990;263:2239–40, 2243.

65. Eddy DM. Clinical decision making: from theory to practice. Anatomy of a decision. JAMA 1990;263:441–3.

66. Eddy DM. Clinical decision making: from theory to practice. Practice policies—guidelines for methods. JAMA 1990;263:1839–41.

67. Eddy DM. Designing a practice policy. Standards, guidelines, and options. JAMA 1990;263: 3077–81, 3084.

68. Woolf SH. Manual for clinical practice guideline development. AHCPR Publication No. 91-0007. Rockville (MD): Agency for Health Care Policy and Research, Public Health Service, U.S. Department of Health and Human Services; 1991.

69. About AHCPR Agency for Health Care Policy and Research, Rockville MD [cited 1999 Feb 1]:[1 screen]. Available from: URL: http://www.ahcpr.gov/about/.

70. AHCPR announces 12 evidence-based practice centers. Agency for Health Care Policy and Research. 1997 June 25 [cited 1999 Feb 1]:[1 screen]. Available from: URL: http://www.ahcpr.gov/news/press/12epcpr.htm.

71. AHCPR Strategic Plan December 15, 1998. Agency for Health Care Policy and Research, Rockville MD. 1998 Dec 15 [cited 1999 Feb 9]:[1 screen]. Available from: URL: http://www.ahcpr.gov/about/stratpln.htm.

72. Ritchie JR, Forrester JS, Fye WB. Practice guidelines and quality of care. Proceedings of the 28th Bethesda Conference; 1996 October 21–22; Bethesda (MD). J Am Coll Cardiol 1997; 29:1125–79.

73. Dalen JE, Hirsh J. Fifth ACCP Consensus Conference on Antithrombotic Therapy. Chest 1998; 114(5 suppl):439S–769S.

74. Konstam M, Dracup K, Bottorff M, Brooks NH, Dacey RA, Dunbar SB, et al. Heart failure: evaluation and care of patients with left-ventricular systolic dysfunction. Clinical practice guideline No.11. AHCPR Publication No. 94-0612. Rockville (MD): Agency for Health Care Policy and Research, Public Health Service, U.S. Department of Health and Human Services; 1994.

75. Parmley WW. Clinical practice guidelines: does the cookbook have enough recipes? [editorial] JAMA 1994;272:1374–5.

76. Phillips WR. Clinical policies: making conflicts of interest explicit. Task Force on Clinical Policies for Patient Care. American Academy of Family Physicians [letter]. JAMA 1994;272:1479.

77. Evans RS, Classen DC, Pestotnik SL, Lundsgaarde HP, Burke JP. Improving empiric antibiotic selection using computer decision support. Arch Intern Med 1994;154:878–84.

78. Evans RS, Pestotnik SL, Classen DC, Clemmer TP, Weaver LK, Orme JF Jr. A computer-assisted management program for antibiotics and other antiinfective agents. N Engl J Med 1998;338:232–8.

79. Guyatt GH, Cook DJ, Sackett DL, Eckman M, Pauker S. Grades of recommendation for antithrombotic agents. Chest 1998;114:441S–4S.

80. National partnership for Quality in Health. Guidelines for Canadian clinical practice guidelines. Ottawa, Ontario: Canadian Medical Association; 1994.

81. Rafuse J. Evidence-based medicine means MDs must develop new skills, attitudes, CMA conference told. CMAJ 1994;150:1479–81.

82. Evidence-Based Care Resource Group. Evidence-based care: 1. Setting priorities: how important is this problem? CMAJ 1994;150:1249–54.

83. Evidence-Based Care Resource Group. Evidence-based care: 2. Setting guidelines: how should we manage this problem? CMAJ 1994;150:1417–23.

84. Evidence-Based Care Resource Group. Evidence-based care: 3. Measuring performance: how are we managing this problem? CMAJ 1994;150:1575–9.

85. Evidence-Based Care Resource Group. Evidence-based care: 4. Improving performance: how can we improve the way we manage this problem? CMAJ 1994;150:1793–6.

86. Evidence-Based Care Resource Group. Evidence-based care: 5. Lifelong learning: how can we learn to be more effective? CMAJ 1994;150:1971–3.

87. Hayward RS, Wilson MC, Tunis SR, Bass EB, Guyatt G. Users' guide to the medical literature. VIII. How to use clinical practice guidelines. A. Are the recommendations valid? The Evidence-Based Medicine Working Group. JAMA 1995;274:570–4.

88. Wilson MC, Hayward RS, Tunis SR, Bass EB, Guyatt G. Users' guides to the medical literature. VIII. How to use clinical practice guidelines. B. What are the recommendations and will they help you in caring for your patients? The Evidence-Based Medicine Working Group. JAMA 1995;274:1630–2.

89. Shaneyfelt TM, Mayo-Smith MF, Rothwangl J. Are guidelines following guidelines? The methodological quality of clinical practice guidelines in the peer-reviewed medical literature. JAMA 1999;281:1900–5.

90. McDonald CJ, Overhage JM. Guidelines you can follow and can trust. An ideal and an example. JAMA 1994;271:872–3.

91. Davis DA, Taylor-Vaisey A. Translating guidelines into practice. A systematic review of theoretic concepts, practical experience and research evidence in the adoption of clinical practice guidelines. CMAJ 1997;157:408–16.

92. Cabana MD, Rand CS, Powe NR, Wu AW, Wilson MH, Abboud PAC, et al. Why don't physicians follow clinical practice guidelines? A framework for improvement. JAMA 1999;282:1458–65.

93. Hunt DL, Haynes RB, Hanna SE, Smith K. Effects of computer-based clinical decision support systems on physician performance and patient outcomes: a systematic review. JAMA 1998; 280:1339–46.

94. Horowitz CR, Golberg HI, Martin DP, Wagner EH, Fihn SD, Christensen DB, et al. Conducting a randomized controlled trial of CQI and academic detailing to implement clinical guidelines. Jt Comm J Qual Improv 1996;22:734–50.

95. Grol R, Dalhuijsen J, Thomas S, Veld C, Rutten G, Mokkink H. Attributes of clinical guidelines that influence use of guidelines in general practice: observational study. Br Med J 1998;317: 858–61.

96. Grimshaw JM, Russell IT. Effect of clinical guidelines on medical practice: a systematic review of rigorous evaluations. Lancet 1993;342:1317–22.

97. Owens DK. Use of medical informatics to implement and develop clinical practice guidelines. West J Med 1998;168:166–75.

98. Duff L, Casey A. Implementing clinical guidelines: How can informatics help? J Am Med Inform Assoc 1998;5:225–6.

99. Zielstorff RD. Online practice guidelines: Issues, obstacles, and future prospects. J Am Med Inform Assoc 1998;5:227–36.

100. Henry SB, Douglas K, Galzagorry G, Lahey A, Holzemer WL. A template-based approach to support utilization of clinical practice guidelines within an electronic health record. J Am Med Inform Assoc 1998;5:237–44.

101. Eddy DM Performance measurement: Problems and solutions. Health Aff (Millwood) 1998; 17(4):7–25.

102. Chassin MR. Is health care ready for six sigma quality? Milbank Q 1998;76(4):565–91, 510.

103. Cook DJ, Mulrow CD, Haynes RB. Systematic review: synthesis of best evidence for clinical decisions. Ann Intern Med 1997;126:376–80.

104. Hunt DL, McKibbon KA. Locating and appraising systematic reviews. Ann Intern Med 1997;126:532–8.

105. Sackett DL. The Cochrane collaboration [editorial]. ACP J Club 1994;May/June, 120(suppl 3):A11.

106. Practice standards of ASHP 1993–1994. Bethesda (MD): American Society of Hospital Pharmacists; 1993.

107. American Society of Health-System Pharmacists. ASHP Therapeutic Guidelines on Angiotensin-Converting-Enzyme Inhibitors in Patients with Left Ventricular Dysfunction. This official ASHP practice standard was developed through the ASHP Commission on Therapeutics and approved by the ASHP Board of Directors on November 16, 1996. Am J Health-Syst Pharm 1997;54:299–313.

108. Cooke-Ariel H. Promoting use of angiotensin-converting-enzyme inhibitors. Am J Health-Syst Pharm 1997;54:264.

109. American Society of Health-System Pharmacists. ASHP therapeutic guidelines on stress ulcer prophylaxis. Am J Health-Syst Pharm 1999;56:347–79.

110. Manolakis PG, editor. APhA guide to drug treatment protocols: a resource for creating & using disease-specific pathways. Washington (DC): American Pharmaceutical Association; 1997.

10

Chapter Ten

Clinical Application of Statistical Analysis

Karen L. Kier

Objectives

After completing this chapter, the reader will be able to:

- Describe the importance of interpreting statistics in completing and evaluating scientific studies.
- Define the various levels of data.
- Determine whether the appropriate statistics have been performed and provided in a study.
- Interpret the statistical results provided in a research study to determine whether the authors' conclusions are supported.

Biostatistics is an area essential to understanding biomedical and pharmacy literature. This chapter provides a basic understanding of biostatistics for the reader who has little or no statistical background. The focus is on describing concepts as they relate to evaluating medical literature rather than discussing the mathematical formulas and various statistical procedures. Understanding statistics will enhance the pharmacist's ability to interpret the biomedical literature and draw conclusions from research studies.

Before discussing many of the types of statistics that are used in medical literature, it may be helpful to review information about the design of studies and type of data collected. When using statistical tests, assumptions are often made that require knowledge of the research design and the methods used by the researchers. The first part of this chapter reviews some basic concepts about populations, samples, data, and variables. The second part discusses specific types of descriptive and inferential statistics. This chapter should be used in conjunction with Chaps 6 and 7 because many of the concepts are interrelated.

Basic Concepts

POPULATIONS AND SAMPLES

A *population* refers to all objects of a particular kind in the universe; a *sample* is a portion of that population. The measurements that describe a population are referred to as *parameters;* those measurements that describe a sample are considered *statistics.* The *sample statistic* is an estimate of the population parameter. When investigating a particular issue, one must describe the population to be studied. In most practical situations, it is impossible to measure the entire population; rather, one must take a representative sample. For example, if one wanted to study the effect that a calcium channel blocker agent has on blood glucose levels in people with insulin-dependent diabetes mellitus, then patients with insulin-dependent diabetes would be the study population. To study this group, the researchers would have to take a representative sample from all insulin-dependent diabetic patients.

To make appropriate and accurate inferences about the study population, the sample must be representative of the population. Samples must be selected from the population appropriately or the data may not actually reflect the population parameters. One of the most common methods for selecting a representative sample is called a simple random sample. When making inferences from the study population by using a sample of the population, it is important that the study sample be selected at random. *Random,* in this case, does not imply that the sample is drawn haphazardly or in an unplanned fashion, but that each member of the population has an equal probability of being selected for the sample. Referring back to the example of diabetes, each insulin-dependent diabetic patient theoretically has an equal chance of being selected into the sample from the population. There are several approaches to selecting a simple random sample; however, the most common is the use of a random numbers table. A *random numbers table* is a set of integers between 0 and 9 that have been selected at random without any trends or patterns. At any point in the table, it is equally likely that any digit between 0 and 9 would be selected. Choosing a number in this fashion is analogous to pulling numbers from a hat. In using a random numbers table, a point is selected within the table as the starting point and the numbers are then used in order from that point.

Depending on the type of study design, a simple random sample may not be the best means for determining a representative sample. Sometimes it may be necessary to separate the population into nonoverlapping groups called *strata,* where a specific factor (e.g., gender) will be contained in separate strata to aid in analysis. In this case, the random sample is drawn within each strata. This method is called a *stratified random sample.* For certain types of research, a certain factor is important in the study group. An example would be when gender or ethnic background are important factors within the study. To ensure that gender or ethnic background are studied, one has to represent these individuals in the sample. By creating the stratified groups based on this factor, the researcher is assured that these groups will be appropriately represented in the sample. In stratified random sampling, a simple random sample is still performed within each group or strata.

Another means of randomly sampling a population is a method that is known as *random cluster sampling.* It may not be practical to sample all pharmacists in the United States about their patient counseling practices; therefore, the researchers may opt to randomly select 5 states from the 50 states; the 5 states would represent the clusters to be sampled. The researchers would then select their sample from the pharmacists within these 5 states, or clusters, for their study.

Another method often used is referred to as *systematic sampling.* This technique is used when information about the population is provided in list format, such as in the telephone book. With systematic sampling, one name is selected near the beginning of the list and every nth name is then selected thereafter. For example, the researchers may decide to take every 10th name from the first name selected. It should be noted, however, that some individuals do not consider this type of sampling to be truly random.

In review, the sample describes those individuals who are in the study. The population describes the infinite number of people to whom the study refers.

VARIABLES AND DATA

A *variable* is a characteristic that is being observed or measured. Data are the values assigned to that variable for each individual member of the population. There are two types of variables: independent and dependent. Some statistical textbooks will refer to a third type of variable called a confounding variable. Within a study, the *dependent variable* is the one that changes in response to the *independent variable.* The dependent variable is the outcome of interest within the study. In the previous example involving a calcium channel blockers effect on blood glucose, blood glucose would be the dependent variable; the independent variable is the intervention or what is being manipulated (the calcium channel blocker in the example). A *confounding variable* is one that can confuse or cloud the study variables. In the calcium channel blocker example, the participants' diets need to be controlled as a confounding variable because of the influence diet has on blood glucose levels.

Discrete versus Continuous Data

Discrete variables can have only one of a limited set of values. Discrete variables can also be described as being able to assume only the value of a whole number. For example, in studying the number of seizures that patients experienced with certain tricyclic antidepressants, it would only be practical to describe seizures as whole numbers. It would not be possible for a patient to have half of a seizure. *Continuous data* may take on any value within a defined range. This would include time, temperature, length, and blood glucose. Blood glucose level is usually only reported in whole numbers, which seems to be a discrete variable. However, blood glucose can be measured in fractions of whole numbers. If using very sensitive laboratory equipment, glucose could be measured as accurately as 80.3 mg/dL. It is important to understand the difference between discrete and continuous variables. The type of variable is a determining factor in selecting the appropriate statistical procedure.

Scales of Measurement

There are four recognized levels of measurement: nominal, ordinal, interval, and ratio scales. Each of these scales has certain distinguishing characteristics that are important in determining which statistical procedure should be used to analyze the data.

A *nominal variable,* sometimes called the classificatory variable, consists of categories that have no implied rank or order. Nominal data fit into classifications or categories such as male or female and presence or absence of a disease state.

An *ordinal variable* is similar to a nominal variable in that the data are placed into categories. However, ordinal variables do have an implied order or rank. It is important to note that the differences between the categories cannot be considered equal. Examples of this type of data include ranks assigned in the military or grade levels in school (sophomore versus senior). In medicine, an example would be a pain scale, where the patient may be able to tell you it hurts more but not exactly how much more. In such a case, the patient may be asked to classify the pain as none, mild, moderate, severe, or unbearable.

An *interval variable* and a *ratio variable* are also similar because they both have constant and defined units of measurement. There is an equal distance or interval between values. Both of these variables imply that a value is greater than, less than, or equal to another variable. For example, blood glucose of 80 mg/dL is the same interval from 70 mg/dL as it is from 90 mg/dL. Each mg/dL is at an equal distance or interval from the next; likewise, each mg/dL is greater than, less than, or equal to all other mg/dL measurements. The difference between interval and ratio variables is that the ratio scale has an absolute zero. Be careful not to confuse an absolute zero with an arbitrary zero point that is set. The classic example of this difference is that the Celsius scale for temperature, which has an arbitrary zero that has been set at the freezing point for water, and the Kelvin scale, which has an absolute zero that represents the absence of molecular motion. This difference is really not essential when determining the type of statistical test to perform. Interval and ratio variables are analyzed using the same statistical procedures.

Descriptive and Inferential Statistics

Statistics can be used in two different ways. One is *descriptive statistics,* which are used to present, organize, and summarize data. Descriptive statistics are usually the basic presentation of the data. This information can give clues as to the appearance of the data. In comparison, *inferential statistics* allow generalization about the population from the sample data.

DESCRIPTIVE STATISTICS

Data and descriptive statistics are often organized, summarized, and presented in tables or graphic form. Some things to consider when reviewing tables and graphs include the following.

1. The table or graph should be easy to read and understand.
2. The title should be clear and concise, as well as accurately describe the data being presented.
3. The units of measure on all scales, axes, rows, or columns should be easily visible and understandable.
4. The scales should be of equal interval or space without exaggerating one part of the scale; if an axis is shown with a break in the intervals, it should be clearly marked. Often a break will be noted by two slash marks at that point.
5. Codes, abbreviations, and symbols should be defined in the text of the paper or explained in a footnote with the graph or table.
6. If comparisons are made between data or groups, the comparison should be done on equivalent scales.

Sometimes when evaluating a graph taken from an article, it can be helpful to graph the information on graph paper using a standard scale. Many times a graph will appear very differently on standard paper.

MEASURES OF CENTRAL TENDENCY

Measures of central tendency are sometimes referred to as measures of location. These descriptive measures are helpful in identifying where a set of values are located. The most common measures of central tendency are the mode, the median, and the arithmetic mean. In a normal distribution of values, the mean is equal to the median and the mode. The central tendency value used depends on the type of measurement scale.

The *mode* is defined as the most frequently occurring value or category in the set of data. A data set can have more than one mode; a data set with two modes is referred to as bimodal, and so on. The mode is the measure of central tendency for nominal data. Remember that nominal data are categories with no specific order or rank. Therefore, the only appropriate measure of central tendency is the category that contains the most values.

The *median* is the middle value in a set of ranked data; in other words, it is a value such that half of the data points fall above it and half fall below it. In terms of percentiles, it is the value at the 50th percentile. The median is the appropriate measure of central tendency when describing ordinal data. Likewise, it can be useful in describing interval or ratio data.

The *mean* or arithmetic mean is the most common and appropriate measure of central tendency for data measured on an interval or ratio scale. It is best described as the average numerical value for the data set. The mean is calculated by adding all the data points and dividing this number by the sample size. In the calcium channel blocker example, the mean would be the average blood glucose value for the study group. For certain types of data, the arithmetic mean is not the best measure of central tendency. If data involve exponential growth, a statistic called the geometric mean is the more appropriate measure.

MEASURES OF VARIABILITY

Measures of variability, another type of descriptive statistic, are also referred to as measures of dispersion. The most common measures of variability are the range, interquartile range, standard deviation, and variance. In analyzing data, the measures of variability are useful in indicating how close the data are to the measure of central tendency. In other words, how scattered are the data from the median and/or mean? Data points that are widely scattered from the mean give a different perspective than data points very close to the mean. The mean value could be equal for two groups, but the variability of the data can give a different picture. In evaluating nominal data, there is no measure of dispersion. The best option is to describe the number of categories studied.

The *range* can be used to describe ordinal, interval, and ratio data. The range is the difference between the highest data value and the lowest data value. In the calcium channel blocker example, if the highest blood glucose was 357 mg/dL and the lowest was 54 mg/dL, the range would be equal to 303 mg/dL. In medical literature, authors often provide the range by indicating the lowest to the highest values without actually calculating the difference for the reader (i.e., the blood glucose range was from 54 to 357 mg/dL). Although the range is an easy number to calculate, the measurement is not very useful in describing or comparing data.

The *interquartile range* is another measure of dispersion that can be used to describe ordinal, interval, and ratio data. This range is a measure of variability directly related to the median. The interquartile range takes the data values within the 25th and 75th percent quartiles. Therefore, the interquartile range deals with the middle 50% of the data. This value is less likely to be affected by extreme values in the data, which plagues the usefulness of the range.

The two best measures of dispersion with interval and ratio data are the *standard deviation* and *variance.* The relationship between the standard deviation and variance is that the standard deviation is the square root of the variance. The standard deviation is often preferred over the variance because it is the measure of the average amount by which each observation in a series of data points differs from the mean. In other words, how far away is each data point from the mean (dispersion or variability) or what is the average deviation from the mean? In medical literature, the standard deviation and mean are often reported in the following fashion: mean ± standard deviation. In comparing two groups with equal means, the standard deviation can give an idea of how much the individuals in each group were scattered from the mean value. It is important when evaluating the literature to look at the standard deviation in comparison to the mean. How much variability existed among the subjects in the study? In the study of calcium channel blocker, a large standard deviation indicates a wide variability in the blood glucose levels and that some patients were more affected by the agent than others.

The coefficient of variation is another measure used when evaluating dispersion from one data set to another. The *coefficient of variation* is the standard deviation expressed as a percentage of the mean. This value is calculated by dividing the standard deviation by the mean and multiplying this value by 100. This index is useful in comparing the relative difference in variability between two or more samples or determining which group has the largest relative variability of values from the mean.

MEASURES OF SHAPE

Two other descriptive measures that refer to the shape of a distribution are the coefficient of skewness and the coefficient of kurtosis; both are used to describe the distribution of interval and ratio data. *Skewness* is the measure of symmetry of a curve. These descriptive measures are usually not described in the biomedical literature but rather are used by researchers to evaluate the distribution properties of their variables. These distribution properties can be helpful in determining the type of statistical tests that best suit the research. Skewness tells how well each half of the curve or distribution relates to the other half of a normal distribution; if each half is equal in shape and size to the other half, they are mirror images of each other. Skewness is an indicator of where the data lie within the distribution. A distribution is said to be skewed to the right or have a positive skew when the mode and median are less than the mean. A distribution that is skewed to the left, or that has a negative skew, is one in which the mode and median are greater than the mean. *Kurtosis* refers to how flat or peaked the curve appears. A curve with a flat or board top is referred to as platykurtic, while a peaked distribution is described as leptokurtic. A normal distribution or curve has a kurtosis value of zero.

RATIOS, PROPORTIONS, AND RATES

Ratios, proportions, and rates are frequent terms used in the medical literature. A *ratio* expresses the relationship between two numbers, such as the ratio of men to women who suffer from multiple sclerosis (MS). A *proportion* is a specific type of ratio in which the numerator is included in the denominator and the value is expressed as a percentage. For example, the percentage of men with MS would be the number of men with MS in the numerator divided by the number of people in the population with MS (this number would include the men in the numerator). A *rate* is a special form of proportion that includes a specific time frame. The rate is equal to the number of events in a specified period divided by the population at risk in a specified period. The rate for MS would be the number of cases during a specified time frame, such as 1 year, divided by the total population in that time frame. The reason the total population is used as the denominator is that the population is the group at risk for the disease.

INCIDENCE AND PREVALENCE

Incidence and prevalence are two measures used to describe illness within the population. Both measures are frequently used in the literature pertaining to epidemiology and public health. The *incidence rate* measures the probability that a healthy person will develop a disease within a specified period. In essence, it is the number of new cases of disease in the population within a specific period. *Prevalence,* on the other hand, measures the number of people in the population who have the disease at a given time. Incidence and prevalence differ in that incidence refers to only new cases and prevalence to all existing cases, regardless of whether they are newly discovered.

$$\text{Incidence rate} = \frac{\text{Number of new cases of a disease}}{\text{Population at risk}} \text{ per a given time frame}$$

$$\text{Prevalence} = \frac{\text{Number of existing cases of a disease}}{\text{Total population}} \text{ per a given time frame}$$

Incidence indicates the rate at which new disease occurs in a previously disease free group over a specified time frame, while prevalence describes the probability of people having a disease within a specified time frame. It is important to look at both incidence and prevalence when describing diseases. Prevalence varies directly with incidence and the duration of the disease. In a disease with a rapid recovery or rapid death, the duration is short and the prevalence low. With a drug treatment that has a profound effect on prolonging life without curing the disease, prevalence will be high but the incidence may be low. A good research article will describe both incidence and prevalence, as well as specify the time frame studied.

RELATIVE RISK AND ODDS RATIO

Relative risk and odds ratio are two measures of disease frequency. Both measures compare the incidence of disease when a specific factor is present or absent. An actual risk (such as relative risk) can only be measured by using a cohort type of study design (see Chap. 6). The *relative risk* is defined as the incidence rate among those exposed to a particular factor divided by the incidence among those not exposed to the same factor. The relative risk is an appropriate measure in a cohort study. Prospective studies allow for defining populations at risk and, therefore, allow calculation of the excess risk caused by exposure to a particular factor.

If a cohort study design is not practical or is not chosen by the researchers, a case-control study design (see Chap. 7) is used and the *odds ratio,* an estimator of relative risk, is calculated. When a retrospective case-control study design is used, the relative risk can be estimated by using the odds ratio. In using the odds ratio as an estimator of relative risk, one must assume that the control group is representative of the general population, the cases are representative of the population with the disease, and the frequency of the disease in the population is small. The odds ratio is calculated by multiplying the number of cases with the disease and exposed to the factor by the number of cases without the disease and not exposed to the factor, and dividing this number by the number of cases with the disease without exposure to the factor multiplied by those cases without the disease but exposed to the factor. The table that follows may clarify this calculation.

		Disease	
		Present	**Absent**
Factor	Exposed factor	A	B
	Not exposed	C	D

$$\text{Odds ratio} = \frac{A \times D}{B \times C}$$

The odds ratio is commonly referred to in the medical literature, as well as in the lay press. When describing that prostate cancer is ten times more likely in tobacco users than nontobacco users, an odds ratio is reported. Remember that the odds ratio is an estimate of relative risk and dependent on good study design and meeting the assumptions previously described.

SENSITIVITY, SPECIFICITY, AND PREDICTIVE VALUES

Sensitivity, specificity, and predictive values are measures of the effectiveness of a test procedure. Sensitivity and specificity are the two indices used to evaluate the accuracy of a test. The following definitions will help in understanding these important measures.

- *True positives* (TP) are individuals with the disease who were correctly identified as having the disease by the test.
- *False positives* (FP) are individuals without the disease who were incorrectly identified as having the disease by the test.
- *True negatives* (TN) are individuals without the disease who were correctly identified as disease free by the test.
- *False negatives* (FN) are individuals with the disease who were incorrectly identified as disease free by the test.

Sensitivity is the probability that a diseased individual will have a positive test result. Sensitivity is the true positive rate of the test.

$$\text{Sensitivity} = \frac{\text{Disease with positive test}}{\text{All diseased}}$$

In other terms

$$\text{Sensitivity} = \frac{\text{True positives}}{\text{True positives} + \text{false negatives}}$$

Specificity is the probability that a disease-free individual will have a negative test result. Specificity is the true negative rate of the test.

$$\text{Specificity} = \frac{\text{Disease free with negative test}}{\text{All disease free}}$$

$$\text{Specificity} = \frac{\text{True negatives}}{\text{True negatives} + \text{false positives}}$$

In designing research studies involving a diagnostic test procedure or a screening test, the authors need to specify their test level. In setting their test level, they determine who is to be identified with the disease and those patients who will be omitted without disease. In making this judgment they need to decide the cost of classifying individuals as false negatives and false positives.

Predictive values are also calculated as a measure of the accuracy of a test procedure. *Predictive value* can be expressed as a function of sensitivity, specificity, and the probability of disease in the general population.

$$\text{Positive predictive value} = \frac{\text{Diseased with positive test}}{\text{All with positive test}}$$

$$\text{Negative predictive value} = \frac{\text{Disease-free with negative test}}{\text{All with negative test}}$$

DISTRIBUTIONS

All types of data can be organized in a manner that allows the observer to view general patterns and tendencies in the data. Data can be organized such that the values construct a frequency distribution (see example following this paragraph). If the variable is continuous, there is an infinite number of possible values that graph as a continuous frequency distribution. Whereas, if the variable is discrete, the frequency distribution is limited in the number of possible values. The type of distribution can be helpful in determining the appropriate statistical test. Probability distributions like the binomial and the Poisson (see a later section) are analyzed using specific formulas that evaluate the probability of an event occurring. This is often referred to as the success or failure of an event.

Blood Glucose Level (mg/dL)	Number of Patients
75	212
125	333
175	401
225	198
275	97
	Total 1241

Probability Distribution

A *probability distribution* is exactly that, a distribution of probabilities. Probability deals with the relative likelihood that a certain event will or will not occur, relative to some other events. The binomial distribution and the Poisson distribution are two forms of probability distributions.

Binomial Distribution

Many discrete objects or events belong to one of two mutually exclusive categories. For example, in describing gender, people can be categorized into either the male or female group. All people belong to one of these two groups, but cannot belong to both (mutually exclusive). The binomial distribution shows the probabilities of different outcomes for a series of random events, which can have only one of two values.

Properties of the binomial distribution include:

1. The event or trial occurs a specified number of times (analogous to sample size).
2. Each time the event occurs, there are only two mutually exclusive outcomes.
3. The events or trials are independent, meaning that one outcome has no effect on the next outcome of events.

Poisson Distribution

The Poisson distribution is another form of a discrete probability distribution. This distribution is used to predict the probabilities of the occurrence of rare, independent events or determine whether these events are independent when the sample size is indefinitely large. For example, the Poisson distribution could predict radioactive counts per unit of time.

Normal Distribution

The frequency distribution histogram of a continuous variable often forms a symmetric, bell-shaped curve referred to as a normal distribution. The normal distribution is one of several continuous probability distributions with the following characteristics:

1. The mean, median, and mode all have the same value (Fig. 10-1).
2. The curve is symmetric around the mean.
3. The kurtosis is zero.
4. The tails of the distribution get closer and closer to the x-axis as the values move away from the mean but the tails never quite touch the x-axis.
5. The distribution is completely defined by the mean and standard deviation.
6. One standard deviation above and below the mean includes 68.26% of the values in the population; two standard deviations above and below the mean include 95.46% of the values; and three standard deviations include 99.73%.
7. The area under the normal curve is by definition 1.

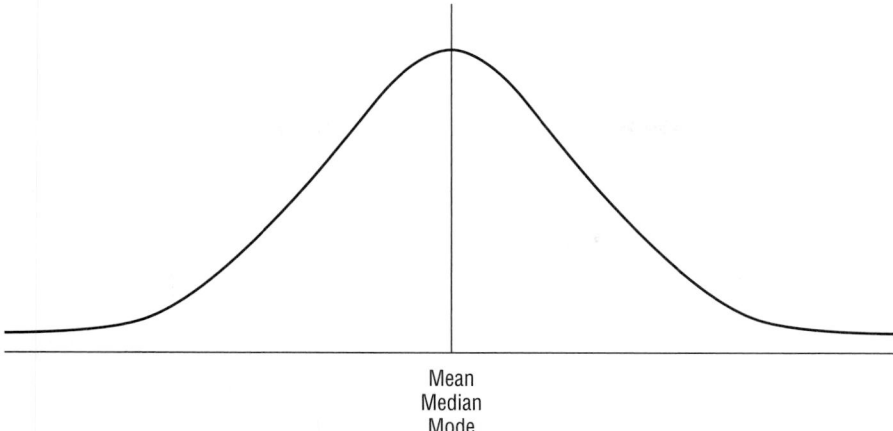

Mean
Median
Mode

Figure 10–1. Mean, median, and mode of normal distribution.

It is statistically very important to know whether a variable is normally distributed in the population or approaches a normal distribution. The type of statistical test that is selected to analyze data often makes an assumption about the variables being normally distributed. This can be a key in interpreting the medical literature, which will be discussed later in this chapter. Did the researchers assume a normal distribution or was their variable normally distributed in the population?

Standard Normal Distribution

Among the infinite number of possible normal distributions, there is one normal distribution that can be compared to all other normal distributions. This distribution is called the standard normal distribution. The standard normal distribution has a mean of 0 and a standard deviation and variance of 1 (Fig. 10-2). The tails of the distribution extend from minus infinity to positive infinity. When converting normal distributions to the standard normal, the variables are transformed to standardized scores referred to as z scores. A standard z score is a means of expressing a raw score in terms of the standard deviation. The raw score is so many standard deviation units from the standard mean score of zero, which would correlate to the number of standard deviation units that the score was from the mean score of the original distribution. Researchers can use the standard normal distribution to take their raw data and put it into standardized scores. Often by doing this the authors can make comparisons between data sets that may be on different scales or have different values. By standardizing the data, a comparison can be made using a standard or equivalent scale. Therefore, differences between the data sets may be more easily detected and understood.

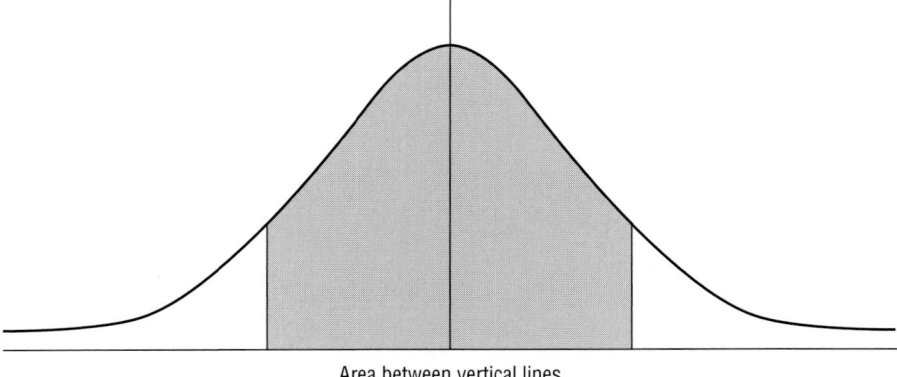

Area between vertical lines
is one standard deviation
(shaded area is 68 percent
of the total area)

Figure 10–2. Area of one standard deviation.

Statistical Inference

Inferential statistics are used to determine the likelihood that a conclusion, based on the analysis of the data from a sample, is true and represents the population studied.

CENTRAL LIMIT THEOREM

To use various statistical tests appropriately, an assumption is made that the variable or item being studied is normally distributed in the population. Many times researchers do not know whether their variable is normally distributed. In addition, the distribution does not always have to be normally distributed to apply certain statistical tests because of the central limit theorem. The *central limit theorem* states that when equally sized samples are drawn from a non-normal distribution, the mean values from those samples will form a normal distribution. With repeated sampling of size *n* samples, the mean value from each one of these samples when plotted will form a normal distribution. Therefore, the central limit theorem states that with a large enough sample size, an assumption can be made about the distribution being normal. A large enough sample size according to the central limit theorem is usually considered greater than 30. For further review of the issues related to sample size, refer to Chap. 6.

When looking at the distribution of the sample means as is done with the central limit theorem, the standard deviation of the sample means can be calculated. This standard deviation of the sample means is referred to as the standard error of the mean (SEM). The *standard deviation* reflects how close the values cluster to the sample mean;

the *standard error of the mean* indicates how close the repeated sample's mean scores are from the population mean. It is important in evaluating the medical literature to distinguish between the standard deviation and the standard error of the mean. Researchers often use the standard error of the mean to show variability instead of appropriately using the standard deviation. The standard error of the mean is the standard deviation divided by the square root of the sample size. Obviously, the standard error of the mean will be a smaller number than the standard deviation, which makes the data look less variable and more appealing. Unfortunately, it is the wrong measure of dispersion.

PARAMETRIC VERSUS NONPARAMETRIC TESTING

After determining whether a variable is normally distributed or the researchers have applied the central limit theorem, it is important to focus on whether the research required a parametric or nonparametric test. Often in the statistical methods used within the medical literature, the use of a parametric or nonparametric test is inappropriately applied. In most cases, a parametric test is used when a nonparametric method should have been applied. The essential aspect is to ensure the assumptions are met for performing that statistical test.

When selecting a statistical test for evaluating data there are several assumptions that one makes about the variable or variables. The type of assumptions made determines whether the data are to be analyzed by parametric or nonparametric statistical testing. If an erroneous assumption has been made, often the inappropriate statistical test has been performed. Basic assumptions for a parametric test include:

1. The variable is normally distributed or an assumption is made based on a large enough sample size to consider the variable normally distributed (central limit theorem).
2. The variable is continuous or, if it is discrete, it at least approximates a normal distribution.
3. The variable is measured on an interval or ratio scale.

If the data do not meet these basic assumptions, a nonparametric test rather than a parametric test should be used to analyze the data. Nonparametric tests are considered to be distribution-free methods and are also useful in analyzing nominal and ordinal scale data. The key to understanding the major differences between parametric and nonparametric tests is that parametric statistical tests require interval or ratio level data and nonparametric tests can be used for nominal and ordinal data. A researcher may have interval or ratio level data, but may still not meet the first assumption for parametric testing. In this case, interval or ratio data would have to be analyzed using a nonparametric test (parametric and nonparametric tests will be described later in this chapter).

HYPOTHESIS TESTING

A *hypothesis* is a contention about some aspect that the researcher is interested in studying. Further information on developing a hypothesis can be found in Chap. 6. A hypothesis may or may not be true, but is assumed to be true until proven differently with evidence; it is a contention about a population. The *null hypothesis* is the hypothesis of no difference, and the *alternate hypothesis* (often referred to as the research hypothesis) is the hypothesis of difference. A study is performed to determine whether this contention is true. A representative sample is drawn from the population to provide estimates of the population parameters. These estimates are then tested to see whether the contention is indeed true or false. In answering this contention, statistical or significance testing is performed.

When establishing the hypothesis, the researcher often needs to determine whether he or she is writing a hypothesis that involves a one-sided or two-sided test. When writing a hypothesis it is necessary for the researcher to determine whether he or she is looking for any difference, whether it is greater or smaller, or whether the difference will only occur in a single direction. If the researcher is looking for any difference, it is considered a two-sided test. A specific difference in only one direction uses a one-sided test. The previous example using a calcium channel blocker would be a two-sided test, because the study is testing whether the calcium channel blocker had either raised or lowered blood glucose. If the researcher had been interested specifically in a calcium channel blocker causing only an increase in blood glucose in insulin-dependent diabetics, this would have been a one-sided test. Two-sided tests are considered to be statistically stronger, because they are harder to prove and are the test of choice for clinical trials.

ERRORS

It is essential that researchers establish how much error they are willing to accept before the initiation of the study. Refer to the Chap. 6 for a review of type I and type II errors and their acceptable values.

SIGNIFICANCE

Once alpha (type I) error has been established and the data collected, a researcher is interested in knowing whether to accept or reject the null hypothesis. Once the appropriate statistical test has been selected, a test statistic is calculated that is compared to a standard for that test. In comparing the test statistic, a *p*-value is calculated. The

p-value for any hypothesis test is the alpha level at which the given value of the statistic would be on the borderline between accepting or rejecting the null hypothesis (generally, .05 is the highest acceptable p-value). The p-value is the probability of obtaining a result as extreme or more extreme than the actual sample value obtained given that the null hypothesis is true. Some statisticians refer to the p-value as the actual probability of an alpha error.

If the p-value is less than or equal to the alpha value established, the null hypothesis is rejected and the difference between the groups is considered statistically significant. If the p-value is greater than the alpha value established, the null hypothesis is accepted and the difference between the groups is not considered statistically significant. The smaller the p-value, the greater the statistical significance. Also, the smaller the p-value, the less likely that the test statistic happened by chance and that a real difference exists. Researchers should include the actual p-value in their reports.

Establishing a confidence interval, which is sometimes used by researchers instead of expressing p-values, can also test significance. The p-value is a probability of the outcome of the study occurring by chance alone, and the confidence interval is a range of values in which there is confidence that the population parameter being measured is actually contained. Generally, either a 95% or 99% confidence interval is re-ported. When a study is measuring the differences between two treatments, a difference in the mean values can be reported by a confidence interval. In theory, if the difference in mean values were calculated between all possible study groups in the population, the 95% confidence interval would contain the true difference 95% of the time. As an example, a study may have reported that drug A decreased blood pressure an average of 8 mm Hg more than drug B with a confidence interval (this could be either a 95% or 99% confidence interval, depending on what the authors set) of a –4 to 16 mm Hg decrease in blood pressure. In this example, because the confidence interval contains a value of zero, it is not possible to reject the null hypothesis (stating there is no difference between the two treatments).

It is important when evaluating significance to keep in mind that statistical significance does not always correlate with clinical significance. What is proven statistically may not make a difference clinically. For example, with a large enough sample size, the researchers may have been able to prove that a calcium channel blocker caused a statistically significant difference in blood glucose in patients with insulin-dependent diabetes mellitus. However, upon examining the data, they may have found that the difference in blood glucose was 5 mg/dL. Clinically is this a significant difference? Probably not. Other things that may be taken into consideration when evaluating clinical and statistical significance include costs, adverse effects, quality of life, and actual morbidity and mortality numbers within the study.

Statistical Tests

Once the basic assumptions have been considered, it is time to determine whether the appropriate statistical tests have been used. The statistical tests will be covered in the order in which they are most commonly seen in the literature. Whenever a parametric test is reviewed, the nonparametric equivalent will also be discussed. Refer to Table 10–1 to help put the statistical tests into perspective.

Most statistical hypothesis testing includes the following sequence of steps. It is essential when evaluating the medical literature to determine whether the researchers have followed these steps.

1. Clearly state the research question.
2. What are the characteristics of the sample and the variables in question? On what scale is the variable measured? What is the distribution of the variable? Is it known or can a normal distribution be assumed?
3. State the null hypothesis and the alternative hypothesis. Do the data require a one-sided or two-sided test?
4. Set alpha and beta errors.
5. Based on your answers to points 2, 3, and 4, what type of statistical test should be used (see the following information)?
6. After data collection, calculate the test statistic.
7. Determine the p-value or the confidence interval in order to accept or reject the null hypothesis.

TABLE 10–1. OVERVIEW OF STATISTICAL TESTS

Type of Data	Two Independent Samples	Two Related Samples (Paired/Matched)	Three or More Independent Samples	Three or More Related Samples (Paired/Matched)
Nominal	Chi square	Chi square (McNemar)		Chi square
Ordinal	Mann-Whitney U	Sign test Wilcoxon signed ranks	Kruskal-Wallis	Friedman
Interval or ratio	Parametric t-test	Parametric paired t-test	Parametric ANOVA	Parametric ANOVA Repeated measures
	Nonparametric Mann-Whitney U	Nonparametric Wilcoxon signed ranks	Nonparametric Kruskal-Wallis	Nonparametric Friedman

COMPARING TWO GROUPS

Parametric Tests

t-*test for Independent Samples*

The *t*-test for independent samples (also referred to as the Student's *t*-test) is a statistical method used to test for differences between the means of the two independent groups. The null hypothesis assumes that the means of the two populations are equal. This test statistic can be used to compare two groups of equal sample size or two unequal sample size groups. The equations differ slightly but both rely on the following assumptions.

Assumptions
1. The two samples are random samples drawn from two independent populations of interest.
2. The measured variable is approximately normally distributed and continuous.
3. The variable is measured on an interval or ratio scale (e.g., the effect on blood glucose levels or a difference in white blood cell counts).
4. The variances of the two groups are similar; this is known as the requirement of homogeneity of variance.

A *t*-test can still be performed if there is a violation of the last assumption. If the variances are shown to be different, a *t*-test that does not pool the variances is used.

t-*test for Matched or Paired Data*

If there is a violation of the first assumption, a different type of *t*-test is performed. In medical research paired or matched data are often used. Matching or pairing data is a good way to control for issues that may confound or confuse the data. In pairing data, the same subject is used to collect data for both groups. In many instances, a cross-over design is used so that the same subject receives all treatments. A good example of paired data is a pretest and posttest design. In matching data, the subjects from one group are matched on certain factors or conditions relevant to the study to a subject in the other group. For example, in the study with the calcium channel blockers and diabetes, the researcher may find it helpful to match age, gender, and age at first diagnosis between the two groups. Therefore, the data from the two groups are no longer independent because they have been matched or paired. In addition to a cross-over design, researchers will sometimes match subjects for certain characteristics and run a paired *t*-test. When the first assumption is violated and the samples are no longer independent, a paired *t*-test is the appropriate statistical test.

A common error often made by researchers is the use of the *t*-test when they are studying more than two groups (comparing two groups at a time). The *t*-test can be used only when comparing two groups. When looking at more than two groups, other tests such as analysis of variance (ANOVA) are appropriate.

Nonparametric Equivalents to *t*-tests
For Independent Samples
Mann-Whitney U Test

The nonparametric Mann-Whitney U test can be used when data are measured on an ordinal scale, are not normally distributed, or when the variable is discrete. Therefore, the *t*-test is not appropriate to compare the samples, but the Mann-Whitney U test can be used in its place.

For Matched or Paired Samples
Sign Test

The sign text is a nonparametric test used with paired or matched data. The sign test involves determining if there is a positive (+) or negative (–) difference between the pairs (i.e., which treatment is better or worse than the other). The test involves determining if the probability of the + and – values actually occurring. If the sign test is statistically significant, it shows that a larger portion of the data was either positive (one treatment was better than the other) or negative (one treatment was worse than the other). Otherwise, if the sign test is not statistically significant, then the treatment groups would be deemed equal.

Wilcoxon Signed-Ranks Matched-Pairs Test

This nonparametric test can be used when data are matched or paired but do not meet assumptions 2, 3, and 4 for the parametric paired *t*-test. When paired or matched data are measured on an ordinal scale or the variable is not normally distributed within the population, the Wilcoxon signed-ranks test can be used as the test statistic. This test is often preferred over the sign test because it reflects the magnitude of difference between the pairs. This test actually requires a rank order of the differences of the pairs and provides a rank order of the positive and negative differences.

COMPARING MORE THAN TWO GROUPS

Parametric
Analysis of Variance

The null hypothesis of ANOVA assumes that the means of the various groups being compared in the study are not different. In testing the null hypothesis, it is not possible to simply compare the mean of each group with every other mean, but rather it is necessary to use ANOVA to partition the variance in a set of data into various components. The test then determines the contribution of each of these components to the overall variation. The components compared include the total variance for the complete data set, the variance within each group of the data set, and the variance between each group within the data set. The error within each group is called the *error variance*. The total variance is compared to the error variance. If there is a large difference in this comparison, it is attributed to a difference between groups, which can be related to the treatment or intervention. In certain types of ANOVA designs, the main effect of a variable can be contrasted with interactions between variables. The main effect is the effect of the variable by itself on the outcome. An interaction is defined as two variables whose interaction or relationship with each other explains the outcome.

The test statistic calculated for ANOVA is the *F* statistic. As with the *t*-test, there are several different types of ANOVA testing that depend on the experimental design. The assumptions for all types of ANOVA remains the same.

Assumptions
1. Each of the groups is a random sample from the population of interest.
2. The measured variable is continuous.
3. The variable is measured on a ratio or interval scale.
4. The error variances are equal.
5. The variable is approximately normally distributed.

The first assumption cannot be violated. If assumptions 2 through 5 cannot be met, one should consider a nonparametric test equivalent such as the Kruskal-Wallis or Friedman's test.

Types of ANOVA Tests

Completely Randomized Design ANOVA with Fixed Effects

This test involves a random assignment of subjects to various treatment groups, but the investigator chooses the treatments for each group. For example, if researchers wanted to compare the cardiovascular side effects of tricyclic antidepressants (TCA), patients would be randomly assigned to groups, but the researchers would assign which TCA each group would receive.

Completely Randomized Design ANOVA with Random Effects

This test includes random assignment of subjects with random treatment effects. Compared to the previous example, the patients would be randomly assigned to groups and the treatment with TCA would be random as well.

Randomized Complete Blocks Design ANOVA

This test is also referred to as a two-way ANOVA without replication. Individuals are blocked or grouped according to the characteristic whose variance one wishes to identify. The treatments are chosen for each group. With the TCA example, individuals in the study would be blocked based on side effect profile such as electrocardiographic changes or increases in heart rate, and then the researchers would again assign treatments with TCA.

Randomized Complete Blocks Design ANOVA with Repeated Measures

With this test, the same individual is used for the repeated measurement. This is similar to the paired *t*-test, but more than two measurements are involved. This test is the same as the preceding example, except each patient receives each treatment. In other words, each patient would serve as his or her own control and receive all treatments.

Factorial Design ANOVA

When two or more factors interact with each other to produce either synergistic or antagonistic effects, the factorial design is appropriate. This test is also referred to as the two-way ANOVA with replication. If the TCA example was taken one step further, the effect that benzodiazepine therapy had on the TCA-induced cardiovascular side effects would be studied using this design.

Types of Post Hoc Comparisons

After getting a significant ANOVA result, a researcher knows there is a difference among the means of the different groups. Sometimes this is all that is necessary for the research. At other times, the researcher may be interested in knowing which group is different from the others. To answer this question, the researcher can do several post hoc comparisons to compare the means of the groups two at a time. This is very different from performing separate *t*-tests between each group (a common error in the medical literature). Rather than using separate *t*-tests, there are several types of post hoc comparison tests that can be used with ANOVA. The reason post hoc tests are used rather than separate *t*-tests is related to the error rate across the multiple tests. The post hoc tests correct for the multiple error rates that would be associated with running the separate *t*-tests. It is important to realize that some post hoc tests are more conservative than others, meaning that they have less error associated with them. The following tests are all post hoc procedures that compare the means of the various groups and may be cited in the literature: Bonferroni Correction, Scheffe's Method, Tukey's Least Significant Difference, and Newman-Kuels.

Nonparametric Tests
Kruskal-Wallis One-Way ANOVA

This is the nonparametric counterpart to the ANOVA with a completely randomized design. The data need to be at least measured on an ordinal scale. The samples must still be drawn from independent populations.

Friedman Two-Way ANOVA

This is the nonparametric counterpart to the randomized complete block design. Like the Kruskal-Wallis, the data need to be of at least an ordinal scale.

DESCRIBING THE RELATIONSHIP BETWEEN TWO OR MORE VARIABLES

Correlation and Regression

Correlation and regression are used when there is an interest in exploring the relationship between two or more variables. These analyses are applied to data to quantify and define the relationship between the variables. An example may be the relationship between estrogen use and cervical cancer. *Correlation* analysis allows for a quantitative measurement indicating the strength of the relationship between two variables. Correlation helps to determine whether there is an association between two variables and also indicates the strength of the association. In this description, association is one way of saying that one variable changes in a consistent manner when the other variable changes. Correlation analysis does not assume a cause and effect relationship. In comparison, *regression* analysis is used to mathematically describe the relationship such as predicting one variable from other variables. Regression analysis or linear regression usually assumes some type of cause and effect relationship. In regression analysis, the independent variable or variables explain the dependent variable. When more than one independent variable is analyzed the technique is known as multiple linear regression.

Correlation

In correlation analysis, the following questions are asked:

1. Are the two variables related in some consistent and linear fashion?
2. What is the strength of the relationship between the two variables?

The measure of the strength of the relationship is the correlation coefficient often referred to as Pearson Correlation Coefficient or Pearson Product-Moment Coefficient. The sample correlation coefficient is usually symbolized by a small **r.**

The null hypothesis for correlation analysis is that **r** will be equal to zero, meaning that there is no correlation or linear relationship. If **r** is not equal to zero, some relationship exists. The value of **r** is important in determining the strength of the relationship and is a dimensionless number that varies from 0 (no relationship) to +1 or −1 (strongest relationship). Therefore, if **r** is close to zero, a weak relationship exists; if **r** is closer to +1 or −1, a stronger relationship exists. A +1 depicts a perfect positive linear relationship indicating that as one variable changes the other changes in the same direction. Likewise, a −1 indicates a perfect negative linear relationship in which as one variable changes the other changes in an inverse fashion.

Assumptions
1. Random sample from the population of interest.
2. Variables are normally distributed.
3. Variables are measured on an interval or ratio scale.
4. If a relationship exists, the relationship is linear.

Remember that correlation does not mean causation. Two variables may be correlated, but that does not mean that one variable can be predicted from the other variable.

Regression

In regression analysis, the hypothesis is that there is a functional relationship that allows prediction of a value of the dependent variable corresponding to a value of the independent variable. Mathematically, a regression equation is developed that indicates that the dependent variable is a function of the independent variable. This concept is frequently seen in pharmacy-related information: for example, the relationship between the dose of gentamicin and the blood level of gentamicin. A graph can be drawn with the data and a linear regression line can be predicted from the graph. Therefore, regression analysis approximates an equation that describes the linear relationship between two variables (regression equation) and constructs a line through the data points in a graphic presentation (regression or least squares line). Regression analysis answers the question, "what proportion of the variance in the dependent variable is explained or described by the independent variable? In regression analysis, the coefficient of determination, also known as r^2 (the square of the correlation coefficient), is the indicator of explained variance. The coefficient of determination describes the proportion of variance in the dependent variable explained by the independent variable. The coefficient of determination varies from 0 to 1, and the closer to 1, the greater the amount that variance in the dependent variable is explained by the independent variable. An example would be how much does hypertension explain the variation in left ventricular hypertrophy (LVH)? In looking at left ventricular size, how much of this size change can be related to or explained by the individual's blood pressure? For example, researchers could discover that 60% of the changes that occur in left ventricular size is directly related to the individual's blood pressure.

Assumptions
1. The independent variable is fixed and does not represent a random variable in the population.
2. The dependent variable is normally distributed.
3. Observations are independent.

Simple Linear Regression

Simple linear regression is used when there is only one dependent variable with only one independent variable being analyzed. Within this test, the independent variable is analyzed to determine how much it explains the change or variance in the dependent variable. The example above of LVH and hypertension is representative of a simple linear regression. It would help answer the question, how much does hypertension explain or predict LVH?

Multiple Linear Regression

Multiple regression is similar to simple linear regression except that there is one dependent variable with more than one independent variable. Multiple regression is used when a more complex problem exists that involves multiple variables to predict the dependent variable. An example of multiple regression would be the effects that stress and vitamin intake have on blood glucose levels. One of the problems to be aware of in multiple regression is the possibility that the independent variables may be intercorrelated such that one independent variable has some relationship with another independent variable. A correlation analysis is often done to determine whether the independent variables are correlated to one another. If a relationship exists between the independent variables, it is often referred to as *multicollinearity*. In the example of LVH, researchers may be interested in more than just the relationship to blood pressure. They may also want to consider the relationship of LDL cholesterol, exercise capacity, and blood pressure. The study may indicate that blood pressure explains 60%, LDL cholesterol 20%, and exercise capacity 8%. This would help the researchers to understand the relationship these variables have in explaining changes in left ventricular size. It would also demonstrate that blood pressure is a stronger factor than LDL cholesterol or exercise capacity. Notice that these numbers do not add up to 100%. This outcome is common in regression analysis, where other factors explain part but not all of the changes. Often the researchers do not know what the other factors are, or additional factors may need to be included in future studies to determine their contributions. Sometimes when doing regression analysis, a certain study variable may not explain any variance or less than 2% of the variance; this variable is considered to be unrelated or not predictive of the outcome (dependent variable).

Nonparametric Tests for Correlation and Regression

Correlation Tests

Nominal Data

There are three nonparametric measures of association for nominal data. These include the contingency coefficient, the phi coefficient, and Cohen's kappa coefficient. When looking at the correlation or association between nominal variables, the tests involve the degree of frequency expressed within categories. The contingency coefficient involves the use of chi-square. It is actually the square root of the chi-square statistic divided by the chi-square statistic added to the sample size. One noted problem with this measure is that even with a perfect relationship, the coefficient will never be 1. The phi coefficient is a ratio of the quantities found in a 2×2 contingency table. The 2×2 contingency table has four cells labeled a to d. The equation for phi is $(ad - bc)/bc$. The kappa coefficient also involves the 2×2 contingency table. This measure adjusts for error in data. So the equation for kappa is equal to the observed agreement (from the table) minus chance agreement divided by 1 minus the chance agreement. The kappa coefficient is often considered the most desirable measure for a 2×2 table.

Ordinal Data

There are three nonparametric measures of association for ordinal data. The three measures are Spearman rank correlation, Kendall's tau coefficient, and Kendall W coefficient. Spearman's **r** or Spearman's rank **r** is the nonparametric equivalent to Pearson's **r.** When data are measured on an ordinal scale or when other parametric assumptions are not met, Spearman's **r** would be the appropriate test. Spearman correlation is based on the differences in the ranks of paired data. Kendall's tau can be used for the same types of data as one would use Spearman's **r.** However, Kendall's tau does not require the mathematical calculations that Spearman's requires. Kendall's tau relies on counting the ranks and comparing them to see if they are in the right order. Kendall's W is utilized when there are multiple observations. For example, if you were looking to see the extent of agreement between three different observers of faculty teaching, you may have observations from the students, the department chairs, and peer faculty members. Kendall's W allows for the sum of the ranks of the different observers.

Nonparametric Regression Tests

Logistic Regression

Logistic regression is similar to linear regression. The difference is that logistic regression does not require the dependent variable or outcome variable to be measured on an interval or ratio scale. In the medical literature, the dependent variable is often measured as an ordinal scale. In this case, logistic regression would be preferred to linear regression. Logistic regression can be used when assumption 2 of linear regression is not met. Logistic regression can be performed as simple logistic regression (one dependent variable and one independent variable) or as multiple logistic regression (one dependent variable and more than one independent variables). Logistic regression also provides odds ratios for the data determining outcome measures of risk.

Log-Linear Analysis

Log-linear analysis is used to analyze categorical variables to determine if an effect exists among the variables. Log-linear analysis treats all variables as categorical variables. Log-linear analysis tries to determine if there is an association between the dependent variable, the independent variables, and the interaction of independent variables. As with certain ANOVA models, log-linear analysis allows the researcher to look at the main effects of each variable and likewise analyze the interaction effects between the variables.

Analysis of Covariance

Analysis of covariance (ANCOVA) is a technique that is used to analyze independent variables that include both categorical data and interval level data. ANOVA and regression are two methods that can be used for interval level data. ANCOVA provides a way to combine ANOVA and regression techniques when research involves categorical independent variables. ANCOVA can be a useful test when researchers want to adjust for baseline differences among the different treatment groups or therapies. An important assumption that must be met prior to doing ANCOVA is that there is *no* relationship between the covariate and the treatment variables. A good example of a study design that would lend itself to an ANCOVA test would be if a researcher wants to determine what effect three different calcium channel blockers may have on left ventricular ejection fraction controlling for the independent variable of gender. Gender would be the covariate and the treatment would be the drug therapy. The assumption would be met that gender was not correlated with the drug therapy of a calcium channel blocker. In addition, ANCOVA can be performed with multiple covariates within a particular study design. In the previous example, the study may have also included ethnic background as a covariate.

OTHER NONPARAMETRIC TESTS

Chi-Square

Chi-square is the most commonly reported nonparametric statistical test. This test can be used with one or more groups and compares the actual number within a group to the expected number for that same group. The expected number is based on theory, previous experience, or comparison groups. Chi-square tests are used to answer research questions related to rates, proportions, or frequencies. Chi-square analysis is an appropriate test for evaluating nominal and ordinal data; however, it is probably most useful in analyzing nominal data. When evaluating ordinal data, other methods that preserve the ranked nature may be preferred over chi-square.

Assumptions
1. Frequency data.
2. The measures are independent of one another.
3. Categorization of the variables or that the variables are best described by placing them into categories.

Contingency Tables

Categorical data are often arranged in a table consisting of columns and rows with individual data fitting into one of the designated squares. The rows represent the categories of one variable and the columns represent the categories of the other variable. The chi-square test is essentially the comparison of the expected frequencies in each cell compared to the actual or observed frequencies in those same cells. If the frequencies from the observed to the expected are significantly different, the independent variable had some effect on the dependent variable. This chi-square test is also known as the chi-square test of association. The most common contingency table is the 2×2 table. An example is cigarette smoking and its effect on lung cancer. The rows would be cases with lung cancer and controls without lung cancer. The columns would be exposure to the risk factor cigarette smoking or nonexposure to the risk factor cigarette smoking. The 2×2 contingency table would appear as the following:

		Lung Cancer	
		Yes	No
Cigarette smoking	Yes	# of patients	# of patients
	No	# of patients	# of patients

The researcher would then compare the expected with the observed to determine whether cigarette smoking contributed to lung cancer.

OTHER METHODS OF INFERENCE FOR CATEGORICAL DATA

Fisher's Exact Test

Sometimes in performing a study, a cell within the matrix will have an expected frequency of less than five or the sample size may be small; the most appropriate type of analysis for this case is called Fisher's exact test. This situation usually occurs when the number of people being studied or the number of individuals who are expected to have a particular outcome is small. It is important to remember that it is the expected cell frequency and not the actual cell frequencies observed that will determine whether Fisher's exact test should be used. A researcher should be able to calculate the expected cell frequency before collecting the data.

McNemar's Test (Paired or Matched Data)

The usual chi-square test cannot be used for paired or matched data, because this violates the assumption of independence. Therefore, when matched or paired nominal data are collected as part of the research design, the appropriate statistical test is McNemar's test. In the lung cancer study, if the subjects were matched for gender, paired data would be placed in the contingency table and McNemar's test could be performed.

Mantel-Haenszel Test

The Mantel-Haenszel test is necessary when analyzing stratified data. In performing research it may often be necessary to stratify data based on some factor that may be confounding or confusing the data. In the lung cancer example, what would the effect be of passive smoke on the rate of lung cancer? Were any of the nonsmokers or smokers also exposed to passive smoke? In this case, the researchers would stratify the data based on exposure to passive smoke. Therefore, the data would be presented as two separate 2×2 contingency tables. One table would be for passive smoke exposure and the other for no exposure to passive smoke.

OTHER NONPARAMETRIC TESTS

Survival Analysis

There are four basic assumptions that must be met prior to doing survival analysis. They are that:

1. each person must have an identified starting point and each subject at this point should be as similar as possible in the diagnosis of the illness (i.e., length of type I diabetes since diagnosis).
2. a clearly defined outcome or end point.
3. drop-out rates should be independent of the outcome (i.e., loss to follow-up).
4. the diagnostic and therapeutic practices did not change during the observational period.

Survival analysis is done with observational studies in which the outcome variable may have significant variability in the time it takes to reach the defined outcome. This outcome could be time period that a subject takes to develop the disease state of interest or it could be an outcome such as death. This outcome could occur at anytime within the study time frame or sometimes may not occur at all within the allocated time for the study. Sometimes within these observational study designs, enrollment may take place over a specified period of time (i.e., 3 months or 3 years). Not all subjects enter at time zero. In addition, subjects may also drop out of the study or be lost to follow-up. Therefore, survival analysis is often done to analyze this specific type of data. Survival analysis will place each subject at time zero and follow them until the designated outcome is met or the study ends, whichever comes first. Some common examples of this type of study analysis include the time frame to develop complications as it relates to diabetes or 5-year survival rates for cancer after treatment with chemotherapy or radiation.

There are two methods of looking at survival data. The first is referred to as the *actuarial method for survival analysis*. This method takes fixed time periods or end points. So a researcher could pick fixed time periods like 6 months, 1 year, and 2 years. With this method, the number of patients who have survived to these end points are counted. This method does not account for actual days, months, or years of survival, just who reaches that end point. So a subject could die at 5 months and 29 days and not be included in the 6-month analysis. The second technique is called the *Kaplan-Meier survival analysis*. The advantage to this method is that the actual length of time is measured for the end point or outcome. In the previous example, the subject who died at 5 months and 29 days would be in the analysis. Kaplan-Meier is considered to be superior to the actuarial method especially when the sample size is less than 50.

Cox's Proportional Hazards Model

Adjusting survival data based on subject differences at the beginning of the study can be accomplished one of two ways. If a researcher is concerned about group differences as they relate to a covariate that is dichotomous (such as gender), then a Mantel-Haenszel test can be performed by stratifying for the variable. If a researcher is concerned about group differences at baseline that relate to a covariate that is measured on a continuous scale, then Cox's proportional hazards model is used. This technique allows researchers to look at survival data and adjust for differences in the groups such as age or blood levels. In many cases, Cox's proportional hazards model can provide a better analysis of survival data by controlling for confounding issues or by showing differences in survival by baseline characteristics. For example, if a researcher was looking at cancer survival, they may want to control for tumor size and staging.

MULTIVARIATE ANALYSIS

Multivariate analysis is a means to study multiple dependent variables simultaneously versus the univariate techniques previously described in this chapter, which allow for only one dependent variable to be analyzed at a time. The multivariate technique is a superior technique for handling multiple dependent variables rather than performing multiple univariate tests to determine the significance of each dependent variable independent of each other. In the calcium channel blocker example, the researcher may be interested in two outcomes of the drug therapy. The outcomes or dependent variables could be systolic blood pressure and blood glucose levels. With the univariate *t*-test, these two dependent variables would be analyzed separately from each other. A multivariate technique, however, would be more appropriate because often the two dependent variables, when measured for the same person, can be correlated to each other.

Hotelling's T

Hotelling's *T* is a modified *t*-test that allows the researcher to look at two or more dependent variables at one time in two different groups. Like the *t*-test, this test is a comparison of two groups. The difference lies in the fact that Hotelling's *T* can analyze multiple dependent (outcome) variables simultaneously. Hotelling's *T* uses a vector of means rather than the means and plots a centroid of data. Hotelling's *T* determines the standard deviation of the data but also determines a correlation among the variables.

Multivariate Analysis of Variance

With ANOVA as the univariate technique, only one dependent variable could be analyzed with more than two groups. Multivariate analysis of variance is the multivariate ANOVA technique for analyzing more than two groups. Like Hotelling's T, multivariate analysis of variance (MANOVA) calculates a vector of means, a centroid for each group, and a grand centroid for all groups. In MANOVA, the within-group variability must also be calculated for each dependent variable. Unlike ANOVA, where the F statistic is considered the statistical test for significance, there have been several test statistics reported for MANOVA. The most common method used for determining statistical significance is Wilk's lambda.

Multivariate Analysis of Covariance

Similar to using ANCOVA when a covariate is identified for a ANOVA test, multivariate analysis of covariance (MANCOVA) is utilized when a covariate is identified as part of a MANOVA test. If there are multiple dependent variables with more than two treatment groups and the researcher would like to control for a covariate or confounding issue or a difference in baseline characteristics, then a MANCOVA could be used.

Discriminate Function Analysis

Discriminate function analysis is used when researchers want to account for differences among the variables. This analysis is also a multivariate technique that has multiple dependent variables. What discriminate function analysis tries to do for the researcher is to indicate which variables are the most important ones in explaining the differences in the groups. Therefore, it tries to find the variables that best discriminate between the groups. This technique can be used with two or more than two groups. As with MANOVA, Wilk's lambda is also used to test for statistical significance. Discriminate function analysis can be done after finding a statistically significant value for data analyzed using Hotelling's T or MANOVA. This type of test can help to discriminate which variables explained the differences noted.

Factor Analysis

Factor analysis is a multivariate technique that can be used to explore patterns in data, confirm researchers' suggested hypotheses, or reduce correlated variables into related factors, a factor being an underlying related phenomena that more than one variable may help to explain. In factor analysis, a model is developed that explores the relationship of the variables to the factors and the factors to the dependent (outcome) variables. This model can be developed a priori by the researcher and then tested for accuracy. The model can also be developed after the factor analysis by the researcher depending on the factor loadings that are reported by the statistical test. For example, a researcher may be trying to identify what factors affect a pharmacist's ability to counsel a patient. Researchers may decide that there are three factors that they feel influence patient counseling by the pharmacist. They title these factors patient demographics, pharmacy setting, and communication skills. The researcher may decide to measure the following variables to help explain the factor described as pharmacy setting: the number of pre- scriptions waiting, FTE technician help, number of phone lines into the pharmacy, loca- tion of the pharmacy within the store, and/or the public's access to the pharmacist. After measuring each of these variables, the statistical program will produce a correla- tion matrix for the variables, and also give what is termed *factor loadings*. This matrix and factor loading table provide a means to determine which variables explain a certain factor. The researcher can then decide if their model is sound or if another model should be constructed and tested.

OTHER TYPES OF STUDY DESIGN WITH STATISTICAL ANALYSIS

Meta-Analysis

Meta-analysis is a technique used to perform a study by combining previously published or unpublished data. The researchers combine data from multiple sources (independent clinical trials) and reanalyze the data hoping to strengthen the conclusions. This study design is used to increase the power of a study or improve the effect size (clinical detectable difference) by combining studies. It can be helpful when clinical trials may conflict in their conclusions.[12] Sacks and associates have published six major quality points for meta-analysis studies. These include looking at the (1) study design, (2) abil- ity to combine the data from the studies selected, (3) control bias within studies, (4) sta- tistical analysis, (5) sensitivity analysis, and (6) application of the results from combined studies.[13] It is essential that the authors of the meta-analysis provide explicit criteria for how a study ended up in their analysis. From a statistical standpoint, meta-analysis involves very complex statistical techniques. When looking at a meta-analysis, it is important to analyze two areas. The first is to determine if they did a test of homogene- ity. This test essentially tells the reader if the outcome variables used in the different studies were very similar. In other words, did each study that was being combined into the analysis have similar characteristics as it related to the outcome variables? The sec- ond area is to determine if the authors performed a sensitivity analysis. As with the test of homogeneity, sensitivity testing is extremely valuable in determining if the meta- analysis was sound. Sensitivity analysis is a means for the researchers to determine if certain trials were excluded or included in the study, how that would change the results they found. How would the inclusion or exclusion of trials affect the outcome variables or would it change the test of significance? It is a means to show the reader that the results would have been the same regardless of the inclusion or exclusion criteria of the related studies. Many types of bias can also adversely affect a meta-analysis design. Refer to the Chaps 6 and 7 for a discussion of bias.

One way that researchers have found to detect and quantify bias in a meta-analysis has been by using funnel plots. A *funnel plot* is a graphing of the trials effect size versus the sample size. The results are then plotted against a measure of precision such as the standard deviation or variance. A funnel-shaped plot will form as the precision or similarity of the studies increase. If a funnel shape does not appear or if there is asymmetry in the plot, this may indicate discordance among the different study results selected for the meta-analysis. In general, a good meta-analysis will present homogeneity tests, sensitivity analysis, and measures of precision.

Conclusion

Statistics are an integral part of evaluating the medical literature. Understanding the various assumptions is essential to the basic foundation of statistical testing. The reader is encouraged to look at the medical literature and determine whether the basic assumptions have been met. Once this issue has been resolved, refer to Table 10–1 and decide whether the appropriate statistical test was chosen. The correct selection of a statistical test is an integral part of assuring that the research conclusions are accurate. Keep in mind that this chapter is by no means comprehensive for all types of statistical tests. The field of statistics is rapidly changing and different techniques continue to be developed and validated.

Study Questions

1. A researcher is looking at the effect that high pH soil has on the color of soybean leaves. The colors are classified as light green, dark green, blue-green, and yellow-green. What kind of measurement variable is leaf color?

2. A researcher is evaluating 60 patients using a cross-over design to determine whether propranolol or hydrochlorothiazide is more effective in managing isolated systolic hypertension. What is the appropriate statistical test to analyze whether there is a difference in the mean blood pressure when using propranolol and hydrochlorothiazide?

3. A researcher has completed a cohort study on the effects of fertilizer on the development of breast cancer in women who live or work on farms. Will the researcher be calculating relative risk or an odds ratio?

4. A study has been performed that evaluates the effect that smoking has on the development of lung cancer. The researcher is looking at smokers versus nonsmokers

who did or did not develop lung cancer. However, the researcher wants to stratify the data to look at the effects of passive smoke. What statistical procedure would be best for this type of research question?

5. A study was performed that evaluated the difference in platelet count after patients were treated with heparin, low molecular-weight heparin, and warfarin. Three hundred patients were enrolled and randomly assigned to one of the three treatment groups. What is the best statistical procedure to evaluate the difference between the mean platelet counts?

REFERENCES

1. Gaddis ML, Gaddis GM. Introduction to biostatistics: part 1, basic concepts. Ann Emerg Med 1990;19:86–9.
2. Gaddis GM, Gaddis ML. Introduction to biostatistics: part 2, descriptive statistics. Ann Emerg Med 1990;19:309–15.
3. Gaddis GM, Gaddis ML. Introduction to biostatistics: part 3, sensitivity, specificity, predictive value and hypothesis testing. Ann Emerg Med 1990;19:591–7.
4. Gaddis GM, Gaddis ML. Introduction to biostatistics: part 4, statistical inference techniques in hypothesis testing. Ann Emerg Med 1990;19:820–5.
5. Gaddis GM, Gaddis ML. Introduction to biostatistics: part 5, statistical inference technique for hypothesis testing with nonparametric data. Ann Emerg Med 1990;19:1054–9.
6. Gaddis GM, Gaddis ML. Introduction to biostatistics: part 6, correlation and regression. Ann Emerg Med 1990;19:1462–8.
7. Daniel WW. Applied nonparametric statistics. 2nd ed. Boston: PWS-Kent Publishing Company; 1990.
8. Munro BH, Page EB. Statistical methods for health care research. 2nd ed. Philadelphia: Lippincott; 1993.
9. Elston RC, Johnson WD. Essential of biostatistics. 2nd ed. Philadelphia: F.A. Davis; 1993.
10. Norman GR, Streiner DL. Biostatistics: the bare essentials. Chicago: Mosby; 1993.
11. Hampton RE. Introductory biological statistics. Dubuque (IA): Wm. C. Brown Publishers; 1994.
12. Mancano MA, Bullano MF. Meta-analysis: Methodology, utility, and limitations. J Pharm Pract 1998;11(4):239–50.
13. Sacks HS, Berrier J, Reitman D, Ancona-Berk VA, Chalmers TC. Meta-analyses of randomized controlled trials. N Engl J Med 1987;316:450–5.

Chapter Eleven

Professional Writing

Patrick M. Malone

Objectives

After completing this chapter, the reader will be able to:

- State reasons both for and against writing professionally.
- Describe the various steps of professional writing.
- Identify the order for authors in a professional paper.
- Describe the importance of "knowing their audience."
- Describe the various writing styles and their differences.
- Explain where to find a publication's requirements for submission.
- Describe what an article proposal consists of and why it is used.
- Explain the need for practice to develop good writing skills.
- List the components of both a research and review paper.
- Explain the general guidelines for writing.
- Explain the absolute importance of revision.
- Describe how to prepare audiovisual materials for a poster or platform presentation and place those items on a web site.
- Describe techniques for creating an abstract for an article.
- Describe how to correctly cite an article in a bibliography.

A common thought when considering the topic of professional writing is "That doesn't apply to me, I'm not writing for a journal." But professional writing is certainly not limited to journal articles or books. It includes writing evaluations of medications for consideration on a hospital formulary, preparing written policies and procedures for the preparation of an intravenous admixture, reporting the results of the latest sale to the home office, preparing a written evaluation of a technician or clerk, writing in a chart, writing a term paper for a class, preparing slides or posters for presentation, and many other things. Essentially any time a professional takes pen, pencil, chalk, typewriter, word processor, or any other writing implement in hand to fulfill professional duties, it is considered professional writing. Although the format changes, the general principles remain the same. So whether the object is to write the ultimate book on the practice of pharmacy or to type a label, a pharmacist must know how to write professionally.

Although some may say the purpose of writing is "to keep my job" or "to pass this course," there are, generally, four larger purposes for the existence of written material. That material serves to inform, instruct, persuade, or entertain. The first three items are those usually considered in professional writing, although including the fourth (whenever possible) will help convince people to read what has been written.

There are also some advantages to professional writing, besides those mentioned above. For example, writing is often good for promotion in many jobs. In academia, there is always the concept of "publish or perish." Even pharmacy technicians are encouraged to write as a means of advancement.[1] Also, writing gives the authors the opportunity to share their knowledge or ideas, obtain gratification or satisfaction, and improve their knowledge. It may even lead to some fame or notoriety in a field.

Unfortunately, there are disadvantages to professional writing, too. The major problem is that any significant amount of writing often involves a lot of potentially frustrating work, because few people are natural writers. The author must practice to become proficient at writing, which will involve false starts, numerous drafts, roadblocks, and other problems. If that is not enough, writing exposes a person to criticism and possible rejection. Although at one time authors were paid to publish articles, today it is not unheard of that authors may actually have to pay to have their article published.[2] At best, the direct financial rewards are likely to be few, unless a best-selling novel is produced. Indirectly, writing may lead to pay increases and promotions. However, because writing is a professional necessity, it can be made easier by following the correct procedures, which will be covered in this chapter.

Steps in Writing

As each of the steps in professional writing are covered in this section, the emphasis will be on writing items likely to be encountered in a practice setting, although additional steps necessary when writing for publication will be mentioned.

PREPARING TO WRITE

The first step in writing is to know the purpose—why something needs to be written in the first place. It is necessary at this time to have a good idea of the expected endpoint, which is a good idea, no matter what is being done. For example, someone learning to plow a field with a tractor may be concentrating on the ground near the tractor and end up wandering all over the field, thinking he or she was going straight. However, by concentrating on going to a specific point on the far end of the field, rather than looking just in front of the tractor, the row will probably be plowed fairly straight. Throughout this whole process it is necessary to keep in mind that endpoint, to keep from wandering all over the place. If the item being written is for publication, rather than something required for work, it will also be necessary to pick the topic. Although the writing is considered to be more important than the idea, it is still important to have a good idea or important topic before starting.[3] The topic should be of interest and/or importance to the prospective readers. It can even cover an old topic, as long as the topic is covered in greater depth, in a new way, or is addressed to a different group.

It is also necessary to decide whether there needs to be a co-author. This may be easy to resolve, depending on who is working on the project. However, even if no one else has been involved, it may be a good idea to look for a co-author. An inexperienced writer would benefit from working with an experienced author, and working with someone will give a different perspective and, hopefully, lessen the work for each person. Finally, it is sometimes a necessity to include co-authors for political reasons (as in "Would you prefer to share the credit or work nights and holidays for the rest of your life?"). Although this last reason should not exist, it does. A variety of other problems with authorship credit are also seen.[4,5] The best that may be fought for under the circumstances may be that everyone must do part of the writing and that authors be listed in the order of their contributions to the project. This does not always happen.[6,7] Although arguments may be made,[8-14] there is no valid reason for people to be listed as an author in excess of their contribution to the writing and submission of the work for publication.[15-18] The only exception would be if the publisher has specific other rules. For example, some journals may want to list "contributors" with an explanation of what they contributed (e.g., writing, origination of study idea, data collection). Generally, all of the following must be met for an individual to be given credit as an author[18]:

- Conception and design of the study, or analysis and interpretation of the data in the study
- Writing or revising the article
- Final approval of the version that is published

Things that do not qualify a person to be listed as an author include[18]:

- Acquisition of funding
- General supervision of the research group

Individuals that do not meet the first qualifications should be listed in the acknowledgments section.

It should also be mentioned that there can be too many authors and acknowledgements.[19] Some scientific papers list many, many authors for a particular paper, and the number of authors has grown over the last few years.[20] It is obvious that 20 authors could not have written a 3-page paper. Some of this may be a result of job requirements that include publishing a certain number of articles, leading to demands by individuals to get their name listed on any article they can. Again, authors should contribute to the written work in some significant way, as defined above. In some cases it may be necessary to just name the group performing the research, with a few of the most responsible individuals specifically named, and list others as acknowledgments, sometimes by group or institution.[19,21]

Before the first word is written, it is necessary to know the audience, which involves knowing the type of person who will be reading the final document and where it will be published. Keep in mind that the word "published" was picked for a specific reason. Whether the final product appears in *New England Journal of Medicine,* the "IV Room Policy and Procedure Book," or even the label on a prescription vial, it is "published." It is necessary to aim the work at the audience. At a broad level, written work should not be submitted for possible publication in a journal that does not cover the topic; it is no more appropriate to submit an article on preparation of cardioplegic solutions to *Journal of Urology* than it is to type a monthly fiscal report on prescription labels.

More specifically, it is necessary to aim both the writing style and depth of information toward the audience. If something is written for physicians, it is not likely to be understood by lay people. Conversely, items written for lay people may not satisfy the needs of physicians. It is certainly appropriate to have a secondary audience in mind. For example, a report written for physicians may be of interest to pharmacists and nurses. However, make sure the secondary audience is not served at the expense of the primary audience.

In regard to writing style, there are three types normally used by pharmacists and other health care professionals: "pure technical style," "middle technical style," and "popular technical style" (Table 11–1).[22]

Pure technical style is used by business or technical professionals when they are writing for other professionals in the same or similar fields. For example, an article published in *American Journal of Health-Systems Pharmacy* would normally be written in this style. There are several characteristics of this style. First, the authors can use technical

ARTICLE PROPOSAL TO PUBLISHERS

Although relatively few professionals write articles for journals or books, those who do need to follow an occasional step in addition to those outlined in the main text of this chapter. One difference is the potential need to write an article proposal to the publisher. This simply is a letter asking the publisher whether he or she would be interested in possibly publishing something on a particular topic written by the person who is inquiring. As might be expected, this step is generally not necessary if writing a description of original research, but would be important when writing a review article or even a descriptive article. The letter should contain certain information, which will be described below, and be addressed to an appropriate editor. If at all possible, it is also a good idea to talk to an editor before submitting your proposal. For example, the proposal for the first edition of this book originated after a discussion with the editor at the Appleton & Lange booth in the ASHP Midyear Clinical Meeting Exhibitor's Area.

In the written proposal, the prospective author should first briefly explain the basic idea that is to be covered in the article or book, including a working title. Similarly, a description of the approach the author wishes to take in covering the subject should be described. Although this description should be kept brief, it must provide enough information for the publisher to determine whether the topic and approach are even appropriate for their journal, etc. In the case of a book, it is important to include a table of contents that is descriptive enough to be useful to reviewers who will be advising the publisher on the need for such a book. Related to that need, it is also necessary to describe why the proposed article or book will be important to the publisher's customers. This is the sales pitch. It is necessary to briefly show that there is nothing similar, or as good, currently available in the literature for the audience being addressed.

Although the above is the meat of the proposal, there are several other items that should be included. These include the time necessary to complete the article/book (be realistic), the approximate length of the work, and a statement of the authors' qualifications, including any previous publications.

There are several good reasons for submitting a proposal. The first is simply to avoid work if the editor decides that there is no need for such a publication (although an author should not hesitate to send the proposal to another publisher, if it still seems that the topic is important). Second, and perhaps most important, it allows the editor(s) to make suggestions. By following those suggestions, an author is more likely to be successful in getting work published. Finally, if the idea is accepted, the acceptance letter will provide motivation.

TABLE 11–1. TYPES OF TECHNICAL WRITING

- Pure technical style—used by professionals addressing other professionals in the same field
- Middle technical style—used by professionals addressing professionals in other fields
- Popular technical style—used by professionals addressing lay people

jargon, because they can expect the readers will understand it. Second, it is written in formal English. Third, it is written in the third person; words such as I, we, us, and you are eliminated. Finally, there is a general lack of slang or contractions. The great majority of writing done by pharmacists will be in this style, because it is usually other pharmacists who will be reading their work.

Middle technical style is very closely related to pure technical style. This style is used by authors when they are writing for readers with a variety of technical backgrounds, with everyone having some unifying factor. For example, a report regarding a Pharmacy Department's quality assurance activities might be presented to the hospital's pharmacy and therapeutics committee. That committee is made up of physicians, nurses, hospital administrators, and other professionals. Although each has a background that makes their membership on the committee appropriate, not all of them would understand what a HEPA filter is, as would most hospital pharmacists. Therefore, it is necessary to better explain, or sometimes avoid, some technical areas. Otherwise, this writing style is very similar in most respects to pure technical style.

Finally, popular technical style is used in anything meant for the general public. Common language is used throughout. For example, a patient information sheet would need to be written in this style. A widely available example would be the "I am Joe's (name your favorite organ)" series that has appeared in *Reader's Digest* over the years. Information that is written in this style will use less complicated words and be less formal in its presentation.

It should be pointed out that usual technical writing differs greatly from what most people learn in high school English class or college composition courses. Although there is often a tendency to protest the formality of professional writing styles at first, the reality of the situation is that those styles must be followed for a piece of written material to be accepted.

The next step is to know the requirements of the publisher. Whether the work is for the department's policy and procedure manual or a journal, chances are that there is a format that needs to be followed. In the case of a journal, directions on the format to follow will be published at least once a year. Also, specific guidelines are followed by a number of professional journals, both for general format and statistical reporting. Many journals have approved those guidelines and expect that all work submitted for publication will follow them. They are referred to as the "Uniform Requirements for Manuscripts Submitted to Biomedical Journals."[18] This standardization makes it easier on the prospective author; one style can be learned and followed, regardless of the journal. Other publications that can be helpful are the *Council of Biology Editors (CBE) Style Manual, The American Medical Association Manual of Style, The MLA Style Manual,* and the *Publication Manual of the American Psychiatric Association.*

In the case of reports, policy and procedure manuals, and similar documents, it is best to see what has been done in the past. If this is the first time a particular item is being prepared, it is advisable to try to see what has been done in other places, and prepare something similar that meets the perceived needs. If writing something for work, do not be afraid to try to improve the format to make it more usable. However, be aware that it may be necessary to get any changes in format approved by the appropriate individual(s) or committee(s). Whenever possible, follow the "Uniform Requirements" format used by the medical journals, because it is the standard for biomedical writing.

GENERAL RULES OF WRITING

Once the preparation is completed, it is time to start writing. Unfortunately, there is no easy way to learn how to write professionally; it just requires a lot of practice. However, a number of rules can be followed (Table 11–2). This section covers some of the general rules, with information on how to prepare specific items (e.g., introduction, body, conclusion, references, abstracts) being covered later. The first step is to organize the information before starting to write. At risk of sounding like a high school English teacher, it is still true that this step should include preparing an outline. In the past, that was an onerous task that few performed. However, with modern word processing software, the

TABLE 11–2. CHECKLIST IN PREPARATION OF WRITTEN MATERIALS

- Do research first.
- Put yourself in the reader's position.
- Use proper grammar and spelling.
- Make the document look "professional."
- Keep things simple and direct.
- Keep the document short.
- Avoid abbreviations and acronyms.
- Avoid the first person (e.g., I, we, us).
- Use active sentences.
- Avoid slash construction (e.g., he/she, him/her).
- Avoid contractions.
- Cite other references wherever appropriate (and get permission to do so where appropriate).
- Cover things in whatever order is easiest.
- Get everything down on paper before revising.
- Edit, Edit, Edit!

outline actually becomes part of the finished product, so it does not amount to any significant extra work. Minimally the different sections should be listed to create some order to the layout of the work (remember, keep in mind the endpoint). Overall, the goal is to prepare a document that is clear, concise, complete, and correct. The two latter items depend, to a large part, on preparation. The former items, however, can be helped by following some simple rules.

The first two rules actually apply to the organization step. First, do sufficient research before getting started. Research in this regard, means obtaining whatever information—whether records, articles, performance evaluations, or anything else—necessary to prepare the item. Although it is likely that additional research will be necessary to fill in the "fine points" at some point in the process, most information should be gathered ahead of time. It is impossible to be organized if there is nothing collected, and a document that is not organized will generally not be worth much. The second rule is to put yourself in the reader's position. What does that reader want and how does he or she want it presented?

Although it should not need to be stated, it is quite important to use proper spelling and grammar. This is easier than in the past, because high-end word processing programs can check both; however, it is still necessary to double check, because the computer is likely to overlook things. For example, a properly spelled, but incorrect, word will be missed (e.g., "two" instead of "to"). Unfortunately for some writers, appearances count greatly. The writer may know more about a particular subject than anyone else, but if poor grammar and spelling permeate the document, it is unlikely that anyone will read or believe the information presented.[23] It will be dismissed as probably wrong, based on grammar and spelling alone. In a case where the finished product will be published in a language other than the writer's native language, the writer should have the work read and edited by someone for whom the language is his or her native tongue. It should also be mentioned that the writing should try to be entertaining. Although professional writing tends to be a bit dry, an attempt should be made to make it as enjoyable and easy to read as possible. It should also be unpretentious, direct, and accurate.[24]

Related to this, the document should look presentable. Some students are well known for turning in papers that are crumpled, creased, torn, dirty, or practically dipped in correction fluid. That is not professional and must be avoided. Fortunately, that problem should be lessened with the use of word processors. The sad truth is that people will assume that if an author was sloppy with the appearance of the document, he or she was probably sloppy with the information. That may not be so, but that assumption will kill a good but sloppy document.

When writing it is best to keep things as simple and direct as possible.[25–27] This has been referred to as the KISS (Keep It Simple, Stupid) principle. There is a temptation to use big words that sound impressive, but doing so is more likely to confuse than impress. Related to that, keep the paper as short as possible.[28] Also, consider whether tables, figures, or graphs would make the document simpler.

When writing, avoid using abbreviations or acronyms. If it is necessary to do so, state the full form of the word or term the first time it is mentioned in the document, followed by the abbreviation in parenthesis (e.g., acquired immunodeficiency syndrome [AIDS]). The only exceptions to this rule are units of measurement (e.g., mL, mg). Units of measurement should be expressed in the metric system. Clinical chemistry and hematologic measurements should be in terms of the International System of Units (SI).

If a document is long, subheadings should be used. This can be part of the outline step, mentioned earlier.

Several rules apply to the wording that is used in professional writing.[22] First, completely avoid writing in the first person, and avoid the second person wherever possible. It is not a bad idea, at least at first, to ask the word processor to find all occurrences of *I, we, us,* and *you.* If those words are found, try to rewrite the sentence to avoid them. Also, it is preferable to avoid using the passive voice throughout[29]; again, a grammar checker can help. Avoid both contractions and slash construction (i.e., *and/or, he/she* [use *he or she*], *this/that*). Finally, in this politically correct era, avoid sexism. That includes words like *he* or *she,* although it is not always appropriate or desirable to delete those terms. It is also inappropriate to use *their* instead of *his or her* to get around the problem.

When writing, be sure to give credit where it is due. This just does not mean making sure the listed authors wrote part of the document. It includes endnoting all information obtained from one or a limited number of sources. If there is extensive quoting, permission to do so should be obtained by writing to the person or organization holding the copyright on the material. Endnoting in the past was something everyone dreaded. They waited until the end, because the articles should be cited in the order they appear in the document. By that time it was difficult to go back and do it. Now, however, it is much easier with modern word processors; it is possible to insert the citations as the document is prepared and let the software worry about making sure they are in the correct order.

Related to the endnoting, everything that is stated should be supported by objective evidence. When writing a paper based on scientific literature, that evidence must be shown in the endnoting. To reemphasize, any unreferenced statement of fact is for all practical purposes worthless. However, it is necessary to make sure information is extracted from the original article and expressed properly. Some writers will improperly twist facts, whether inadvertently or not, to support their assertions.[30]

Finally, work through the document in whatever order seems easiest. In preparing a drug evaluation for a Pharmacy and Therapeutics Committee, a stack of 50 articles might be used. At first, the stack may look impossible, but after sorting the articles into groups that correspond to the sections, start with the shortest stack or the easiest information. By the time the document is finished, the writer may be surprised to find out that they were all fairly short, easy stacks.

At first, a writer should simply try to make sure that all of the information is down on paper. Once that occurs, go back and revise, and perhaps reorganize the document. Waiting a few days before revising the document can be very beneficial. After some time away from the project, errors practically jump off the page. It is also a good idea to have someone else who has not been involved with the writing, read the document. Something that seems quite clear to the author may not actually be clear at all. Also, the author may be mentally inserting words or even sentences that were inadvertently omitted. Having someone edit the document can be humbling but helpful. Be sure to provide the product in a format that will make things easier for the person reviewing the document. A typed, double-spaced manuscript will make it easy to read and provide room for comment. Even better, it is now possible to send electronic versions of a document out for review directly from the word processor. The reviewer can put in comments or suggested wording changes electronically and then return the document. The writer can then go through the document making changes or simply accepting proposed changes with the click of a mouse. Often, the use of the electronic reviewing mechanism will be quicker, easier, and provide much clearer suggestions.

The three most important things in real estate may be "location, location, location," but the three most important things in writing are "edit, edit, edit." It is not sufficient to settle for "good enough"—do your best. Look at it this way: the boss or editor is only going to do so much editing before giving up. The trick is to make sure that the document is well prepared and does not need that much editing.

SPECIFIC DOCUMENT SECTIONS

A typical document consists of three main parts—the introduction, body, and conclusion. Other parts, such as references, tables, figures, and abstracts may also be necessary. These will be discussed in later sections and in the appendices of this chapter. It should also be noted that a number of the points in Chaps 6 and 10 are applicable to writing, and should be considered along with this material. An example question layout is show in Appendix 11–1.

Introduction

With the probable exception of policy and procedure documents, the two most important paragraphs in any document are the first and last. It is vital to start out strong, to encourage the reader to continue reading. Otherwise, the work will end up in that stack of articles everyone has that they "intend to read someday." That first paragraph should also inform the reader of what they can expect in the rest of the document; it should be similar to a road map that shows what is to be accomplished in the document. The introduction should have a clear objective for the existence of the document. Many people neglect the need for a clear objective, which leaves the reader to flounder and wonder whether there really is a purpose to the document. In a research article, the introduction will also contain the hypothesis being investigated. In a policy and procedure document, it may simply be a description of what the remainder of the document will cover. The introduction should also contain background information about the topic that provides a good information base for the reader. The amount of background information has to be a balance—enough to show the reader that the writer has done an appropriate amount of research, but yet not so exhaustive as to bore or overwhelm the reader with unnecessary details.[31] Overall, the introduction should be short but contain properly referenced background material and show the reader where the document is headed.

The introduction should generally not be a conclusion; some people are so anxious to jump to the end that they put the conclusion first. Admittedly, the BLOT concept (bottom line on top) has its purpose in some documents (e.g., policy and procedures, formulary monographs), but that should be a conscious decision. If the introduction amounts to a conclusion, many people will read no further, making the remainder of the document a waste of time and paper.

Body

The body of the document contains all of the details. In a research article, the body may be divided into the methods, results, and, possibly, discussion sections, although the latter section may be incorporated into the conclusion. Details of what should be included are covered in Chap. 6. In other documents, the body will probably be divided into whatever sections are appropriate or logical. A number of rules can be followed in preparing the body of a document.

The first rule is that, while it is important to be concise, all necessary information must be presented. Again, keep an eye on the desired endpoint, and do not stray from the subject unless it is absolutely necessary. Including unnecessary information, even if it is interesting, will tend to confuse or obscure the important points.

It is important to cover the information in a logical order, so that it flows easily from one point to another. A common mistake, when learning to write professionally, is to skip back and forth between subjects. For example, someone might insert a point about dosing in the middle of indications, when dosing is discussed at another point in the document.

The writer should also put the information in his or her own words. Perhaps out of lack of confidence, a number of professionals are tempted to simply quote other authors word for word. However, by presenting the information in their own words, writers demonstrate that they actually understand the topic. Remember, though, that if the information is taken from a particular source, even if it is reworded, the original author should be given credit via endnotes.

It is necessary to expand on the topic discussed in the previous paragraph, because there seems to be much confusion about it and there are many cases where the rules against copyright infringement and plagiarism are broken. Plagiarism can be considered the copying of another's words or ideas, without properly giving credit. Copyright violations consist of copying another's work, even with appropriate quotations and citation, without permission. They are similar; however, it is possible to commit either plagiarism or copyright violations without committing the other.

Sometimes those infractions are rather blatant, such as the cases documented in the newspapers about students downloading papers from the Internet and presenting them as their own or simply retyping a previously published article. (Interestingly, an attempt to prevent this can be seen on the Internet at <<http://www.plagiarism.com>>).[32] Other times, the infringement is quite accidental. For example, it was once brought to the attention of the famous science fiction writer, Isaac Asimov, that a short story that he wrote was similar to an article that had been published 10 years previously.[33] Dr. Asimov went back and found the article and read it, realizing as he did so that he had read it when it first came out and had forgotten about it. When he wrote his story 10 years later, he did not at all realize that portions of it could be considered plagiarism. Although he had no intention of infringing upon the other author's work, Dr. Asimov made sure that the story was never reprinted and even wrote an article discussing the problem. This shows how easy it is to inadvertently cross the line into copyright infringement or plagiarism, and there are many examples that would fall in between the extremes given above. Therefore, it is necessary for the author to be on guard and to try to prevent the problem in the first place. A few general rules can act as a guide.

- When copying wording directly from another's work, it should be in quotations (or otherwise shown to be a quote) and a citation should appear to give credit to the original author(s). Also, if a significant amount of a work published in the last 100 years is quoted, it is probably necessary to get permission from the copyright holder, which may require paying a fee.[34] Exactly what is a "significant amount" is debatable; however, it would be best to err on the side of asking for permission if a quotation is more than a few sentences. Reproducing an entire chart, table, figure, and so on should normally require asking for permission. A letter to the copyright holder will solve problems; publishers often also have forms to request permission. A couple of special cases need to be mentioned. U.S. government documents are not copyrighted, so only quotation marks and citations are necessary. Second, if it is impossible to locate a copyright holder (e.g., the publisher went out of business without transferring copyrights), the writer should at least be able to document a thorough effort to obtain permission.

- Extensive quotations should be avoided. After all, if a writer cannot put something in his or her own words, does that person truly understand the material?
- Paraphrased information should have the original publication(s) cited, if it comes from one or a limited number of sources.
- Extensive paraphrasing, particularly without citations, may be considered plagiarism (i.e., copying the ideas of others).
- When citing an article, cite the one that the material comes from. If the material came from a review article, cite that article, not the original study that was not consulted. It is worth mentioning that in the case of unusual information, reading and citing the original study is preferable to just using a review article, because the review may be inaccurate.
- Be sure to follow publishers' rules, which may be stricter and may not allow any reproduction of material.

In preparing certain documents (written answers to questions for example), there may be very little information available. Perhaps only one or two research articles will have been written on the topic. If so, it will often be desirable to summarize the articles in detail, including most of the information presented in an abstract (see Appendix 11–2). In general, the information presented will summarize how many and what type of patients (i.e., inclusion and exclusion criteria), the drug or procedure being investigated, the results (e.g., efficacy, adverse effects), and the author's conclusions. It is also important to point out any noticeable flaws in the paper. An example would be:

Smith and Jones performed a double-blind, randomized comparison of the effects of drug X and drug Y in patients with tsutsugamushi fever. Patients were required to be between 18 and 70 years old, and could not have any concurrent infection or disorder that would affect the immune response to the disease (e.g., neutropenia, AIDS). Twenty patients received 10 mg of drug X, three times a day for 15 days. Eighteen patients received 250 mg of drug Y, twice a day for 10 days. The two groups were comparable, except that the patients receiving drug X were an average of 5 years younger ($p < .05$). Drug X was shown to produce a cure, both in terms of symptoms and cultures in 85% of patients, whereas drug Y only produced a cure in 55.5% of patients. The difference was statistically significant ($p < .01$). No significant adverse effects were seen in either group. Although it appears that drug X was the better agent, it should be noted that drug Y was given in its minimally effective dose, and may have performed better in a somewhat higher or longer regimen.

TABLE 11–3. ITEMS TO INCLUDE IN WRITTEN REVIEW OF A JOURNAL ARTICLE

Items to Include	Examples
Main author of article and a reference number	Johnson et al.[2] Smith and associates[24]
Type of article	Clinical study, case report, case series, review, meeting abstract
Research design (if appropriate)	Blinding, randomization, experience report, descriptive report
Purpose of the report	
Description of group studied	Size of groups, age, sex, disease state(s), other pertinent demographic characteristics
Any important confounding factors	Smoking, age, general health
Description of treatment being studied	Drug, dose, administration route, dosing interval, treatment duration
What was measured as an indicator of effect	
Results	Efficacy, adverse effects
Author conclusions	
Strengths and weaknesses of the study	See Chaps 6 and 7

A list of material to be covered in a review of an article similar to that above is found in Table 11–3.

Conclusion

A conclusion should be placed at the end of the body of the document, except for certain documents (e.g., policy and procedures). This conclusion should follow logically from the information presented and should serve to summarize that information. Remember, the conclusion should also correspond with the objective stated in the introduction.[35] It is also worth noting that in clinical consultations, a common mistake is to write the conclusion in a general manner, rather than addressing the specific patient in question, which is what the reader wants to hear about.

Many writers are tempted to avoid formulating a conclusion. Various reasons include not feeling qualified to make a conclusion for the reader, not wanting to restate what has already been stated, laziness, and so on. This is improper. The readers need something to bring their thoughts together at the end, and the author is in the perfect position to provide this closure. However, the author should also be careful to avoid extrapolating beyond the information available.

Other Items

If items are endnoted, the references should be found following the conclusion (see Appendix 11–3 for more information on how to prepare a bibliography). Other items may also be necessary, depending on the document, such as tables, graphs, figures, and so forth. They will not be dealt with here, other than to say that those items should supplement or clarify (not distort or misrepresent!), and not duplicate material in the text portion of a piece of written work. Also, it is worth mentioning that many computer programs make the preparation of professional-quality graphs and figures easy and often allow embedding the artwork in the word processing document itself, when allowed by the circumstances.

SUBMISSION OF THE DOCUMENT

Once the document is completed, proofread, and edited, it is ready to be submitted, whether that is to a boss or a journal. In the latter case, you will need to include a cover letter that serves as an introduction to the document. In the former case, it will be possible to be less formal. Also, it should be noted that when submitting an item to a journal it may be necessary to include transfer of copyright forms, conflict of interest disclosures (including financial)[36] or other items, which will be found in the directions for authors for that journal (usually found in the first issue of each year). The conflict of interest may be reported by the publisher in the final publication, but that is variable.[37] In addition, be sure to precisely follow the journal's "Instructions for Authors" to improve chances for acceptance.[38] It is also worth a word of warning that articles should very rarely, if ever, be submitted to more than one journal at the same time. If duplicate submission is felt to be appropriate and/or necessary, the rules outlined in the "Uniform Requirements" must be followed. Also, the article should not be broken down into many small articles and submitted over time, unless submission as a whole would result in a publication that would be too long or complex.[39]

REVISION

In many cases, revision of the document will be necessary. This may be due to a difference in opinion or different perception of need. Although an author should never change a document to say something he or she believes is wrong, minor revisions are often necessary. The comments given with the request for revision are likely to be helpful,[40] and they should be taken seriously. Even if it is felt that the person who read and commented on the paper is wrong, all concerns should be addressed. If a comment is truly wrong, it may still indicate that the work was not clear in a particular area. Changes should be made, based on the comments and completed within the time limits necessary.

Sometimes, however, a document may be rejected entirely. This can be for any of the following reasons[22]:

- The document is not up to standards (too much work for the boss or editor to correct).

- The idea or research the document is based on is too weak.
- The idea is inappropriate for that forum of publication.
- A similar article has been prepared (and possibly published) by someone else in that forum recently.

In the case of the first item, major revisions would be necessary before resubmitting to the boss or a journal. The second reason may also prompt major revisions, or even cause an author to stop working on the document. An article submitted to a journal but rejected for the last two reasons is not necessarily bad. It may be possible to submit it to another journal after only minor changes.

GALLEY PROOFS

A term well known to authors who have published articles or books is galley (or page) proofs. This is a copy of the final article, as it is to appear when published. It is the responsibility of the author(s) to carefully check to make sure there have been no mistakes made in typesetting. Although it may seem like a lot of work, everything must be checked, including the references, which frequently contain errors.[41-46] This step is necessary to prevent problems later. Although documents ready for the copy machine at work are generally not referred to as galley proofs, it is still necessary to carefully check those items.

Referees

Although this term is more familiar to sports fans, referees (also referred to as reviewers) are used in writing. These are the individuals to whom journals send submitted articles for review and comment. On a local level, they are the people that a writer may ask to look at a report before the boss gets it. Whatever arena, whether local or international, a person should also be willing to be a reviewer at that level. To be a reviewer for a journal, a person usually can simply write a letter stating interests, qualifications, and experience, and ask to be considered for the journal's reviewer list. If the person has adequate credentials, the journal will usually be happy to have that person as a reviewer.

Anyone who is a reviewer should be up front about such things as lack of expertise, conflict of interest, or inability to complete a review within a reasonable time, and should be willing to step aside as a reviewer of a particular paper if those are problems.[47] Also, a reviewer should treat anything submitted to him or her as a confidential document.

It should be pointed out that people who act as a reviewer for a paper should follow the procedures discussed in Chaps 6 and 7. Specific directions will also be received from the editor and may involve preparing comments for both the editor (to discuss matters, such as ethics, with the editor alone) and for the author (which is also used by the editor). It may be required that the latter be signed or unsigned. Also, as with any quality assurance procedure, the reviewer should treat it as an opportunity to provide constructive, as opposed to destructive, criticism.[48]

Specific Documents

NEWSLETTERS AND WEB SITES

Newsletters can be considered to be an aspect of any pharmacy practice, but are probably encountered most frequently in hospitals as a method for communicating Pharmacy and Therapeutics Committee actions and other drug-related topics to the medical, pharmacy, nursing, and other health care provider staffs. Newsletters are also seen from community pharmacies[49,50] (addressed to patients and/or physicians), nursing homes, drug companies, pharmacy organizations, and government or regulatory bodies. Wherever newsletters are found, their reason for existence is likely to be one or more of the following reasons: to communicate information to a target group, advertisement, and/or compliance with legal/accreditation standards.

In many cases, a newsletter can now be replaced by a web site. Such sites can serve the same purposes, but can also have some specific advantages and disadvantages. For example, web sites take very little effort for distribution, because all they take is a computer on the Internet, which can actually be provided by an Internet service provider (ISP) for a few dollars a month. Also, the material can take a greater variety of forms, including audio and video. The web site can actually be used to sell products, including prescriptions. Within institutions, the material can be kept available for health care providers to review for an indefinite time period, thereby preventing problems when somebody wants another copy of some old article or when the nurses are trying to make sure they have all of the publications for an accreditation visit. In regards to disadvantages, it does have to be noted that consulting a web site does take more effort, because it does not just fall into people's hands when they open their mailboxes. Also, some people do not use the Internet and would, therefore, not be able to consult the site.

Whatever the reason for the existence of a newsletter or web site, the same set of steps generally apply to their preparation.[51-55] These steps will be covered individually in the remainder of this section.

Define the Audience

Who will, or at least should, be reading the newsletter or accessing the web site? It may be physicians, pharmacists, nurses, other health care professionals, the lay public, other groups, or some combination of these. The target group(s) will have an effect on decisions made in the other steps.

Define the Goals of the Newsletter

The goal can be any of the reasons mentioned previously, but generally includes informing and educating the reader, and also to report news (including changes in policies and procedures, laws, etc.). With web sites, it can also be to directly sell products or gather information.

Identify Constraints

No matter what kind of newsletter or web site is produced, there are always going to be constraints that will limit what it can contain and how good it will be. One of the first constraints is time. It seems like every year people are busier and have less time to do things that they want or need to do. This includes preparing a newsletter or keeping up a web site (must be done continuously), which can take a significant amount of time if it is done right. It will be necessary to have time to write, type, edit, typeset, and perform other functions in publishing the newsletter—and all of those things have to be done in time to get the finished result to the printer, so that it can be ready for distribution on time. With a web site, it is necessary to write the material, figure out the layout or organization, and prepare it on the computer.

It is generally best, when beginning publication of a newsletter, to have it come out at longer intervals. If the newsletter is well received, it is found that there is enough time, and there is sufficient material, publication frequency can be increased. Overall, it is better to find it necessary to speed up publication frequency, rather than spread it out (people might get the idea the newsletter ceased publication).

Another constraint is the people that can or will be involved with publishing the newsletter or web site, particularly the editor-in-chief and/or webmaster. This is a case where the phrase, "many hands make light work" may be applicable. If a group of dependable people are willing to work together to make sure the articles get written and so forth the job may be easier. Generally there are two extremely hard parts to publishing a newsletter or web site, neither of which is the actual writing. One of them is coming up with topic ideas; the other is to make it look good. If others are at least willing to help here it can be a great aid to the editor of the newsletter. If at all possible, people from all groups served by the newsletter should be asked for topics, if not entire articles. If a pharmacist is in charge of the newsletter, some other possible places for help include an institution's public relations department, if available, and clerical help (to do the typing, formatting, copying, distribution, etc.). Keep an eye on the time necessary for pharmacy staff to produce the newsletter or web site, because this is likely to be the most costly item.

The third constraint is financial. As has been said, "There is no such thing as a free lunch." This also applies to newsletters and web sites. There is always some cost involved. Although personnel costs are likely to be the largest expense, the computer equipment and printing or duplication charges (for newsletters) can be significant. If the printing is to be done by an outside agency it is best to check on such items as the effect of order size (number of copies) and type of paper (e.g., plain vs. glossy, 8½ × 11 vs. 11 × 17 vs. A4, colors), stapling or binding on the cost. It is preferable to get bids from at least three printers. Another item to consider is method of delivery (e.g., personal vs. first-class mail vs. second-class mail). All of these items do add up and, depending on the budget, it may be necessary to sell advertising space to cover the costs.

Finally, it is necessary to look at what equipment is available. In the past it was necessary to either typeset or have a somewhat amateuristic cut and pasted typewritten newsletter; however, most places now have a computer and letter quality output device available. If at all possible, the use of a high-end word processing program or desktop publishing program with a laser or inkjet printer will allow production of a high-quality, professional newsletter quicker and at a lower cost. This equipment may be all that is necessary for a web site, assuming that the computer has some type of Internet connection. Although a number of web programs are now available for little cost, many times it is possible to just use a word processor or web browser to create and maintain the web site.

Newsletter/Web Site Design

As a child of the 1960s, it was easy during and shortly after college to believe substance was more important than appearance. Being older and (hopefully!) wiser (or at least more cynical), it now is noticeable that many people do not bother looking at the substance if the appearance is poor or unprofessional. Therefore, one of the most important things is to make the publication look appealing.[56,57] People tend to throw away newsletters that look sloppy or unprofessional, and do not bother with web sites that are not exciting and "neat." Even if the publication looks good it may[58–60] or may not[61,62] have any impact on physicians; but without looking professional it is highly unlikely to even have a chance.

A few general rules can help to make a newsletter or web site more appealing. These will be covered in the remainder of this section. However, for a more in-depth look at this subject, the reader is directed to references specializing in the subject.[63–65]

One of the first rules is to keep the publication consistent. This means not only from month to month, but also from page to page. This does not mean that improvements cannot be made from time to time. Nor does it mean that each page has to look exactly like the previous one. Instead, it means that it should have its own style that is recognizable by the reader, and that the various pages must fit with one another. The easiest way to do this, with either a newsletter or web site, is to create a template, style sheet, or theme (these terms overlap somewhat). Many pieces of software make this possible for either type of publication. A *template* is a file that contains material that appears the same from issue to issue—the term is often associated with a newsletter. Examples of this can be the newsletter's masthead (first page heading), the listing of editors, footers at the bottom of each page, number of columns, and so on. A *theme* should be similar to a template, but may be used more frequently when discussing a web site. *Style sheets* are a definition of how specific paragraphs or other parts of the newsletter or web sites will look (they would often be incorporated into the template or theme). For example, a style might be called "Heading 1," and by using this style for each article's title, the look remains the same from page to page, and issue to issue. This style can include such items as what the font looks like (e.g., typeface, font size, bold, italic, underlined, superscript, subscript, etc.), and what the paragraph looks like (e.g., left justified, right justified, centered, line spacing, space before or after, etc.), in addition to other items (e.g., whether the section is to be located in a particular part of the page, borders, etc.). A style manual should be established or at least a commercially available style manual, such as the *American Medical Association Manual of Style,* should be used. Whatever the editor(s) establish should be reasonably simple and elegant (i.e., don't get carried away—a couple of fonts on a page are fine, but 10 fonts look terrible). In the case of web sites, it might be useful to consult the publication *Elements of E-text Style,* which is available at <<http://wiretap.spies.com/ftp.items/Library/Classic/estyle.txt>>.

A second rule is to use appropriate software and equipment. A high-end word processor or desktop publishing program and a laser printer can be used to produce the master copy of the newsletter for reproduction.[66,67] This can allow a pharmacy to turn out a product that looks typeset at a fraction of the cost. As mentioned, there are a variety of low (or no) cost web site software tools. Some are specific (Microsoft FrontPage is probably the most popular and highest rated), whereas others are incorporated into word processors, web browsers, or other software. Also, just using a text editor is possible, although that tends to be much more difficult.

A third rule is to make the newsletter or web site look "good." For example, use "white space" properly. Do not just crowd in as much material as possible on the page. The reader will have a hard time following if it is too crowded, and just give up. Layout really is a difficult problem, and requires at least a little artistic ability to do well. If lack of artistic ability is a problem, it is probably a good idea to look over other newsletters or web sites from various sources to try to come up with ideas concerning what looks good. Minimally, most newsletters should at least be set up in two columns to allow easier reading. Other, more artistic, items to consider are asymmetrical layout (not having the two sides of each page look the same from a distance, perhaps using a narrow column for graphics or titles along one edge), different column widths, "teasers" (statements taken from the text that may pique the curiosity of the reader enough to read the article), surrounding boxes and columns with rules, and artwork/graphics.[68]

Next on the list for newsletters is to design a masthead. As mentioned, the masthead is essentially the part of the first page of the newsletter that gives the name of the publication, volume, issue, date, and so on. This may be at the top of the page or down one side of the first page. It is a good idea to consider having this done professionally, because it is a one-time expense and can be a major factor in the appearance of the newsletter. Sometimes it is good to have a multicolored masthead that is preprinted on blank stock paper. The newsletter text can then just be photocopied onto the paper and look much more professional. Material to be put into the masthead, or at least be included somewhere in the newsletter includes the newsletter name (be descriptive, but do not get cute—remember this is a professional newsletter), name and address of the pharmacy/organization, names of editor and editorial staff (give credit or blame where it is due), and frequency of publication. The name of the publication, along with some way of identifying the issue and page, should be placed on every page of the newsletter, so that the source of information can be identified if the page is photocopied or torn out.

Much of the material in a masthead should also be contained on the home page, if not every page, of a web site. Again, getting professional design help, at least at first, may be of value. Also, following the guidelines of the Health on the Net Foundation Code of Conduct (<<http://www.hon.ch/HONcode/Conduct.html>>) in designing the web page is appropriate.

In general, software themes available will help create a professional looking site, if professional help is not available. However, some specific items that need to be considered for a web site include[69,70]:

- Provide information that is good, credible, timely, and original. Share everything possible.
- Custom tailor information to take into account user preferences.
- Break up tables for readability.
- Use graphics effectively, but sparingly (they may take too long to download, annoying the reader). Graphics should be no more than 20 kilobytes in size.
- Related to the previous item, optimize the other aspects of the page to improve download times.
- Make the page easy to read—good contrast between the text and background, not too busy.
- Use self-generating content—make the site interactive.
- Web pages should be well organized—both the pages by themselves and how the pages are interconnected on the site.

- Consider selling things, if appropriate.
- Make sure everything works, from all likely browsers

In designing the newsletter or web site, effort should also be placed in deciding on a name. A local or institutional newsletter will often have a name related to the organization and the purpose of the newsletter. A web site may be similarly named, but there is an opportunity to go farther. In this case, the Uniform Resource Locator (URL) should be considered. This is the address of the web site on the intranet and/or the Internet. An institution may already have a registered URL, and the pharmacy web page may simply be under that name (e.g., <<http://www.yourorganizationname.org/pharmacy>>). However, independent community pharmacies can also register an unused name on the Internet and have that address (e.g., <<www.johnspharmacy.com>>).

It has been alluded to, but it is necessary to make a very specific decision on how the newsletter is to be printed. While typesetting still produces the best looking newsletter, it is quite easy to get a good-looking final product using a good photocopy machine. Also, even if the pharmacy produces the original copy on its computer, the file can be taken to a service bureau that can essentially produce a typeset copy. It is necessary to determine the paper to be used (glossy paper is not going to be used if you are photocopying). Most newsletters are 8½ × 11 inches in size, but that does not mean the paper is that size. It is better to use 11 × 17 paper for multipage newsletters and just fold the sheets. That looks much better than simply stapling the corner. Also, it is possible to take a disk with the newsletter file on it to some professional printers for them to print good-looking final copies.

Newsletter/Web Page Content

Before getting into items that a newsletter or web site should or can contain, it is necessary to discuss some general rules that deal with any article.[71]

First, it is a good idea to have a number of short articles, rather than one long article.[57,72] People will take a look at a short article and mentally decide they have the time to read it, whereas a long article may be dismissed immediately ("If I'm going to read something that long, it will be out of *New England Journal of Medicine!*") or put aside to read "when I have time." (A personal theory is that house dust actually comes from publications on the bottom of that "read someday" pile disintegrating from old age.) As a matter of fact, some recommend that newsletters should not exceed two pages (one sheet, front and back)[71] and one hospital cut their newsletter to one page (for P&T News) and replaced the remaining articles with a page to fit into a Drug Therapy Pocket Guide that consisted of useful tables (e.g., sodium content and neutralizing capacity of different antacids).[73]

Related to the above, use catchy titles to draw the reader into reading the article right then.

TABLE 11-4. NEWSLETTER OR WEB SITE TOPICS[51,53,57,71]

- Adverse drug reactions
- Calendar of events
- Clinical "Pearls"
- Effects of external events on jobs
- Job-related information
- New information sources
- New legal or regulatory requirements
- New services
- News from other departments
- Organization's stand on issues
- Personnel policies
- Pharmacoeconomics
- Pharmacy and Therapeutics Committee actions and news (major area to be covered)
- Productivity improvement
- Professional announcements
- Review of drugs/drug classes
- Quality assurance

Use proper writing techniques, as described earlier in this chapter. Be clear, concise and complete—do not waste the reader's valuable time. Also, be unbiased—support the article with facts. Be positive—talk about 90% compliance, rather than 10% noncompliance.

Finally, be sure the newsletter or web site is properly edited. Have multiple people read and edit the newsletter or web pages before publication. Having more people read it makes it more likely that dumb mistakes will be noticed and corrected. In particular, the editors should check for spelling, grammar, and readability. Also, it is a good idea to have people from each target group as editors, particularly physicians.[74]

The actual content of a newsletter or web site is one of the two most difficult areas for the editor that were mentioned (the other being that the newsletter should look good). Coming up with new ideas on a regular basis can be rather difficult. A list of possible areas to cover are included in Table 11-4.[51,53,57,71] If at all possible, material that was prepared for a different audience can be recycled for the newsletter or web site readers. For example, material from the Pharmacy and Therapeutics Committee meeting might be turned into a short review of a drug. Whenever possible, the material presented should be topics not available from another source, or material that is prepared in a format that will be of greater value to the readers than that same topic area as presented by other publications. Whatever the topics used, it is a good idea to survey the readers on a regular basis to make sure their needs are being met.

Newsletter Distribution

All of the above work will be for nothing if the readers do not get the newsletter. A good distribution system must be developed. Sometimes it can be as simple as sticking the newsletters in individual mailboxes, setting out piles of newsletters, or using interorganizational mail systems. If it is necessary to use the post office, it would be a good idea to check on the possibility of second class or bulk mail, which can save money. Newer innovative distribution methods are by electronic mail[75] or other computerized methods.[76] Community pharmacies may also distribute their newsletters by providing copies to physician waiting rooms or noncompeting businesses (e.g., banks, barber shops, beauty shops, day-care centers), or even including them with monthly statements.[50] Whatever method used, it is important to make sure the readers actually get the newsletter. Also, make sure they get the newsletters on a regular "cycle," so that they know when to anticipate the arrival of the publication.

PRESENTATIONS

Some time during a pharmacist's career, he or she may have the opportunity to give a formal presentation. This could be simply where he or she works or at a national meeting. Although it is well known that fear of public speaking is an extremely common occurrence, a speaker who prepares should do well. The problem may simply be fear of the unknown. Having some simple directions may be of immense help. Overall, the main concern should be to know the topic. If someone knows enough to be asked to talk, chances are that person will know quite a bit about a topic, or will be able to learn enough about the topic. Alternately, the potential presenter may volunteer to give a presentation on a topic he or she is interested in or has done a lot of work about (e.g., a new method to practice or a new practice area). After that, most of the concern will deal with looking good. This includes a variety of items, many of which involve professional writing, and will be dealt with in the remainder of this section.

In cases where a person is asking to speak, a proposal will need to be submitted. This describes the proposed topic, which should be of interest to the target audience. The directions given by the organization preparing the meeting will need to be followed. Beyond that, the skills described earlier in this chapter or appendicies will need to be used.

Next, it may be necessary to write an abstract that the organization providing the presentation forum will use to inform potential attendees about the presentation. Each organization may have a format to be followed in creating the abstract, which should be followed. As to what should appear in the abstract, the writer might use the information presented in Appendix 11–2. Admittedly, an abstract should usually be prepared after the presentation is done to best reflect what will be said. However, abstracts may be requested more than 6 months before the presentation, so in this case it will serve more as a planning document. Actually, it is probably best to create a brief outline of the presentation (at least the topics to be covered) and then write the abstract.

Along with the abstract, it may be necessary to prepare learning objectives to describe what the attendee will be able to do as a result of participating in the program. The objective should state that behavior in objective, measurable terms. For example, the objective may state that the attendee can "explain," "list," or "identify" something. It will not say that the attendee "knows," "understands," or "learns," because those are not measurable. The objectives should relate directly to the program and should be adequately broken down to cover the different areas of the presentation. Refer to the beginning of any of the chapters of this book for examples of objectives.

Occasionally, the presenter may be requested to provide self-assessment questions. Often these will be multiple choice or true/false, to simplify assessment. Those questions should be clearly stated and measure that the attendee has met the objective. Efforts should be made to make the questions clear. Also, they should avoid the use of "not" or "except," because these terms can lead to confusion. Writing good questions can be extremely difficult, so testing the questions out on others before the presentation may help improve the quality.

The speaker may also have to prepare a brief biography to be used in his or her introduction. This includes a few items about his or her background, such as title and current position. Also, some information that gives the audience an idea of why that speaker is qualified to make a presentation is useful. Typically, the information given in the biography will be rather brief.

Presentations can usually be broken down into platform or poster presentations. The former is a more formal, oral presentation that typically requires some sort of audiovisual component and is often presented in a room set up for an audience. The latter requires the presenter to place a summary of the material to be presented on a poster (or series of small posters) that will be displayed on a bulletin board–type display (usually provided by the organization) that will be 3 to 4 feet high and 6 to 8 feet wide. In that situation, the attendees can walk through a group of such presentations, stopping to look at any that appeal to them and ask the presenter questions.

Many of the rules described in the main part of this chapter relate to preparing the information to be presented, including slides, posters and other audiovisual materials. However, a few other rules need to be mentioned.

- The presenter should learn the circumstances under which the presentation is to be given. That includes whether it is a platform or poster presentation.
- The presenter should learn what equipment is to be provided (e.g., slide projector, overhead projector, microphone, size of poster presentation).
- If the presenter needs other items, they should be made clear to the organization. For example, it is becoming common for presenters to want to use computer slide projection equipment, which may present certain technical requirements for both

the equipment and support people. Also, the presenter may need such things as power outlet strips, extension cords, wireless microphones (many good speakers "wander" and would be frustrated by a podium microphone), Internet connection, connections from a computer to the room sound system, videotape player, cables, and other items. The presenter should take into account his or her own needs and desires, in addition to those of the audience. It is necessary to be very specific, since the people organizing the meeting may not understand the requirements. For example, if the speaker requests an Internet connection, he or she may think he or she is getting a T1 connection that will work well with a graphics-intensive presentation, but may arrive to find a phone line that will be totally inadequate. Also, even the resolution of a computer projector or type of connector for a network will need to be specified.

- The audience should be taken into account. One common complaint when a speaker flies in for a presentation is that they may not know anything about local circumstances, including simple social skills that are expected (e.g., foreign countries). It is best if the speaker tries to find out more about the audience and the situation, adjusting the presentation to take those items into account.[77]
- If necessary, the set up of the room should be specified.

All of the above should be double checked at the location of the presentation after arrival, but in plenty of time to correct any problems. As a side note, checking in with those arranging the presentation is necessary so that they will not be worried about your arrival and they will be able to clear up any last minute items.

The speaker then needs to prepare the presentation, doing appropriate research and preparation, using skills described earlier in this chapter and in the following sections. The presentation should also be rehearsed adequately. The next steps will discuss preparation of audiovisual materials, which can enhance the audience's ability to understand and retain the material.[78,79]

Platform Presentations

When giving platform presentations it is usually necessary to prepare audiovisual materials and, possibly, handouts. This was once rather difficult and expensive. Often a graphic artist would be necessary to prepare good-looking slides. Presenters might have settled for slides prepared by a drug company or may have tried to type and photograph simple slides. In some cases, simple handwritten overhead projector transparencies would be used. However, the availability of presentation programs has made the preparation of professional quality audiovisual materials a much easier task. Overhead slides should only be used to allow recording of items during a discussion; there is little, if any, reason to use them in a formal presentation.

Most office software suites (e.g., Microsoft Office) have very powerful tools to create slides and other materials. These also have professionally designed "templates" that provide good layouts for materials, including color and background choices. The programs may also guide the user to follow general rules, such as avoiding a "busy" slide that will be unreadable from the back of a large room. Also, the programs can be used to do everything from creating simple slides to multimedia extravaganzas—the former being learned in a few minutes, with the more advanced features available for those who need or desire them.

When starting to prepare audiovisuals, it is necessary to determine what type of equipment and situation will be found at the presentation. The most desirable type of audiovisual is rapidly becoming the use of a computer with a projector and appropriate software to give the presentation. This poses various advantages, including lower cost for the presenter, the ability to make last minute changes to slides before the presentation, the ability to include audio and video in the presentation slides, and the capability to embed Internet links into the presentation. When information or software is available on the network or the Internet, it can be demonstrated. Also, in cases where a discussion ensues, it is possible for the presenter to use a word processor, presentation program, or other software to record items on the screen for users to read during or after the session. It is even possible, using a web creation program (e.g., Microsoft Front-Page) to not only record the information on the screen during the presentation, but to also make it immediately available on the Internet at the end of the program. Some disadvantages include the cost of the equipment for the organizing group, the need for greater technical skills by both the presenter and organizing group, the potential for technological problems (e.g., a computer that refuses to boot, a corrupted data disk, an Internet connection that does not work), and it may be necessary for the presenter to bring his or her own notebook computer with appropriate software and data. Fortunately, the technical support people for professional meetings are becoming much more familiar with the equipment and the equipment itself is often more dependable.

When preparing the slides themselves, the presenter will have to prepare an outline to guide what is to be presented and determine the information to be presented in each slide. Some general rules can be mentioned.

- Limit each slide to a particular topic. Sometimes this will be an overview, but specifics should be limited to a discrete topic. One or two minutes of presentation material per slide is appropriate. If it is necessary to refer back to a previous slide, just make a duplicate that is inserted at the appropriate location.
- Keep things simple. The program may be able to do many things (e.g., 20 fonts in 16 million colors), but they may not be desirable. Typically use one font (perhaps with bold or underline in a few specific places for emphasis) and limited graphics.

- Limit the amount of information presented on each slide. A rule of thumb is no more than about five bulleted points per slide and no more than about five words per bulleted point. Any more than that quickly becomes confusing or unreadable. Generally, if someone in the back of the room has to squint or it takes more than 10 seconds to take in a slide, there is too much information on it.[80]
- Consider using a "theme" in the program that will provide colors that go together well and contrast enough to be legible. Colors and color combinations have to be carefully considered, because they may have emotional overtones or, in cases of color-blind attendees, may not even be distinguishable.[81]
- Consider graphics. They can make the slide more pleasing to the eye, but they also need to be as simple as possible. If cartoons are included to entertain the audience, make sure they are related to the talk and, preferably, help to make a point. Also, pictures of landscapes or the presenter's institution may be desired by the presenter, but serve only to distract from the presentation and should be avoided.
- Consider embedding sound or video in the presentation. That sounds difficult, but may be done with a few clicks of the mouse.
- Embed links to appropriate web sites in the presentation.
- Save the presentation several ways. Even if it is on the computer hard drive, it may become corrupted or the computer can break. Perhaps also bring it on a floppy disk, so that someone else's computer can be borrowed if necessary. It may be preferable to consider "burning" the presentation to a recordable (or read/write) CD-ROM or DVD, which will not be sensitive to magnetic fields that might have affected the original disk. Also, in case the computer to be used in the presentation does not have presentation software, it might be necessary to use the feature in many presentation software packages that creates a run-time presentation that does not require the actual software. In some cases, putting the slides on a web server in presentation format may work, although accessing the slides and web pages over the Internet can be a risky proposition.

Other items to consider include the following.

- When presenting, if traditional 2×2 slides are used, bring them in a projector carousel tray that is labeled with the name and address of the speaker, and with the title of the presentation. Check the slides before the meeting to make sure they are in the correct order and are in the correct orientation.
- Try to make the presentation interactive—ask the audience questions and take input.
- Keep to the slides, if at all possible, but do not read the slides—use the slides as a jumping point to your oral presentation information and to organize your thoughts.

- Do not read a prepared script. Actors and politicians can read such scripts and sound natural, but most speakers cannot do so. Instead use the slides (preferable) or a simple outline. The presentation program will allow easy preparation of handouts and speakers notes that can be used.
- Be prepared for technological disaster. Even when using something as simple as an overhead projector, the bulb can burn out. When using more equipment and more complex equipment, the potential for equipment failure rapidly increases. Whenever possible, have backup equipment, but also have a backup plan so that the presentation can proceed without any equipment.

It may be desirable to prepare a handout for the audience, in which case, the presenter can consider the following styles[82]:

- *Outlines*—a reference document that gives the audience a guide to where the speaker is going in text form. This can often be prepared by importing the slide content from the presentation software to a word processor. Some presentation programs will also prepare the document itself.
- *Full text handouts*—This is essentially a transcription of the speech. While helpful as a reference document, it is probably of more use to politicians when they wish to avoid being misquoted. This is seldom seen in pharmacy, because the presenter will not be able to make last minute changes and the audience will likely read ahead and become bored. Interestingly, a comment heard when such documents are presented is that "the speaker did not know the material, because all she (or he) did was read the handout," even though the speaker was the one who wrote it!
- *Slide reproductions*—This is becoming more popular and easy; presentation programs allow easy slide handout preparation. This does give the attendee all of the information, including graphics, but will likely require more paper.
- *Partial text handouts*—This can be something of a combination of the above, where only a portion of the talk is on the handouts.

In any of the above, it is good to consider the following.[82]

- Consider whether it is necessary to provide references or supplemental readings.
- Make sure the handout follows the order of the presentation. If it doesn't, the attendee may become confused and annoyed.
- Make it look good, using skills mentioned elsewhere in this chapter. By all means, allow plenty of room for the attendee to take notes.

The speaker may also use the handout as a set of speaker notes, but care should generally be taken to avoid just reading the handout to the audience, except in the case of full text handouts, for the reasons previously mentioned.

The skills necessary to give the presentation itself are beyond the scope of this chapter that deals with the preparation and distribution of written material. New presenters may wish to read a book or pamphlet on how to give effective talks. Also, Toastmasters International (<<http://www.toastmasters.org>>) is a group that will help individuals develop their speaking skills. Many organizations have a chapter of this organization. These aids will provide guidance on such skills as what level of sophistication to use in speaking, how to stand (e.g., "do not hide behind the podium," making eye contact), what language to use, how to use humor and other techniques to entertain the audience, how to address questions, and so forth. Also, some of the references used in preparation of this chapter provide many additional suggestions.[78,82]

Poster Presentations

Preparing a poster requires the presenter to first determine what is to be included. Typically, the information will be similar to that found in an abstract, but with an expansion of the various sections. There are likely to be tables, bulleted points, and figures. Overall, the information to be presented must be brief, so that it can be read within a couple of minutes by an individual passing by the display. Therefore, large amounts of text are undesirable. A poster presentation will not likely contain nearly as much information as a formal journal article, but will contain many of the same sections. It will serve as a place for discussion to begin between the presenter and interested individuals.

Preparing posters was at one time a very difficult prospect. A good-looking poster required either the use of graphics services or many hours using rub-on letters. This has changed with the availability of presentation and high-end word processing software on computers.

Some people prefer to use essentially the same presentation programs as would be used for slides. The individual "slides," which may be longer than could possibly fit on a typical 2 × 2 slide, will then be printed on a color printer and mounted on poster board. An assortment of these "slides" will then be pinned to the board provided at the meeting. This is easy to do, but does require carrying and mounting many individual pieces. Also, it tends to limit the size of items on the presentation and may not lend itself to allowing the most professional looking presentation. A final disadvantage is that any 1-page handouts will have to be prepared separately.

Another possibility is the preparation of a large, 1-piece poster that is typically about 3 × 6 feet. Although the final poster must be printed by a graphics firm (e.g., printer, architectural drawing firm), the cost can be reasonable to produce a very good-looking poster. The initial preparatory work can also be done by such firms, but it is less expensive to do this yourself. The software necessary would be either a desktop publishing software (e.g., Adobe PageMaker, Microsoft Publisher) or a high-end word processor (e.g., Microsoft Word, WordPerfect). Essentially, what needs to be done is to lay out the page in these programs so that it is in landscape format (i.e., sideways from the normal typed page). The top of the page will have a centered title in large print, with the author names, institution, city, and so on centered in a smaller font below the title. Often, it is desirable to place graphics to one or both sides of that information, such as the symbol for the authors' institution(s). Under that, the page may be divided up into three or so columns and the information laid out in a logical order, including tables and figures. It may be desirable, once finished, to print out the final copy in two sizes. One can be a copy that fits on typical 8½ × 11 inch paper, which can be reproduced and distributed to interested individuals at the meeting. The second may be on larger paper (e.g., 11 × 17 inch) if there is a suitable high-quality printer available. The graphics firm can use then this and/or the data file on a disk to create the final poster. Using the data file may be less expensive, but it will be necessary to contact and work with a graphics firm before preparing the file to make sure that the file is prepared with a program and in a format that can be used by the graphics firm.

Whatever method is used, the final product will need to be transported to the meeting (poster tubes are available for little or no cost from many graphics firms). It is preferable to carry such posters on airplanes, because they may be crushed in the baggage areas. The presenter should also remember to bring pushpins to mount the presentation at the meeting. The presenter should show up early enough for the presentation to have the material mounted to the bulletin board before meeting attendees are allowed in the area and will be expected to remain with the presentation to answer questions for the assigned time. Although many people may be the authors of a presentation, it is not uncommon that only one or two actually attend the meeting and give the presentation.

Web Posting

After a presentation, consider making the material available on the Internet. Some organizations are now making at least some presentation materials available that way. Of course, copyright restrictions may prevent individuals from posting the material, but technology makes it easy. Text documents, such as posters, are easily placed on a web site. However, even full slide presentations can be placed on a web site, using streaming audiovisual. A variety of software, such as RealVideo or Microsoft PowerPoint and Windows Media, can be used to prepare such streaming presentations that can include slides and an audiovisual recording of the presenter. This can even be done concurrently with the presentation (live streaming), with a recording being made for later viewing. The equipment needs are relatively minor (i.e., modern computer, presentation software, microphone, inexpensive computer video capture device [e.g., Logitech QuickCam] for recording). For the actual Internet streaming, the appropriate streaming software, running on a file server, is necessary. For those who do not have the appropriate streaming software, just placing the slides themselves, as a downloadable file or in presentation format, can be an easy process using the original software used to prepare the slides. Even the simplest web site can then be used to give access to the material.

Conclusion

Professional writing is a skill necessary for every pharmacist. It simply consists of following the accepted rules for writing that have been established by the profession to prepare a written item that is clear, concise, complete, correct, and in the appropriate format.

REFERENCES

1. Thordsen DJ. Preparing an article for publication. J Pharm Technol 1986; Nov/Dec:268–75.
2. Fye WB. Medical authorship: traditions, trends, and tribulations. Ann Intern Med 1990;113: 317–25.
3. Nahata MC. Publishing by pharmacists. DICP Ann Pharmacother 1989;23:809–10.
4. Wilcox LJ. Authorship. The coin of the realm, the source of complaints. JAMA 1998;280:216–17.
5. Hoen WP, Walvoort HC, Overbeke AJPM. What are the factors determining authorship and the order of the authors' names? A study among authors of the Nederlands. Tijdschrift voor Geneeskunde (Dutch Journal of Medicine) 1998;280:217–18.
6. Shapiro DW, Wenger NS, Shapiro MF. The contributions of authors to multiauthored biomedical research papers. JAMA 1994;271:438–42.
7. Flanagin A, Carey LA, Fontanarosa PB, Phillips SG, Pace BP, Lundberg GD, et al. Prevalence of articles with honorary authors and ghost authors in peer-reviewed medical journals. JAMA 1998;280:222–4.
8. Peterson AM, Lowenthal W, Veatch RM. Authorship on a manuscript intended for publication. Am J Hosp Pharm 1993;50:2082–5.
9. Carbone PP. On authorship and acknowledgments. N Engl J Med 1992;326;1084.
10. Hart RG. On authorship and acknowledgments. N Engl J Med 1992;326;1084.
11. Pinching AJ. On authorship and acknowledgments. N Engl J Med 1992;326;1084–5.
12. Canter D. On authorship and acknowledgments. N Engl J Med 1992;326;1085.
13. Rennie D, Yank V, Emanuel L. When authorship fails. A proposal to make contributors accountable. JAMA 1997;278:579–85.
14. Fathalla MF, VanLook PFA. On authorship and acknowledgments. N Engl J Med 1992;326;1085.
15. The International Committee of Medical Journal Editors. Statement from the International Committee of Medical Journal Editors. JAMA 1991;265:2697–8.
16. Hasegawa GR. Spurious authorship. Am J Hosp Pharm 1993;50:2063.

17. Rennie D, Flanagin A. Authorship! Authorship! Guests, ghosts, grafters, and the two-sided coin. JAMA 1994;271:469–71.

18. International Committee of Medical Journal Editors. Uniform requirements for manuscripts submitted to biomedical journals. Med Educ 1999;33:66–78.

19. Kassirer JP, Angell M. On authorship and acknowledgments. N Engl J Med 1991;325:1510–12.

20. Drenth JPH. Multiple authorship. The contribution of senior authors. JAMA 1998;280:219–21.

21. Kassirer JP, Angell M. On authorship and acknowledgments. N Engl J Med 1992;326;1085.

22. McConnell CR. From idea to print: writing and publishing a journal article. Health Care Supervisor 1984;2:78–94.

23. Burnakis TG. Advice on submitting papers. Am J Hosp Pharm 1993;50:2523.

24. Higa GM. Scientific publications and scientific style. W V Med J 1995;91:198–9.

25. Crichton M. Medical obfuscation: structure and function. N Engl J Med 1975;293:1257–9.

26. Jones DEH. Last word. Omni 1980;2(12):130.

27. Hamilton CW. How to write effective business letters: scribing information for pharmacists. Hosp Pharm 1993;28:1095–1100.

28. Baker SJ. Getting published. Aust J Hosp Pharm 1994;24(5):410–15.

29. Hamilton CW. How to write and publish scientific papers: scribing information for pharmacists. Am J Hosp Pharm 1992;49:2477–84.

30. Ingelfinger FJ. Seduction by citation. N Engl J Med 1976;295:1075–6.

31. Talley CR. Perspective in journal publishing. Am J Hosp Pharm 1993;50:451.

32. Ware J. Cheat wave. Yahoo! Internet Life 1999;5(5):102–3.

33. Asimov I. Gold. The final science fiction collection. New York: HarperPrism; 1995.

34. Ardito SC, Eiblum P, Daulong R. Conflicted copy rights. Online 1999 May/June:23(3):91–5.

35. Gousse G. Advice on submitting papers: I. Am J Hosp Pharm 1993;50:2523.

36. International Committee of Medical Journal Editors. Conflict of interest. Am J Hosp Pharm 1993;50:2398.

37. Krimsky S, Rothenberg LS. Financial interest and its disclosure in scientific publications. JAMA 1998;280:225–6.

38. Laniado M. How to present research data consistently in a scientific paper. Eur Radiol 1996;6:S16–S18.

39. Stead WW. The responsibilities of authorship. J Am Med Inform Assoc 1997;4:394–5.

40. Garfunkel JM, Lawson EE, Hamrick HJ, Ulshen MH. JAMA 1990;263:1376–8.

41. Evans JT, Nadjari HI, Burchell SA. Quotation and reference accuracy in surgical journals. JAMA 1990;263:1353–4.

42. Roland CG. Thoughts about medical writing. XXXVII. Verify your references. Anesth Analg 1976;55:717–18.

43. Biebuyck JF. Concerning the ethics and accuracy of scientific citations. J Anesthesiol 1992;77:1–2.

44. McLellan MF, Case LD, Barnett MC. Trust, but verify. The accuracy of references in four anesthesia journals. Anesthesiology 1992;77:185–8.

45. de Lacy G, Record C, Wade J. How accurate are quotations and references in medical journals. Br Med J 1985;291:884–6.

46. Doms CA. A survey of reference accuracy in five national dental journals. J Dent Res 1989; 68:442–4.

47. Hasegawa GR. How to review a manuscript intended for publication. Am J Hosp Pharm 1994; 51:839–40.

48. Hoppe S, Chandler MJJ. Constructive versus destructive criticism. Am J Health-Syst Pharm 1995;52:103.

49. Seltzer SM, Desktop publishing in a drug store? Am Druggist 1987:196:64, 66.

50. Srnka QM, Scoggin JA. 10 ways to distribute newsletters to build sales volume. Pharm Times 1984:50;71–2, 74.

51. Making the media. The pharmacy newsletter. Hosp Pharm Connection 1986;2(3):11–12.

52. Kaldy J. Effectively creating a pharmacy newsletter. Consult Pharm 1992;7(6):700, 697–8.

53. Goldwater SH, Haydon-Greatting S. How to publish a pharmacy newsletter. Am J Hosp Pharm 1991;48:2121, 2125.

54. Almquist AF, Wolfgang AP, Perri M. Pharmacy newsletters—the journalistic approach. Hosp Pharm 1988;23:974–5.

55. Schultz WL, Dendiak ST. Pharmacy newsletters: a needed service. Hosp Pharm 1975;10(4): 146–7.

56. Plumridge RJ, Berbatis CG. Drug bulletins: effectiveness in modifying prescribing and methods of improving impact. DICP Ann Pharmacother 1989;23:330–4.

57. Appearance and content attract newsletter audience. Drug Utilization Review 1988;4(4):45–8.

58. Lyon RA, Norvell MJ. Effect of a P&T Committee newsletter on anti-infective prescribing habits. Hosp Formul 1985;20:742–4.

59. Fendler KJ, Gumbhir AK, Sall K. The impact of drug bulletins on physician prescribing habits in a health maintenance organization. Drug Intell Clin Pharm 1984;18:627–31.

60. May JR, Andrusko KT, DiPiro JT. Impact and cost justification of a surgery drug newsletter. Am J Hosp Pharm 1984;41:1837–9.

61. Ross MB, Volger BW, Bradley JK. Use of "dispense-as-written" on prescriptions for targeted drugs: influence of a newsletter. Am J Hosp Pharm 1990;47:2519–20.

62. Denig P, Haaijer-Ruskamp FM, Zijsling DH. Impact of a drug bulletin on the knowledge, perception of drug utility, and prescribing behavior of physicians. DICP Ann Pharmacother 1990;24:87–93.

63. Parker RC. Looking good in print. A guide to basic design for desktop publishing. 2nd ed. Chapel Hill (NC): Ventana Press; 1990.

64. Baird RN, McDonald D, Pittman RK, Turnbull AT. The graphics of communication. Methods, media and technology. 6th ed. New York: Hartcourt Brace Jovanovich College Publishers; 1993.

65. Pfeiffer KS. Word for Windows Design Companion, 2nd ed. Chapel Hill (NC): Ventana Press; 1994.

66. Don't let cost prohibit publication of pharmacy-related newsletter. Drug Utilization Review 1988;4(4):48–9.

67. Utt JK, Lewis KT. Using desktop publishing to enhance pharmacy publications. Am J Hosp Pharm 1988;45:1863–4.

68. Pfeiffer KS. Award-winning newsletter design. Windows Magazine 1994;5(8):208–18.

69. What makes a great web site? [cited 1999 May 13]:[1 screen]. Available from: URL: http://www.webreference.com/greatsite.html.

70. Tweney D. Don't be a slow poke: keep your site up to speed or lose visitors. InfoWorld 1999; 22;21(12):64.

71. Tullio CJ. Selecting material for your newsletter. Hosp Pharm Times 1992;Oct:12HPT–16HPT.

72. Journalism pro offers editing tips for effective pharmacy newsletters. Drug Utilization Review 1988;4(4):49–50.

73. Mitchell JF, Cook RL. Pharmacy newsletters: time for a new approach. Hosp Formul 1985;20: 360–5.

74. Ritchie DJ, Manchester RF, Rich MW, Rockwell MM, Stein PM. Acceptance of a pharmacy-based, physician-edited hospital Pharmacy and Therapeutics Committee newsletter. Ann Pharmacother 1992;26:886–9.

75. Craghead RM. Electronic mail pharmacy newsletters. Hosp Pharm 1989;24:490.

76. Mok MP, Castile JA, Kowaloff HB, Janousek JR. Drugman—a computerized supplement to a hospital's drug information newsletter. Am J Hosp Pharm 1985;42:1565–7.

77. Speaking abroad. How to prepare when you're presenting over there. Presentations 1999;13(6): A1–A15.

78. Spinler SA. How to prepare and deliver pharmacy presentations. Am J Hosp Pharm 1991;48: 1730–8.

79. Simons T. Multimedia or bust? Presentations 2000;14(2):40–50.

80. Endicott J. For the prepared presenter, fonts of inspiration abound. Presentations 1999;13(4): 22–3.

81. The psychology of presentation visuals. Presentations 1998;12(5):45–51.

82. Engle JP, Firman SC. Perfecting pharmacist presentation skills. Am Pharm 1994;NS34(7):60–4.

12

Chapter Twelve

Legal Responsibility for the Provision of Drug Information

Martha M. Rumore

Objectives

After completing this chapter, the reader will be able to:

- Describe the legal issues related to the provision of drug information.
- Determine the applicability of various legal theories that impose liability on pharmacists providing drug information.
- Describe recent case law expanding the legal responsibilities of pharmacists.
- Describe how pharmacists can help protect themselves from malpractice claims resulting from the provision of drug information.

An understanding of the legal aspects of drug information can help the practitioner to better understand the scenarios that can occur in day-to-day practice, as well as some possible ways to protect himself or herself in the legal system. This chapter is intended to examine legal issues and should not be considered legal advice.

More than 30 years after the genesis of drug information services, the legal duties of pharmacists providing drug information are still evolving. Today, most pharmacy curriculums include drug information (DI), realizing that whether a student specializes in DI or not, it is an integral part of pharmaceutical care. Pharmacists can and will be held liable for their conduct relating to DI. This chapter begins with an examination of the expanded liability of the DI specialist, which is defined as those pharmacists who either work in drug information centers (DICs) or who spend the majority of their working day providing DI. The liability inherent in the provisions of DI to patients as an integral component of pharmaceutical care is then examined. The liability of the DI specialist versus generalist differs for a number of reasons, the most obvious of which are the nature of the information provided and the recipients of the information. In the provision of pharmaceutical care, pharmacists are providing information to patients, whereas the DI specialist is often providing DI to other health professionals. The chapter then explores copyright and some unique legal issues, as well as case law. Finally, recommendations for prevention and mitigation of liability are provided.

The Drug Information Specialist

Drug information practice is a specialized discipline of pharmacy. Despite the clear prevalence of pharmacist-staffed DICs, the legal obligations of the DI specialist remain unclear. Specialists are held to the highest degree of care by the law. Because of the DI pharmacists' greater expertise in the area of DI, it is likely that the courts would expand their legal and professional liability beyond that of other pharmacists. Functions such as on-line searching, monitoring or recommending drug therapy, patient counseling, participation in clinical studies and pharmacy and therapeutics (P&T) committees, drug use evaluation, and identifying adverse drug experiences entail legal obligations of proper performance. Willig has stated[1]:

> If you voluntarily offer and create a higher standard of careful practice, the public has a legal right to assume that pharmacists can and will consistently perform according to that standard.

Minimal practice standards for specialists have been put forth to delineate functions and activities that may be considered essential to the provision of DI services and the expected competencies of DI specialists. Position papers and standards of the American Society of Health-System Pharmacists (ASHP) and Joint Commission on Accreditation of Healthcare Organizations (JCAHO), as well as DI curriculum standards, remove any doubt about the level of expertise needed for DI specialists and standards for DICs.[2,3] Minimal standards of performance and a consistent level of competence must be assured by pharmacists promoting or offering this service regardless of the practice site. Although there are no standards to "accredit" DICs, professional standards of performance may be used by courts as an objective measuring tool for the standard of care.

In the latter part of the nineteenth century the "locality rule" or "community rule" was followed. This doctrine stated that the local defendant practitioner would have his or her standard of performance evaluated in light of the performance of other peers in the same or similar communities.[4] This is no longer the case and a DIC in New York City will be held to the same standard as one in a rural area. Creation of standards of practice and the disappearance of the "locality rule" have made it easier for plaintiffs to prevail.

Drug Information in Pharmaceutical Care

In addition to the DI specialist, the pharmacy profession is assuming an increased legal responsibility to provide DI in daily practice. Although the physician has been considered the "learned intermediary," responsible for communicating the manufacturer's warnings to the patient, the Omnibus Budget Reconciliation Act of 1990 (OBRA '90) may be shifting this responsibility to the pharmacist. Failure to counsel or warn cases are showing an increasing trend in pharmacist liability.[5] Recent cases demonstrate the pharmacist's duty to warn of foreseeable complications of drug therapy is becoming a recognized part of the expanded legal responsibility of pharmacists.

Where the patient is at higher risk than the general population, the courts have uniformly found liability. There are many such cases against physicians for failure to disclose material risks of medical procedures or treatments to their patients.[6–8] Today, there is some question as to whether, in providing DI, pharmacists are held to the same standards as physicians when determining standard of care. Traditionally, physicians remain responsible for their patients and must exert "due care"; that is, a physician who knows or should have known that the information provided was improper may be held liable for negligence. Recent cases against pharmacists have held that pharmacists who gain information about the unique susceptibility of a patient are liable for failure to warn of the risks. In *Dooley v. Everett,* the court held the pharmacist liable for failing to warn a patient on theophylline of the interaction with erythromycin that produced seizures and consequent brain damage.[9] Similarly, in *Hand v. Krakowski,* the pharmacist failed to alert either the patient or physician of the drug interaction between the patient's psychotropic drug and alcohol.[10] The fact that the medication profile indicated that the patient was an alcoholic created a foreseeable risk of injury and, therefore, a duty to warn on the part of the pharmacist.

In *Baker v. Arbor Drugs, Inc.,* the court ruled that by advertising its drug interaction software, the defendant pharmacy voluntarily assumed a duty to use its computer technology with due care. The pharmacy technician had overridden the drug interaction between tranylcypromine sulfate (Parnate) and clemastine fumarate/phenylpropalamine hydrochloride (Tavist-D) that the system detected from the patient's medication profile. The patient committed suicide after suffering a stroke from the combination.[11]

Is the pharmacist liable when the DI provided is incomplete? Should the pharmacist provide all the medication information, via a DI sheet or patient package insert (PPI)? There have been several cases against pharmacists for failure to dispense mandatory PPIs for certain drugs that later caused harm. In *Farkas v. Saary,* the court addressed the issue of whether the pharmacist's failure to dispense the FDA-mandated PPI for progesterone was the proximate cause of the congenital eye defect that occurred.[12] Because congenital defects, but not eye deformities, were specified in the PPI, failure to provide the PPI could not be proven to be the proximate cause. Therefore, judgment was in favor of the pharmacy. In *Frye v. Medicare-Glaser Corporation,* the pharmacist counseled the patient regarding drowsiness with Fiorinal, but failed to provide a warning not to consume alcohol. The patient died presumably as a result of combining the drug with beer. Here, the DI provided was incomplete. The trial court did not find the pharmacist had a duty to warn in this instance.[13] It is important to realize that this case was decided before OBRA '90 was in effect; today, the decision may be different.

While pharmacists are in a position to provide drug information, providing the patient with all information may have a detrimental effect. In fact, it is the Food and Drug Administration's (FDA) position that the information contained in professional labeling can be safely used only under the supervision of the licensed prescriber. It has, therefore, been the practice not to provide the patient with the "professional labeling" unless the patient specifically requests it. With regard to the duty to disclose to the patient low percentage risks, the court rulings have been inconsistent.

One court has allowed strict liability against a pharmacy. In *Heredia v. Johnson,* the pharmacist dispensed an otic solution without warning of the risk of tympanic membrane rupture and the need to discontinue the drug if certain symptoms appeared. The plaintiff claimed that because of the lack of warning he suffered from severe and permanent injury including brain damage.[14] However, in *Marchione v. State,* a prison inmate alleged lack of informed consent based on the failure of the prison doctor to inform him about the side effects of prazosin (Minipress), which caused permanent impotence. The physician argued that his duty was only to warn of severe or frequent side effects. The *Marchione* court concluded that the physician need not disclose a laundry list of 31 remote drug side effects. The side effect had a reported incidence of only two or three cases out of several million prescriptions and was, therefore, rare. The plaintiff also did not have any unique risk factors that would increase the likelihood of the reaction occurring.[15] The courts seem to look at risk factors unique to the patient in deciding whether the health professional is required to indicate the likelihood of occurrence of the risks.

Brushwood and Simonsmeier[16] delineate two responsibilities with regard to patient counseling: risk assessment and risk management. *Risk assessment* is judgmental and occurs before prescribing when a decision is made to accept or forego drug therapy. It remains the responsibility of the physician. *Risk management* occurs after prescribing, is nonjudgmental, and assists the patient in proper drug use to maximize benefits and minimize potential problems.[17,18] Drug risk management, but not drug risk assessment information, should be provided to patients. The drug management information provided to patients should be accurate and in a form that the patient understands.

Hall[19] divided the risks associated with a particular drug as inherent or noninherent. *Inherent risks* are unique to the drug and usually identified in the package insert, but do not include probable or common side effects. *Noninherent risks* are created by the particular drug in combination with some extrinsic factor about which the pharmacist should reasonably know, and include maximum safe dosages, interactions, and probable or common side effects. It is the responsibility of the pharmacist to provide DI about noninherent risks that is expanding.

What liability does the pharmacist incur for information outside of the package insert? Physicians may prescribe drugs as they see fit, without adhering to the specific therapeutic indications or dosing guidelines within the labeling. The FDA regulates the manufacture and promotion of drugs, not the practice of medicine. However, it has been held that a physician's deviation from the package insert was prima facie evidence of negligence (i.e., not requiring further support to establish validity, on its face value) if the patient's injury resulted from the failure to adhere to the recommendations.[20] However, the states appear to be split on whether recommendations in a package insert are prima facie evidence of the standard of care. It would be prudent for the pharmacist to consult the package insert when responding to an inquiry and include such information in the response, especially if the response is contrary to what is contained in the package insert.

A recent disciplinary action by a state pharmacy board highlights the importance of checking the package insert or literature concerning the proposed use of a product. In *re Michael A. Gabert,* a pharmacist received a prescription for 5% silver nitrate for bladder instillation. The pharmacist contacted a DIC and was told there was no literature supporting the proposed use of the product. The pharmacist then asked the physician what support he had for such use and the physician referred to a letter from the Mayo Clinic. The pharmacist did not ask to see a copy of the letter, or have a copy of it for the pharmacy records. Significant patient harm resulted when the solution was instilled into the patient's bladder. The Mayo Clinic letter pertained to silver argyrol, not silver nitrate.[21]

The Negligent Provision of Drug Information

It has long been recognized by law that false information provided to another could result in harm to the recipient if the recipient acted in reliance on the false information. Although negligent misrepresentation has not been applied to DI, there is no guarantee that it will not be in the future.[22] The relevant law is the Restatement (Second) of Torts, §311, Negligent Misrepresentation Involving Risk of Physical Harm, which states:

> One who negligently gives false information to another is subject to liability for physical harm caused by action taken by the other in reasonable reliance upon such information. . . . Such negligence may consist of failure to exercise reasonable care in ascertaining the accuracy of the information, or in the manner in which it is communicated.[23]

The DI itself may be faulty for one or more reasons: it may be dated; it may simply be wrong; it may be incomplete and, therefore, misleading; or none may have been provided because of an incompetent search.[19] Information negligence may occur because of (1) parameter negligence (failure to consult the correct source) or (2) omission negligence (consulting the correct source, but failure to locate the correct answer[s]). A recent study evaluated the accuracy of a drug identification response by 56 DICs. Only approximately 30% correctly identified the investigational drug product; 67% could not make the identification; most importantly, 3.6% (two DICs) made an incorrect identification. The study found inconsistencies in responses of DICs.[24]

The responsibility of pharmacists providing DI goes beyond that of mere information intermediary, the person in between the information producer and the user. Published studies for DICs have reported that 41% to 83% of requested information is patient specific or judgmental in nature.[25] In addition to liability for the negligent information retrieval and dissemination, the pharmacist's role involves information interpretation, evaluation, and giving advice. This role falls into a "consultative model" and differs greatly from that of librarians. Librarians are not equipped to give advice. The pharmacist's role as evaluator and interpreter of the information creates a duty sufficient to sustain liability.

Currently, most litigation concerning pharmacists involves negligence. Therefore, it is safe to assume that a legal cause of action pertaining to the provision of DI will be founded on the theory of negligence as the direct or proximate cause of personal injury or death. Malpractice liability based on negligence refers to failure to exercise the degree of care that a prudent (reasonable) person would exercise under the same circumstances. Elements of negligence case include the four Ds (1) duty breached, (2) damages, (3) direct causation, and (4) defenses absent. To establish a negligent failure, actual conduct must be compared to what is considered standard professional conduct.[4] Typically, this is accomplished by introducing evidence of the relevant professional standards or testimony from expert witnesses such as pharmacy school faculty or other DI practitioners. Once the duty of care is established, the plaintiff would need a preponderance of evidence to prove that (1) the information provided was materially deficient, (2) the deficient information was a proximate cause of injury suffered (or at least a substantial contributing factor), (3) the recipient reasonably relied on the information provided, (4) the information deficiency was due to failure to exercise reasonable care, and (5) the pharmacist knew or should have known that the safety or health of another may have depended on the accuracy of the information provided.[19]

It is necessary to expand on the fourth element of negligence, which is reasonable care. *Reasonable care* is that which would be considered acceptable and responsible. Suppose a patient develops a reaction that is believed to be caused by a drug, and the pharmacist is consulted to find any case reports of this drug causing the reaction. If the case is available on-line, but not in print, and the pharmacist had access to on-line data bases, but did not consult them, was the pharmacist required to do so? Did the pharmacist exert reasonable care? What if the pharmacist searched MEDLINE but not *Exerpta Medica* data bases, or vice versa, and thereby failed to retrieve the case? Should the pharmacist have searched both? There are no clear answers here. Who can say what a reasonable search might have been on a given day? However, using outdated references or old editions of textbooks would more likely constitute an inadequate search. In a German case, a court held a patent information service to be responsible for not having used updated materials.[26]

Expanding on the first element of negligence, duty breached, it is important to be aware of the fact that the duty must be a legal duty, not a moral or ethical duty. Although there are many ethical dilemmas pertaining to the provision of DI by pharmacists and they can sometimes give rise to a cause of action, an ethical breach is not necessarily a legal breach. Similarly, conduct that is considered "unprofessional" in the broad sense (e.g., rudeness) is distinct from legal duty. An example of an ethical breach that could result in liability for the pharmacist would be a breach of patient confidentiality, if that disclosure caused damages (e.g., loss of employment or the misuse of information gained in the course of employment). In a study of DI requests, calls from consumers raised more ethical issues than calls from health professionals.[27] For example, should a pharmacist respond to a drug identification request for someone else's medication? Is the situation different if the medication is a drug of abuse and the inquiry is from a parent, relative, teacher, or police officer? Current law provides little guidance for disclosure of DI for questionable purposes and pharmacists must exercise independent professional judgment and assume legal responsibility for that judgment when exercised.

Other Causes of Action

Can pharmacists providing DI be held responsible for retrieving information that is itself inaccurate? What responsibility does the information producer incur for errors in information sources? Although very few cases have been brought before courts concerning the liability of print or on-line information sources, there is some case law to guide. The issue concerns strict liability. Strict liability applies where a defective product proximately causes physical harm. Where the service rendered is deemed to be a professional service, the courts exhibit a reluctance to impose strict liability. With exceptions, persons physically injured because of their reliance on defective and unreasonably dangerous information have only negligence as a cause of action, and only against the author, not the publisher[28]; only if the publisher is negligent or offers intentionally misleading information could it be held liable. This was tested in *Jones v. J.B. Lippincott Co.,* where a nursing student was injured after consulting and relying on a nursing textbook that recommended hydrogen peroxide enemas for the treatment of constipation. The courts rejected the plaintiff's claim that strict liability should be applied to the publisher.[29] Similarly, in a German case, a misprint in a medical textbook resulted in the injection of 25% rather than 2.5% sodium chloride solution, injuring a patient. Again, the court rejected strict liability for the publisher on the basis that any medically educated person should have noticed the misprint.[30] In *Roman v. City of New York,* the plaintiff sued for an alleged misstatement in a booklet distributed by a planned parenthood organization that resulted in a "wrongful conception." The court found that "a publisher cannot assume liability for all misstatements, said or unsaid, to a potentially unlimited public for a potentially unlimited period."[31] In *Winter v. G.P. Putnam's Sons,* two persons required liver transplants after collecting and eating poisonous wild mushrooms. They had relied on an *Encyclopedia of Wild Mushrooms* in choosing to eat the mushrooms that caused this severe harm.[32] The court refused to hold the publisher liable and found that a publisher has no duty to investigate the accuracy of the information it publishes.

In *Delmuth Development Corp. v. Merck & Co.,* the plaintiff claimed lost sales because of the publication of erroneous information in the *Merck Index.* The court considered the duty of a publisher to a reader to publish accurate information in a compendium.[33] The court noted a publisher's right to publish without fear of liability is guaranteed by the First Amendment and societal interest. It further held that even if it had a duty to publish with care, the plaintiff could not claim it suffered damages because of reliance on this information. Summary judgment in favor of the publisher was granted.[29]

In *Libertelli v. Hoffman La Roche, Inc. & Medical Economics Co.,* the plaintiff became addicted to diazepam (Valium) and sued the publisher of the *Physician's Desk Reference* (PDR).[34] The claim was based on the absence of warnings in the PDR regarding the addictive nature of the drug. The court dismissed the case against the publisher. Under a long line of cases, a publisher is not liable for matters of public interest if it has no knowledge of its falsity. Although some effort should be made to verify search results, the pharmacist cannot be held responsible for knowing and verifying the contents of all sources, whether in print or online.

Pharmacists providing DI should be aware of computer-related lawsuits that have arisen involving defects (or "bugs") in software that caused erroneous results. These cases are resulting in greater damage awards based on consequential (i.e., special as opposed to actual) damages suffered. An example of consequential damages would be damage to a firm's reputation. In one particularly relevant case, the court held that the National Weather Service was liable for the deaths of four fishermen off Cape Cod, Massachusetts. The Weather Service had forecasted calm weather because of faulty software. Although the verdict was overturned on technical grounds, the U.S. District Court let stand the precedent holding an entity liable for information it provides.[35] In another case, Jeppesen, an information provider, was held liable for an airplane crash caused by faulty data from the Federal Aviation Administration on flight patterns. A pilot used one of the faulty charts and crashed into a mountain, killing the crew and destroying the plane. The company paid $12 million in damages.[36] The court held the information provider strictly liable because the charts were considered a "product." In *Jeppesen*, the mass production and mass marketing of the charts rendered them a product. Similarly, in *Greenmoss Builders v. Dun & Bradstreet,* the issue involved the erroneous listing of Greenmoss Builders as a company in bankruptcy in Dun & Bradstreet Business Information Report database. A jury awarded $350,000, including $300,000 in punitive damages. The case was appealed all the way to the Supreme Court, where Dun & Bradstreet lost the case.[37]

In *Daniel v. Dow Jones & Co., Inc.,* where a subscriber brought action against a provider of a computerized database alleging that he relied on a false news report in making investments, the court found that the subscriber did not have a "special relationship" with the database provider necessary to impose liability for negligent misstatements. First Amendment guarantees of freedom of the press also protected the provider from liability.[38]

What about information obtained from the Internet? Is there a possibility of pharmacist liability occurring via cyberspace? Although there have been several lawsuits for false information on on-line bulletin boards (e.g., USENET News, CompuServe),[39,40] the basis of these lawsuits has been defamation, not malpractice. The offering of general medical advice and judgments on line (e.g., in chat rooms) does not appear to be creating a formal physician–patient relationship. Nor does it appear that the giving of generic advice will generate liability for either the provider or the publisher. If, however, the information is fraudulent or quackery, then courts do have authority under both state and federal computer statutes to stop the activity.

The legal questions facing networked health information providers who are providing very sensitive material using a relatively new medium are emerging. As telemedicine, which is defined as the use of telecommunications technology to provide health care services to patients who are at a distance, expands, questions regarding liability for pharmacists providing DI on the Internet will need to be addressed. For example, health professionals are licensed by states. Which state law applies when the pharmacist is located in New York, the patient is in Florida, and the web site is maintained by a company in California? Who is liable for technical problems that make it impossible for the information to be received in a timely manner or for breaches of confidentiality caused by those who would invade private files? Already some sites offer fee-based live physician offices and "nurse" triage services (e.g., Optum Online) for self-diagnosis and health screening. Although the courts have yet to test liability for medical malpractice involving the practice of medicine on the Internet, such a case is bound to surface soon. Hard copy printouts of Internet discussions would be discoverable before trial and could be uncovered in the defendant's computer files by a plaintiff's attorney. If the Internet discussion resembles an academic conference rather than a formal consultancy, liability is lessened. Similarly, the issuance of a disclaimer in writing with the original subscription and with each message written can help to insulate from any liability.[41]

Currently, there is inadequate law and no means for ensuring the accuracy of information posed on the Internet.[42] Because the Uniform Commercial Code does not seem to apply, legislation may be necessary. It is possible for information to be false, misleading, corrupted by an outside source, or otherwise harmful to the persons reading to apply it to their specific situation.[43] The Health Summit Working Group, which consists of professional societies including ASHP, and the Health on the Net Foundation are currently working to improve the quality of DI on the Internet.[44] The Health Summit Working Group is developing an interactive tool to use in evaluating quality of drug information on the web (<<http://hitiweb.mitretek.org/hswg>>). Also, the application of the National Information Infrastructure to consumer health information is one of the priorities of the federal government.[45] Perhaps with the coming millennium, health insurers will cover calls made to on-line pharmacists providing DI, much the same way as Medicare now covers for teleconferencing. The Internet is at the forefront of future practice, where pharmacists will consult with each other, thereby learning from one another and benefiting their DI clients and patients.

Copyright

Pharmacists providing DI must have a working knowledge of copyright law both to avoid liability and to protect their own literary works. Under the 1976 Copyright Act, an author is protected as soon as a work is recorded in some concrete way.[46] The process of registering for a copyright involves depositing material with the Copyright Office to be reviewed by an examiner followed by publication with a copyright notice, usually the symbol ©. Under the Copyright Term Extension Act of 1998, such work is protected until 70 years after the death of the author.[47] The author or copyright owner has the exclusive right to make copies of the work, control derivative works or adaptations, and sue for damages and injunctive relief against infringers.[48] Public domain works may be copied and distributed without copyright permission.[49] Works of the U.S. government (e.g., General Accounting Office [GAO] reports, Congressional Record, FDA releases) are considered part of the public domain.

Since the Berne Convention in 1989, the copyright formalities of registration and notice have lost almost all their legal significance.[50] Registration, although not mandatory, affords the copyright claimant certain advantages. For example, it prevents an infringer from pleading "innocent infringement." Similarly, the only substantive legal effect of copyright registration is that attorney fees and statutory damages are only recoverable for postregistration infringements. That is, U.S. authors must register before bringing suit.[51] But for works prior to 1989 and the Berne Convention, copyright can be lost if notice was omitted and that omission was not cured within 5 years of publication by registration and affixation of notice to the remaining copies.[52]

Under the fair use provision of the 1976 Copyright Act, if a use is fair, permission of the copyright owner need not be received, nor royalties paid.[53] Fair use is determined by a four-pronged test: (1) nature and character of use, (2) nature of the work, (3) the proportional amount copied, and, most importantly, (4) the effect on the market for the copied work.[54] Uses for research, teaching, scholarship, and news reporting are more likely to be considered fair than strictly commercial uses. In addition, there is a narrow special exemption for educators. However, the mere fact that the use is educational and not for profit does not insulate the use from a finding of infringement.

Although the statute itself does not set the maximum standards for educational fair use, Classroom Guidelines have been agreed upon by educational, author, and publisher organizations.[55] Multiple copies for classroom use, but not to exceed in any event more than one copy per pupil in a course, are permissible, provided each copy bears a copyright notice and meets the test of (1) brevity, (2) spontaneity, and (3) cumulative effect. For example, to meet the test of brevity the Classroom Guidelines prohibit multiple copying of complete articles longer than 2500 words. They prohibit copying excerpts longer than 1000 words or 10% of the work, whichever is shorter. For motion media, up to 10% or 3 minutes, whichever is less, in the aggregate of a copyrighted motion media work may be reproduced or otherwise incorporated as part of an educational multimedia project.[56] To meet the test of spontaneity, the copying must be at the instance and inspiration of the individual teacher, where the teacher's decision to use the work in class does not allow for a timely reply to request for permission.[55] To meet the cumulative effect requirement, the copying must be for only one course in the school, and except for current news periodicals, newspapers, and current news sections of periodicals, only one article or two excerpts therefrom, may be copied from the same author, or three excerpts from the same collective work or periodical volume, during one class term; and no more than nine instances of such multiple copying for one course during one class term.[57] Students may not be charged for the copy beyond the actual cost of photocopying. In *Association of American Publishers v. New York University* the issue was the production and distribution of custom-made anthologies sold to students. Although the classroom guidelines allow students to make single copies for personal use, the court found infringement when anthologies were sold for profit.[50]

Fair use is determined by the courts on a case-by-case basis. Unfortunately, in court decisions on educational photocopying to date, the ruling in almost every case has been against fair use. Copying by nonprofit medical libraries has been held to be a fair use where the photocopying of medical journals by federal nonprofit institutions was made solely for the purpose of medical research.[58] In this case the library was copying a single copy for each request and the court found that "medical science would be seriously hurt if such library photocopying were stopped."[58] Where the photocopying of medical journals by scientists occurred in a large for-profit company, the court decided the making of unauthorized copies of copyrighted articles published in scientific journals for use by research scientists was not fair use.[59] The court determined that the publishers had created through the Copyright Clearance Center, Inc., a viable market for institutional users to obtain licenses to allow photocopying of individual articles. However, in *Princeton University Press v. Michigan Document Services, Inc.,* the court held that a copy shop selling "course packs," which are compilations of various copyrighted and uncopyrighted materials such as journal articles, sample test questions, course notes, and book excepts, infringed the copyrights of several publishers. In deciding this was not a fair use, the court noted that the copying was substantial and commercial.[60] Similarly, in *Basic Books v. Kinko's Graphic Corp.,* the court held that a copy shop's reproduction and sale of course packs to students was not a fair use of the copyrighted material.[61]

Although the Act allows for damages of as much as $100,000 per infringement, "innocent infringers" (e.g., educators, universities) may be entitled to a remission of statutory damages. They are only liable for actual damages, such as profits earned by the infringer or profits denied to the copyright holder. This provision lowers the incentive for the publishing industry to sue.[62] Recently, publishers have resorted to unsavory tactics in their attempts to control educational copying, such as the sending of letters threatening to sue copy shops for infringement unless they agree to pay royalties.[63]

Newsletter copying is strictly prohibited and violators risk not only the statutory damages ($100,000) but can be subject to criminal penalties. These newsletters require a fee to be paid to the Copyright Clearance Center even for internal or personal copying and offer rewards to those who report violations. Washington Business Information, Inc., has won major payments in infringement actions against pharmaceutical manufacturers for photocopying its *Food & Drug Letter.*[64]

The most effective way for any DI facility to protect itself against copy infringement lawsuits is to copy the page with the copyright notice and stamp the first page of the copies with a statement that the enclosed document is protected by copyright, thus putting the burden of responsibility on the recipient of the one copy.[65] Such a notice might state, "This material is subject to the United States Copyright Law (17 U.S. Code): unauthorized copying may be prohibited by law."

The Computer Software Act of 1980 amended the Copyright Act to extend protection to computer software. However, copyright laws do not provide sufficient protection for information transmitted over the Internet and other information networks. The havoc that cyberspace can wreak on copyright owner's rights cannot be overestimated.[66] Access to works on the Internet does not automatically mean that these can be reproduced and reused without permission or royalty payment and, furthermore, some copyrighted works may have been posted on the Internet without authorization of the copyright holder. Dissemination of DI electronically cannot only be accessed by thousands of computer users, but also readily recovered by the copyright holder. Publishers who did not previously press for royalty payments of small segments of works can now trace the borrowing of snippets of text and create systems of payment and collection.[67] Research downloading, with deletion of material after use, appears to be a fair use of the material. However, downloading to create a personal database and avoid payment of connect fees and higher user fees is illegal unless covered under special agreements between the database owner and subscriber.[68]

Case Law

Is liability for drug information a rhetorical supposition or a real possibility? The paucity of case law in the area does not negate liability. The issue deserves consideration because of the potential for harm caused by the DI pharmacist. There have only been two cases and both involved poison information centers, one of which also was a DIC. In *Reben v. Ely,* the plaintiffs filed suit against the DIC for injuries sustained by inadvertent administration of cocaine solution instead of acetaminophen to a 10-year-old patient. The local pharmacy had colored the 10% cocaine solution red and labeled it "red solution" to thwart abuse. When the nurse realized the mistake she contacted the Arizona Poison and Drug Information Center. The DI pharmacist described the symptomatology of cocaine overdose, but did not go far enough in recommending that the patient seek emergency room care. The patient developed seizures and cardiopulmonary arrest with brain damage that will require lifetime nursing care. At the trial, the expert witness testified that the DIC operated below the standard of care. The issue was not erroneous information, but whether the center went far enough in its responsibility in handling the call. The plaintiff was awarded $6.5 million; the DIC was held liable for $3.6 million.[69]

In another case, a lawsuit named a poison information center that was called for assistance when a student died after swallowing a toxic substance during a laboratory experiment. The poison center was named in the $2.5 million suit because it refused to release proof of its claim that the person who called had given the wrong name for the solution that the student drank.[70]

From a liability standpoint, there are disadvantages to the formal combination of poison control and DI centers. For example, poison inquiries usually require immediate answers without written documentation and sometimes without supporting references.[71,72] The outcomes of poisonings (e.g., overdoses, suicide attempts) are more likely to result in patient morbidity and mortality and require medical backup for acute treatment decisions. Some states (e.g., Arkansas, Oregon, Washington, Arizona, New Jersey) have statutory provisions for joint poison control and DICs. In several of these states, such as Arkansas, immunity from personal liability in judgment (in contrast to carelessness or inadvertence) would not be actionable as malpractice unless a lack of due care can be shown. However, not all DICs are so protected from liability.

Defenses to Negligence and Malpractice Protection

Even if the plaintiff can establish all the necessary elements of negligence, legal defenses can avoid or reduce liability. Some defenses might include a statute of limitations, comparative or contributory negligence, informed consent, or governmental immunity. It is important to keep in mind that there may be differences in both types of defenses to negligence and insurance coverage for individuals and employers. Further information on defenses will be described in the following sections.

DEFENSES FOR INDIVIDUALS

Under informed consent, the defendant could assert that the patient knowingly assumed the risk for a new or experimental therapy or regimen. However, the risks that the patient assumes do not include negligence on the part of the physician or pharmacist. Delegation of authority does not mean abdication of responsibility. Under vicarious liability, a pharmacist who has not been personally negligent could be held responsible for the negligence of others. Supervision and adequate training of subordinates (e.g., interns, externs, residents, other employees) are essential. Incompetence and substandard training of these individuals can lead to liability. An example might include a breach of confidentiality (e.g., revealing someone has a loathsome disease) by one of these employees.

Comparative negligence is the allocation of responsibility for damages incurred between the plaintiff and defendant, based on the relative negligence of the two. *Concurrent negligence* is the wrongful acts or omissions of two or more persons acting independently, but causing the same injury. Under comparative or concurrent negligence, the pharmacist may also be held liable either alone or together with the information requestor (e.g., physician, nurse) for inaccurate information or information that does not ensure maximal protection for the patient. *Vicarious liability* is the imputation of liability upon one person for the actions of another. Through the doctrine of vicarious liability, a pharmacist could become associated with professional liability actions as part of a case against a hospital or physician. In the landmark case *Harbeson v. Parke Davis,* a federal court ruled that the doctrine of informed consent required a physician to furnish a patient contemplating pregnancy with information concerning the teratogenicity of the phenytoin she was taking. The physician had a duty to provide information reasonably available in the medical literature, but failed to do so. Even though the physician was not aware of the potential effects of phenytoin, studies were reported in the medical literature.[73] Cases of vicarious liability are not new to medical malpractice. Physicians have been found negligent for the negligence of nurses, therapists, and others working under their supervision. If a physician requests DI, the physician would also be held liable if a patient suffers because the search was deficient or the information incorrect. For example, in the *Harbeson* case, if the physician had requested the pharmacist to search for information about the teratogenicity of phenytoin and no references were found because of a faulty search, the pharmacist would share in the negligence together with the physician. The institution would probably also be named as a party in such legal action.

From a legal standpoint, does charging a fee increase liability for the DI provider? Fee-based providers would appear to be at greater malpractice risk, especially if the relationship is a contractual one. If any of the contractual expectations are not met, the client has a contractual cause of action against the DIC. The courts will look to the terms of the agreement and the reasonable expectations of the parties. However, where bodily injury results, tort law may impose liability even where the defective information is given gratuitously and the DI provider derives no benefit from giving it.

Does providing DI services to consumers increase liability exposure? Many DICs provide services to consumers; some via a hot line. Health information lines via the Inter-

TABLE 12–1. LEGAL QUESTIONS PERTAINING TO DRUG INFORMATION PRACTICE

Should the DI consult be placed in the patient's chart?

Does the theory of warranty apply to therapeutic recommendations?

How should oral responses to DI inquiries be handled?

What is an unreasonable delay in responding to the DI inquiry?

Does providing DI services to the public open the door to liability?

What is the liability for discontinuing DI services?

What is the liability of drug choice decisions based on economic criteria?

Is the pharmacist providing DI responsible for soliciting information necessary to properly consider the question?

net have been discussed. Several studies have reported that more ethical questions to DICs arise from consumers than any other group.[74-76] Such ethical questions may involve drug abuse and toxicologic effects, the safety of drugs in pregnancy or nursing, experimental therapy, or the appropriateness of prescribing decisions. Decisions to comment on a physician's therapeutic recommendations, even if factually correct and in the patient's best interest, may result in a legal liability. Answers to this and other questions that the pharmacist providing DI encounter (Table 12–1) are not found in the legal precedent.

DEFENSES FOR EMPLOYERS

The vast majority of DICs are located in hospitals and universities. In addition, many pharmaceutical companies have DI departments staffed by pharmacists who handle inquiries on the company's products. There also exist independent information brokers who have liability under contract law, as well as tort law. The employer–employee relationship is a significant factor under either common law *respondeat superior* doctrine or, alternatively, a theory of negligent hire or supervision. *Respondeat superior* refers to the proposition that the employer is responsible for the negligent acts of its agents or employees.[4] The injured party may also sue the employer for its negligence in hiring or supervising the employee. Under a negligent hire theory, it must be shown that the employee was unfit for the position and that a reasonable, pre-employment interview or postemployment supervision would have discovered this fact.[77]

Is the provider the hospital or university where the DIC is located or the pharmacist providing the DI? Although the person who provides the information is liable for the harm caused by it, the employer may also be held liable in the absence of sovereign or charitable immunity. For pharmacists providing DI employed by the government (e.g., Veteran's Administration [VA] or Public Health Service), there are statutes providing governmental immunity, also called sovereign immunity, from civil liability. Such immunity, however, will not protect an intentionally or grossly negligent person.

Even if the lawsuit is nonmeritorious, DICs affiliated with hospitals or universities provide another "deep pocket" for contribution to the settlement. With exceptions, suing the pharmacist alone would fail to provide a windfall settlement for plaintiffs. The board of directors/trustees of the hospital or university or director of the DIC or pharmacy department where the DIC is located would be jointly liable. *Joint and several liability* refers to the sharing of liabilities among a group of people collectively and also individually. If the defendants are jointly and severally liable, it means that the injured party may sue some or all of the defendants together, or each one separately, and may collect equal amounts or unequal amounts from each.[4] In states where joint and several liability applies, the pharmacist provides additional assurance that there will be sufficient assets to recover. The DI provider will be held responsible for the standard of care in the response to DI inquiries and may be found negligent.[65,70]

Protecting Against Malpractice

Methods to protect against lawsuits include contracts covering financial arrangements, adequate documentation, disclaimers, and insurance.[78] For example, a disclaimer can be placed on results of on-line searches stating that the data being provided are from a source believed to be reliable and factually correct.[78] The best way to avoid omission negligence is to learn from experience, anticipate mistakes that may appear in databases, and keep abreast of changes in DI sources. Even if the delivery of false information is the result of inaccurate information itself, the pharmacist would likely be named as a defendant if the database producer were sued.[79]

Adequate documentation may spell the difference between refuting or not refuting an unfounded claim of malpractice. Such documentation includes responses to inquiries, as well as a record of steps taken in a search. Designing and following procedures to document the research process can help avoid negligence. In *Fidelity Leasing Corp. v. Dun & Bradstreet, Inc.,* the court looked at the operation procedures and adherence to them in the particular instance to determine liability for providing false information.[79,80]

Quality assurance (QA) standards for the timeliness, thoroughness, and accuracy of information could also insulate against liability. QA programs, although they exist, are inconsistent among DICs. Problem areas common to DICs regardless of practice site include files not updated and incomplete documentation of responses to requests. DICs should address at least some of the items in Table 12–2.

Insistence on a good educational background for entry-level positions followed by the continuing education of DI professionals, certification in on-line training courses, and good interpersonal communication skills may also protect against malpractice.[78] It

TABLE 12–2. QUALITY ASSURANCE AS A LIABILITY-REDUCING FACTOR

Identification of scope of activities and personnel requirements.

Develop and follow policies and procedures or formal call triaging protocols; keep standard operating procedure manual available for consultation; avoid violations of statutes and regulations; do not recommend an unapproved use or dose; if a use differs from the labeling, the requestor must be so notified.

Do not recommend a use or dose of a drug based solely on foreign literature or animal studies.

Never extrapolate pediatric dosages from adult dosages.

Maintain knowledge of the current literature, new drug applications and supplemental approvals, labeling changes, new warnings.

Do not present inadequate data or ignore contrary data.

Avoid overly enthusiastic or exaggerated efficacy and safety claims; do not attempt to diagnose or treat acute poisoning—direct such inquiries to a poison control center or an emergency room.

Know the circumstances of the case and appropriate background information (e.g., knowledge of causality criteria, laboratory findings, concurrent drugs are necessary for adverse drug reaction inquiries; special care is needed for drug identification questions, especially in view of the surge of counterfeit drugs).

Responses of new employees, students, residents should be checked—document, document, document.

Maintain reasonable response time; if necessary prioritize requests.

Obtain peer concurrence or outside professional consultation, if necessary.

Develop a QA mechanism to ensure that service is maintained at a high level of quality (e.g., periodic audits or surveys).

Maintain up-to-date files and reference texts (e.g., files should be randomly checked to be sure they contain articles at least as recent as 2 years old).

is important to keep abreast of changes in sources of DI via regular advanced training, conferences, and reading. All courses in DI should teach situations in ethical conflict that will assist in the decision making and value judgments encountered in the provision of drug information.

Under the tort law doctrine of *respondeat superior,* both the pharmacist providing DI and the employer are jointly and severally liable for the damages. This enables the plaintiff to have access to the pharmacist's personal assets where the employer's assets are not sufficient to cover an adverse judgment. Professional liability insurance provides protection to cover exactly this kind of liability. Most policies now provide coverage on either an occurrence or claims-made basis. Occurrence means any incident that occurs during the policy period, no matter when the claim is filed, within the applicable statute of limitations. Claims-made policies cover only claims that are filed while the policy is active. To cover claims that are filed after a claims-made policy is terminated, the DI pharmacist can purchase "tail" coverage from the insurer. It is important to be aware of the limitations and exclusions in these policies. Many do not require the carrier to obtain the consent of the insured before settling a claim. In these policies the right to protect one's reputation may conflict with the economic interest of the insurer to dispose of the claim as inexpensively as possible. Therefore, it is imperative that individuals obtain insurance coverage policies separate from those of their employers. Most common exclusions are coverage for dishonest, fraudulent, criminal, or malicious acts; property damage; and personal injury coverage. In these cases, the pharmacist faces such liability alone, and in certain situations can be ruined financially.

Finally, limiting language in subscriber contracts (i.e., exculpatory clauses) may serve to restrict monetary awards in certain circumstances. Such clauses could be included in either contracts for subscribers or signed on acceptance of responses to inquiries. A provision could be included that specifically disclaims any responsibility to a third party who might rely on the information. An attorney could draft a standard agreement providing that the application of the research by the recipient would not be subject to any implied warranty of fitness for that purpose. However, certain jurisdictions have held that contracts that purport to exculpate a party from negligence will be subjected to strict judicial scrutiny. Courts in certain jurisdictions have declared contracts that attempt to exempt a party's willful or grossly negligent conduct to be void. Further, no exculpatory clause will protect a pharmacist who is grossly or intentionally negligent.

Conclusion

To date, pharmacists providing DI have only speculated about and not actually faced malpractice lawsuits. Hopefully, this chapter has shed some light on how courts would react to malpractice suits against pharmacists for negligent provision of DI. What can be done to avoid malpractice and other causes of action? First, be good at what you do. Second, have good relations with requestors and make sure they are aware of vagaries or information systems and sources. Third, make no outrageous claims about the accuracy and thoroughness of the information provided. Finally, carry your own malpractice insurance policy.[81]

The future of DICs clearly lies in their ability to provide consultative DI services. While in the past most of the reported appellate decisions against pharmacists have involved routine dispensing errors, not mistakes in drug information or other expanded practice, in the future this situation may change. Pharmacists should not be preoccupied with the risk of incurring liability, but should take the necessary steps to limit exposure and develop an appreciation of modern legal philosophy. Definitive guidelines need not emerge only through court decisions. It remains most important that DI be recognized as a liability-reducing factor for the institution and personnel who provide health care to patients.[82]

Study Questions

1. What is negligence and what are the four elements of a negligence case?

2. Is a pharmacist liable if he or she does not provide a drug information sheet or PPI?

3. Can a drug information pharmacist be held liable for errors in on-line databases?

4. Describe methods to protect against malpractice.

5. Under what circumstances is written work protected by copyright?

REFERENCES

1. Willig S. Legal considerations for the pharmacist undertaking new drug consultation responsibilities. Food Drug Cosm Law J 1970;25:444–452.
2. American Society of Health-System Pharmacists. ASHP supplemental standard and learning objectives for residency training in drug information practice. Practice standards of ASHP. 1995–1996. Bethesda (MD): American Society of Health-System Pharmacists, 1995.
3. Southwick AF. The law of hospital and health care administration. 2nd ed. Ann Arbor: Health Administration Press; 1988.
4. Dobbs DB, Hayden PT. Torts and compensation. 3rd ed. St. Paul: West Publishing Co.; 1997. p. 336.
5. Kenneth Baker, OBRA '90 Mandate and its impact on pharmacist's standard of care. Drake L R 1996:44:503, 508.
6. Rosenberg v. Equitable Life Insurance Society of the United States, 595 N.E.2d 840 (N.Y. 1992).
7. Keller v. Manhattan Eye, Ear & Throat Hospital, 563 N.Y.S.2d 497 (1990).
8. Kashkin v. Mt. Sinai Medical Center, 538 N.Y.S.2d 686 (Sup. Ct. 1989).
9. 805 S.W.2d, 380 (Tenn. Ct. App. 1991).
10. 453 N.Y.S.2d 121 (1987).
11. 544 N.W.2d 727, 731 (Mich. Ct. App. 1996).
12. 191 A.D.2d 178, 594 N.Y.S.2d 195 (1st Dept. 1993).
13. 579 N.E.2d 1255 (Ill. App. 1991) reversed by 605 N.E.2d 557 (Ill. 1992).
14. 827 F. Supp. 1522 (D. Nev. 1993).
15. 598 N.Y.S.2d 592 (App. Div. 1993).
16. Brushwood DB, Simonsmeier LM. Drug information for patients. J Leg Med 1986;7:279.
17. Abood RR, Brushwood DB. Pharmacy Practice and the law. 2nd ed. Gaithersberg (MD): Aspen; 1997.
18. Berry M. The Canadian pharmacist's duty to counsel. Pharm Law Annual 1992;19–75.
19. Hall M, Honey W. The evolving legal responsibility of the pharmacist. J Pharm Market Manage 1994;8:27–41.

20. Brushwood DB. The pharmacist's drug information responsibility after McKee v. American Home Products. Food Drug Cosm Law J 1993;48:377–410.
21. In re Michael A. Gabert, No. 92 PHM 21 (Wis. Pharmacy Examining Bd., Dec. 14, 1993).
22. Rees W, Rohde NF, Bolan R. Legal issues for an integrated information center. J Amer Soc Info Sci 1991;42:132–6.
23. Restatement (Second) of Torts, Section 311, 1982.
24. Beaird S, Coley R, Blunt JR. Assessing the accuracy of drug information responses from drug information centers. Ann Pharmacother 1994;28:707–11.
25. Amerson AB. Drug information centers: an overview. Drug Info J 1986;20:173–8.
26. Doppelparker Case, OLG Karllsrule GRUR 1979 P267.
27. Kelly WN, Krause EC, Krowinski WJ, Small TR, Drane JF. National survey of ethical issues presented to drug information centers. Am J Hosp Pharm 1990;47:2245–50.
28. Gray JA. Strict liability for the dissemination of dangerous information? Law Lib J 1990;82: 497–517.
29. 694 F.Supp. 1216 (D. Md. 1988).
30. Bundesqe Richtsaf. NJW 1970; 1973.
31. 110 Misc.2d 799, 442 N.Y.S.2d 945 (N.Y. Sup. 1981).
32. 938 F.2d 1033 (9th Cir. 1991).
33. 432 F. Supp. 990 (E.D.N.Y. 1977).
34. Prod. Liab. Rep (CCH). Section 8968 (S.D.N.Y. Feb. 20, 1981).
35. Cuzamanes PT. Automation of medical records: the electronic superhighway and its ramifications for health care providers. J Pharm & Law 1997;6:19.
36. Brocklesby v. Jeppesen, 767 F.2d 1288 (9th Cir. 1985), cert. denied, 474 U.S. 1101 (1986).
37. 472 U.S. 749 (1985).
38. 137 Misc.2d 94, 520 N.Y.S.2d 334 (N.Y. Civ. Ct. 1987).
39. Cubby v. Compuserve Inc., 776 F.Supp. 135 (S.D.N.Y. 1991).
40. Zeran v. America Online, Inc., 129 F.3d 327 (Va. 1997).
41. Tyler BJ. Cyberdoctors: The virtual housecall—the actual practice of medicine on the Internet is here: is it a telemedical accident waiting to happen? Ind L Rev 1998;31:259, 280, 282.
42. Cate FH. Intellectual property and networked health information: issues and principles. Bull Med Libr Assoc 1996;84:229,234.
43. Keltner KB. Networked health information: assuring quality control on the Internet. Fed Comm L J 1998;50:417, 418.
44. Ling CA. Guiding patients through the maze of drug information on the Internet. Am J Health-Syst Pharm 1999;56:212–14.
45. Consumer Health Information Subgroup, Information Infrastructure Task Force, White Paper Working Draft. Available from URL: http://nii.nist.gov/pubs/chi.html.
46. 17 U.S.C.A. §102(a).
47. H.R. 2589, 105th Cong. (1998).
48. 17 U.S.C.A. §302(a).

49. Denis S, Poullet Y. Questions of liability in the provision of drug information services. Online Rev. 1990;14:21–32.

50. Miller AR, Davis MH. Intellectual property. 2nd ed. St. Paul: West Publishing; 1997.

51. 17 U.S.C.A. §411, 412.

52. 17 U.S.C.A. §405.

53. 17 U.S.C.A. §107.

54. Wagner EN. Time to end confusion over copying. Academe 1992;78:27–9.

55. House Rep. No. 94-1476, p. 68.

56. Wasoff LF. Fair use guidelines for educational multimedia. Practicing Law Institute. No. G0-0002U 1998;517:111,118.

57. Schiffres IJ. Copyright and literary property. Fair use doctrine. Am Jur 2d 1985 (current through 1998); Vol. 18 §80–87.

58. Williams & Wilkins Co. v. United States, 487 F.2d 1345 (Ct. Cl. 1973), affirmed by 420 U.S. 376 (1975).

59. Miller ML. Corporate copyright infringers beware: systematic unauthorized photocopying by for-profit corporations does not constitute fair use: American Geophysical Union v. Texaco, Inc., Creighton L R 1997;30:1521

60. 855 F. Supp. 905, 907 (E.D. Mich. 1994), affirmed in part, vacated in part, 99 F.3d 1381 (6th Cir. 1996) (en banc), cert. denied, 117 S. Ct. 1336 (1997).

61. 758 F. Supp. 1522, 1534 (S.D.N.Y. 1991).

62. Association of American Publishers v. New York University, 133 F.2d 889, 891 (1983).

63. Busby G. Fair use and educational copying: a reexamination of Princeton University Press v. Michigan Document Services, Inc. Ky L J 1998;86:675, 677.

64. Drug firm pays out in photocopying suit SCRIP No. 1795, Feb. 16, 1993:14.

65. Clark TT, White BD, Hammer MB. Liability of drug information centers. U.S. Pharmacist 1992;7:39, 42, 56.

66. Kuhn BR. A dilemma in cyberspace and beyond: copyright law for intellectual property distributed over the information superhighways of today and tomorrow. Temp Intl Comp L J 1996;10:171.

67. Gorman RA. Intellectual property: The rights of faculty as creators and users. Academe 1998;84:14–15.

68. Mika JJ, Shuman BA. Legal issues affecting libraries and librarians. Amer Libr 1988;19:108–12.

69. 705 P.2d 1360 (Ariz. Ct. App. 1985).

70. Rumore MM, Rosenberg JM, Costa JG. The pharmacist and the law: legal aspects of providing drug information. Wellcome Trends in Hosp Pharm (Dec) 1989;6–8.

71. Gough AR, Healey KM, Rupp SR. Poison control centers, from aspirin to PCBs and the scarlet runner beam: a study of legal anomaly and social necessity. Santa Clara L R 1983;23:791–809.

72. Brushwood DB, Simonsmeier LM. Drug information for patients—duties of the manufacturer, pharmacist, physician, and hospital. J Leg Med 1986;7:279–341.

73. 746 F.2d 517 (9th Cir. 1984).

74. Sigell LT, Bonfiglio JF, Siegel EG et al. The role of drug information centers with consumers. Drug Info J 1987;21:201–8.

75. Arnold RM, Nissen JC, Campbell NA. Ethical issues in a drug information center. Drug Intell Clin Pharm 1987;21:1008–11.
76. Okasas RM. Hospital drug information centers: a new role in patient counseling. PharmaGuide to Hospital Medicine 1988;2:1–4.
77. Gray JA. The health sciences librarian's exposure to malpractice liability because of negligent provision of information. Bull Med Libr Assoc 1989;77:33–37.
78. Mintz AP. Information practice and malpractice. Libr J 1985:38–43.
79. Fidelity Leasing Corp. v. Dun & Bradstreet, Inc., 494 F. Supp. 786 (E.D. Pa. 1980).
80. Pritchard T, Quigley M. The information specialist: a malpractice risk analysis. Online 1989;13:57–62.
81. Verett JH. Independent information professionals and the question of malpractice liability. Online 1989;13:65–70.
82. Fink JL. Some legal issues presented in clinical pharmacy practice. Drug Intell Clin Pharm 1976;10:444–7.

13

Chapter Thirteen

Ethical Aspects of Drug Information Practice

Linda K. Ohri

Objectives

After completing this chapter, the reader will be able to:

- Identify examples of ethics rules, principles, and theories.
- Describe characteristics that differentiate an ethical dilemma.
- Present examples of ethical dilemmas that may arise for pharmacists when providing drug information, in various practice settings and for various types of clients and circumstances.
- Utilize a process of ethical analysis in order to choose the best course of action available in a given situation.

What Ethics Is and What It Is Not

The Ethics Course Content Committee of the American Association of Colleges of Pharmacy (AACP) described ethics as "the philosophical inquiry of the moral dimensions of human conduct."[1] They mentioned that Aristotle taught ethics as "an eminently practical discipline" ... dealing ..."with concrete judgments in situations in which action must be taken despite uncertainty." These authors indicated that the term ethical is often used synonymously with the term moral to describe an action or decision as "good" or "right." They further stated that ethics is not values clarification, it is not the study of moral development, and it is not the law.

Veatch[2] indicated that ethical deliberations may be differentiated from other endeavors by three characteristics: (1) They are ultimate or fundamental; there is no higher standard against which to measure the rightness of the decision or action. (2)

They are universal; the parties in disagreement do not consider it simply a difference of opinion or taste—each party believes there is a right or wrong answer, even if they are not sure what the answer is. (3) The deliberation takes into account the welfare of all involved or affected by the judgment at hand. Veatch stated that "an ethical, or moral, issue involves judgments between right and wrong human conduct or praiseworthy and blameworthy human character."

Professional ethics has been defined as "rules of conduct or standards by which a particular group in society regulates its actions and sets standards for its members."[3] By contrast, *law* might be defined as rules of conduct imposed by society on its members. Professional ethics focuses on explicit or implicit rules and standards set by a professional subgroup of society, and addresses the responsibilities of only those who are members of that subgroup. Law involves written rules set by the whole society (or its representatives), that address responsibilities of that society's members. Certain ethical standards of a given profession may be institutionalized as law by the whole society. However, professional ethical standards (e.g., "do no harm" or "preserve life"), are often impossible to fully regulate by law. As will be discussed further, law represents one aspect of the culture within which ethical decisions are made. Therefore, relevant legal requirements must be identified and considered when making ethical decisions.

Ethical Issues in Pharmacy Practice

This chapter presents case scenarios that identify what might constitute an ethical issue; they are also used to demonstrate a method of analyzing ethical dilemmas confronted by the pharmacist providing drug information. Although some examples will be drawn from the experiences of drug information "specialists," the discussion will also address ethical dilemmas encountered by other generalist, or specialist, pharmacy practitioners providing drug information. All pharmacists provide drug information and must address the ethical dilemmas that arise in the course of providing this service. Such dilemmas may arise in a wide variety of settings and circumstances where pharmacy is practiced, such as:

- The community pharmacist who is asked by a patient at the counter to critique a physician's prescription
- The home health care pharmacist who is recommending a therapeutic plan to a physician, and who must consider payment constraints imposed by a third-party payer
- The pharmacist working for a managed care system who assesses the literature, and subsequently must approve or deny coverage of a drug used for an unlabeled indication

- The hospital practitioner who is confronted by a physician or an administrator demanding a certain formulary recommendation that may not be appropriate
- The drug information specialist who is asked by a layperson or another health professional to provide information that could be misused.

These ethical dilemmas tend to relate to the perceived rights and/or responsibilities of the pharmacist, relative to the rights and responsibilities of the client, other directly affected "clients" (e.g., a child, other relatives, or "significant others" affected by the client), other health professionals, society at large, and of any "higher power" recognized by the pharmacist.

The next section provides a brief overview of terminology and definitions used in the field of ethics, as well as a discussion of those levels of analysis that are generally used in assessing ethical dilemmas. In the final section, specific examples of case scenarios and a process for analyzing these scenarios are demonstrated.

Basics of Ethics Analysis

DEFINITIONS USED IN THE FIELD OF ETHICS

Beauchamp and Childress[4] define ethics as "a generic term for several ways of examining the moral life." These authors describe a process of deliberation and justification that is necessary when confronting a moral dilemma. They state, "When we deliberate . . . we are considering which judgment is morally justified. . . ." They indicate that "Particular judgments are justified by moral rules, which in turn are justified by principles, which ultimately are defended by an ethical theory." Beauchamp and Childress present a hierarchical diagram that depicts this approach to analysis:

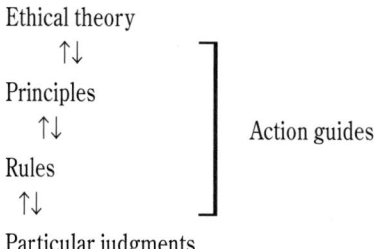

Beauchamp and Childress refer to these hierarchical levels of analysis (particularly rules and principles) as action guides, which may be used in an upwardly directed process to justify a "particular judgment." They also note that attention to particular judgments contributes to an evolving understanding of existing and even new ethical rules, principles, and theories. Hence these action guides function both to assist with particular judgments and to inform evolution of ethical theory.

These authors describe a *rule* of ethics as specific to context and relatively restricted in scope; for instance, the moral rule about confidentiality that specifically addresses a patients' right to consent prior to release of privileged information.[4] *Principles* are more broad and fundamental in scope; for example, the principle of respect for autonomy, that is the patient's right to decide on personal issues. They describe *ethical theories* as "integrated bodies of principles and rules . . . that may include mediating rules that govern cases of conflicts." For example, two cardinal principles of consequentialist theory are beneficence (do that which promotes a good outcome) and nonmaleficence (do that which minimizes bad outcomes). A mediating rule utilized by many advocates of this theory is to hold nonmaleficence as more important, or more foundational, than beneficence. These action guides can help pharmacists assess ethical dilemmas that arise in the course of providing drug information.

OVERVIEW OF A PROCESS OF ANALYSIS TO BE USED WHEN AN ETHICAL DILEMMA ARISES

Veatch[2] indicates that often we may reach a particular ethical decision without a great deal of conscious deliberation, through our moral intuition, and without subsequent challenge from any external party. However, on occasion, when pondering a certain ethical judgment, we are called on (internally or externally) to analyze and justify the basis for our conviction. He suggested progression through four process stages by which we may identify, analyze, and present reasons for our judgment, reasons that are evermore fundamental and universal. The following steps of ethics analysis are derived from the writings of Veatch, Beauchamp, and Childress, as well as other authors.[2,4–6]

Identification of Relevant Background Information

The first process step requires identification and evaluation of pertinent background information to ensure that the facts of the specific case are understood. This first step deserves careful consideration and research. Once we know the facts of a case, our moral concerns may be resolved. This step can be divided into three parts: (1) data gathering, (2) identifying all involved parties, and (3) considering the cultural perspectives of all involved parties.

Pharmacists already use the data gathering process when they apply a "systematic approach" to answering any drug information question (see Chap. 2). The pharmacist must learn about the factual details of the issue, who is directly involved, and whether there is conflict in factual understanding among the involved parties in the issue. For example, does the parent who calls to ask about the medication recently prescribed for her teenager already know that the teenager is taking a birth control pill, prescribed by a gynecologist rather than a dermatologist, and simply wants to know the name of the product?

If the matter remains an ethical issue once data gathering clarifies the facts, the pharmacist should consider the rights and responsibilities of all affected parties. As mentioned, Veatch describes this as an essential characteristic of any ethical deliberation.[2] The pharmacist, the direct client, other indirect but individual "clients" (i.e., an unborn child), other health professionals (i.e., a patient's physician), other societal groups (i.e., patients who might be harmed by an incompetent practitioner), and any higher power recognized by the pharmacist may all have rights and/or responsibilities that should be considered.

When considering any ethical issue, the pharmacist should also take into account the cultures of the affected parties.[5] In his review of the foundations of modern medical ethics theories, Veatch[6] describes how the cultural perspectives of Western, Chinese, Hindu, Jewish, Catholic, Protestant, and other groups have affected the formulation of their dominant medical ethics traditions. It should be noted here that the religious affiliation of an individual is an important component of their cultural perspective.

In a very interesting case study, Carrese and associates[7] discussed the ethical obligations of medical professionals in caring for those of a different culture. In this case, a young Laotian mother had utilized a traditional Mien folk cure to treat her infant. The treatment involved placing several small burns on the child's abdomen to treat *gusia mun toe,* an apparently transient but very distressing colic-like ailment. The cure resulted in several small scars, but no other obvious ill effects. The mother indicated that the cure worked. The physician was aware of the positive impacts of the woman's attachment to her cultural support group. However, the physician was confronted with the dilemma of how to respond to this mother's revelation of a culturally promoted treatment measure that was not scientifically supported and could be dangerous. Sometimes culturally based actions may conflict with the professional's goal to avoid harm and promote benefit. However, failing to consider cultural perspective may have its own harmful effects. An extended discussion of how awareness of a differing cultural perspective might affect the ethical decision making process is beyond the scope of this chapter; however, the pharmacist should strive to be aware and respect the cultural perspectives of the affected parties when contemplating an ethical dilemma.

One final issue should be addressed relative to cultural considerations. The legal requirements of the society within which an ethical dilemma occurs are part of the culture and must be identified. A specific ethical decision will not always exactly conform to the existing legal requirements of society. The ultimate nature of ethical deliberations may result in decisions that are more demanding than the legal requirements, and unfortunately, may even occasionally involve perceived or true conflict with specific legal requirements. This may involve, for instance, a decision not to divulge confidential communications between a professional and client, which may or may not be acceptable within law. In another case, the pharmacist may decide not to provide information related to abortion or capital punishment, even though these activities are acceptable within the law. Obviously, legal requirements cannot be ignored or dismissed lightly when making a specific ethical decision.

Use of Action Guides in Analysis of an Ethical Dilemma

If necessary, once the necessary background information has been identified and considered, the process of full ethical deliberation can proceed. Veatch suggests that the involved party or parties can proceed as far as necessary through successive stages of general moral reflection: the level of moral rules, the level of ethical principles, and the level of ethical theory.[2] These are the action guides also referred to by Beauchamp and Childress.[4] The second process step of analysis looks at moral rules that may apply to the specific case and at more general ethical principles. Definitions are provided at the end of this section for a number of ethical rules and principles that are considered particularly relevant to decision making by pharmacists. Examples of moral rules within biomedical ethics include a confidentiality rule that dictates that patient-entrusted information should not be disclosed, and an informed consent rule that addresses the individual's right to information before agreeing to a specific medical procedure. In general ethics inquiry, there are moral rules that dictate that one should not inflict suffering or death. Unfortunately, there is no definitive list of such rules and sometimes multiple pertinent rules can be in conflict. Furthermore, there are acceptable exceptions to most moral rules. For instance, disregarding the informed consent rule might be justifiable to acutely protect the life of the client, suffering may be necessary to achieve cure of serious disease, and some may consider killing justified under certain circumstances. Therefore, there may not be a specific rule that resolves a particular ethical dilemma.

At this point the involved party may need to begin a more general level of analysis by looking at the ethical principles that apply to the case. Sometimes, the involved parties can reach an acceptable resolution to an ethical dilemma once they recognize the relevant ethical principles. In a given dilemma, the professional may decide that the primary principle is to respect the autonomy of the client, and that this requires providing complete information that enables the client to make an informed decision. In another dilemma, if the sanctity of human life is considered the most fundamental ethical principle, decisions or acts that deny this principle would be considered unethical. It immediately becomes obvious, however, that the relevant ethical principles may also be in conflict. This problem can be demonstrated by the following example: The pharmacist may believe that full disclosure will result in noncompliance by the patient, with significant risk of resultant harm. The pharmacist therefore confronts two conflicting principles: respecting client autonomy versus the duty to do no harm.

It should be noted that specific action guides may be considered a rule within one ethical theory and a principle within another; for example, veracity (truth telling) may be considered by some ethicists to be a specific moral rule and by others to be a general principle, depending on which ethical theory is followed. For the practitioner immediately involved in analyzing a specific ethical dilemma, defining the relevant action guides as rules or principles is important only to the extent that this helps in assessing which are more fundamental to the issue at hand. Therefore, in this chapter, both rules and principles will be included within the same process step of ethical analysis.

Ethical Theory as the Means to Examine Conflicting Rules and Principles

When confronted with conflicting ethical rules or principles, the professional will need to examine the ethical theories that describe how they should be prioritized or balanced. This third step of ethical analysis helps to further reveal how the relevant moral rules and principles interact within a given dilemma. According to Veatch,[2] this can lead to more rational and honest decision making or action taking. Those dilemmas that cannot be fully resolved can at least be viewed with greater clarity. Veatch suggests that these ultimate deliberations at the level of ethical theory will be affected by our most basic religious and/or philosophical commitments.

The prominent rules and principles guiding ethical decision making by health care professionals can be generally placed within one of two broad ethical theories: consequentialist theory or deontological (derived from the Greek word *deon,* meaning "duty") theory.[4] Multiple versions exist of each of these broad categories. *Consequentialist theories* could be defined as those moral theories that describe actions or decisions as morally right or wrong based on their consequences, rather than on any intrinsic features they may have. Consequentialist theory focuses on one feature of an act—its consequences. For example, the informed consent rule can be of value within consequentialist theory because consent generally results in improved compliance and outcome—good consequences. However, if informed consent were likely to result in a bad outcome, it would not be justifiable within consequentialist theory.

Deontological theories look more to intrinsic qualities of an act or decision to assert its moral rightness or wrongness. Deontological theory considers inherent features of an act, besides consequences, as relevant and often of greater importance. For example, the act is considered wrong if it involves dishonesty, or if it does not respect the sanctity of human life.

Veatch[6] states that, "The components of a complete theory will answer such questions as what rules apply to specific ethical cases, what ethical principles stand behind the rules, how seriously the rules should be taken, and what constitutes the fundamental meaning and justification of the ethical principles." He reviews the foundations of consequentialist, deontological, and other ethics theories particularly relevant to health professionals, including the Hippocratic tradition; the Judeo-Christian traditions; the philosophies of the modern secular West; and medical ethics theories outside the Anglo-American West, including Socialist, Islamic, Hindu, Chinese, and Japanese traditions. Versions of the broad consequentialist and deontological theories are expressed in various ways within each of these traditions. Particular note will be given here to Veatch's description of what he considers the core of the various Hippocratic Oaths, because this has been the central ethical tradition of Western medicine: "Those who have stood in that (Hippocratic) tradition are committed to producing good for their patient and to protecting that patient from harm." In Hippocratic tradition, there is also a special emphasis placed on the responsibility of the medical professional to the specific patient versus obligations to other less directly affected parties or to society in general. The reader is referred to the writings of Veatch as well as those of Beauchamp and Childress for more in-depth discussions of the various medical ethics theories.[2,4,6]

Veatch[6] also discusses what he calls a Contract Theory of medical ethics, which describes an implicit (unwritten) contract between professionals and patients. This modern theory is of special relevance to the pharmacist providing drug information as a service within an implicit pharmaceutical care "contract."[6,8]

Section Summary

This section addresses the application of a process of ethical analysis in identifying, analyzing and resolving ethical dilemmas that may arise during the provision of drug information by pharmacists. This process of analysis may be summarized as follows.

I. Identification of relevant background information
    A.   Factual details of the issue at hand
    B.   Identification of who is affected by the ethical issue
    C.   Determination of the cultural perspectives and legal requirements for those affected by the dilemma
II. Identification and justification of the relevant moral rules and principles pertinent to the case
III. Deliberation on how to rank or balance the rules and principles pertinent to the case through the use of moral intuition and application of ethical theory to resolve the ethical dilemma

RULES AND PRINCIPLES (ACTION GUIDES) APPLIED IN MEDICAL ETHICS INQUIRY

The following rules and principles of ethical conduct are described, and subsequently used in the analysis of case scenarios provided in the third section. Their description will necessarily be brief. The reader is referred to Beauchamp and Childress[4] and Veatch[6] for more about these rules and principles.

    1. *Nonmaleficence*—A basic principle of consequentialist theory; encompasses the duty to "do no harm." This tenet has a long history as part of the Hippocratic tradition, where it has often been described in terms of the health care provider's

duty to the individual patient. The principle is also cited as justification for actions benefiting all. Sometimes, application of the principle requires addressing conflicts between the needs of one and all.

2. *Beneficence*—Another basic principle of consequentialist theory that expresses the duty to promote good. Again, conflict can arise between what constitutes good for one individual versus the larger societal group. Good or bad consequences are also of importance within deontological theories, but are evaluated along with other principles that may be considered of equal or greater importance.

3. *Respecting the patient–professional relationship*—A moral rule, often referring to respect for the physician–patient relationship, but also applicable to other professional–patient relationships. This rule has been mentioned in published reports of ethical dilemmas arising during the provision of drug information.[9–11] It is expressed in the Hippocratic tradition, which usually indicates that the physician's primary duty is to the patient. Traditional interpretations of this rule have tended to give the physician, rather than the patient, control in the relationship. This rule supports consequentialist theory because it suggests that good outcomes are enhanced through a committed relationship between professional and patient.

4. *Respect for autonomy*—A principle described particularly within deontological theory. This principle is founded on a belief in the right of the individual to self-rule. It speaks to the individual's right to decide on issues that primarily affect self.

5. *Consent*—A moral rule related to the principle of autonomy, which states that the client has a right to be informed and to freely choose a course of action (e.g., informed consent to receive a therapy or procedure).

6. *Confidentiality*—A moral rule, also related to the principle of autonomy, which specifically addresses the individual client's right to give or refuse consent relative to release of privileged information.

7. *Privacy*—Another rule within the principle of autonomy, more generally relating to the right of the individual to control his or her own affairs, without interference from or knowledge of outside parties. This rule has been addressed in deliberations on the rights of women considering abortion or the rights of individuals with AIDS versus those of their potential contacts.

8. *Respect for persons*—A principle expressing duty to the welfare of the individual, particularly described within religion-based deontological theories. This principle may also be partially expressed within dignity of life or sanctity of human life principles. It has common elements with the respect for autonomy principle, but addresses more directly a belief in the inherent value of human life, independent of characteristics or abilities of the specific human being.

9. *Veracity*—This term has been described as either a rule or a principle; it addresses the obligation to truth telling or honesty. Veracity is considered an ethical principle within deontological theory. However, it is considered a useful rule within consequentialist theory to the extent that it promotes good.

10. *Fidelity*—Another principle of moral duty in deontological theory that addresses the responsibility to be trustworthy and keep promises. This principle also relates to a duty of reciprocity—consideration of the other's point of view. Recent descriptions of "Pharmaceutical Care" have spoken of the need to develop an "ethical covenant" between pharmacist and client.[8] This covenant details the characteristics of a relationship requiring fidelity and reciprocity, in which each party takes on certain responsibilities and gives up certain rights to achieve specific good outcomes (consequentialist theory); success of this contract depends in good measure on consideration by each party of the other's point of view.

11. *Justice*—This concept has been presented within various principles that relate to the concept of fairness and tendering what is due; providing that to which the individual is entitled. A number of justice theories have also been developed to connect and justify these various principles.[4]

These are certainly not the only relevant rules or principles, nor are they necessarily universally accepted definitions. However, these action guides seem particularly pertinent to medical ethics inquiry. Furthermore, several of these rules and principles have been specifically discussed in published reports that describe ethical dilemmas encountered by drug information specialists.[9,10] In particular, such dilemmas have been described in situations where pharmacists are providing drug information directly to patients, either from a formal drug information center or during the process of providing patient care.

Demonstration of a Process for Analyzing Ethical Dilemmas

EXAMPLES OF ETHICAL DILEMMAS ARISING DURING THE PROVISION OF DRUG INFORMATION

The following examples demonstrate ethical dilemmas that might arise for a pharmacist providing drug information to consumers or to other health care personnel. These two cases will be used to demonstrate the aforementioned process of analysis for the pharmacist encountering an ethical dilemma. Appendix 13–1 provides additional examples of case scenarios describing ethical dilemmas that might arise for pharmacists who are providing drug information.

Case #1

Mrs. Green, a new patient, calls the drug information center and asks Dr. Smith, the drug information specialist, a question. She is concerned about whether she should take the metronidazole just prescribed for her by Dr. Mack, her family practitioner (who practices at the center where the drug information center is located).

ANALYSIS

Step #1

  I. Identification of relevant background information.
  - A. Factual details of the issue at hand: The pharmacist learns the following information through discussion with the patient.
    1. Mrs. Green is approximately 8 weeks pregnant; she wonders if this medication is safe for the baby.
    2. She says she is being treated for a recently acquired vaginal infection.
    3. She states that this is the first vaginal infection that she has had in several years.
    4. She mentions that she has only recently begun seeing Dr. Mack as her family just moved into town about 3 months ago.
    5. Mrs. Green indicates that Dr. Mack knows she is pregnant; he is managing her pregnancy.
    6. She states that she asked him about the drug's safety, but he rather impatiently brushed off her questions by asking, "Don't you trust me?"
    7. The pharmacist may decide that it is necessary to consult professional resources to evaluate whether the therapy appears to be appropriate. The pharmacist should not hesitate to ask the patient for some reasonable time period in which to investigate the pertinent information before providing an answer.
    8. The pharmacist will need to consider whether any identified risks are likely to be known to the physician.
    9. The pharmacist may decide that further facts must be obtained through direct discussion with the prescriber.
  - B. Identification of who is affected by the ethical issue: As the pharmacist reflects on this patient's inquiry, it is helpful to consider who might be impacted by his response.
    1. Dr. Smith, relative to his own desire to do right; the relationship between him and his patient, the relationship between him and the physician.

2. Mrs. Green, relative to the consequences of any harm to her fetus or of inadequate treatment of the infection, and relative to her future relationships with both the physician and the pharmacist.

3. Mrs. Green's fetus, relative to the consequences of any teratogenic effects of the drug, or of inadequate treatment of the mother's infection.

4. Dr. Mack, relative to the consequences of prescribing a potentially inappropriate therapy during the woman's pregnancy, and relative to the effects of any drug information provided on the patient–physician relationship.

5. Mrs. Green's family, significant others, and society in general, relative to the impacts of either delivery or abortion of a child with birth defects, or of inadequate treatment of the woman's infection.

C. Consideration for the cultural perspectives of those affected by the dilemma.

The pharmacist will consciously or unconsciously act within his own cultural and religious framework, and his understanding of his legal obligations. Awareness of his own perspective, as well as consideration of the cultural perspectives of others who may be affected, is important if he is to pursue a truly ethical course of action. To repeat Veatch's words differentiating ethical deliberations, "The deliberation takes into account the welfare of all involved or affected."[2] Each involved party's welfare is affected by his/her cultural perspective. Cultural, religious, and legal perspectives that the pharmacist must be aware of in this case might include the following.

Step #2

- Perspectives regarding parental responsibility to the unborn fetus versus self
- Perspectives and legal requirements relative to both the pharmacist's and physician's obligations to the patient and to her fetus
- Perspectives about the role and authority of the physician

Identification and justification of the relevant moral rules and principles ("action guides") pertinent to the case at hand.

If the background facts of Mrs. Green's inquiry do not dismiss the pharmacist's ethical concerns, Dr. Smith will find it helpful to consider the various rules and principles discussed above to clarify the dimensions of his concern. It is most useful to first identify all potentially pertinent action guides, and seek an understanding of how fundamentally each applies to the situation, Ethical action guides that seem pertinent to this inquiry include the following.

1. Informed consent—A moral rule supporting Mrs. Smith's right to be informed and freely choose whether to take the metronidazole in relation to other available options.

2. Respect for the patient–professional relationship—This rule addresses Dr. Smith's obligation to support the professional relationship between Mrs. Smith and Dr. Mack. It also requires Dr. Smith to respect his own professional relationship with the patient. Increasingly, pharmacists are interpreting this ethical rule to define their obligation to the patient as primary. Such an interpretation represents a departure for many pharmacists from a historical orientation of primary obligation to the physician.

3. Veracity—Addresses Dr. Smith's responsibility to tell the truth to Mrs. Smith. This may be considered a basic principle of obligation within deontological theory, or a useful rule within consequentialist theory (to the extent that it promotes "good").

4. Nonmaleficence—A basic principle of consequentialist theory that would found a decision to divulge information on minimizing the potential for harm.

5. Beneficence—This consequentialist principle would base the decision regarding what information to divulge on the potential to promote "good." Beneficence and nonmaleficence can be considered together in judging the ethical response to Dr. Smith's dilemma.

    Dr. Smith must consider the potential benefits of the prescribed therapy for Mrs. Green, and address the potential harm resulting from exposure of her fetus to the metronidazole. Consideration of other available alternatives for therapy is also pertinent. Frequently such consideration takes place, at least initially, in the face of inadequate and conflicting information. Dr. Smith will also need to decide what constitutes "harm" and "good" for Mrs. Green versus all others who may be affected.

6. Fidelity/reciprocity—A principle of obligation to an "ethical covenant" between Dr. Smith and Mrs. Green (within deontological theory), which may suggest a requirement for full disclosure of information. However, to the extent that this covenant asks that each party take on certain responsibilities and give up certain rights in order to achieve specific "good" outcomes full disclosure of potentially harmful information may not be required. For instance, if Dr. Smith were concerned that Mrs. Green may decide to forgo any treatment and this could have strong potential of negative consequences for both her and her infant.

7. Justice—This principle is considered of intrinsic value within certain deontological theories, and addresses Mrs. Green's (and other affected parties') right to be given what is due—entitlement to information may be considered justice in this case. Certainly Dr. Smith's time and expertise might be legitimately considered due to his patient.

8. Autonomy—This principle is directly applicable to Dr. Smith's dilemma, as was the related rule of informed consent, based on a belief in Mrs. Green's right to decide on issues that primarily affect her. The principle of autonomy has support within both deontological (as an intrinsic good) and consequentialist (if it is

likely to promote good consequences) theories. However, competing interests (for example, Mrs. Green's and her fetus'), and the individual's capability to be truly autonomous (for example, the fetus in this case), are factors that often complicate the application of this principle in medical ethics.

The reader may believe that other ethical rules or principles are pertinent to this case. If so, they should also be considered as the analysis proceeds.

Step #3

How should these rules and principles be ranked or balanced against each other in order to resolve the ethical dilemma?

This step may sometimes be accomplished rather easily through the use of moral intuition. At other times, careful consideration of ethical theory can suggest which are the more fundamental "action guides" to be applied. In some cases, it may be necessary to balance similarly weighted principles against each other, identifying when the weight of one versus another might be considered greater.

The rules and principles that Dr. Smith considers pertinent in his dilemma over how to respond to Mrs. Green's inquiry could be ranked in the following manner:

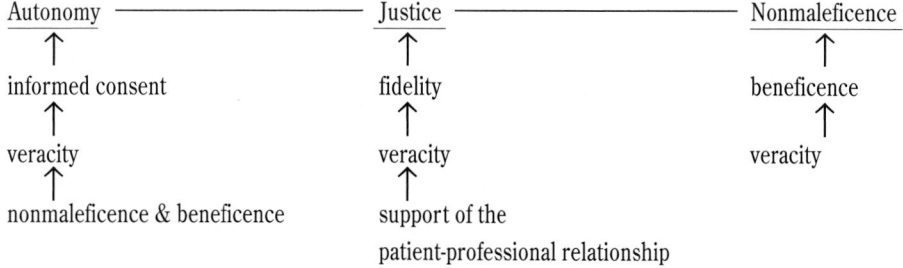

SUMMARY

In the case of Dr. Smith and Mrs. Green, autonomy, justice, and nonmaleficience could be considered the primary principles that must be balanced against each other. Autonomy and justice are both valued principles within various deontological theories. Nonmaleficence and beneficence are the cornerstone principles of consequentialist theory. The principle of justice also seems to be inherent in the contract theory of medical ethics described by Veatch.[6] The other relevant rules and principles above support these primary principles and inform how they apply to specific ethical dilemmas. The Code of Ethics for Pharmacists approved in 1994 provides further support for these fundamental principles and clearly indicates that Dr. Smith's primary obligation is to Mrs. Green rather than to Dr. Mack.[12,13] It may be surmised that all of the fundamental principles seem to support honestly discussing the benefits and risks of the therapy with the patient. However, if there were no good alternative therapies for Mrs. Green's infection and Dr. Smith was concerned that probable noncompliance constituted a greater risk to her, her baby, or both of them, the decision would become more difficult. Once Dr. Smith has considered the facts of the case, who will be affected by his action, the cultural perspectives and legal requirements for the affected parties, and the relevant action guides, he should have more clarity on what constitutes the ethical action. Finally, Dr. Smith's personal beliefs and values relative to these principles of patient autonomy, promotion of justice, and the importance of potential consequences will all affect his ultimate ethical decision. It must be emphasized that he will make some response, even if only by avoiding the patient's question.

It is not likely that all will agree on this ranking or balancing of the pertinent rules and principles in this case, nor will there be universal agreement about what constitutes the right resolution to the ethical dilemma presented. It is necessary to remember that an ethical issue has been defined as one where most agree that there is a right answer, but cannot always agree on what that answer is.

Case #2

Dr. Rich, a drug information pharmacist working for a managed care organization, is asked to review and strongly encouraged to deny coverage for an expensive drug therapy intravenous immune globulin (IVIG) used to treat asthma.

ANALYSIS

Step #1

Identification of relevant background information.

I. Factual details of the case: Dr. Rich learns the following information through literature research and expert consultation, as well as through discussion with colleagues and supervisors.

    A. IVIG is not FDA indicated for treating asthma.

    B. A single dose will cost the payer several hundred dollars.

    C. There is limited study and experience literature that documents therapeutic benefits of the therapy in treating asthma.

D. Relatively few and nonserious adverse events were associated with use of the agent in the limited literature available for all studied indications.

E. The case manager has identified that the claimant patient has been tried on virtually all standard therapies with poor control over the past year; there are some other experimental therapies that have not been tried.

F. The prescribing rheumatologist is a faculty member and researcher at the state medical university.

G. The medical record showed that the claimant patient had been informed and agreed to the IVIG being prescribed for this unapproved indication.

II. Identification of who is affected by the ethical dilemma: Dr. Rich is aware that the following parties may be affected by this issue.

A. Herself

B. The claimant patient and his or her significant others

C. The payer organization

D. Other groups and individuals covered by the managed care organization whose rates may be affected by increased costs related to the drug therapy

E. The prescriber

F. Other potential patients who may be prescribed this drug or who may benefit from the knowledge gained by specialists first prescribing the agent

III. Consideration for the cultural perspectives of those affected by the dilemma: Dr. Rich is cognizant of the following cultural perspectives of the involved parties.

A. The financial and cost-benefit perspectives of the organization for which she works

B. Her own scientific perspective relative to the appropriate volume and weight of evidence relative to safety and benefits of new agents

C. The legal interpretation that allows physicians to prescribe approved products for unapproved uses

D. The research perspective of specialists who conduct exploratory evaluation of new agents for alternative indications

E. The typical cultural perspective of patient reliance on the recommendations of experts in the field that manages a particular disease

F. A fairly typical cultural perspective that research costs should not be born by the research subject (this perspective may or may not also be applied to the subject's insurer)

Depending on the authority of published and other accepted expert sources, the discovered facts of this case may resolve any supervisory conflict and/or ethical concerns. If Dr. Rich still feels that she is confronted by a moral dilemma, she may go on to the following steps in the process of ethical analysis.

Step #2

Identification and justification of the relevant moral rules and principles (action guides) pertinent to the case at hand. Action guides that seem pertinent to this inquiry include the following.

1. Veracity—There seems to be a clear obligation on the pharmacist's part to tender a truthful recommendation based on her professional evaluation of the available resources. It may be hoped that the organization has guidelines in place that support and protect this employee responsibility.
2. Fidelity—This principle of moral duty also appears applicable; the question the pharmacist must answer is, to whom does she most owe her fidelity? To the claimant patient? To the organization for which she works? To the entire patient population served by the organization?
3. Nonmaleficence—and
4. Beneficence—Both of those principles will probably be pertinent in the face of limited data on this drug indication. Potential dangers and benefits for both the patient and the other involved parties must be considered.
5. Justice—Dr. Rich may believe that this principle obligates her to consider what is fair to the claimant patient, but also to other insured groups and individuals. She will need to resolve any conflicts in these interests.

Step #3

How should these rules and principles be ranked or balanced against each other to resolve the ethical dilemma?

The pharmacist must consider the interests of all those affected parties she has identified previously. She will need to decide if she has greater obligation to certain of the affected parties. It is hoped that, as Dr. Rich prioritizes and balances these applicable action guides, she gains more clarity about the appropriate course of action. One possible way to address these relevant rules and principles follows.

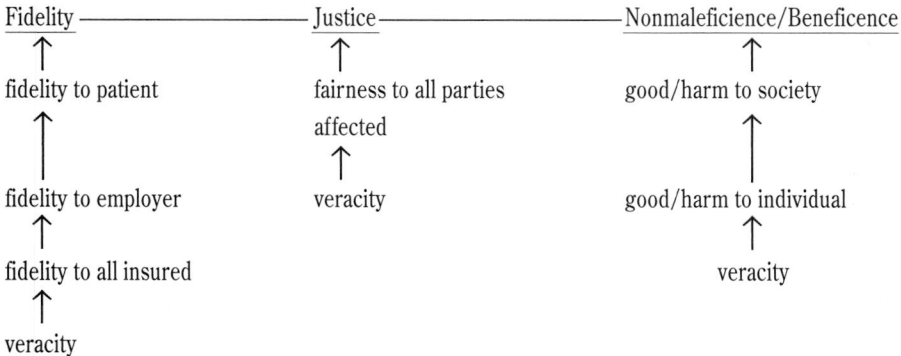

SUMMARY

It is hoped that Dr. Rich will find that this process of analysis has helped her to reach better clarity about where her primary obligations lie, and to sort out the benefits and problems that should be considered in making the recommendation she decides is most appropriate. Her decision will be affected by a general orientation either toward a consequentialist theory of ethical obligation or toward deontological theory. Consequentialist theory judges on the basis of good versus bad outcome. Deontological theory places more importance on certain foundational principles such as fidelity, with perhaps a greater emphasis on responsibility to the individual, or justice, which particularly emphasizes responsibilities to all involved parties and groups. In this example, the alternative ways of balancing or prioritizing the pertinent rules and principles helps to clarify for the pharmacist that she must decide about her obligations to the individual client involved versus a larger group. The larger group could be her employer, organization, all plan participants, or even larger societal groups.

Again, it is unlikely that all will agree that this issue constitutes an ethical dilemma or on how to balance any pertinent rules and principles in this case. Ultimately, Dr. Rich will need to decide what constitutes the best resolution she can reach in this ethical dilemma.

Brief Review of Medical Ethics Resources for Use by Pharmacists

The first goal in learning about analysis of ethical issues is to become aware of opportunities for ethical deliberation when they confront us. Situations will arise where ethical judgments will be made that have moral consequences, with or without the conscious understanding of the parties involved.

Formal coursework, inservices, or continuing education opportunities can teach skills that will aid pharmacists in handling ethical dilemmas related to work responsibilities. Thornton and co-workers[5] discuss what should be taught in basic ethics education that takes place within and outside the academic environment. Their review of important elements to be included in ethics education is worthwhile reading for anyone who may desire to participate in such activities. They also refer the reader to other useful resources on the topic. Haddad and associates[1] provide comprehensive guidelines on ethics course content that is also valuable reading for those wishing to address ethics topics in the continuing education of the pharmacist. This guideline describes examples of educational methods including case presentation and debate; scenario building, with identification and discussion of potential ethical issues; and role-playing activities. The authors indicate that such educational methods should involve group participation to conduct the analysis of the ethical issue being discussed. Writing techniques, such as a "5-minute write" exercise prior to discussion, can serve to focus the participant's ideas and facilitate the resultant discussion.[14] The guideline also provides an extensive bibliography of resource materials. Pirl[3] describes the use of role-playing assignments for undergraduate pharmacy students. This article also lists case scenarios that could be used in continuing education programs for practitioners who are exploring ways to resolve ethical dilemmas arising in pharmacy practice.

Smith and colleagues[15] have written a book on pharmacy ethics that also provides background discussion and case examples that relate to many target areas of pharmacy practice. This resource can be very useful for the pharmacy practitioner who wishes to address ethical issues in a particular area of practice.

An Organizational Structure That Supports Ethical Decision Making

Something should be said about establishment of an organizational structure that supports the pharmacist (providing drug information in any setting) when he or she is faced with an ethical dilemma. Some formal structures (Ethics Committees, Consultation Teams, Codes of Ethical Conduct) are increasingly available in larger institutional health care organizations, but are also needed within the chain pharmacy setting or in smaller organizations such as the independent community pharmacy. On a day-to-day basis, practitioners generally have to conduct such analysis very rapidly and often alone to decide or act in a timely manner. Prior knowledge of structures and processes that exist to support the clinician in overall client interactions, and in analysis and decision making, can better prepare the pharmacist to address the real-life dilemmas he or she will encounter.

Berger[8] describes the need for an "ethical covenant" between the pharmacist and the patient who is being provided pharmaceutical care. This term suggests an implicit contract between client and health care provider that broadly describes the relationship involved whenever a pharmacist provides drug information. Within this contract, the service recipient has a right to receive competently provided information as well as respectful treatment, and has the obligation to provide the background information needed by the pharmacist. Likewise, the provider pharmacist has the right to adequate background information (and respectful treatment as well), and the obligation to give competent, trustworthy, and caring service. Recognition of this implicit contract can occasionally suggest corrective action to resolve or avoid perceived ethical dilemmas, especially those that arise out of a failure to adequately communicate, or out of a lack of mutual respect in the interaction. Pharmacists also have a revised Code of Ethics for Pharmacists available to them since 1994, which may serve as a general guide to those obligations implicit to the patient–pharmacist relationship. This code, which took several years to develop, has been published in the *American Journal of Health-System Pharmacists* and has received final approval from the membership of the American Pharmaceutical Association.[12,13] The text of this Code is provided in Appendix 13–2.

The organization can also assist professionals by creating explicit policies addressing some issues with potential ethical dimensions. For example, a written policy stating that pharmacists are not required to answer questions from a client who refuses to provide required background information could avoid the dilemma of the unidentified client who wanted to know how long amphetamine can be detected in the urine. A second policy might address adequate staffing requirements to ensure the community pharmacist of adequate time to perform counseling services. A third example might be a policy that states that pharmacists may refer questions where provision of an answer would violate their personal ethics, which could at least partially resolve a potential dilemma for the pharmacist who has been asked to provide advice on the use of a drug to induce abortion. Of course, the legal and ethical rights of clients have to be recognized during development of such policies. As professionals, pharmacists should reserve the right to have a major role in such policy development, preferably with input from client or patient representatives. To be useful, policies must be developed with attention to avoiding what constitutes infringement on the domain of personal ethics (e.g., a personal prohibition against euthanasia).

Appropriate institutional policies can support the pharmacist in recognizing and addressing true ethical dilemmas. Such policies can also serve to define the breadth and limits of the client's right to the requested drug information.

Summary

All pharmacists will be called upon to provide drug information. On occasion they will encounter ethical dilemmas regarding what information, if any, should be provided. It is important that the pharmacy professional approach such moments prepared to (often quickly) identify the pertinent circumstances, and analyze and rank or balance the pertinent ethical rules and principles that are involved. The individual pharmacist must recognize his or her rights and responsibilities relative to the client, to other involved individuals, to society as a whole, and to any higher power to whom the pharmacist feels accountable. Organizations can assist the employee pharmacist by formal recognition of certain implicit and explicit policies. Furthermore, deliberate study and rehearsal of important analytic steps that may be used to address ethical dilemmas can be of great help to every pharmacist who will provide drug information.

Study Questions

One of the family practice physicians located in the medical building next to your pharmacy calls. He asks you for information about the combination regimen of two prescription medications that has been promoted as a "morning-after" contraceptive. He indicates that he has a patient who had an unplanned/undesired sexual encounter the previous evening and is concerned about becoming pregnant.

1. Assess whether this drug information request constitutes a potential ethical dilemma, based on three characteristics that differentiate such a situation.

2. What background information might you want to obtain to clarify this information request?

3. For pharmacists for whom this question constitutes an ethical dilemma, consider what moral rules and principles are likely to apply to this issue.

4. Assuming that some of these relevant action guides conflict with each other, and describe further deliberations by which the pharmacist might prioritize or balance these conflicts to reach a decision on how to respond to the information request.

5. What organizational strategies might best prepare this pharmacist to most effectively respond to ethical dilemmas such as this one?

REFERENCES

1. Haddad AM, Kaatz B, McCart G, McCarthy RL, Pink LA, Richardson J. Report of the ethics course content committee: Curricular guidelines for pharmacy education. Am J Pharmaceut Ed 1993 (Winter Supple); 57:34S–43S.
2. Veatch RM. Hospital pharmacy: What is ethical? (Primer) Am J Hosp Pharm 1989;46:109–15.
3. Pirl MA. An ethics laboratory as an educational tool in a pharmacy law and ethics course. J Pharm Teach 1990;1(3):51–68.
4. Beauchamp TLC, Childress JF. Principles of biomedical ethics. 4th ed. New York: Oxford University Press, 1994. p. 15.
5. Thornton BC, Callahan D, Nelson JL. Bioethics education: Expanding the circle of participants. Hastings Cent Rep 1993;23(1):25–9.
6. Veatch RM. A theory of medical ethics. New York: Basic Books; 1981.

7. Carrese J, Brown K, Jameton A. Culture, healing, and professional obligations. Hastings Cent Rep 1993; Jul-Aug:15–17.

8. Berger BA. Building an effective therapeutic alliance: Competence, trustworthiness, and caring. Am J Hosp Pharm 1993;50:2399–403.

9. Arnold RM, Nissen JC, Campbell NA. Ethical issues in a drug information center. Drug Intell Clin Pharm 1987;21:1008–11.

10. Kelly WN, Krause EC, Krowsinski WJ, Small TR, Drane JF. National survey of ethical issues presented to drug information centers. Am J Hosp Pharm 1990;47:2245–50.

11. Schools RM, Brushwood DB. The pharmacist's role in patient care. Hastings Cent Rep 1991; Jan-Feb:12–17.

12. Vottero LD. Code of ethics for pharmacists. Am J Health-Syst Pharm 1995;52:2096, 2131.

13. Code of ethics adopted. Am Pharm 1994;NS34(11):72.

14. Coach R. Five minutes to monitor progress. Teaching Prof 1991;5(9):1–2.

15. Smith M, Strauss S, Baldwin HJ, Alberts KT. Pharmacy ethics. New York: Pharmaceutical Products Press; 1991.

16. Uretsky SD, Kelly WN, Veatch RM. Pharmacist's responsibility for providing drug information to be used for questionable purposes. Am J Hosp Pharm 1992;49:1725–30.

14

Chapter Fourteen

Pharmacy and Therapeutics Committee

Patrick M. Malone

Objectives

After completing this chapter, the reader will be able to:

- Describe where and how the pharmacy and therapeutics committee fits into the organizational structure of a health care institution.
- Describe the functions of the pharmacy and therapeutics committee.
- Describe how the pharmacy department participates in pharmacy and therapeutics committee activities.
- Describe and explain the concepts of drug formularies and drug formulary systems, and how pharmacy participates in those areas.
- Describe and perform an evaluation of a drug product for a drug formulary.
- Describe how to develop policies and procedures.

Concept and Organization

When considering how a clinical pharmacist can have an impact on a patient's drug therapy, it is common to consider the individual practitioner dealing with a specific patient or, perhaps, a small group of patients. Certainly the clinician can have a deep impact this way, but it does have the disadvantage of dealing with a very limited number of patients. For pharmacists to efficiently impact a great number of patients, a different approach is necessary. Fortunately, one way pharmacists have that opportunity is through participation in the activities of the pharmacy and therapeutics (P&T) committee or its equivalent. It should be pointed out that P&T committees are normally associated with institutional pharmacy. Although this has often been the case, other organizations have increasingly used P&T-type committees in an attempt to improve drug therapy while lowering costs. Some places where such committees are seen include managed care organizations (MCOs),[1] insurance companies, state Medicaid boards, and even community pharmacies.[2] Although much of this chapter will use examples from institutional pharmacy, simply because most of the published literature deals with that area of practice, the concepts covered are applicable to any P&T-type committee and comply with recommendations of the American Medical Association (AMA),[3] American Society of Health-System Pharmacists (ASHP), and the Joint Commission on Accreditation of Healthcare Organizations (JCAHO).[4]

Although it is easy to assume from its name that the P&T committee is organizationally a part of the pharmacy department, such is not the case. Instead, it is usually a medical staff entity and, perhaps, only one or two pharmacists may actually be members of the committee (possibly ex officio members without voting privileges). Commonly the pharmacy director, serving as the committee's secretary (taking minutes, collating and arranging the agenda, etc.), may be the sole official pharmacy representative. Other pharmacists may also attend to act as consultants to the committee—often having great impact on the committee's decisions, even if they cannot officially vote. Fortunately, in larger hospitals, it appears that more pharmacists are now becoming members of the P&T committee.[5] Hospitals can have different organizational structures, however. Figure 14–1 shows a typical structure. On first glance, hospitals seem to be unique because they have two parallel organizational structures. On the left, clinical functions are overseen by the medical staff. This is different than a typical business because the medical staff often does not directly work for the hospital, even though they have a great impact on how the hospital is run. On the right is a typical business organizational chart, much the same as would be seen in any business. This right side generally oversees the business aspects of the hospital. The two sides of the chart really are not separate, because their cooperation is certainly necessary for the success of the hospital and the medical staff may be directly employed by the hospital.

Although the medical staff as a whole is ultimately in charge of the clinical aspects of care in the hospital, in places other than very small institutions, this is unworkable without an administrative structure of some kind. Therefore, the medical staff may elect officers and elect or appoint some body to oversee all aspects of patient care. In this example, the term medical executive committee is used for that body, although the name and exact function may vary.

In modern medicine, there are so many clinical areas to consider that it is unrealistic for one committee to adequately oversee all aspects of patient care, except in very small institutions. For that reason, various subcommittees of the medical executive committee are usually necessary (Fig. 14–1). One of these may be the P&T committee, which is charged with overseeing all aspects of drug therapy. Membership is mostly

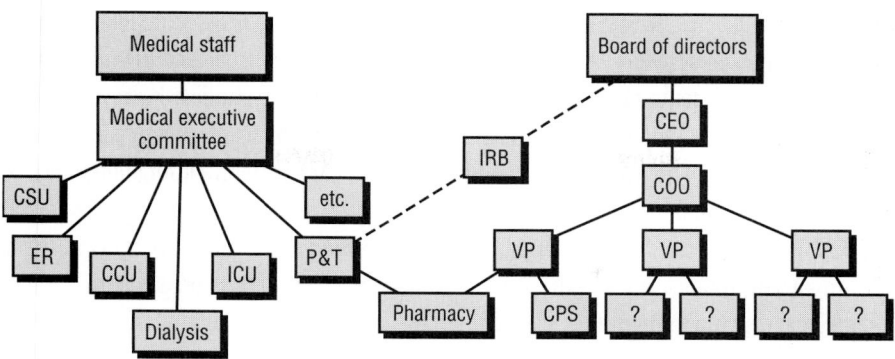

CCU   Coronary care unit committee
CEO   Chief executive officer
COO   Chief operating officer
CPS   Central processing and supply
CSU   Cardiac surgery unit committee
ER   Emergency room committee
ICU   Intensive care unit committee
IRB   Institutional Review Board
P&T   Pharmacy and Therapeutics Committee
VP   Vice president
?   Other hospital departments

Figure 14–1. Hospital organization.

physicians (preferably a wide variety of physicians from various areas of practice), but usually includes at least one pharmacist and often members from other areas of the hospital (e.g., nursing, administration, quality assurance, medical records, laboratory, risk management). A pharmacoeconomicist also can be extremely helpful. In some cases, pharmacy is asked to recommend physicians for the committee. If possible, pharmacy should suggest physicians who are committed to rational drug therapy.[6] Also, efforts should be made to ensure the physician chosen as chairman of the committee is an advocate of the pharmacy department.

Although the P&T committee has been referred to in JCAHO accreditation standards in the past, it is no longer required and may be replaced by some other committee or body.[4,7,8] In some cases the name or some of the functions of the committee will change; for example, this committee is referred to as the Drug and Therapeutics Committee (DTC) in Australia.[9]

Typically, P&T committee functions include determining what drugs are available, who can prescribe specific drugs, policies and procedures regarding drug use (including clinical guidelines; see Chap. 9), quality assurance activities (e.g., drug utilization review/ drug usage evaluation/medication usage evaluation; see Chap. 15), adverse drug reaction reporting (see Chap. 16), and education in drug use.[4,10] Many of those functions are quality assurance–type activities, because they are designed to improve the quality of drug therapy.[11] The functions can also include investigational drug studies; however, that is often delegated to the Institutional Review Board, which oversees all investigational activities in the hospital (see Chap. 17). In addition, some P&T committee functions may be delegated to subcommittees (e.g., quality assurance subcommittee, antibiotic subcommittee)[12]; however, this can be cumbersome and is often avoided, except in larger institutions. It is important to point out that the P&T committee may act only as an advisory body to the medical executive committee. Decisions of the P&T committee may not be considered final (and therefore not be implemented) until they are reviewed and approved by the medical executive committee.

According to the JCAHO, the medical staff, pharmacy, nursing, and others are to cooperate in carrying out the previously mentioned functions.[4] Although the medical staff normally takes overseeing drug therapy very seriously and expects to approve all activities of the P&T committee, it is common for the pharmacy department to do much of the preparation work for the committee. Although it is tempting to say the reason pharmacy is charged with all of the work is that they are the "drug experts," which is often true, it is probably more realistic that the reason is that pharmacists are paid to do this as part of their salary, whereas physicians often do not obtain any direct monetary compensation for this committee's preparatory work.

Pharmacy Support of the Pharmacy and Therapeutics Committee

Although it is not uncommon for pharmacists to downplay or misunderstand the importance of P&T committee support in comparison to other clinical activities, these activities are vital for pharmacy to impact patient care. P&T committee support and participation can have far-reaching effects on the overall quality of drug therapy in an institution and must be given a great deal of attention. Although such attention is time consuming,[13] it can be valuable to the pharmacy. It must also be stressed that P&T committees most often accept pharmacy recommendations[14,15] and, therefore, pharmacy departments can have a great impact on drug therapy through this mechanism.

Some pharmacists who participate in P&T committee activities feel they are serving their function by providing information requested by physicians and considering drugs for formulary approval only following physician requests. This can rapidly deteriorate into "crisis management," where the pharmacy department reacts to problems, fighting each fire as it occurs. It is much better for a pharmacy to be proactive,[11,16] seeking to address issues (e.g., changes in drugs carried on the formulary, new policies and procedures, quality assurance activities, etc.) before they become problems. Through such actions it is possible for the pharmacy to better get physician support for all of its clinical activities.

In the specific instance of P&T committee support, one or more pharmacists must be identified to conduct the necessary planning. This can include administrators, purchasing agents, or clinicians, particularly drug information specialists. These people must develop and regularly evaluate data sources to anticipate physicians' needs[17] (Table 14–1). For example, it is necessary to find out what drugs have recently been approved by the Food and Drug Administration (FDA) to identify drugs for possible formulary inclusion. Approval often comes about three months before commercial availability and is published on the FDA web site (<<http://www.fda.gov/cder/drug/default.htm>>). Therefore, there is time for the drug to be considered for formulary addition before the first orders arrive from the nursing units. In a case where it is not possible to consider a drug before it is commercially available, it has been suggested by some that drugs rated "P" (priority) by the FDA be made available to physicians until the drug can be considered.[18] This latter procedure may be effective, but considering the drug before commercial availability is preferable, because if the ultimate P&T committee decision is to leave the drug off the drug formulary, there may be difficulties. It is also a good idea to track older drugs. For example, the use of nonformulary drugs may be tracked within the hospital.[19,20] If patterns of increased use are noted, it is best to identify a reason for that use. If the use is inappropriate, the physician(s) should be contacted and given information about alternative formulary agents. In some cases, new information may be available showing a new advantage or use for an old agent, which can lead to its reconsideration for formulary adoption. Related to this is the necessity to regularly consider the material being promoted by drug company representatives. It is worth mentioning that some hospitals will restrict drug representa-

TABLE 14–1. AREAS WHERE PHARMACISTS SHOULD BE SUPPORTING A PHARMACY AND THERAPEUTICS COMMITTEE

- Planning future agendas (including medications, policies and procedures, and quality assurance subjects to be addressed)
- Gathering data and creating drug monographs
- Evaluating medications for formulary adoption or deletion
- Preparing and conducting quality assurance programs (including drug usage evaluation and monitoring of adverse effects and medication errors)
- Preparing policies and procedures
- Communicating information from the P&T committee to other areas of the institution
- Creating hard copy and electronic versions of the formulary

tive access to the institution or restrict the drugs that may be promoted to items approved for use in the hospital to prevent this problem. There may also be new indications or other information that will increase demand for nonformulary items. If there are sufficient changes noted in the use(s) of a particular class of drugs, it is useful to review the class as a whole to decide which drug(s) are to be retained on the formulary. Most likely, class reviews should be regularly scheduled because there may be new information not otherwise noted that necessitates changes in formulary items in a particular class—both additions and deletions. Other items, such as trends in reported adverse drug reactions in the institution, or published data for new products with little information in the literature on first approval, may also be useful in determining products for P&T committee consideration or reconsideration.[21] Although there must be a mechanism by which physicians can request that drugs be added to the formulary, all of the above methods and others can help the pharmacy anticipate physician needs, allowing time for information gathering, evaluation of products, and P&T committee consideration before the need becomes too urgent to permit proper consideration.

To guide physicians into considering the logic of requesting items to be added to the drug formulary that have not been evaluated by the P&T committee, via the prospective mechanisms mentioned above, a specific request form may be useful. Items that a physician may be required to fill out or attach to the form can be seen listed in Table 14–2.[22]

The P&T committee should be kept advised by this pharmacy-based steering committee of future plans, so that they can be aware that a rational planning process is governing their agenda. Also, it is a good idea for one or more representative(s) of this steering committee to meet with the pharmacy director, chairman of the P&T committee, and a representative of the hospital administration on a regular basis to assist with planning and ensure their concerns are addressed. This meeting could be held shortly before the P&T committee actually meets to present preliminary formulary evaluations,

---

TABLE 14–2. ITEMS THAT MAY BE ON A REQUEST FOR FORMULARY CONSIDERATION FORM

- Date and time of request
- Name of product (e.g., generic, trade, chemical)
- Source of product (e.g., manufacturer, distributor)
- Specific information about drug product (e.g., class of drug, mechanism, adverse effects, clinical studies)
- Anticipated use of drug (e.g., what type of patient, how often)
- Comparable drugs already on the formulary
- Why the product is needed
- What drugs could be removed from the formulary
- What restrictions, policies, cautions, etc., are necessary
- How the drug fits into any clinical guidelines
- Action requested (e.g., addition, deletion, restriction)

---

quality assurance material and policy and procedure documents for an initial review, allowing modifications addressing physician and administration concerns to be made before formal committee review and action. During this meeting, plans for future months can be made or adjusted as the circumstances dictate. Other appropriate physicians or groups should also be consulted to assure that their concerns are addressed. For example, if changes to the cephalosporins carried on the drug formulary are considered, the infectious disease specialists should be contacted to provide input.

In regard to quality assurance activities, the pharmacy department should obtain data to guide the selection of upcoming quality assurance programs. This is covered in greater detail in Chap. 15. The pharmacy should also investigate what drugs may need specific policies and procedures developed. This may be done when the drug is first being evaluated for formulary addition, or later if problems (e.g., increased adverse drug reaction reports, medication errors, overuse) are noted. For example, concerns about a new thrombolytic agent leading to increased morbidity and mortality through improper use might prompt the P&T committee to approve specific protocols for the use of the agent.

Finally, it is extremely important for the pharmacy to inform physicians about activities of the P&T committee. While a great deal of effort is placed on communication with the committee itself, it is also necessary to keep the entire medical staff informed. This may be accomplished through newsletters and web sites (refer to Chap. 11) or other mechanisms.

Drug Formulary System

Drug formularies can be defined as a continually revised list of medications that are readily available for use within an institution that reflect the current clinical judgment of the medical staff.[23] This physical or electronic list can be a very simple publication, or can have a great deal of information on how to use drugs (doses, indications, policy and procedures, etc.), but in either case must be readily available to the staff who use it. An example of a web-based drug formulary may be seen at <<http://www.intmed.mcw.edu/drug.html>>.

A related term, the *formulary system,* can be thought of as a method for developing the list, and sometimes even as a philosophy. In theory, a well-designed drug formulary can guide clinicians to prescribe the safest and most effective agents for treating a particular medical problem.[24] Some people argue that the formulary system itself does not work because it is not properly applied and recommend replacing it with counterdetailing by pharmacists or computers at the time a prescription order is written[25]; however, whether or not that is true has yet to be determined. The most well-known article indicating that formularies may ultimately result in higher patient costs was written by Horn and associates.[26] Although this may be one of the best articles on the topic and the author has defended criticism of the article,[27] there are nevertheless various deficiencies in the study that make it uncertain whether it was truly the drug formulary or other factors that led to increased costs.[28–31] Horn and associates[32] also published a similar study conducted in the ambulatory environment, which appears to have similar results and deficiencies. Further research is needed before a definite conclusion may be reached on the effectiveness of formulary management.[33] For now, a well-constructed formulary is still believed to improve patient care while decreasing costs.

The formulary system as a whole is often associated with hospitals; however, it is also applicable in many other places, such as nursing homes,[34] health maintenance organizations (HMOs),[35–37], health care systems,[38] states,[39] long-term care facilities,[40,41] community pharmacies, chain pharmacies,[42] and as part of insurance companies' benefit plans.[43,44] Some entire countries also have instituted formulary systems in an attempt to cut medical costs.[45] National and third-party payer formularies, however, may be based more on economics than a traditional institutional formulary.[46] The formulary system is the method by which the medical staff, through the P&T committee, evaluates, appraises, and selects the drug products most useful in patient care for availability through the pharmacy.[23,47] Whether the formulary system is specific to one institution or a large health care group, the process is approximately the same, although the politics and the necessity to take into account many environments may slow formulary development to a greater extent in large health care groups (e.g., hospital chain) as each individual institution fights for what is best for its specific circumstances. The ASHP does suggest standardization of formularies within and, possibly, between health care systems to simplify matters for the prescribers and patients.[48] To integrate formularies between hospitals, a facilitator may be helpful to ensure the process remains unbiased.[49] Also, overlap with other third-party payers has to be evaluated, because that may affect reimbursement.

The goal of the formulary system is to provide a group of high-quality drugs for the situation. There needs to be an effort to ensure that drugs are available for any disease states likely to be treated. Those drugs should be the most efficacious agents with the fewest side effects and lowest cost.[8] Other factors should also be taken into consideration, such as dosage forms, estimated use, convenience, dosing schedule, compliance, abuse potential, physician demand, ease of preparation, and storage requirements.[50] Typically, only two or, perhaps, three drugs from any drug class are added to the formulary. Some people would argue that only one agent is necessary from any class; however, some individuals will not respond to and/or tolerate certain agents, so at least one secondary agent is usually desirable. Therapeutic redundancy must be minimized, however, by excluding superfluous or inferior preparations. This should improve the quality of prescribing and also lead to improved cost effectiveness, both by eliminating expensive agents that do not improve patient care and by assisting patients to become well faster.

Whether an institution has a very strict formulary with a minimum number of items, or a looser formulary that excludes items that are significantly inferior is sometimes a matter of philosophy. The former will cut down the pharmacy department's inventory and often save money through avoidance of highly priced products, but may only be practical in closed HMOs where the same formulary is used in both the inpatient and ambulatory environments. In cases where physicians are free to prescribe whatever products they prefer in the ambulatory environment, the increased time necessary for pharmacists to contact physicians for order changes and the disruption to patient care may make a less restrictive formulary more practical. An example where the latter situation could cause problems would be when a patient on a nonformulary antihypertensive is admitted for hip replacement surgery. Although there would be other satisfactory antihypertensives on the formulary, it may be best to simply allow use of the other product, rather than adding another complicating factor to the patient's hospital treatment by attempting to change therapy to one of the formulary products. Pharmacist and physician time would also be saved.

Even in cases where an institution has a strict and enforced drug formulary, it should be noted that there are occasions when it is necessary to prescribe a drug that is not on the drug formulary. This might be due to a patient with a rare illness, a patient that does not respond or has intolerable side effects to the formulary drugs, a patient stabilized on a nonformulary medication where it would be difficult or dangerous to change, a conflict between the institutional formulary and the patient's insurance company formulary,[51] or some other valid reason. A mechanism must be in place to promptly obtain the particular drug when it is shown to be necessary (the National Committee for Quality Assurance [NCQA] requires such a mechanism for HMOs,[52] as does JCAHO for other hospitals[4]),[8] but it must try to prevent physicians from ordering nonformulary drugs "because I said so!" Some institutions require specific request forms to be filled out, sometimes with a co-signature from the physician's department head, or at least require a consultation between a pharmacist and the physician before the drug is obtained. Also, patients may be charged more for the nonformulary medications. In some HMOs and insurance company plans, the physicians or pharmacies may be financially penalized for use or overuse of nonformulary medications.[43] Whatever mechanism is used, it is important to make it easy to obtain necessary nonformulary medications, but difficult to obtain unnecessary medications. Otherwise, the benefits of the formulary system may be negated.[19] Also, it is necessary to track which nonformulary drugs are being used regularly and why that is happening, because it may be worthwhile to add some of those agents to the drug formulary.[53]

Some physicians feel that a drug formulary serves only to keep costs down, at the expense of good patient care.[54] These physicians must be reassured that there is evidence to support that a good formulary does keep expenses down[34] without negatively affecting care,[55] although in some cases the costs are merely transferred to other hospital expenses.[45,56] One study demonstrated that a well-controlled formulary or therapeutic substitution (substituting a different medication that is effective for the disease being treated for the one ordered by the physician) results in 10.7% lower drug costs per patient day, and both a well-controlled formulary and therapeutic substitution together could cause 13.4% lower drug costs per day.[57] Some physicians do not like formularies because they consider them to be a limitation to their "authority."[54] It is necessary to keep in mind that when physicians become a part of a medical staff or sign up to partici-pate in some managed care group they are given privileges not rights. The privileges generally do include limitations on what medications they can prescribe, and when and how they can prescribe them. If a drug formulary system is run well there is little reason to feel there are inadequate drugs available; however, it does take some effort for the physician to learn to use the drugs available rather than the drugs they normally prescribe. An effort must be made to help physicians in this regard and to reassure them that every effort is being made to ensure the best drugs are available for the patients. Additionally, all changes to the drug formulary must be quickly and effectively communicated to the physicians to avoid confusion. A lack of such communication can negate some of the benefits of the formulary and lead to poor physician–pharmacist relations.[45] Also, it is important for physicians to be aware that it is the medical staff that makes these decisions, to avoid pharmacy being perceived as the policeman who is waiting to jump on the unsuspecting physician.[58] In the future, physicians will enter prescription orders into the computer, which can quickly inform the physician of formulary drug choices and guide therapeutic decisions. Currently, however, pharmacists may have to tactfully contact the physician about nonformulary drugs to make a formulary system work. Similarly, pharmacies filling prescriptions for an HMO must be kept informed of formulary status of drugs. One suggestion is to have a "help desk" to answer pharmacist questions and to provide information.[59]

FORMULARY DEVELOPMENT

The formulary itself is developed under the auspices of the P&T committee, which evaluates the drugs or drug classes. In addition to traditional marketed products, it is now becoming necessary to similarly evaluate herbal or other alternative medicine products,[60–62] although some institutions may instead handle them as nonformulary requests or investigational drugs.[63] Although alternative and herbal medications seem somewhat unusual to the P&T committee, they can still be treated much the same way, perhaps with additional evaluation of the purity and composition of the products.[64]

To perform adequate evaluations, the committee needs a membership that can address many aspects of drug therapy. It is best to have the physician membership composed of individuals from the major disciplines in the hospital. Although internal medicine and family practice should certainly be represented on the average P&T committee, it is good to have members from such specialties as infectious disease, oncology, cardiology, surgery, and any other area that may be particularly important for the specific institution. In some cases, consultants from other unrepresented areas may be invited for specific meetings in which drugs they would commonly use are being evaluated.

When setting up a drug formulary there are several things to consider. First is whether there will be an open or closed formulary. The former essentially means any drug on the market is available, and some would argue that the term "open formulary" is really an oxymoron.[24] One exception to this definition is that the NCQA states that an open formulary for an MCO can be a list of recommended drugs, as long as there are no requirements concerning their use.[65] A closed formulary means that only a limited number of agents are available. This is certainly preferable, because such agents should be chosen by objective evidence in the scientific literature that supports the superiority of the agents over other similar drugs. Closed formularies are becoming much more common in HMOs.[66,67] The closed formulary can also be broken down into what is referred to as positive or negative formularies. This is the method by which the formulary is developed. A positive formulary effectively starts with a blank sheet of paper and specifically adds agents. Although this is probably the best method to limit the number of drugs available, it is often not very popular when first implementing the formulary because every agent must be considered. That means the physicians must even make specific decisions on whether they should add such things as acetaminophen and amoxicillin to the formulary. Therefore, in hospitals just establishing a formulary it is often more popular and easier to use a negative formulary system. This essentially starts with the current hospital drug stock, with each drug class being considered to eliminate agents that are not necessary.[68] First steps in this process may be as simple as eliminating multiple salts/esters of the same drug. Then classes of drugs with multiple similar products could be addressed (e.g., analgesics, antacids, laxatives, vitamins, topical steroids). Although in some ways this process is easier, it is also likely to result in a much bigger formulary, because the decision will be made as to what drugs are definitely not needed, rather than which drugs the institution definitely needs. However, the specific institution's situation will need to be assessed before the method of determining the formulary items can be decided on. Overall, the goal is to provide the optimal agents; it is easy to end up with too many duplicative agents; however, having a greater number of agents to choose from can lead to better patient care in some areas.[69,70]

Drug Evaluation Monographs

The establishment and maintenance of a drug formulary requires that drugs or drug classes be objectively assessed based on scientific information (e.g., efficacy, adverse effects, cost, other appropriate items), not anecdotal physician experience. When a P&T committee considers a drug for formulary adoption, it is quite common for the discussion to include statements such as "In my clinical experience . . .", which leads the discussion into rather subjective areas. It must be kept in mind that physicians are most likely to request drugs if they have met with the pharmaceutical company representative or received money from the drug company (e.g., speaking fees, travel funds to a meeting).[71] Valid formulary decisions should be based on objective evidence, rather than a few cases of "clinical experience." Efforts must be made to guide discussions to scientific information when it wanders into vague subjective areas.[24] In some cases this is rather difficult, because many new drugs have limited published information when they are first commercially available. In situations such as this, the decision on formulary addition may need to be postponed until adequate information is available. Although there is a temptation to think that anything new is better (and that attitude is certainly pushed by drug company representatives with new products to sell), that cannot be assumed and must be proven. Some places have even tried computerized methods to make more objective decisions[72]; however, there does not seem to be any data demonstrating the superiority of such a method. Similarly, there is a process called System of Objectified Judgement Analysis (SOJA) that uses a computer program to score different aspects of drugs in the same class to determine the best product.[73,74]

Also, it is necessary to determine whether people involved with the discussion and decision about a drug's formulary status have some conflict of interest (i.e., would receive some direct or indirect compensation from having a drug available; e.g., stock in a company, honoraria for speaking, consulting fees, gifts or grants from a company[75]) and avoid that biasing factor. Perhaps a conflict of interest policy, requiring regular disclosure of any possible conflicts (e.g., drug company stock, honoraria, professional travel expenses, gifts above a certain amount) would be necessary.[76,77]

The way to decide what drug is best for formulary addition is to rationally evaluate all aspects of the drug in relation to similar agents. In particular, it is necessary to consider need, effectiveness, risk, and cost—often in that order. It is expected that in the future there will be more emphasis on evaluating clinical outcomes, continuous quality assurance information, and quality of life.[78] An in-depth monograph can be prepared to assist in this process as described below. Commercially prepared monographs can also be obtained from several sources that can be used "as is" or with modifications to suit the needs of the institution. If this latter method is used, be aware that the quality of the commercial monographs vary, even from the same publisher, and that they may need extensive updating. Often, writing a new drug evaluation monograph may be easier than improving a commercial monograph. Drug class reviews prepared for the Veterans Administration are also available on the Internet at <<http://www.dppm.med.va.gov/pbm/reviews.htm>>. Whether or not the monograph is commercial or local, the material should reflect the local conditions and should be sent to P&T committee members a reasonable time before the meeting to allow full consideration of the information. To prevent drug company representatives or others from obtaining the material, however, some institutions only distribute this material for review during the meeting.

Although there are recommendations concerning monograph contents,[79] information is commonly missing.[80] An outline of a sample monograph is found in Appendix 14–1. Each of the sections of this monograph will be discussed below. An example of some of the information found in the various parts of a monograph is seen in Appendix 14–2. This sample monograph meets or exceeds ASHP recommendations,[79] and should serve as a good example for most circumstances. Nonetheless, the precise monograph should be tailored to the institution, clinic, and so on. Several sections not recommended by ASHP have been added to increase the utility of the monograph for other sites of practice, including ambulatory clinics. Also, in some cases the information has been divided into multiple sections or subsections to increase clarity. This format can also be used to evaluate whole classes of drugs. In most cases, a specific drug is compared to others in the same class. The only difference in a class review is that one drug is not receiving the greatest attention; all drugs are being compared with equal attention.

Specific formats, differing some from the one presented here, may be required by organizations or governments. For example, both Australia (<<http://www.health.gov.au/haf/docs/pharmpac/gusubpac.htm>>) and Ontario, Canada (<<http://www.gov.on.ca/health/english/pub/drugs/drugpro/dsguide.html>>) have very specific published guidelines that need to be followed for a drug product to be considered for their formularies.

Before discussing details about monograph preparation, it should be emphasized that the drug monograph is a powerful tool for pharmacy to guide the rational development of a drug formulary. Although pharmacy may have few, if any, votes in the ultimate adoption of a formulary agent, the monograph guides the evaluation process and is likely to be a major factor in the final decision. While monograph preparation can be very time consuming, it is extremely important and should be given proper attention.

SUMMARY PAGE

The first page of the monograph is essentially a summary of the most important information concerning the drug, and includes a specific recommendation of the action to be taken on the product. Some P&T committees only review this first sheet; however, the remainder of the document should be prepared to completely evaluate a drug product. The summary and recommendation could be placed at the end of the monograph, but it is probably best to keep it on the front to make it easier to refer to during the meeting.

The generic name, trade name, and manufacturer are self-explanatory, but the classification may require some explanation. This is meant to give the readers a very quick way of classifying the agent in their heads. It includes the prescription/controlled substance status, American Hospital Formulary Service (AHFS) classification, and FDA classification. It may also contain other classification schemes used by a particular organization, such as the Veterans' Administration.

The AHFS classification can be found in the *AHFS Drug Information* book, which is published by ASHP. This classification can help the reader determine where this new agent falls in therapy. Most of the time drugs will be evaluated for possible formulary addition before they are actually placed in that book, so it will be necessary to consult the therapeutic classification table in the front of the *AHFS Drug Information* book to decide where the product fits. The classification of similar products listed in *AHFS Drug Information* can also be checked before deciding where to categorize the new product.

The FDA classification is given to nonbiological products during the review process and is finalized when the new drug application (NDA) is approved. This classification gives some idea of the importance of the product. The classification consists of Chemical Type classification (see Table 14–3) and Therapeutic Rating classification (see Table 14–5). An FDA classification of 1P (or 1A prior to 1992) would indicate a drug that is quite an important advance and probably deserves to be on many formularies, whereas a classification of 3S (or 3C prior to 1992) is probably a "me-too" product that is not likely to be a priority item for the P&T committee. A supplementary designation (see Table 14–6) may be added to the two-character designation previously discussed. For example, a new AIDS drug might be classified 1P,AA.

The similar drug section would indicate those agents that are used for the same uses. It will usually make clear what drugs are being compared throughout. It may also just list drug classes.

TABLE 14–3. FDA CLASSIFICATIONS BY CHEMICAL TYPE

Type	Definition
1	New molecular entity not marketed in the US
2	New salt, ester, or other derivative of another drug marketed in the US
3	New formulation or dosage form of a active ingredient marketed in the US
4	New combination of drugs already marketed in the US
5	New manufacturer of a drug product already marketed by another company
6	New indication for a product already marketed
7	Drug that is already legally marketed without an approved NDA
	• First application since 1962 for a drug marketed prior to 1938.
	• First application for Drug Efficacy Study Implementation (DESI) related products that were first marketed between 1938 and 1962 without an NDA.
	• First application for DESI-related products first marketed after 1962 without NDAs. In this case, the indications may be the same or different from the legally marketed product.

SOURCES: Sanborn MD, Godwin HN, Pessetto JD. FDA drug classification system. Am J Hosp Pharm 1991;48:2659–62; Crawford SY. Changes in FDA drug classification and priority review policy. Am J Hosp Pharm 1992;49:2383, 2386; and FDA drug approvals list. <<http://www.fda.gov/cder/da/da.htm#definitions>>. Accessed 6/3/99.

TABLE 14–4. EFFECTIVENESS SUPPLEMENTAL CODE DEFINITIONS

Type	Definition
SE1	New indication or significant modification of an existing indication. Includes removal of a major limitation to use.
SE2	New dosage regimen, including an increase or decrease of daily dose, or change in administration frequency.
SE3	New route of administration.
SE4	Comparative efficacy or pharmacokinetic claim naming another drug.
SE5	Change in any section other than *Indications and Usage* that would significantly alter the patient population being treated (e.g., addition of pediatric dosing information).
SE6	Switch from prescription to over the counter (OTC).

SOURCES: Sanborn MD, Godwin HN, Pessetto JD. FDA drug classification system. Am J Hosp Pharm 1991;48:2659–62; Crawford SY. Changes in FDA drug classification and priority review policy. Am J Hosp Pharm 1992;49:2383, 2386; and FDA drug approvals list. <<http://www.fda.gov/cder/da/da.htm#definitions>>. Accessed 6/3/99.

TABLE 14–5. FDA CLASSIFICATIONS BY THERAPEUTIC POTENTIAL

Type	Definition
P	Priority handling by FDA—before 1992 this was two categories: A—Major therapeutic gain B—Moderate therapeutic gain
S	Standard handling by FDA—before 1992 this was referred to as class C, which indicated the product offered only a minor or no therapeutic gain

TABLE 14–6. FDA SUPPLEMENTARY DESIGNATORS

Type	Definition
AA	Drug used for Acquired Immunodeficiency Syndrome (AIDS) or complications of that disease
E	Drug developed or evaluated under special procedures for a life-threatening or severely debilitating illness
F	Drug under review for fraud policy; validity of data submitted being assessed
G	Drug originally given Type F designation, once its data is found to be reliable
N	Product with nonprescription marketing for some indication
V	Orphan Drug

SOURCES: Sanborn MD, Godwin HN, Pessetto JD. FDA drug classification system. Am J Hosp Pharm 1991;48:2659–62; Crawford SY. Changes in FDA drug classification and priority review policy. Am J Hosp Pharm 1992;49:2383, 2386; and FDA drug approvals list. <<http://www.fda.gov/cder/da/da.htm#definitions>>. Accessed 6/3/99.

The summary is a brief overview of the important aspects of the drug product. If there are similar products or different drugs used for the same indication, it is important to state how the drug being reviewed compares to those products. If a comparison between the agent in question and some other treatment is possible, that comparison must make up the bulk of the section, just as the comparison must be a prominent feature in every other section of the document. The summary will include efficacy, safety (e.g., adverse effects, drug interactions[81]), cost, and other factors, such as the likelihood patients would be more compliant with one agent or another[82,83] or how the therapy fits into published clinical guidelines. Information should be limited in this section to those items where a drug has a definite advantage or, if products are similar, where there would be concern about the possibility of a clinically significant difference. Items that are not clinically significant and not likely to be of concern should be left out of the summary to avoid distractions. In cases where the new drug under evaluation is indicated for a disease that has normally received nondrug treatment (e.g., surgery, radiation, physical therapy, etc.) the drug should be compared to that standard treatment. It is worth pointing out that the summary should be just that—a summary of the material presented in the body of the document. Like a conclusion of a journal article, this is not the place to put new material or, for that matter, to provide citations; both of those items belong in the body.

Finally, a definite recommendation must be made based on need, therapeutics (including outcome data and the use of evidence-based clinical guidelines), side effects, cost (full pharmacoeconomic analysis, if possible), and other items specific to the particular agent (e.g., dosage forms, convenience, dosage interval, inclusion on the formulary of third party payers, hospital antibiotic resistance patterns, potential for causing medication errors,[21] etc.), usually in that order.[84,85] Quality of life information and patient preferences should be considered, if possible. Recommendations should be specific to the circumstances in the institution in which it is being considered. Recommendations to conduct drug use evaluation on the drug (see Chap. 15), clinical guidelines to be followed (see Chap. 9), how physicians are to be educated about the new drug, and other items may also be necessary. Education may range from a simple newsletter or web page to a specific educational program and certification required before a physician can prescribe a drug product.[86]

Some people strongly object to the presence of specific recommendations being placed in the document. This may be because they do not feel it is appropriate for them to make these decisions; however, this should not be a concern if adequate research was done in preparing the evaluation. Sometimes, they have a philosophy that an unbiased decision should be reached only through a group consensus after discussing the matter in the P&T committee meeting; however, that too should not be a concern. For one thing, the person preparing the document, who also obtains input from other appropriate individuals, is in the best situation to advance a logical recommendation. Second, without a recommendation, the discussion does not have a foundation to begin, allowing the discussion to wander aimlessly to some conclusion that may not make optimal sense. Third, the lack of a specific recommendation allows emotion and "loudness" to more easily overcome logic and science. The provision of a specific recommendation is one of the best opportunities for pharmacists to have a deep and wide-ranging impact on patient care, and should not be neglected.

The recommendation must be supported by objective evidence (presented in the summary). Subjective factors that are likely to be significant from the point of view of all involved parties (i.e., physicians, pharmacists, nurses, etc.) should also be considered. Decision analysis can be used to show the best drug at the least cost (effectively pharmacoeconomic analysis; see Chap. 8).[87–90] Other factors may also be considered and given weight to indicate importance (e.g., multiattribute utility theory[91]). These methods are commonly seen in HMOs.[92] They look at the possible decisions and their likely outcome, allowing a decision to be made that is likely to lead to the most desirable outcome. Meta-analysis may also find a place in the decision making process[93]; however, it seems unlikely that most individuals evaluating products for formulary addition would have the skill or time to use that method. Tentative recommendations should be discussed with appropriate physicians and any clinical pharmacists specializing in that area of therapy before the recommendation is finalized. For example, if a cardiac medication is being evaluated, one or more cardiologists should be consulted to identify their concerns and desires. That does not mean the recommendation should necessarily be changed to what a physician wants. If the objective evidence supports the original recommendation, that is the one that should be made; however, it is necessary to demonstrate that the physicians' concerns were addressed.

Overall, the items most likely to be added to the formulary include those that are unique, those that serve the specific population of a hospital and, unfortunately, those with the biggest marketing drive by the marketer. Multiple ingredient products are least likely to be added.[94]

The recommendation should be whatever logical conclusion is supported by the objective evidence and the needs of the institution, including medical staff needs, distribution concerns, and drug availability. Whenever possible, it is best to follow the ASHP guidelines for recommendations, which would place the drug into one or a combination of the following groups.[79]

- Added for uncontrolled use by the entire medical staff
- Added for monitored use—No restrictions placed on use, but the drug will be monitored to determine appropriateness of use. This is a tie-in to the quality assurance process.[11] *Please note:* this category does not mean that the patient is monitored, because that is necessary for every drug. It means that the quality of how the drug is used is monitored.
- Added with restrictions—The drug is added to the drug formulary, but there are restrictions on who may prescribe it and/or how it may be used (e.g., specific indications, certain physicians or physician groups, certain policies to be followed).

- Conditional—Available for use by the entire medical staff for a finite period of time.
- Not added/deleted from formulary.

Note that there may be different recommendations presented for specific strengths, forms, sizes, and so forth of a drug being reviewed; however, such detail sometimes does not result in real benefit.[95]

Most drugs should be added for uncontrolled use or not be added, simply because the three other categories cause greater work for the pharmacy or other departments. As a side point, if a recommendation to not add the drug to the formulary is approved, it is often good to require a time period before the drug can be considered again (typically 6 months) to prevent heavy political action pushing through approval of a less than desirable drug, just because the P&T committee gets tired of having it requested every month. Monitored use is occasionally needed if there is concern that a drug might be used in some inappropriate manner or has a great risk for adverse events. A limited quality assurance evaluation would be conducted until it is evident that the drug is being appropriately used or not causing adverse events. One example where monitored use might be considered is an expensive biotechnology product that only has one or two approved indications, but multiple investigational uses, where it could be inappropriately prescribed without an investigational protocol. Also, a very toxic product might be monitored to see if adverse effects are appropriately addressed by the prescriber. As electronic quality assurance methods become standard, monitoring may be used to a greater extent, but is seldom justified in systems requiring the pharmacist to manually collect data. Conditional addition to the formulary is a recommendation of last resort, simply because it is much easier to keep a drug off the formulary rather than try to delete an inappropriate drug that is being used by physicians. This type of approval might be used when it is very difficult to clearly determine whether an agent will benefit the institution or if available data are limited at the time of the P&T meeting. If conditional approval is given, it is absolutely necessary to specify when the P&T committee will reconsider whether the drug should be retained on the formulary.

The added with restrictions choice deserves more explanation. Occasionally there are drugs that should be added to a drug formulary, but are dangerous,[96] or prone to misuse or overuse. This could include agents such as antineoplastics, thrombolytics, and third or fourth generation cephalosporins.[97] In such cases it may be desirable to limit the use of the drugs in some manner.[98] For example, the antineoplastics might be limited to prescriptions from oncologists or a defined group that might include a few nononcology physicians (e.g., rheumatologists using methotrexate). Specific antibiotics might be limited to either infectious disease physicians or to specific, culture-proven diagnoses. Often antibiotics may be restricted to a specific length of therapy, after which a new order must be written or the original order will automatically be discontinued. Other restrictions could include specific floors or areas of the institution where the drug may be prescribed or requiring that the physician must receive counterdetailing by the pharmacist before the drug is dispensed.[99] Relatively new methods of restriction involve formularies for MCOs, where there may be a cap on how many times a patient may receive a drug (e.g., one time use for nicotine patches to quit smoking), how much a patient may receive at one time (e.g., 3-month ambulatory supply) or whether the practitioners (e.g., physicians, pharmacists) may receive financial or other incentives to cut back on the use of specific products.[28] Whenever possible, restrictions should be based on objective data, such as that obtained from DUE or medication use evaluation (MUE). Some physicians will object to restrictions, but remember that the physicians are given privileges to prescribe drugs and not rights. Usually, this is not much of a problem because good physicians realize there is a reason for the restrictions.

The real problem, however, is the desire to use this category much to often in an attempt to ensure proper use of all drugs. Although restrictions can be effective in changing usage of specific formulary agents,[100] every time a restricted drug is prescribed, more time and effort by the pharmacy, MCO, and perhaps the physician is required to ensure compliance with restrictions. At the very least, a policy and procedure, and probably appropriate forms, will need to be developed or adapted, and be presented as part of the drug recommendation to the P&T committee. Therefore, unless a computer system can eliminate much of the effort, there needs to be great restraint used when deciding to recommend a drug be added to the drug formulary with restrictions. Oftentimes, adding with monitoring may be a viable alternative. A relatively new twist to the "restrictions" or "monitoring" types of approval is the use of critical or clinical pathways.[101,102] In this case, a drug may be approved for use in a particular manner for the treatment of a particular disease. These "critical pathways" may be established for several target populations or target diseases, where additional guidance of patient treatments can result in significant improvement in patient care and/or significant decreases in costs. Because a great deal of time is necessary to develop and manage these critical pathways, they will most likely only be seen in a few areas of any institution at any given time. The recommendation should state that whether a drug is to be used as part of some clinical guidelines or disease state management (DSM) program (see Chap. 9).[103]

While the decision to add or delete a drug from the formulary is seldom black or white, a general rule of thumb may be helpful. If the drug is less expensive or the same price as others, and more efficacious or safer, add it to the formulary. If the drug is more expensive without added benefit, do not add to the formulary (or delete it from the formulary if it is already on it). The problem comes when the drug is more expensive and also has more benefits. In that case, careful analysis of the literature and weighing of the institution's needs must be carried out. This is the gray area that has no "right" answer, but a most "appropriate" decision must be found. This latter decision may also involve "conditional" or "monitored" use.

Whenever a recommendation is made to add a new agent, consideration should be given to the possibility of removing agents that will no longer be necessary. This whole process can be used as a way of cleaning up extraneous agents on the formulary; however, removal of agents can be difficult if the products are frequently prescribed (*note:* it is often worthwhile to annually review a list of products that have seen little or no use in the previous year in an attempt to remove these products from the formulary). Whether removing agents individually or through a review of an entire therapeutic class, there needs to be adequate information presented to the P&T committee to show the product is no longer necessary. The reasons for removal may include superior agent(s) on the formulary, safety, low or no use, and high cost.[50] A timetable for deleting these agents from the formulary must then be developed and the physicians must be informed when the agents will no longer be available. Use should be monitored and follow-up is necessary to ensure that formulary deletions proceed smoothly.[104]

Finally, therapeutic interchange or substitution must be considered.[105] If these concepts are acceptable to the institution and legal in the state, it may be appropriate that the new drug be used to substitute for a less desirable agent, or vice-versa. The AMA[3] defines therapeutic interchange as "authorized exchange of therapeutic alternatives in accordance with previously established and approved written guidelines or protocols within a formulary system." An example would be the use of cefazolin in specific doses whenever any other first generation injectable cephalosporin is ordered. The reasons for therapeutic interchange could be to save money,[106,107] improve patient outcomes, decrease adverse effects, or obtain other benefits. Therapeutic interchange has been shown to decrease costs without adversely affecting patient outcomes.[16,108]

Therapeutic interchange is considered acceptable to the AMA, unlike therapeutic substitution, which they define as the "act of dispensing a therapeutic alternative for the drug product prescribed without prior authorization of the prescriber" (*please note:* prior authorization may be a blanket authorization, not a specific authorization for each case[109]). Therapeutic interchange has also been found to be acceptable by other organizations, including the American College of Clinical Pharmacy (ACCP), American College of Physicians (ACP) (they require immediate prior consent by the physician),[110] ASHP, American Pharmaceutical Association (APHA), American Association of Colleges of Pharmacy (AACP), Academy of Managed Care Pharmacy (AMCP),[111] and the American Society of Consultant Pharmacists (ASCP).[12,113] The ACCP spells out the concept in great detail and suggests that it not only be conducted under the auspices of a P&T-type committee, but also that it specifically include DUE, a set method for informing the physicians and other staff that interchange is taking place (should be well planned and thorough[114]), and a mechanism under which the therapeutic interchange policies may be overridden in specific cases. Other practical aspects, such as communication forms, policies and procedures, medical staff bylaw changes, and other items may need to be addressed by the institution.[115] Electronic means to provide authorization for interchange may be seen more in the future.[116] Outside of an institution (e.g., ambulatory environment) therapeutic interchange may not be as easy to implement due to practical procedure methods and because patients are not as closely monitored; however, it may still be possible.[117,118]

Generic substitution is also considered by the P&T committee in some cases, but many pharmacies consider generic substitution to be one of their responsibilities and do not take such decisions to the P&T committee for approval. The one exception may be drugs with narrow therapeutic indexes (e.g., anticonvulsants), where a P&T committee may determine a list of products where generic substitution is not allowed,[119] although the FDA insists that such precautions are unnecessary.[120]

All of the material on recommendations presented above may be confusing. Simply the most logical decision to benefit the patient and the institution should be recommended to the P&T committee.

BODY OF THE MONOGRAPH

Many parts of the body of the monograph are self-explanatory, and will not be discussed further. Some specific points, however, do need to be made about the body. First, the body may not always be reviewed by the P&T committee and, even if presented, may be covered only briefly. The body needs to be written as a means to compile the information for reference and further information. Importantly, it serves as a way of bringing all of the information together in a logical order for preparation of the summary. Some P&T committees will want to review the data presented in the body of the monograph, but all need to know that the clinical data was reviewed adequately.

Second, effort must be made to ensure that the drug in question has been adequately compared to other therapies (whether drug, surgical, radiation, or something else). The person preparing a monograph must go through each section and ask themselves "Have I compared this drug to the gold standard?" If not, there should either be a good reason for the lack of comparison or some explanation must be put in the section. Sometimes, there will be no published comparison with other drugs or therapies. For example, when anistreplase was first marketed there were only comparisons to streptokinase available, but physicians wanted to know how the drug compared to alteplase. In that case, information comparing both drugs to streptokinase was used to discern how the drugs would compare to each other. Scientifically, this leaves much to be desired, but sometimes there is no choice. Other indirect methods of comparison may also be necessary. If at all possible, studies directly comparing the drug being evaluated to the standard of therapy should be used. Also, data from outcome studies can be very important to put in the evaluation, including such hard to quantify items as quality of life.[121]

Third, every item should be addressed, even if only to state that information was not available or that it is not applicable (absorption of IV drugs for example). This follows the rule that "if it was not written down, it was not done," or in this case was not reviewed.

Finally, the source of the information should be mentioned; any important statement of fact must be referenced, or must be suspected of being inaccurate. The package insert (now often available from <<http://www.fda.gov/cder/approval/index.htm>> for newly approved products) will serve as a basis for some of the information, particularly to define what is the FDA-approved information, but other references must be used to fill in the gaps and to back up that information.

The Pharmacologic Data section is often one of the briefest. A simple one-paragraph explanation of the proposed mechanism of action and how it differs from the comparator agent(s) usually will suffice for the drug in question. More may be needed if the agent is being compared to a drug with an entirely different mechanism of action (e.g., comparing a new ACE inhibitor to a calcium channel-blocking agent). If the agent under consideration is an antibiotic, the spectrum of activity should be discussed, which will be much longer.

The Therapeutic Indications section normally requires the most work. This section may be broken into three main subsections. The first is a brief coverage of what indications the drug has been used to treat. It is necessary to clearly indicate which uses are FDA approved, non-FDA approved but reasonably supported and likely to be seen, and those that are early in investigation. The second subsection explains how the product and any comparison products fit into any published clinical guidelines. The third subsection consists of abstracts of clinical studies supporting the various uses (see Chap. 11). In the rare case where a product only has one use, data from several studies on that use should be reviewed in the monograph. If there are multiple uses, one well-conducted study for each FDA-approved or likely to be seen indication is usually reviewed (more can be added, but may be redundant and provide no added benefit). If there are several similar studies, one may be covered in depth with a statement at the end of the paragraph that the use is supported by other studies (giving their citations). If one well-conducted study for a use cannot be found, several less desirable studies may be needed to provide sufficient information. Whenever possible, clinical comparison studies should be used. When reviewing newly approved drugs, it is not unusual to find that no comparison studies have been published. In that case, a simple efficacy study should be used. In cases where no published human trials are available, unless there are extenuating circumstances, the drug should generally not be added to a drug formulary until sufficient published information is available. An example of extenuating circumstances would be when a new drug is available for a previously untreatable illness. In that case, the philosophy of anything is better than nothing may apply.

The Bioavailability/Pharmacokinetics section is similar to what would be found in most publications, but the information may be difficult to find for some new drugs. In some cases, a new dosage form may be considered in a drug evaluation. For example, when a drug is released in IV form, its use may be entirely different from the oral form, so the P&T committee might separately consider it. A change in route, however, does not necessarily mean that elimination is significantly different in the same patient population. Therefore, oral data may be more useful than no information. Whenever possible, a table comparing the drug in question to other products may be helpful.

The Dosage Form section is a good place to point out both the limitations in dosage forms available for some drugs (perhaps the drug in question is available only as an oral solid, but the gold standard is available in oral solid, oral liquid, and injectable forms). This section can also be used to discuss unusual preparation directions or pointing out which product would be easier, quicker, and less expensive to prepare.

A problem often develops in the Known Adverse Effects/Toxicities section. Quite simply, some drugs have so many adverse effects listed that pages could be written. Instead concentrate on the serious adverse effects, common adverse effects or both for the specific drug and the drug class. Whenever possible, incidence and severity should be included. An incidence comparison table listing the agent under consideration and other similar agents may be an efficient and informative method to show the material. If there are many rare, minor adverse effects, a statement to that effect can be listed at the end of the discussion. Conversely, other agents may have very little information available on adverse effects, simply because they are too new. In that case, it may be necessary to discuss adverse effects common to that class of agent, making it clear that they have not yet been seen with the new drug, but are possible. In any case, the new agent should be compared to other agents used for the same indication to determine whether there are any advantages. Keep in mind that older agents may have 20 years of side effect reports, whereas a number of adverse effects of the new agent may not have yet been discovered.

The Patient Monitoring Guidelines and Patient Information sections listed are items not suggested by ASHP. These sections were added for use in the ambulatory environment, although they can be quite informative in any practice area. The Patient Information section complies with the OBRA '90 standards for prospective drug use review (DUR).

The final section to be discussed is the Cost Comparison section, where the product being reviewed is compared in price to other similar products. Typically, three or four medications (possibly including both trade and generic products) are compared, although sometimes it is necessary to compare a dozen or more products or dosage forms. Preferably, a pharmacoeconomic analysis should be prepared[122] (see Chap. 8), because the seemingly more expensive agent may turn out to be less expensive overall because it decreases the length of hospitalization, degree of monitoring, or number of adverse events that would otherwise occur.[123] Often, a full pharmacoeconomic review is not practical because of lack of time or expertise, although most large hospitals do report doing a formal economic analysis of some kind for each drug reviewed for possible formulary addition.[5] With particularly expensive products, a comprehensive pharmacoeconomic analysis becomes more necessary.[35,124] Even when a full pharmacoeconomic analysis is not practical, any pertinent information that could be used in a full analysis should be included.

In some cases, a simple price comparison can be prepared using just the cost of the drugs and the frequency of administration. Such a price comparison must consider that the patient may be getting medications both within an institution and after returning home, because institutional pharmacies may get considerable discounts. Therefore, both the institution's cost for the medication and the average wholesale price (AWP) should be considered. Some medications are extremely inexpensive to the institution, making it tempting to include those agents on the formulary instead of similar therapeutic agents; however, if the AWP is quite high, the patient may not be able to afford the product in the community. In those cases, it may not be a good item to carry on the formulary. Also, the differences in package sizes and frequency of administration must be considered. In most cases, products can be compared on the cost of a typical day's therapy at a relatively normal dose; however, in some cases, a different approach may be necessary. For example, an antineoplastic agent may need to be compared with other agents based on a per cycle or per cost of therapeutic regimen basis. Another example encountered by some in the past was Norplant (an implantable contraceptive agent effective for 5 years). The cost of both the drug and the implantation procedure needed to be compared to a five-year supply of other contraceptive agents (in cases like this, over a period of years, it may be necessary to include calculations of inflation or other factors likely to change over the years[125]). Other costs should also be considered when possible, such as drug preparation costs, administration costs, laboratory tests, monitoring requirements, and changes of length of stay or therapy; after all, it is not a savings overall if costs are simply shifted from the pharmacy (i.e., drug price) to the laboratory (i.e., monitoring costs).[126] Some pharmacies even include such items as the cost to order and hold the drug and the cost of preparing the evaluation of the drug for the P&T committee.[127] Also, it is becoming more common to take into account some more difficult to assess items, such as the probability and cost of therapeutic failure in comparison to other similar agents, impact of specific drug therapy on other health care costs (a drug may be cheaper, but require an increase in the cost of other nondrug therapies for the patient), and the cost of adverse drug effects.[17] Because these items may depend on the characteristics of the patients (e.g., age, socioeconomic status, education level, etc.), the figures used are necessarily going to be uncertain. In some cases, however, they will be very important in the final formulary decisions; a drug that at first glance seems more expensive, may be found to actually cost the institution less in the end.[128] Also, it is necessary to consider nondrug therapy (e.g., surgery, radiation therapy, physical therapy) in the comparison when they are legitimate alternatives to drug therapy. Overall, the goal is to ensure that the comparison makes sense and takes into consideration all of the relevant economic factors. Although some people think that cost is emphasized too much in formulary decisions, it is still an extremely important item. Some drugs cost thousands of dollars per dose, which can quickly deplete a pharmacy department's budget and significantly affect the economic status of an institution.

Drug Formulary

Wherever a drug formulary system is in place, there is usually a drug formulary published, as a hard copy "book" and/or in electronic format (e.g., web site). In its simplest form, the drug formulary contains a list of drugs that are available under that formulary system. This list will be arranged alphabetically and/or by therapeutic class (AHFS classification usually), and usually contains information on the dosage forms, strengths, names (e.g., generic, trade, chemical), and ingredients of combination products. Many of these publications contain a great deal more material related to the drugs, including a summary of indications, side effects, dosing, use restrictions, and other clinical information.[129]

Often, drug formularies will have a number of other sections that may include information about the P&T committee and pharmacy department, policy and procedure information (e.g., how to obtain nonformulary drugs, how to request a drug be placed on the formulary), laboratory test information, dietary supplement charts, kinetics information, approved abbreviations, sodium content, nomograms, dosage equivalency charts, apothecary/metric equivalents, drug–food interactions, skin test directions, cost data, antimicrobial therapy charts, and any other brief clinical information tables felt to be necessary. Use of linking in web sites can make such information much more readily available and usable, because users can hop back and forth between these tables and the drug list. MCOs may need to include the procedure they use to limit choice of drugs by physicians, pharmacists, and patients.[65]

In institutional pharmacies, a hard copy book is normally published once a year. Often it was published in a pocket-sized format that could be carried in lab coats by physicians, pharmacists, and nurses. There may also have been a larger loose-leaf binder published that could be updated regularly throughout the year. Such a book is no longer justified. It is now becoming more common for this reference to be available electronically. The electronic form can be made more widely available and can be kept continually up to date by making changes, as necessary, at one central location (an example can be found at <<http://www.intmed.mcw.edu/drug/antibiotics.html>>). Also, the electronic formulary coupled with physician order entry may lead to the most efficient and effective way to encourage or enforce the use of formulary items,[130–132] although there is some evidence that electronic messages may be ignored by physicians.[133] Other directions can also be embedded to improve drug therapy.

The publication of a hard copy drug formulary can be a very time-consuming process. If at all possible it is best if the pharmacy can download the information about drug products carried in the institution from their computer system or a separate database management program to a word processing program.[134] This list can then be manipulated to a more readable and understandable format without a big problem in transcription errors, and the other clinical information can easily be placed into the document (particularly if it is just being updated from a previous year). Almost any high-end word processing program or desktop publishing program can be used to do this, producing a printer ready copy that can be more inexpensively reproduced, in both time and dollars, than a typeset copy. Later, use of colored paper and an edge index can make use of the final product easier. Even with the availability of computer technology, the production of a drug formulary is a very time intensive effort, requiring a few weeks to several months of work. Fortunately, technical and clerical personnel can do much of the work. One or more pharmacists, however, should carefully proof all material to ensure it is correct. Often this task will be divided up so that somebody involved with purchasing will check the drug list, an administrator will review the policies and procedures, and a clinician will update the clinical information.

Pharmacies can also use commercial vendors who will take their drug lists and prepare a professional looking formulary (hard copy and/or electronic). These commercial formularies can also include condensed monograph information (e.g., indications, dosing, side effects, etc.), which can be of value to the prescriber.

Preferably, the pharmacy can use the information on its computer system to create a formulary that is constantly up to date. The information can be accessed as part of the prescription order software and/or it may be interfaced with web software. The latter makes it possible to embed other information easily, but may take further work by the pharmacist. In any case, this information should be available to the physician and other health care professionals wherever necessary, potentially even by wireless connection. As a side note, many institutions do not want information about their formularies readily available to individuals not directly associated with the institution (e.g., pharmaceutical manufacturers), but this should not be a problem using Virtual Private Network (VPN) software and firewalls to secure the data, allowing access to only qualified individuals.

Policies and Procedures

Occasionally, policies and procedures must be developed to support the rational use of medications. While the pharmacy department may decide it needs to have its own policies and procedures for internal functions, that is not the focus of this discussion.[135] Instead, policies and procedures for the use of medications in an institution, clinic, or other institution will be discussed.

To begin, the definitions for policies and procedures should be considered.[136] A *policy* is a broad general statement that describes the goals and purposes of the document. *Procedures* are specific actions to be taken. In some ways, policies and procedures may resemble a cookbook-type approach, in that a set of steps to be accomplished are described in order. Taken together, these policies and procedures may be a logical, step-by-step explanation of why and where a product may be used and how to use it, along with a brief introductory statement describing why the process is necessary.

Before developing specific policies and procedures, the first step should be deciding whether they are necessary at all. In other words, is there a good reason for the existence of the particular policies and procedures, and are they likely to be used? This can be looked at as a risk-benefit decision. For example, is there sufficient risk that a particular medication will be used incorrectly (i.e., prepared wrong, administered wrong, used for an inappropriate indication, etc.) to make it worthwhile to develop policies and procedures? Generally, the answer will be "no," but in a certain number of cases, policies and procedures may be necessary. Examples of where policies and procedures may be necessary include thrombolytic agents (where the drug can cause serious or fatal effects if used improperly), antibiotics (where it is found that expensive, broad-spectrum anti-biotics are being used where amoxicillin should suffice), injectable drugs (where specific individuals who will administer the medication and the process will be defined),[137] or even for drugs where reimbursement may be a problem.

Once a decision is reached to develop the policies and procedures, a logical and orderly course should be followed. It is undesirable to wait until after problems occur before deciding that policies and procedures are necessary. This process should follow the drug formulary process, where a mechanism is set up to help determine that policies and procedures are necessary. In many cases, policies and procedures for use of drugs likely to be misused may be developed in conjunction with consideration for addition to the drug formulary.

As in any process, it is first necessary to decide who will be coordinating the effort and the likely endpoint. That person, or designee, will then need to investigate various sources for background material necessary to develop the policies and procedures. This might include doing a literature search, talking to experts in the field, talking to other institutions that have already developed policies on the same topic, reviewing published professional (e.g., <<http://www.ashp.org/bestpractices/intro.htm/>>) or clinical guidelines (e.g., <<http://www.guideline.gov>>), and checking the institution's requirements for developing policies and procedures. In particular, it is necessary for the person developing the policy and procedure to have good communications with those who will be affected. After all, if the final product is looked at as being more trouble than it is worth, it is not likely to be followed. Where the policy and procedures fit into other institutional policies and procedures will also have to be evaluated. Finally, a document should be written, reviewed, and revised, using many of the skills outlined in Chap. 11.

Once the policy and procedure is finished, it will need to be approved by the same mechanism that drug formulary changes go through (i.e., P&T committee, medical executive committee, etc.). The approval and/or effective date for the policy and procedures should be recorded on the document itself to ensure they are not confused with earlier or later documents. A plan for implementing the policy and procedures will need to be developed. Forms may need to be prepared and distributed. Copies of the policy and procedures will have to be distributed to those affected (preferably on the computer network), and inservices will need to be planned and given. At that point, the policy and procedures can be implemented, perhaps in conjunction with the first appearance of a particular agent on the drug formulary. That is not the end of the process, however. At some point, the policy and procedures should be evaluated to determine if it is being properly followed and having the desired effect as a part of a quality assurance plan. Also, the policy and procedures will need to be reviewed, revised (if necessary), and reapproved on a regular basis (probably once a year). As part of that process, the actual need for the policy and procedures should be reconsidered. The policy and procedures should be eliminated if no longer needed. One way to determine whether the policy and procedures are consulted is if they are on a web server, where the number of times the specific page is opened is recorded. Superseded copies (i.e., previous versions) of the policies and procedures should be kept on file for background and for legal purposes.

It is also necessary to have policies and procedures for the operation of the P&T committee itself. For example, how are new drugs requested for addition to the formulary, how can nonformulary drugs be used, what procedure is used to evaluate new drugs, the composition of the committee, and other committee functions (e.g., conflict of interest)? These have been discussed elsewhere in the chapter and will not be dealt with further at this point.

Clinical Guidelines

P&T committees may be involved with the development, alteration (to fit local circumstances), and/or approval of evidence-based clinical guidelines. The reader is directed to Chap. 9 to obtain further information.

Conclusion

The pharmacy department can have a major impact on the quality of drug therapy in an institution through participation in P&T committee functions and activities described in this chapter. Although there are many "right" ways that may be used in addition to those outlined above, those described can be successfully used to improve drug therapy.

Study Questions

1. What is the P&T Committee, what are its functions, and how does the committee relate to a pharmacy department?

2. How should a pharmacy/pharmacist be involved in supporting a P&T Committee?

3. Define drug formulary and formulary system. How do those items relate to one another?

4. Describe how a drug may be evaluated objectively for formulary addition.

5. Define policy. Define procedure.

6. What are the steps in preparing policies and procedures?

REFERENCES

1. Redman RL, Mays DA. Data analysis. Drug information services in the managed care setting. Drug Benefit Trends 1997;9:28–40.
2. Jenkins A. Formulary development by community pharmacists. Pharm J 1996;256:861–3.
3. AMA Board of Trustees. Drug formularies and therapeutic interchange. Recommendations adopted at the American Medical Association (AMA) House of Delegates Interim Meeting 1993. Chicago: American Medical Association; 1993.
4. CAMH Comprehensive Accreditation Manual for Hospitals. Oakbrook Terrace, IL: Joint Commission on Accreditation of Healthcare Organizations; 2000.
5. Mannebach MA, Ascione FJ, Gaither CA, Bagozzi RP, Cohen IA, Ryan ML. Activities, functions, and structure of pharmacy and therapeutics committees in large teaching hospitals. Am J Health-Syst Pharm 1999;56:622–8.
6. Miller WA. Making the Pharmacy and Therapeutics Committee more effective. Curr Concepts Hosp Pharm Manage 1986; Summer:10–15.
7. Doherty EC. The JCAHO Agenda for Change: what changes in pharmacy and P&T activities do you need to prepare for in 1994. Hosp Formul 1994;29:54–68.

8. The Joint Commission on Accreditation of Healthcare Organizations. 1995 Comprehensive Accreditation Manual for Hospitals. Oakbrook Terrace, IL: Joint Commission on Accreditation of Healthcare Organizations; 1994.

9. Plumridge RJ, Stoelwinder JU, Rucker TD. Drug and therapeutics committees: the relationships among structure, function, and effectiveness. Hosp Pharm 1993;28:492–3, 496–8, 508.

10. ASHP statement on the Pharmacy and Therapeutics Committee. Am J Hosp Pharm 1992;49: 2008–9.

11. Chase P, Bell J, Smith P, Fallik A. Redesign of the P&T committee around continuous quality improvement principles. P&T 1995 Jan;20(1):25–6, 29–30, 32, 34, 37–8, 40.

12. Mutnick AH, Ross MB. Formulary management at a tertiary care teaching hospital. Pharm Pract Manage Q 1997;17(1):63–87.

13. Butler CD, Manchester R. The P&T Committee: descriptive survey of activities and time requirements. Hosp Formul 1986;21:89–98.

14. Chi J. When R.Ph.s talk P&T Committees listen. Hosp Pharm Rep 1994;8(5):1, 7–8.

15. Gannon K. More power to you. Pharmacists flex their muscles and exert greater influence on P&T committees. Hosp Pharm Rep 1998;12(2):18–20.

16. Croft CL, Crane VS. Redesign of P&T Committee functions and processes: a model. Formulary 1998;33:1105–22.

17. Crane VS, Gonzalez ER, Hull BL. How to develop a proactive formulary system. Hosp Formul 1994;29:700–10.

18. Poirier TI, Vorbach M, Bache T. Linking a policy on nonformulary drugs to the FDA's therapeutic-potential classification system. Am J Hosp Pharm 1994;51:2277–8.

19. Green JA, Chawla AK, Fong PA. Evaluating a restrictive formulary system by assessing nonformulary-drug requests. Am J Hosp Pharm 1985;42:1537–41.

20. Hailemeskel B, Kelvas M. Nonformulary drug requests as a guide in formulary system management. Am J Health-Syst Pharm 1999;56:818, 820.

21. Adding drugs to the formulary: your work is never done. Hosp Pharm 1999;34(7):828.

22. Shea BF, Churchill WW, Powell SH, Cooley TW, Maguire JH. P&T committee overview: Brigham and Women's Hospital. Pharm Pract Manage Q 1998;17(4):76–83.

23. ASHP statement on the formulary system. Am J Hosp Pharm 1983;40:1384–5.

24. Rucker TD, Schiff G. Drug formularies: myths-in-formation. Med Care 1990;28:928–42.

25. Chi J. Hospital consultant foresees dim future for drug formularies. Drug Topics 1999;19:67.

26. Horn SD, Sharkey PD, Tracy DM, Horn C, James B, Goodwin F. Intended and unintended consequences of HMO cost-containment strategies: results from the managed care outcomes project. Am J Manage Care 1996;2:253–64.

27. Horn SD. Unintended consequences of drug formularies. Am J Health-Syst Pharm 1996;53: 2204–6.

28. Goldberg RB. Managing the pharmacy benefit: the formulary system. J Managed Care Pharm 1997;3(5):565–73.

29. Formulary effectiveness: many questions, but few clear answers. Consult Pharm 1996;11(7):635.

30. Curtiss FR. Drug formularies provide a path to best care. Am J Health-Syst Pharm 1996; 53:2201–3.

31. Formularies and generics drive up health resource use, study suggests. Am J Health-Syst Pharm 1996;53:971–5.

32. Horn SD, Sharkey PD, Phillips-Harris C. Formulary limitations and the elderly: results from the managed care outcomes project. Am J Managed Care 1998;4:1105–13.

33. Hepler CD. Where is the evidence for formulary effectiveness. Am J Health-Syst Pharm 1997;54:95.

34. Palmer MA, Hartman SK, Gervais S. Introducing a formulary system in long-term care facilities: initial experience. Consult Pharm 1994;9:307–14.

35. Shepard MD, Salzman RD. The formulary decision-making process in a Health Maintenance Organisation setting. PharmacoEconomics 1994;5:29–38.

36. Kreling DH, Mucha RE. Drug product management in health maintenance organizations. Am J Hosp Pharm 1992;49:374–81.

37. Zachary R. Formulary management from a health maintenance organization (HMO) perspective. J Pharm Pract 1994;VII(2):68–73.

38. Meszaros E. Unification: from mirage to reality. Managed Healthcare 1995;5(Suppl):S18,S28–S29.

39. Fiorello SJ. Developing and implementing a statewide formulary system: one state's experience. Formulary 1995;30:808–11.

40. Babington MA. Use of a geriatric formulary in long-term care. Medical Interface 1997;10(1): 87–8, 115.

41. Navarro RP. Formularies in long-term care. Medical Interface 1997;10(1):81, 84.

42. Fleming H Jr. Formulary flap. Should chains create their own drug lists. Drug Topics 1998; 142(1):44.

43. Bruzek RJ, Dullinger D. Drug formulary: the cornerstone of a managed pharmacy program. J Pharm Pract 1992;V(2):75–81.

44. Muirhead G. Learning to live with formularies. Drug Topics 1994;138(4):38–43.

45. Pearce MJ, Begg EJ. A review of limited lists and formularies. Are they cost-effective? PharmacoEconomics 1992;1:191–202.

46. Langley PC. Meeting the information needs of drug purchasers: the evolution of formulary submission guidelines. Clin Ther 1999;21(4):768–87.

47. ASHP guidelines on formulary system management. Am J Hosp Pharm 1992;49:648–52.

48. Hitchens K. Formulary integration: can it be accomplished? Hosp Pharm Rep 1996 July; 10:52–3.

49. Gannon K. The right elements can ease strain of formulary integration. Hosp Pharm Rep 1996; 10(1):1, 8, 11.

50. Kelly WN, Rucker TD. Considerations in deciding which drugs should be in a formulary. J Pharm Pract 1994;VII(2):51–7.

51. Muirhead G. When formularies collide. Hospitals vs. health plans. Hosp Pharm Report 1994;8(10):1, 8.

52. 1999 accreditation standards address public concerns, says NCQA. Am J Health-Syst Pharm 1998;55:2221, 2225.

53. North GLT. Handling nonformulary requests for returning or transfer patients. Am J Hosp Pharm 1994;51:2360, 2364.

54. Davis FA. Formularies: a dangerous concept for patients. Private Practice 1991;Sept:11–17.

55. Shulkin DJ. Enhancing the role of physicians in the cost-effective use of pharmaceuticals. Hosp Formul 1994;29:262–73.

56. Sloan FA, Gordon GS, Cocks DL. Hospital drug formularies and use of hospital services. Med Care 1993;31:851–67.

57. Hazlet TK, Hu T-W. Association between formulary strategies and hospital drug expenditures. Am J Hosp Pharm 1992;49:2207–10.

58. Pickette S, Hanish L. Dealing with demands for nonformulary drugs. Am J Hosp Pharm 1992;49:2920, 2923.

59. Corliss DA. Computer-assisted help desk for handling drug benefits. Am J Health-Syst Pharm 1977;54:1941–2, 1945.

60. Cardinale V. Alternative medicine: the law, the marketplace, the formulary. Hosp Pharm Rep 1999;13(7):15.

61. Is alternative medicine poised for hospital formularies. Drug Utilization Review 1999 May; 15(5):65–8.

62. Brubaker ML. Setting up the herbal formulary system for an alternative medicine clinic. Am J Health-Syst Pharm 1998;55:435–6.

63. Beal FC. Herbals and homeopathic remedies as formulary items. Am J Health-Syst Pharm 1998;55:1266–7.

64. Johnson ST, Wordell CJ. Homeopathic and herbal medicine: considerations for formulary evaluation. Formulary 1997;32:1166–73.

65. NCQA draft accreditation standards for 2000 address formularies. Am J Health-Syst Pharm 1999;56:846.

66. Survey reveals continued HMO shift toward closed and partially closed formularies. Formulary 1997;32:781–2.

67. Survey Finds HMOs, PBMs still moving to restricted formularies, quickly advancing in informatics. Formulary 1998;33:622, 625.

68. Abramowitz PW. Controlling financial variables—changing prescribing patterns. Am J Hosp Pharm 1984;41:503–15.

69. Open formularies improve oncology outcomes in capitated care system. Formulary 1996;31: 878,881.

70. TennCare formulary restrictions hurt patient care, survey says. Formulary 1996;31(6):443.

71. Chren M-M, Landefeld CS. Physicians' behavior and their interactions with drug companies. JAMA 1994;271:684–9.

72. Senthilkumaran K, Shatz SM, Kalies RF. Computer-based support system for formulary decisions. Am J Hosp Pharm 1987;44:1362–6.

73. Janknegt R, Steenhoek A. The system of objectified judgement analysis (SOJA). A tool in rational drug selection for formulary inclusion. Drugs 1997;53(4):550–62.

74. Janknegt R, van den Broek PJ, Kulberg BJ, Stobberingh E. Glycopeptides: drug selection by means of the SOJA method. Eur Hosp Pharm 1997;3(4):127–35.

75. Berghelli JA. Conflict of interest policy approved. P&T 1995;20:497.

76. Palmer MA. Developing a conflict-of-interest policy for the pharmacy and therapeutics committee. Am J Hosp Pharm 1987;44:2012–14.

77. Fredrick DS, Maddock JR, Graman PS. Hashing out a policy on conflicts of interest for a P&T committee. Am J Health-Syst Pharm 1995;52:2791–2.

78. Wade WE, Spruill WJ, Taylor AT, Longe RL, Hawkins DW. The expanding role of pharmacy and therapeutics committees. The 1990s and beyond. PharmacoEconomics 1996;10(2):123–8.

79. ASHP technical assistance bulletin on the evaluation of drugs for formularies. Am J Hosp Pharm 1988;45:386–7.

80. Majercik PL, May JR, Longe RL, Johnson MH. Evaluation of pharmacy and therapeutics committee drug evaluation reports. Am J Hosp Pharm 1985;42:1073–6.

81. Chan L-N. Consider potential for drug interactions during formulary review. Am J Health-Syst Pharm 2000;57:391.

82. Feldman JA, DeTullio PL. Medication noncompliance: an issue to consider in the drug selection process. Hosp Formul 1994;29:204–11.

83. Sesin GP. Therapeutic decision-making: a model for formulary evaluation. Drug Intell Clin Pharm 1986;20:581–3.

84. Hedblom EC. Pharmacoeconomic and outcomes data in the managed care formulary decision-making process. P&T 1995;20:462–4, 468, 471–3.

85. Klink B. Formulary influences. Drug Top 1998;142(20):72.

86. Dedrick S, Kessler JM. Formulary evaluation teams: Duke University Medical Center's approach to P&T committee reorganization. Formulary 1999;34:47–51.

87. Kresel JJ, Hutchings HC, MacKay DN, Weinstein MC, Read JL, Taylor-Halvorsen K, et al. Application of decision analysis to drug selection for formulary addition. Hosp Formul 1987;22:658–76.

88. Szymusiak-Mutnick B, Mutnick AH. Application of decision analysis in antibiotic formulary choices. j Pharm Technol 1994;10:23–6.

89. Basskin L. How to use decision analysis to solve pharmacoeconomic problems. Formulary 1997;32:619–28.

90. Kessler JM. Decision analysis in the formulary process. Am J Health-Syst Pharm 1997;54(Suppl 1):S5–S8.

91. Schumacher GE. Multiattribute evaluation in formulary decision making as applied to calcium-channel blockers. Am J Hosp Pharm 1991;48:301–8.

92. Barner JC, Thomas J III. Tools, information sources, and methods used in deciding on drug availability in HMOs. Am J Health-Syst Pharm 1998;55:50–6.

93. Gibaldi M. Meta-analysis. A review of its place in therapeutic decision making. Drugs 1993;46:805–18.

94. Gannon K. Uniqueness of a drug key to formulary inclusion. Hosp Pharm Rep 1996 April;10:27.

95. Ain KB, Pucino F, Csako G, Wesley RA, Drass JA, Clark C, et al. Effects of restricting levothyroxine dosage strength availability. Pharmacotherapy 1996;16(6):1103–10.

96. Limit potential dangers by restricting problem drugs on formulary. Drug Utilization Review 1997;13(4):49–51.

97. Anassi EO. Ericsson C, Lal L, McCants E, Stewart K, Moseley C. Using a pharmaceutical restriction program to control antibiotic use. Formulary 1995;30:711–14.

98. Berndt EM. Drug expenditures. A medical center's experience with antibiotic cost-saving measures. Drug Benefit Trends 1997;9:32–6.

99. McCloskey WW, Johnson PN, Jeffrey LP. Cephalosporin-use restrictions in teaching hospitals. Am J Hosp Pharm 1984;41:2359–62.

100. Hayman JN, Sbravati EC. Controlling cephalosporin and aminoglycoside costs through pharmacy and therapeutics committee restrictions. Am J Hosp Pharm 1985;42:1343–7.

101. McCaffrey S, Nightingale CH. The evolving health care marketplace. How to develop critical paths and prepare for other formulary management changes. Hosp Formul 1994;29:628–35.

102. Dana WJ, McWhinney B. Managing high cost and biotech drugs: two institutions' perspectives. Hosp Formul 1994;29:638–45.

103. Armstrong EP. Disease state management and its influence on health systems today. Drug Benefit Trends 1996;8:18–20, 25, 29.

104. Lemay AP, Salzer LB, Visconti JA, Latiolais CJ. Strategies for deleting popular drugs from a hospital formulary. Am J Hosp Pharm 1981;38:506–10.

105. Boesch D. Formularies and therapeutic substitution: gaining ground in long-term care. Consult Pharm 1994;9:284–97.

106. Bowman GK, Moleski R, Mangi RJ. Measuring the impact of a formulary decision: conversion to one quinolone agent. Formulary 1996;31:906–14.

107. Chase SL, Peterson AM, Wordell CJ. Therapeutic-interchange program for oral histamine H_2-receptor antagonists. Am J Health-Syst Pharm 1998;55:1382–6.

108. Frighetto L, Nickoloff D, Jewesson P. Antibiotic therapeutic interchange program: six years of experience. Hosp Formul 1995;30:92–105.

109. Reich P. Therapeutic drug interchange. Medical Interface 1996;9(5):14.

110. American College of Physicians. Therapeutic substitution and formulary systems. Ann Intern Med 1990;113:160–3.

111. AMCP position statement on therapeutic interchange. 1997 Sept 13 [cited 2000 Feb 4]:[1 screen]. Available from: URL: http://www.amcp.org/public/legislative/position/therapeutic.html.

112. American College of Clinical Pharmacy. Guidelines for therapeutic interchange. Pharmacotherapy 1993;13(2):252–6.

113. Massoomi F. Formulary management: antibiotics and therapeutic interchange. Pharm Pract Manage Q 1996;16(3):11–18.

114. Heiner CR. Communicating about therapeutic interchange. Am J Health-Syst Pharm 1996;53:2568–70.

115. Rosen A, Kay BG, Halecky D. Implementing a therapeutic interchange program in an institutional setting. P&T 1995;20:711–17.

116. Kielty M. Improving the prior-authorization process to the satisfaction of customers. Am J Health-Syst Pharm 1999;56:1499–1501.

117. Carroll NV. Formularies and therapeutic interchange: the health care setting makes a difference. Am J Health-Syst Pharm 1999;56:467–72.

118. Nelson KM. Improving ambulatory care through therapeutic interchange. Am J Health-Syst Pharm 1999;56:1307.

119. Banahan BF III, Bonnarens JK, Bentley JP. Generic substitution of NTI drugs: issues for Formulary Committee consideration. Formulary 1998;33:1082–96.

120. FDA comments on activities in states concerning narrow-therapeutic-index drugs. Am J Health-Syst Pharm 1998;55:686–7.

121. Lewis BE, Fish L. Drug approvals. Formulary decisions in managed care: the role of quality of life. Drug Benefit Trends 1997;9:41–7.

122. Sanchez LA. Pharmacoeconomics and formulary decision making. PharmacoEconomics 1996;9(Suppl 1):16–25.

123. Heiligenstein JH. Reformulating our formularies to reflect real-world outcomes. Drug Benefit Trends 1996;8:35, 42.

124. Johnson JA, Bootman JL. Pharmacoeconomic analysis in formulary decisions: an international perspective. Am J Hosp Pharm 1994;51:2593–8.

125. Basskin L. Discounting in pharmacoeconomic analyses: when and how to do it. Formulary 1996;31:1217–27.

126. Macklin R. Understanding formularies. Drug Store News for the Pharmacist 1995;5:82–8.

127. Myers CE, Pierpaoli P, Smith MA. Measurement of formulary inclusion costs. Hosp Formul 1981;16:951–3, 957–8, 967–8, 970–1, 975–6.

128. Heiligenstein JH. Reformulating our formularies to reflect real-world outcomes. Drug Benefit Trends 1996;8:35, 42.

129. ASHP technical assistance bulletin on drug formularies. Am J Hosp Pharm 1991;48:791–3.

130. Navarro RP. Electronic formulary control. Medical Interface 1997;10(8):74–6.

131. Drug czars, electronic formulary systems increase formulary compliance. Formulary 1997;32: 171–2.

132. Ukens C. Hospital finds computer carrot can save drug dollars. Hosp Pharm Report 1994; 8(6):20.

133. Computerized drug cost information fails to sway physician prescribing. Am J Health-Syst Pharm 1999;56:1183–4.

134. Sateren LA, Sudds TW, Tyler LS. Computer-based system for maintaining and printing a hospital formulary. Am J Hosp Pharm 1987;44:1367–70.

135. Steinberg SK. The development of a hospital pharmacy policy and procedure manual. Can J Hosp Pharm 1980;XXXIII(6):194–5, 211.

136. Ginnow WK, King CM Jr. Revision and reorganization of a hospital pharmacy and procedure manual. Am J Hosp Pharm 1978;35:698–704.

137. Piecoro JJ Jr. Development of an institutional i.v. drug delivery policy. Am J Hosp Pharm 1987;44:2557–9.

Chapter Fifteen

Quality Improvement and the Medication Use Process

Mark A. Ninno • Sharon Davis Ninno

Objectives

After completing this chapter, the reader will be able to:

- Explain the evolution of quality management in industry and health care.
- Describe the processes used to assess and improve quality.
- Define the role of the pharmacist in modern health care quality improvement initiatives.
- Describe the expectation of quality in health care as outlined by the Joint Commission on Accreditation of Health Care Organizations (JCAHO).
- Define ORYX and its role in health system accreditation.
- Define the role of National Committee for Quality Assurance (NCQA) on quality measures in managed health care.
- Describe the role of medication use evaluation as a component of an organization's quality improvement program.
- Outline the general process of medication use evaluation.
- Describe the role of pharmacists and other health professionals in the medication use evaluation process.
- Discuss quality improvement techniques applied in drug information practice.

Quality Improvement

Probably no initiative has had a bigger impact on the delivery of health care in the United States during the past decade than the emphasis being placed on quality. For many years, it was accepted that the quality of the American health care system was second to none and the consumer public was rather passive in its belief that the standard of health care in the United States was exceptionally high.[1,2] However, quantification of this "perceived" level of quality remains difficult as the standard of care varies from state to state, institution to institution, practitioner to practitioner, and even patient to patient. Increasing competition in the health care market place, decreasing dollars with which to treat patients, and greater access to the availability of medical information through media outlets and the Internet, have served to increase the public's awareness about the need to be more actively involved in the management of its health. As a result, there is an increasing demand for quality health care services at more affordable costs.[3] This demand is coming from all sectors of the community including health care providers, institutions, third-party payers, the government, and, most importantly, the consumer public. More and more consumers are seeking information to compare health care providers and payers, and are "shopping" for health care services. Similarly, employers are seeking the best health care coverage for their employees while trying to reduce the costs associated with expanding medical technology. Balanced against all of this is an effort to ensure that all individuals, regardless of payer status, receive the same level and quality of health care, which has resulted in an unprecedented focus by governmental, consumer, and private health care organizations to quantify and regulate the quality of health care in the United States.

For the profession of pharmacy, the new focus on quality of health care comes as both a great opportunity and a large challenge. While in the past, the assessment of quality was the domain of only a few pharmacy practitioners, today it has become an integral part of every pharmacy practice setting.[4] The use of quality management techniques in assessing therapy and influencing outcomes blends well with pharmacy's initiative to shed its traditional role in medication dispensing and become more involved in the provision of patient-focused care; however, determining "what is quality" and how it is measured has provided many hurdles in achieving this goal. Complicating matters are the numerous national, state, local, private organizations, and regulatory bodies, that each define quality in their own terms. As a result, a survey that asks the question "what is quality health care?" may be greeted with as many different responses as responders.

DEFINING QUALITY

The term *quality* has meant different things to different groups for as long as the term has been defined. Compounding the confusion in defining quality has been the multitude of terms used to express the process of assessing quality in providing a good or service. Terms such as quality control, quality assurance, quality improvement, continuous quality improvement, total quality management, and performance improvement have all been used, sometimes interchangeably, to define the process of determining and improving quality. In its most basic definition, *quality* is "a degree or grade of excellence" and can be applied to goods, services, processes or even people (although often in a biased fashion).[5] Measures of quality can be applied to any service or good, but is most often associated with a physical product such as an automobile, computer, appliance, or other product. Often the association of quality is made with the service of a product and not the product itself (e.g., we may not be as aware of the quality in the construction of a dishwasher as we are the dishwasher repair service). More often, quality is associated with intangible items, such as friendliness or timeliness (e.g., we may not be as aware of the quality of the construction of the dishwasher or the repair service as we are of the friendliness of the repairman).

Quality measures have been used for years in the industrial sector. Some quality assurance programs can be traced back to JC Penney and Company in 1913.[6] Walter Shewart is often viewed as the "founding father" of the American quality improvement initiative. Shewart and others at Bell Laboratories during World War II used quality improvement techniques in its zero-defect program.[7,8] Shewart, a statistician, recognized that quality could be best improved by preventing the defects that can be expected with any process. To prevent defects, one had to first identify them through a continuous analysis of data produced by the process. By continually reviewing these data, variations and defects can be anticipated and prevented thus improving quality.[1,8] Shewart developed the simple model of "plan, do, check, and act" (PDCA); a model frequently employed in quality management today. This view of quality control as a statistical process is at the heart of modern quality management initiatives. The first real use of quality assurance techniques in large-scale industry can be traced back to the Japanese in the 1950s.[7,8] In an effort to rebuild their economy after World War II, the Japanese began to compete in markets traditionally dominated by the United States and Western Europe, such as automobile manufacturing. The Japanese had a limited infrastructure and few resources with which to begin manufacturing goods. Gaining insight from early quality pioneers such as Deming and Juran, the Japanese employed quality improvement techniques to manufacturing. The Japanese recognized that to be competitive they needed to prevent defects because they did not have the resources to correct them after they had occurred, as was the practice in American manufacturing.[8] Early Japanese automobiles had a notorious reputation for being inferior in design and construction, and were held with little regard in the marketplace. Utilizing quality management techniques outlined by Shewart and others, the Japanese soon began to revolutionize the automotive industry with higher quality cars at competitive prices, much to the chagrin of many U.S. automobile manufacturers. Application of similar quality techniques ultimately lead to Japanese dominance in other industrial fields and, to some degree, to the revitalization of the U.S. automobile industry.[7]

Having access to quality management techniques has not always proven to be the key to successful quality improvement. Many U.S. industries started to adopt quality assurance techniques when faced with stiff competition from abroad.[2,7] Unfortunately, many of these quality programs focused on measures of productivity and financial profitability without much regard to the final product or customer satisfaction. In this environment, individuals involved in the production of a good or service focused on identifying and changing the work habits of problematic departments or workers in an effort to improve quality. This practice is known as *quality assurance* or *quality control* and differs in practice from quality improvement. In most situations, quality assurance is retroactive, seeking to identify problems and those responsible for allowing problems to occur.[1,9] Additionally, quality assurance tends to focus only on the quality of a particular component within the process, but not the entire process. For example, individuals building the engine of a car may focus only on the quality of the engine production, but not be involved with those responsible for bolting the engine to the chassis. Although it may have resulted in a top quality engine, it does little good when the engine falls out of the car! Unfortunately, many quality assurance programs took on an accusatory and punitive aspect for those individuals or departments that did not meet the established expectation of quality.[1] This short-sighted view of quality lead to the demise, or near-demise, of many facets of the American industrial sector.

More recently, the focus has been shifted away from quality assurance and quality control to embrace a new discipline in the search for quality—total quality management (TQM). TQM takes a more investigative approach to identifying barriers to quality in the processes of providing goods or services.[1,8,9] TQM works under the basic principle that individuals are committed to quality; however, the processes under which they operate may not be conducive for allowing them to achieve that level of quality. In TQM, all participants are involved in the search for more cost-effective ways to improve services, products, and processes. TQM is a statistical, data-driven process that strives to improve quality by limiting variation in the processes involved in providing a good or service.[1] This contrasts with *quality assurance,* in which the assessment of quality and the plan to improve quality were managed by a limited few and focused on standards that may or may not be driven by data. A table comparing and contrasting the differences in approach and methodology between TQM and quality assurance is provided in Appendix 15–1.

Continuous quality improvement (CQI) is the term given to the methodologies used in the process of TQM. By using a systematic approach to identify internal and external factors that influence processes and functions, CQI seeks to remove the subjectivity from the assessment of quality and provide an ongoing mechanism for improving quality. CQI uses tools such as brainstorming, Pareto charts, scatter diagrams, fishbone diagrams, run charts, control charts, and other statistical and investigational tools to provide insight into which barriers are decreasing quality (or which processes are improving quality) and to what extent those barriers exist.[9] Examples of these tools are provided in Appendix 15–2.

The shift in the global workplace from quality assurance to TQM has revolutionized many industries. Many companies now embrace these practices very zealously and have incorporated these techniques into their daily routine. Although this change has come more quickly to some industries, health care is just now beginning to embrace these philosophies. Accrediting organizations such as the Joint Commission on Accreditation of Health Care Organizations (JCAHO) and the National Committee for Quality Assurance (NCQA) have been instrumental in bringing these philosophies to the forefront of contemporary health care. Despite this, many obstacles remain in place as health care seeks to improve quality. In the following sections of this chapter, changes and barriers to quality in health care as well as the expectations of quality set forth by some of the national health care accrediting bodies are reviewed. TQM as it pertains to the medication use process is discussed, and the steps to implement a medication quality program are outlined.

QUALITY IN HEALTH CARE

In the industrial setting, assuring quality has often focused on materials, people, and processes to achieve a common goal of a quality product.[8] The measure of quality is usually associated with the final product and is often very tangible (e.g., car has no defects, functions, and has a low repair record). Health care is not different in that quality also focuses on materials, people, and processes; however, the end product or service is often much more difficult to quantify than a physical product.[10] Differences in diseases, treatments, facilities, and health providers all impact the level of quality. More importantly, differences in patients, their expectations, and their response to a given therapy significantly influence the perception of quality. Unlike the industrial sector, health care is also hampered by the complexity of its health systems and payer structure. While an automobile manufacturer may recognize the need to improve quality and can call on all of its employees to contribute to obtain the desired goal, health care has many autonomous practitioners seeking to meet the expectation of quality of numerous institutions, governmental agencies, third-party payers, and patients.

Problems associated with quality in health care fall into one of three categories: overuse, underuse, and misuse.[11] *Overuse* occurs when a service is provided but is not needed, and thus the risk of harm from that service outweighs the potential benefit. *Underuse* results when a needed service is unavailable or not provided. *Misuse* occurs when the correct service is provided so poorly that the full benefit is not seen. In the past, health care addressed these problems through quality assurance techniques. Traditionally, a committee or group would identify a standard that was thought to reflect quality (e.g., infection rate after surgery, cart fill errors, readmission rates) and would establish an acceptable threshold for performance of that standard. A review of the performance of a particular group or individual would be compared against the standard and some corrective action taken if variations existed. Often, such programs had a limited effect on quality and were perceived as punitive or judgmental.[1] In an effort to avoid the drawbacks of quality assurance techniques, many health care practices are employing the principles of TQM. However, utilizing these techniques is difficult work and still faces many barriers in the health care setting.

Many health practitioners take an isolated view of their role in providing care and do not consider how their actions and processes affect others involved in the care of the patient. For example, the pharmacy may only focus on decreasing the number of missing doses by getting the right drug into the right medication drawer, whereas it may be more appropriate to assist nursing in improving the documentation on the medication administration record to achieve the same goal. Additionally, a physician may view the delay of medication delivery as a quality issue among pharmacy and nursing, and not address the role that his or her illegible handwriting contributes to the process. This compartmentalized (or "departmentalized") view is a barrier to quality in many health care systems and has unfortunately become entrenched in many practices.[9] The classic battle between pharmacy and nursing over missing doses is an excellent example of a systems breakdown. While it is easier to blame nursing for misplacing the dose or to lay blame on pharmacy for not sending the dose, it is more effective to apply the principles of TQM and systematically identify those process problems that contribute to poor quality (i.e., missing doses). The role of the pharmacist in the TQM process is varied and determined by his or her role within the department and the institution. Most importantly, pharmacists must be willing to work within multidisciplinary groups and serve as leaders in identifying barriers to quality within pharmacy processes as well as in other processes that impact patient care.

The process of quality improvement must involve all practitioners involved in the aspect of care under assessment.[8,12] Within health care organizations, quality improvement functions are often coordinated through the Pharmacy and Therapeutics (P&T) Committee or other similar multidisciplinary groups. The approach to quality improvement varies among organizations and is often specific to the opportunities for improvement identified. The section of this chapter discussing medication use evaluation outlines an example of how quality improvement activities can be conducted. Regardless of the process involved there are some aspects of multidisciplinary group dynamics that are important to consider.

Working within multidisciplinary groups can pose significant challenges. Busy schedules, politics, and poor communication and planning can contribute to dysfunction. Often, physicians or other health practitioners are left out of quality improvement initiatives for a variety of reasons. Perceptions of aloofness or disinterest, fear of reprisal or admission of guilt, or previous conflicts may result in the exclusion of individuals or groups that are essential to the quality improvement process. Likewise, it is important when interfacing with a group charged with resolving quality issues that one go about the process with an open mind. Understand where current practices may provide a barrier to others and how those practices can be changed without creating barriers. All groups or individuals involved in the process should be included as early as possible, preferably from the beginning.[13] One of the single greatest barriers to effective quality improvement is the addition of a new group or individuals once work has begun. This not only delays the process, but is likely to leave that group feeling "slighted" and they are less likely to be cooperative.

Leadership is one of the most important aspects of a successful quality management initiative.[13] Most of us can recall a committee that has seemingly met forever, always covering the same ground, seldom reaching closure on any issues. Strong leadership is essential to help keep working groups focused on the task at hand. It is important to establish which systems are contributing to the majority of problems and address only those that will have the biggest impact. It is of little benefit to expend a great deal of time and resources on a process that contributes little to the problem. Establishing clear goals, a timeline for completing tasks, and routine follow-up on progress will facilitate involvement and assist in bringing closure and documenting results. Although strong leadership is needed to facilitate any large working group such as a committee or quality improvement team, the leadership of that group should not override the group's ideas or present an accusatory or punitive image.[1,8,11,13] It is important that all involved with quality initiative feel free to speak their minds and contribute to the process. The approach to developing and implementing a successful quality management program is varied and complex; however, some time-tested approaches such as FOCUS-PDCA, SMART, and the Ten-step method can be employed. Appendix 15–3 outlines the key components of these quality management tools.

The application of quality management techniques in health care is not very different than in other industries. Strong leadership, an open mind, willingness to put past differences or processes behind, and most importantly, a willingness to improve the existing system, are required to assure that quality goals are met. Often, it is most beneficial to examine programs or processes that work well and determine what makes them successful. Flowcharts are useful in describing a process and can illustrate how a system is designed to work well. An example of a flowchart appears in Appendix 15–2. Applying these successes to processes that need improvement (e.g., problematic or high-risk processes) will often result in additional successes while making the most efficient use of time and resources. Determining the expectation of quality can often be the largest challenge facing a quality improvement initiative. For this reason, many national organizations and accrediting bodies have set forth to establish benchmarks for quality in health care. This will be discussed in the next section of this chapter.

QUALITY AND JCAHO

Undoubtedly, the single most influential group directing quality improvement in the health system setting is the JCAHO, (<<http://www.jcaho.org>>). Established in 1951 as the Joint Commission on the Accreditation of Hospitals, JCAHO has been a leader in assessing and promoting quality in the health care setting.[14] The JCAHO currently oversees the accreditation of more than 5000 hospitals and 15,000 health care organizations including laboratories, home-care organizations, long-term care organizations, behavioral health organizations, and integrated health systems.[14] Accreditation by JCAHO is an important component in maintaining eligibility for reimbursement from Medicare and Medicaid and often serves as a means for comparison to similar health systems. The importance of JCAHO accreditation to many health systems is so great that a significant amount of resources are committed on an ongoing basis to meet their standards.

Prior to the early 1990s, JCAHO took a fairly standard stance on quality in the health care setting. The JCAHO standards were divided into departmental areas, outlining the roles of those departments and the quality measures that should be expected from activities governed by those departments.[14] This departmental approach to quality focused more on function than outcome and did not meet the needs of modern health systems that were looking to improve quality and contain costs. As a result, JCAHO initiated its *Agenda for Change* in 1986, shifting the focus of quality away from departments and departmental roles to process oriented quality.[15] For example, there are no longer standards for pharmacy or specific mention of P&T committees, drug use evaluation, or formulary management in the current standards. However, traditional activities that pharmacy has been closely associated with are now contained in other standards.[14] This initiative was designed to remove the responsibility of a particular activity away from a particular group or department, and increase the responsibility of all practitioners within the system to all aspects of patient care. The *Agenda for Change* reflects the shift from quality assurance to TQM and CQI.

Defining quality in terms of the JCAHO's standards is not an easy task. Because the standards reflect quality in the process of providing care, there are few specific mandates to be found. This leaves the specific system for defining, assessing, and documenting quality to be established by each institution or health system. The revised JCAHO accreditation standards are divided into three main sections, further subdivided into chapters relating to aspects of organizational activity.[16] Within these chapters, the specific standards are detailed. The sections, chapters, and a brief description of the chapter's goals are provided below.

Patient-Focused Care

- *Patient's Rights and Organization Ethics (RI)*—improve patient outcomes by supporting each patient's rights and conducting business relationships with patients and the public in an ethical manner.
- *Assessment of Patients (PE)*—determine what kind of care is required to meet a patient's initial needs as well as his or her needs as they change in response to care.
- *Care of Patients (TX)*—provide individualized care in settings responsive to specific patient needs.
- *Education (PF)*—improve patient health outcomes by promoting healthy behavior and involving the patient in care and care decisions.
- *Continuum of Care (CC)*—define, shape and sequence processes and activities to maximize coordination of care within the continuum of care.

Organization-Focused Functions

- *Improving Organization Performance (PI)*—ensure that the organization designs processes well and systematically monitors, analyzes, and improves its performance to improve patient outcomes.
- *Leadership (LD)*—hospital's leaders use a framework to establish health care services that respond to community and patients' needs.
- *Management of the Environment of Care (EC)*—provide a safe, functional, and effective environment for patients, staff members, and other individuals in the hospital.
- *Management of Human Resources (HR)*—identify and provide the right number of competent staff to meet the needs of patients served by the hospital.
- *Management of Information (IM)*—obtain, manage, and use information to improve patient outcomes and individual and hospital performance in patient care, governance, management, and support processes.
- *Surveillance, Prevention, and Control of Infection (IC)*—identify and reduce the risk of acquiring and transmitting infections among patients, employees, physicians, and other licensed independent practitioners, contract service workers, volunteers, students, and visitors.

Structures with Functions

- *Governance (GO)*—sets the organizational policy that supports patient care.
- *Management (MA)*—covers the responsibilities of the chief executive officer and executive management and the relationship between the governing body and the chief executive officer.
- *Medical Staff (MS)*—medical staff leadership and participation in assessing and improving the quality of care delivered in health care organizations occurs at the various levels within the organization.
- *Nursing (NR)*—covers the provision of nursing services to patients.

While each of the chapters addresses the expectation of quality associated with the particular aspect it covers, the chapter on Improving Organizational Performance outlines JCAHO's expectation of how a health system or hospital improves performance in order to improve patient care. Within this chapter are JCAHO's standards outlining its vision of quality. JCAHO defines *performance improvement* in terms of the "Dimensions of Performance."[16] In essence, the "Dimensions of Performance" asks two very basic questions: (1) "Are you doing the right thing?" and (2) "Are you doing the right thing well?" These questions seek to determine important aspects of any therapy, test, or interaction with the patient that the health system may have. "Doing the right thing" can be viewed in terms of the efficacy and appropriateness of any given procedure or therapy. For example, in a patient undergoing treatment for cancer, it may be asked, "Is this therapy efficacious for the patient's condition?" That is to say, will it achieve the desired outcome? Additionally, it may be asked, "Is this therapy appropriate?" or "Is this the right service or therapy considering the patient's clinical needs?" These are basic questions asked when making care decisions for patients. It is always hoped that, based on the best scientific knowledge and in accordance with the patient's desires, efficacious and appropriate therapies or diagnostic tests are selected for patients. The measure of quality, or performance, comes into play when the question, "Are we doing the right thing well?" is considered. In this light, initiatives that go beyond simply selecting the best services for patients must be considered, but more importantly the circumstances with which those services are provided. When examining how "well" a service is provided, aspects such as availability must be considered. In this example, it may be asked, "Is the cancer treatment that is best suited to this patient's needs readily available?" Similarly, the timeliness, effectiveness, and safety with which desired therapy is used must be considered. These factors address those measures of quality that maximize the benefit of the therapy. For example, even though the best chemotherapy regimen may have been selected for the patient in terms of efficacy, that efficacy will be diminished if the treatment is not delivered in a timely fashion or at all before the patient's condition worsens.

Additionally, when considering how well a service is provided, the continuity of that service with respect to other services and practitioners, as well as the respect and caring that is afforded to the patient must be considered. Obviously, if excellent care is provided within the facility, but aftercare cannot be coordinated with other practitioners, the efficacy and quality of the care can be expected to suffer in the long run. Similarly, if excellent care is provided in terms of efficacy and safety, but without caring or respect for the patient's wishes, the quality of the service (and its continued existence) is certainly in doubt.

This view of quality and performance improvement is not new; however, JCAHO's approach is somewhat revolutionary in the health care setting. In essence, JCAHO has mandated that it is no longer sufficient to only "do the right thing," but more importantly, to "do the right thing well." To this end, JCAHO has developed a system by which to assess the level of performance improvement a health system has achieved and to compare that to a national benchmark. This initiative is known as ORYX and it has been called the "next evolution in accreditation."

The ORYX initiative is the first attempt by JCAHO to mandate the use of performance measurement tools to monitor outcomes and to integrate this data into the accreditation process.[17] The goal of ORYX is to establish a data-driven survey that compliments the accreditation process, allowing institutions to use their own performance data in comparison to national benchmarks to ultimately improve care. Currently, ORYX requirements are only applied to health care organizations and home care organizations. Eventually, the ORYX initiative will affect all organizations seeking JCAHO accreditation including long-term care providers, behavorial health centers, laboratories, and other integrated health systems.

In 1997, JCAHO mandated that all hospitals and home care organizations that were currently being accredited by JCAHO identify, by the end of 1998, the performance measurement system they would use to report performance improvement data.[18,19] JCAHO contracted with more than 60 different vendors of performance measurement systems including JCAHO's own Indicator Monitoring System (IMS). Performance measurement systems provide a format by which organizations can collect and report data and compare their performance to similar organizations.

By the end of the same year, JCAHO had also required that each institution undergoing accreditation determine at least two clinical measures to be monitored and reported. Clinical measures assess a wide variety of functions. Common clinical measures include the rate of Caesarian section births at the institution, patient satisfaction surveys, postoperative infection rates, diabetes education, and perioperative mortality. Other clinical measures may be used and are often specific to the health system. Selection of clinical measures is often based on the population of patients seen by that health system. For example, a facility providing acute and long-term care services may wish to select clinical measures reflective of practice in these areas (e.g., perioperative mortality and diabetes education). By collecting data on these measures and submitting them to JCAHO via ORYX, the health system will be able to compare itself to similar institutions collecting the same data. This can be used to obtain benchmarking data. Additionally, tracking these clinical measures over time will assist in identifying when and where improvements in these services may be needed.

The number of clinical measures to monitor and report will increase by two over a 3-year period and be capped at six measures.[17] This stepped approach is intended to allow organizations to become familiar with the process and to assure the quality of data. Health systems may collect data on more measures, but need only submit data for six. These clinical measures must relate to a minimum of 20% of the health system's or home care's base population and be submitted monthly to the measurement system.[17] For example, a 300-bed institution with 200 pediatric beds, 80 obstetrical beds, and 20 gynecology/oncology beds could not report data only on care provided to the oncology patients. These data are then sent to JCAHO on a quarterly basis once the measurement system and the institution clarify any erroneous or missing data. Failure to select a measurement system or submit data may result in loss of accreditation.

Initially, JCAHO was flexible in allowing institutions to use a wide variety of quality measurement tools to satisfy the needs of ORYX. Quality management initiatives such as the Maryland Hospital Association's Quality Indicator Project and others met the requirements for quality data collection outlined by JCAHO.[20] The Maryland Hospital Association's Quality Indicator Project is a state-wide system developed to measure and compare outcomes data in acute care hospitals. Many of the measures in this system have been previously mentioned (e.g., perioperative mortality and Caesarian section rates). However, the multitude of different quality measurement tools and indicators now being employed has made the development of a national benchmarking database nearly impossible. To this end, JCAHO has developed "core" indicators to collect data on specific aspects of care related to specific disease states (e.g., patients with congestive heart failure and low left ventricular ejection fraction prescribed an angiotensin converting enzyme inhibitor at discharge) or health system activities (e.g., timing of prophylactic antibiotic administration during surgery). Use of these indicators would increase the number of institutions collecting data on a particular indicator. In turn, this would increase the data pool size and be used to develop national benchmarks. Currently, JCAHO has announced the initial set of core indicators in therapeutic areas including acute myocardial infarction, heart failure, community acquired pneumonia, surgical procedures and complications, and pregnancy and related conditions.[17] More detailed information about the specific core measures can be obtained from JCAHO and is available at <<www.jcaho.org/oryx_frm.htm/>>.

With the implementation of ORYX, JCAHO hopes to provide a more valuable accreditation process by enabling health care systems to select the measurement tools and clinical measures best suited to their needs and most applicable to their particular setting.[17] Additionally, the development of a national database of performance improvement data will allow JCAHO the ability to detect trends and establish standards of care, thus influencing the quality of care on a larger scale. To some degree, this initiative comes in response to criticism that JCAHO was not flexible enough in its accreditation standards and did not take into account the differing patient populations, and clinical and social issues that vary among health care institutions.[19] The ultimate value of ORYX remains unknown; however, its role in the JCAHO accreditation process has already begun and is likely to expand with further development.

QUALITY AND MANAGED CARE

The increasing role of managed care in the United States has created the need to assess the quality of care provided by these organizations. Depending on who is providing the analysis, health maintenance organizations (HMOs) either represent the best or worst quality that health care has to offer.[21] The expectation of quality as it relates to managed care is not always a function of the care provided and the outcome, but rather a function of financial considerations (i.e., price of coverage of care) and the provider network (i.e., which physicians or institutions participate in the plan). As a result, selecting a quality managed care provider, whether as an employer or an individual, can be confusing at the very least.

As the number of individuals enrolled in managed health plans continued to grow throughout the 1980s and 1990s, several staff- and group-model HMOs recognized the need to collect and report quality measurement data among managed care providers.[22-24] To this end, the NCQA was formed in 1990.[22] The NCQA (<<http://www.ncqa .org/>>) is a nonprofit organization dedicated to assessing and reporting on the quality of managed care plans. The NCQA surveys and accredits managed care organizations much like JCAHO accredits hospitals.[22] The NCQA's mission is "to provide information that enables purchasers and consumers of managed health care to distinguish among plans based on quality, thereby allowing them to make more informed health care decisions."[22] Since its first survey in 1991, NCQA has been refining its performance measurement and survey/accreditation process and has grown steadily. Approximately 50% of the HMOs in the United States are currently involved in the NCQA accreditation process.

Accreditation from NCQA is a vigorous and voluntary process that includes both on- and off-site surveys. The NCQA reviews five broad categories of quality in the survey process. Within these five broad categories, there are over 60 NCQA standards that must be met.[22]

1. *Access and service*—Assesses access and availability of care and services.
2. *Qualified providers*—Assesses the qualifications of health care providers in the system.
3. *Staying healthy*—Assesses the managed care provider's programs and systems for promoting wellness and provision of preventative care.
4. *Getting better*—Assesses quality of care provided to patients who become ill.
5. *Living with illness*—Assesses the managed care provider's ability to care for patients with chronic or debilitating illnesses.

In addition to the survey and accreditation process, MCOs seeking NCQA accreditation must also submit performance improvement data. The Health Plan Employer Data and

Information Set (HEDIS) is a set of more than 50 performance measures used to compare managed health care plans.[22–24] Since its inception in 1992, HEDIS has been regularly updated to include new advancements in medical practice and changes in the standard of care. Data from HEDIS are included into NCQA's Quality Compass, a large, national database of NCQA accreditation and HEDIS data. These data are made available to the consumer public for use as a comparison between managed care providers. In recent years, however, the number of managed care providers opting to allow NCQA to release their HEDIS data to the public has decreased.[25,26] A review of HEDIS data has shown that the level of quality is lower among those managed care providers that do not release their HEDIS data than for those managed care plans that do.[21,25,26] This change in the willingness to make HEDIS data publicly available has concerned some in the industry who feel this may be the only system for measuring the quality of managed care providers. The managed care plans who have restricted access to their data counter that the HEDIS system does not take into account the poor quality of documentation that often occurs in physician-based practices.

For 2000, the latest release of HEDIS will include specific drug use performance measures.[23] Specific drug use measures include (1) outpatient drug use (carried over from an earlier HEDIS release) including costs and number of prescriptions, (2) beta-blocker treatment following acute myocardial infarction, (3) appropriate medication for the treatment of asthma, and (4) antibiotic treatment for otitis media in children.[23] These performance measures will be used to assess medication use in patients enrolled in managed care programs. None of the measures address the impact or role of pharmacy; however, they do represent the first specific measures of drug use to be collected as part of the HEDIS system. The pharmacist's role in meeting HEDIS requirements should include development of performance criteria, assessment and analysis of data, and involvement in institutional performance improvement initiatives.

The ultimate impact of NCQA and the HEDIS performance monitoring program has yet to be determined; however, it is reasonable to assume that as the number of patients receiving their health care through managed care providers increases and competitive market forces demand higher quality service for the dollar, accreditation and benchmarking data such as HEDIS will become increasingly important in the selection process for care providers, provided, of course, that such information is routinely available to the consumer public.

DRUG REGIMEN REVIEW AND DRUG USE REVIEW

The next section of this chapter discusses medication use evaluation (MUE) and includes examples of quality improvement activities occurring as part of the MUE process. Although MUE is generally conducted in organized health systems, two other processes with similar names, drug regimen review (DRR) and drug use review (DUR), focus on therapy provided within nursing facilities and for outpatients. DRR is a requirement of the Health Care Financing Administration (HCFA) mandating pharmacist review of drug regimens for patients in nursing facilities. The intent of this regulation is to ensure that the drug therapy provided for each resident is reviewed monthly and that pharmacists are making appropriate recommendations to health care professionals to improve drug therapy. This requirement was implemented in 1974 through Medicare (Title XVIII) and Medicaid (Title XIX) regulations and was expanded in 1987 to include intermediate care nursing facilities.[27,28]

The Medicare Catastrophic Coverage Act of 1988 required DUR in outpatient settings. It was rescinded in early 1990. The Medicaid Anti-Discriminatory Drug Price and Patient Benefit Restoration Act ("Pryor II"), enacted in 1990, includes similar requirements. This bill mandates prospective and retrospective DUR and requires that each state establish educational outreach programs for outpatient pharmacy services. The intent of this provision is to ensure that prescription drugs are "appropriate, medically necessary, and not likely to result in adverse medical results." This legislation requires that DUR programs be designed to educate physicians and pharmacists in identifying and reducing the frequency and patterns of fraud, abuse, gross overuse, or inappropriate or medically unnecessary care. DUR is typically retrospective in nature and utilizes claims data as its primary source of information. Long-term care facilities meeting the DRR requirements of the Department of Health and Human Services are exempt from this provision.[27-31]

Medication Use Evaluation

Medication use evaluation is the component of a health care organization's quality improvement program that should examine all aspects of medication use and most often requires direct involvement of pharmacists.[32,33] The goal of MUE is to provide all patients with the most rational, safe, and effective drug therapy through the assessment and improvement of specific medication use processes. MUE may focus on a specific medication (e.g., alteplase), a class of medications (e.g., thrombolytics), medications used in the management of a specific disease state or clinical setting (e.g., thrombolytics in acute myocardial infarction), medications related to a clinical event (e.g., drug therapy within the first 24 hours for patients admitted with acute myocardial infarction including aspirin, beta blockers, thrombolytics, etc.), a specific component of the medication use process (e.g., time from admission to administration of thrombolytic), or can be based on specific outcomes (e.g., vessel patency following thrombolytic administration). It has become an important function mandated to a large extent by JCAHO performance improvement standards. Unfortunately, the standards related to MUE remain among the most challenging for many institutions. Lack of resources or authority, politics, difficulty in identifying issues (e.g., high use, high risk, or problematic medications or processes), reporting, and acting upon data to improve performance can all contribute to ineffective MUE programs.

THE MEDICATION USE PROCESS

In 1989, a multidisciplinary task force was organized by JCAHO to describe the medication use process as a component of its effort to develop tools to assess medication use. The original definition of the medication use process included prescribing, dispensing, administration, monitoring, and systems and management control (Table 15–1). This description serves as the basis for contemporary MUE.[34,35]

It is important to note that this description outlines a process more multidisciplinary than the categories might imply. For example, while the prescribing category may imply a physician function, pharmacists are often involved because they assist in drug selection and individualization of the therapeutic regimen.

MEDICATION USE EVALUATION AND JCAHO

The terminology used to describe MUE has changed over time and can be confusing. MUE, DUE, DUR, and antibiotic utilization review (AUR) are often used interchange-

TABLE 15–1. DESCRIPTION OF THE MEDICATION USE PROCESS

Prescribing	Assessing the need for/selecting the correct drug
	Individualizing the therapeutic regimen
	Designing the desired therapeutic response
Dispensing	Reviewing the order for correctness of dosing and indication for use
	Processing the order
	Compounding/preparing the drug
	Dispensing the drug in a timely manner
Administering	Administering the right medication to the right patient
	Administering the medication when indicated
	Informing the patient about the medication
	Including the patient in administration
Monitoring	Monitoring and documenting the patient's response
	Identifying and reporting adverse drug reactions
	Reevaluating the drug selection, drug regimen, frequency, and duration
Systems/management control	Collaborating and communicating among caregivers
	Reviewing and managing the patient's complete therapeutic drug regimen

ably, but are different in their approach and application. This section will attempt to provide some background as to how these terms developed and changed over time. Table 15–2 summarizes several key events in the development of MUE as it relates to JCAHO and governmental activities in the United States.[27,28,36,37]

One of the first calls for a process to evaluate the use of medications appeared in the final reports of the Task Force on Prescription Drugs (DHEW).[36] This 1969 report called for development of programs to monitor drug use. A retrospective evaluation process referred to as *drug use review* (*DUR*) was suggested.

The Joint Commission on Accreditation of Hospitals (JCAH), as JCAHO was known at the time, required AUR beginning in 1978. A retrospective assessment was performed to evaluate antibiotic use at the institution. This assessment was largely retrospective, quantitative, and evaluated trends in antibiotic use. The number and specific type of evaluation was not specified and patterns of drug use (versus a qualitative evaluation of individual cases) were often the focus. The requirement was expanded to include all drug therapy and the terminology was changed to DUE in 1986. The 1986 standards implied that concurrent evaluation of drug use was required. The responsibility for this function was shared by the medical, pharmacy, nursing, and other staff (as appropriate) and was assigned to the medical staff as a P&T Committee activity. The activity was to be ongoing, planned, systematic, and criteria based using current knowledge and experience. Data from these activities were also to be used in the process of medical staff reappointment and recredentialing within the organization.[37,38]

An initiative called the *Agenda for Change* was adopted by the JCAHO in 1986.[15,39] It was intended to improve standards by focusing on key functions of quality of care, monitor the performance of health care organizations using indicators, improve the rele-

TABLE 15–2. SUMMARY TIMELINE: THE EVOLUTION OF MEDICATION USE EVALUATION

1969	Task Force on Prescription Drugs (DHEW) Report calls for development of programs to monitor drug use
1974	HCFA regulation mandate pharmacists' monthly review of medication for all residents of skilled nursing facilities, this was later (1987) expanded to include residents of intermediate care nursing facilities
1978	Antibiotic utilization review standards included in Accreditation Manual for Hospitals
1980	Quality Assurance Standard included in Accreditation Manual for Hospitals
1986	Drug Usage Evaluation Standard included in Accreditation Manual for Hospitals Agenda for Change initiated
1987	Omnibus Budget Reconciliation Act (OBRA) requires states to develop retrospective and prospective DUR programs
1994	Medication Use Evaluation Standard included in Accreditation Manual for Hospitals
1996	Indicator Monitoring System (IMS) initiated
1997	Medication Use Evaluation Standard included in PI.3.2.2 and TX.3.9 in the Accreditation Manual for Hospitals

vance and quality of the survey process, and enhance the accuracy and value of JCAHO accreditation. The revised process was to focus on actual performance versus the capability to perform well. Within this initiative, the JCAHO endorsed the concept of CQI and included it within its standards beginning in 1994. As part of this process, the Accreditation Manual for Hospitals (AMH) was significantly modified and much of the definition of expectations was deleted. Multidisciplinary involvement in MUE was emphasized. Eventually, the standards were moved from the medical staff chapter of the AMH to the care of patients and performance improvement chapters. In 1992, the terminology was also changed to MUE to reflect that all medications (including vaccines, biotechnology derivatives, etc.) and all medication-related functions are included in the standard. This terminology is also consistent with the medication use process as delineated by a group of practitioners who were developing medication use indicators as described in the *Agenda for Change*. Previously, the evaluation of medication use typically focused on only the prescribing and outcome components of the process. With this change, dispensing and administration were specifically included. MUE standards first appeared in the 1992 AMH and were required of all institutions beginning in 1994.

Current standards focus on quality improvement but no longer require that a specific approach be used.[16] The organization is allowed to select, based on its characteristics and structure, a performance improvement approach (e.g., FOCUS-PDCA, SMART, the Ten-step method, etc.) that best meets its needs and that of its patients. Appendix 15–3 briefly describes these approaches. Standards state that MUE should be a systematic, multidisciplinary process focusing on continual improvement in the medication use process and patient outcomes. The use of data for reappointment/recredentialing is still required but the emphasis is on CQI. Priorities should be established based on

- effect on performance and improved patient outcomes.
- selected high-volume, high-risk, or problem-prone processes.
- resources and organizational priorities.

The pharmacist plays a key role within the multidisciplinary MUE process. Although not always involved in specific initiatives, all pharmacists should actively identify opportunities for improvement in processes.[3,40] Pharmacists participating in the coordination and implementation of MUE initiatives are often those with drug information or quality improvement responsibilities as well as those with specialized knowledge or experience in the component of medication use under assessment. Many of these pharmacists are self-taught using continuing education opportunities or the literature.[41] The American Society of Health-System Pharmacists (ASHP; <<http://www.ashp.org>>) has developed guidelines for pharmacists' participation in DUE and MUE.[33,42] These guidelines can serve as a resource to those developing or revising a MUE program or for practitioners new to the process.

THE MEDICATION USE EVALUATION PROCESS

Figure 15–1 outlines the process of medication use evaluation. This figure is an adaptation of the Ten-step process described by JCAH in 1989.[43,44]

Responsibility for the Medication Use Evaluation Function

Organizations must define which group or groups will participate in and be responsible for the evaluation of medication use. Although the JCAHO standards no longer assign the responsibility for MUE to the P&T Committee, nor do they require a P&T Committee at all, the function is well suited to this group as well as to a Performance/Quality Improvement Committee. Some organizations have formed a MUE subcommittee to the P&T group, whereas others have distributed the responsibility for MUE along patient population or product lines. The entire committee may participate in evaluations or working groups consisting of committee members and nonmembers may be appointed to address specific issues. The size, scope, and makeup of the health care organization and its approach to quality improvement should determine the approach to be used. The participants in the group charged with overseeing MUE must have a clear understanding that the purpose is that of improving the quality of the medication use process and that each member is expected to actively participate.[13] Newly formed groups may benefit from an overview of the organization's overall approach to quality improvement and how MUE contributes to overall goals.

Topic Selection

Topic selection should be based on the scope of care of the organization and should focus on high-volume, high-risk, or problem-prone medication-related processes. Topics may also focus on institutional priorities (e.g., initiation of new clinical programs or services). Several sources of information are commonly used to identify these agents and issues. They include medication error reports, adverse drug reactions (ADRs), advances in patient care modalities that involve changes in optimal pharmacotherapy, Diagnosis-Related Groups (DRG) length of stay or cost outliers within an organization, purchasing reports indicating a significant increase in the use of an agent without a shift in patient population, and medications that are a key component of a process or procedure (e.g., thrombolytics, 2b3A inhibitors), etc. Many organizations emphasize antibiotics within their MUE programs. It is essential that the topics selected reflect the overall scope of medication use throughout the organization, including inpatients, outpatients, emergency care, short-stay settings, and so on.

Ideally, the group charged with MUE should establish an annual plan that will set goals for new topics to be assessed and follow-up on previous evaluations. Priorities should be reevaluated and the scope and breadth of recent evaluations should be assessed relative to the scope of care provided within the organization. For example, if

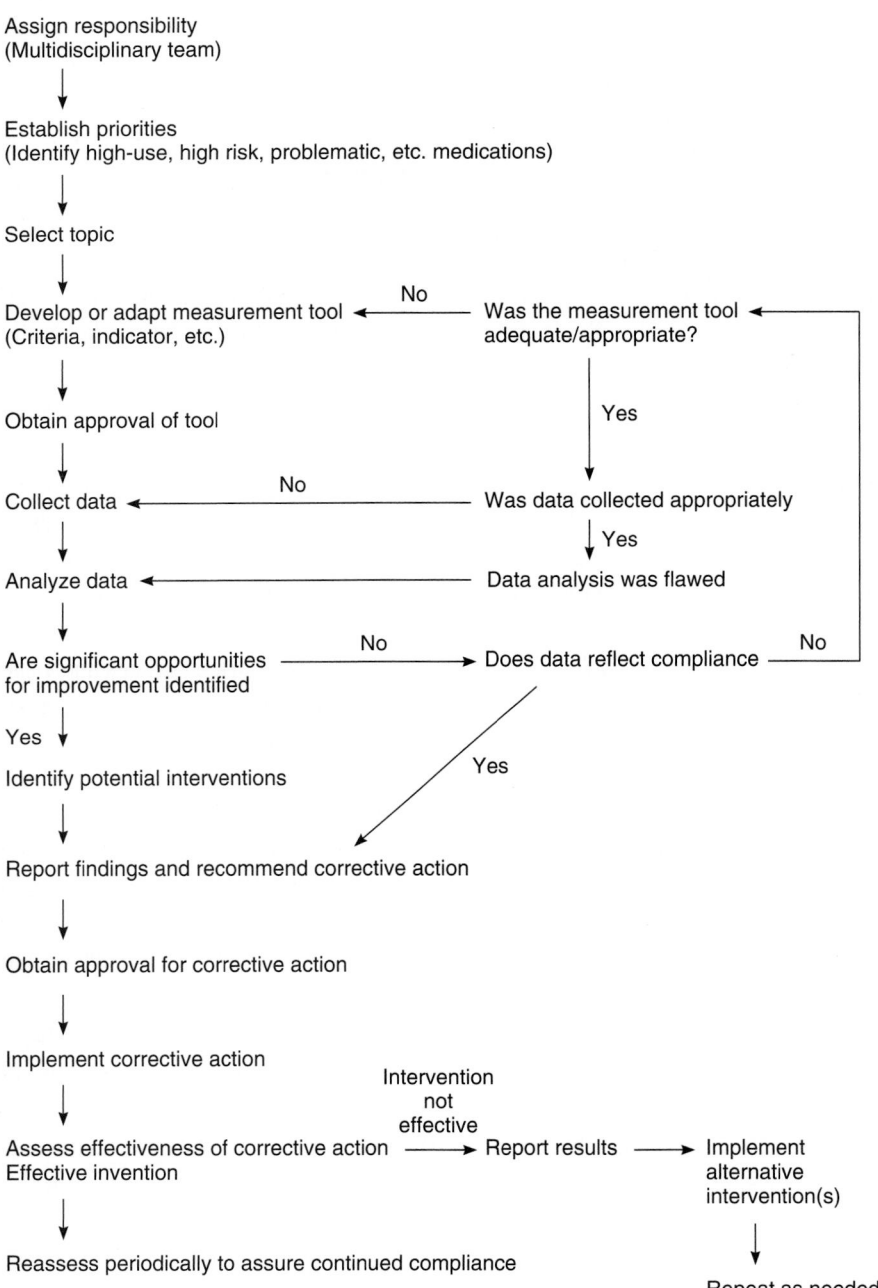

Figure 15–1. Medication use evaluation process.

recent MUE efforts focused primarily on issues related to antibiotic use, the plan for the upcoming year should deemphasize assessment of this class in favor of a more balanced topic selection. The planning process can identify follow-up assessments (used to assess and document that previous efforts were successful in improving performance) that remain to be performed. The failure to perform and document these follow-up evaluations is problematic in many organizations, but is a key component of the quality improvement process. Development of an annual plan also allows an opportunity to discontinue activities that are no longer useful such as an ongoing assessment that has demonstrated sustained improvement and can now be replaced by periodic rechecks to ensure continued compliance.

Criteria, Standards, and Indicators

Criteria are statements of the activity to be measured and standards that define the performance expectations. (See Table 15–1 and Appendix 15–4 for examples.) Criteria should be based on current best or at least accepted practice, appropriate for the target patient population(s), and be supported by current literature. Ideally, a multidisciplinary group develops the criteria. The membership of this group (e.g., prescribers, nurses, pharmacists, respiratory therapists, social workers, clinical laboratory and information systems personnel, discharge planners, etc.) should be determined by the nature of the process under evaluation. A flow diagram (see Appendix 15–2 for example) outlining the process is often useful. Based on this diagram, additional disciplines should be invited to participate in the evaluation process as appropriate. Respiratory therapists, discharge coordinators, and social workers are a few of the disciplines not routinely represented as core members of medication-related committees. Inclusion of all involved disciplines initially will also facilitate implementation of corrective actions. However, criteria are most often developed by one or two of the involved disciplines and are subsequently approved by a multidisciplinary group with representation from all applicable practice groups (e.g., prescribers, pharmacists, nurses, etc.). Explicit (objective) criteria are preferred in that they are clear cut, based on specific parameters, and are better suited for automation. Implicit (subjective) criteria require that a judgment be made and require appropriate clinical expertise to be effective. Table 15–3 compares implicit and explicit criteria statements. It is imperative that the appropriate oversight group approve the criteria prior to initiation of data collection.

Criteria should be phrased in yes/no or true/false formats and should avoid interpretation on the part of data collectors. They should assess important aspects in the use of the medication or therapy under evaluation and focus on aspects most closely related to outcomes. Definition of *outcome* should also be established within the criteria based on the scope of care provided within the organization. For example, in a truly acute care setting, the outcome assessment of antibiotic management of pneumonia may be limited

TABLE 15–3. EXAMPLES OF IMPLICIT AND EXPLICIT CRITERIA STATEMENTS

Explicit Criteria Statements	Implicit Criteria Statements
Blood work ordered	Pretreatment WBC with differential ordered and completed within 48 hours prior to the initiation of therapy
Renal function assessed routinely	Serum creatinine evaluated every 3 days
Neutropenic patients	Patients with WBC <1000/mm^3

WBC, white blood count.

to a decrease in clinical signs and symptoms indicating a response to therapy and the ability to be discharged on an oral antibiotic(s). However, in an integrated system, outcome could be assessed at the conclusion of therapy. It is helpful to consider how opportunities for improvement identified via a criteria statement could be addressed. If the corrective action would involve participation of a group not represented in the development process, it may be wise to include them in the development and assessment process. Table 15–4 summarizes criteria for the validity of criteria or indicators.[45,46]

Criteria are available from a variety of published sources.[47-57] The advantages to using predeveloped criteria include prior expert review and assessment and time savings. However, criteria developed outside the organization must be adapted to the practice setting and patient population as appropriate and must be approved by the designated multidisciplinary group prior to data collection. For example, criteria intended for use in a general adult population may not be appropriate for geriatric patients without modification. Also, criteria may include uses of medication not applicable to certain settings (e.g., criteria for the use of benzodiazepines, including use in conscious sedation in a setting where conscious sedation is not performed). Criteria may also be derived from guidelines for use developed or adopted within the organization. For example, the P&T Committee may agree to add a medication to the formulary for specific indications and require that the use of the agent and patient outcomes be concurrently evaluated based on these guidelines.

Performance indicators can also be used within the medication use evaluation process. An indicator is a screening tool used to detect potential problems in quality.[48,58] Table 15–5 provides some examples of indicators. They can assess structure, process, or outcome. *Structure* refers to the resources, tools, and other established attributes of the setting in which care is provided. *Process* refers to the activities that take place in giving and receiving care. *Outcome* denotes the effects of care on the health status of the patient or population. Indicators can be used as mechanisms to monitor the overall medication use system, to screen for potential problems in a specific component, or confirm that performance improvement is sustained following the completion of an evaluation.[33] For example, the first indicator listed in Table 15–5 involves the estimation of creati-

TABLE 15–4. CRITERIA FOR THE VALIDITY OF CRITERIA OR INDICATORS

Face validity	Importance to patient outcome
	Assess problematic area
	Have some utility in improving patient care
	Reflect system-wide performance
	Accurate based on current practice standards or literature
External validity	Thoroughly reviewed by practitioners with expertise in the use of the drug
	Applicable within organization
	Criteria should be clarified and improved as appropriate, but not weakened, in review process
Feasibility of data collection and retrieval	Clarity
	Availability of data
	Numerator size
	Difficulty or complexity of data collection
	Benefits versus effort of data collection
	Variability of data collection methods

nine clearance in patients older than 65 years of age. If an estimation of a patient's renal function is performed (e.g., if a creatinine clearance is calculated or measured) and is available to caregivers, it can be used by caregivers to adjust therapy accordingly. The availability of an estimated creatinine clearance in the medical record of patients over the age of 65 indicates that the organization is systematically taking steps to adjust drug therapy in this population based on organ function. Of course, it cannot be certain that the information is used appropriately or even if it is used at all. However, the lack of this information may indicate that the organization is not routinely making these assessments as part of their medication use system. Organizations using this indicator have taken a variety of steps to make this information available as part of the routine medication use process. Some organizations have assigned the responsibility to the clinical laboratory with estimated creatinine clearances appearing within laboratory

TABLE 15–5. EXAMPLES OF INDICATORS

Patients >65 years old in whom CrCl has been estimated

Patients undergoing surgery who receive prophylactic antibiotics >2 h before the first incision

Frequency of pharmacy stock outages

Frequency of discrepancies in automatic dispensing units

Patients with a diagnosis of acute myocardial infarction that are prescribed daily aspirin therapy at discharge

Patients with a diagnosis of congestive heart failure receiving an angiotensin converting enzyme inhibitor

Patients discharged on $>X$ number of prescription medications

CrCl, creatinine clearance.

reports. Others have assigned the responsibility to pharmacy, with some organizations automating calculations and screening within the dispensing information system and others requiring that pharmacists document calculations in the medical record.

Standards are used to define performance expectations and are usually set at 0% (should never happen) or 100% (should always happen). Thresholds specifying an acceptable level of compliance or performance are usually set higher than 0% or lower than 100% based on acceptable variation, standards of practice, or benchmarks.[59] Thresholds should not be used to avoid intervention but should allow limited noncompliance with the criteria when the clinical impact of noncompliance is felt to be of low risk. Control limits define the limits of allowable or expected variation in performance (often two to three times the standard deviation from the mean initially) and may be used to assess the results with ongoing monitoring. Control limits should narrow with ongoing process improvements.[48] An example of a control chart with limits appears in Appendix 15–2.

Performance not meeting the defined standard or threshold or falling outside the control limits indicates that intervention to improve performance is necessary. In some cases, performance outside the defined parameters may, upon review, be acceptable to the oversight group. This usually results from expectations being set too high (e.g., that the rate of adverse effects with any agent will be 0%) or when the criteria fail to include the appropriate exceptions. When this occurs, the multidisciplinary oversight group must agree that the level of performance is acceptable and that intervention is not necessary. These decisions must be clearly documented in meeting minutes or summaries of results.

Data Collection

Prior to the initiation of data collection, the multidisciplinary oversight group must approve the topic selection, criteria, patient selection process, sample size and method (e.g., all consecutive patients, intermittent sampling, random sampling, etc.), evaluation time frame, data collection method, and standards of performance.[33] It may be appropriate to distribute the approved criteria as an educational tool prior to data collection. Although this may address some quality issues prior to data collection and result in less dramatic results, it may support the ultimate goal of improving care and may do so in a timelier manner. In this situation, if there is a need to document the overall impact of a MUE effort, collection of baseline performance data even as criteria are being finalized and approved can provide a more accurate representation of before and after. If at any point problems are identified in the criteria or indicators or with any component of the evaluation, the issue should be brought back to the oversight group and modifications made as appropriate.

The timing of data collection can be influenced by seasonal variations in the types of care provided (e.g., increased frequency of pneumonia in the winter months), systems issues (e.g., construction, implementation of new computer systems, initiation of new services), and personnel issues (e.g., the influx of new health professional graduates and medical housestaff that occurs during the summer months, staff absences during vacation or flu seasons). The time frame for data collection, both in duration and time of year, should also be considered in the planning process. For example, an assessment of care provided to patients with pneumonia is usually best performed during the winter months when this diagnosis is more frequent while an assessment of the management of near-drowning may be more appropriate during the summer months. The longer the data collection period, the more likely various fluctuations in quality of care will be identified.

Retrospective data collection was used primarily in the era of AUR and DUR. This method involved reviewing the patient's medical record after discharge. It allowed data collection to be scheduled when convenient or when staff was available, but was totally dependent on documentation in the medical record. If an opportunity for improvement was identified, there was no opportunity to improve that patient's care.

Concurrent data collection occurs while the patient is still actively receiving the medication but after the first dose is dispensed or administered. Data sources other than the medical record are available (e.g., staff or patient interviews) and there is an opportunity to improve patient care. Based on more complete information, results may be more complete as well as more accurate.[60] However, the need for data collection is constant and must occur within a specific time frame, which is not always convenient. This often results in an increased number of personnel being involved in the data collection process and increased inconsistency.

Prospective evaluation occurs before the patient receives the first dose of medication and is initiated whenever an order for the medication is generated. Simple prospective evaluations can be at least partially automated and are likely to become more common. An example of this is a computerized pharmacy system that generates a warning to the pharmacist or prescriber if the dose of a drug is outside the normal limits based on a patient's organ function. Clinical judgment must also be applied in many of these settings. Prospective evaluations that are not automated are the most cumbersome to implement because the evaluation must occur promptly every time an order is initiated to avoid therapy delays. They require that personnel be available to collect data and report results at all times and force immediate interaction between practitioners. This approach offers the greatest opportunity for intervention and education but also increases the risk for potentially negative interactions with prescribers and other health professionals, and can result in therapy delays. Furthermore, it is essential that the interventions made as part of the prospective evaluation are documented in order to evaluate workload, and effectiveness of interventions, and that outcome is assessed in some manner.

Limiting the number of data collectors or automating data collection is valuable in maintaining consistency. When multiple data collectors are involved, it becomes even more important to have clear criteria not subject to interpretation.

The selection of patients or cases for inclusion in the evaluation should be determined and approved by the oversight group prior to data collection. It is essential that the selection be unbiased, consistent, and representative of the care provided. Sample size should be based on size of the patient population. It has been suggested that for frequently occurring events a sample of at least 5% of cases be used, and for events occurring less frequently that a minimum of 30 cases be assessed.[61]

The term *target drug program* is often used to refer to programs that evaluate the use of a medication or group of medications on an ongoing basis. Within these programs, interventions are usually made at the time of discovery based on established criteria or guidelines. It is important that these interventions be documented by practitioners, and periodically assessed by the multidisciplinary oversight group to determine the continued need for and appropriateness of the program.

Confidentiality is a key component of all quality improvement initiatives, including MUE.[13] It is important that the entire MUE program be identified as a performance improvement activity. This helps to ensure that the information collected as part the program is "protected" and/or not "discoverable." Although regulations vary from state to state (check with attorneys in your area), in most cases this means that a plaintiff's lawyer pursuant to a case cannot request the information, nor can this information be available for review to identify potential plaintiffs. Within the program, individual patients and practitioners should be identified in some manner other than their actual name to ensure anonymous review. Many institutions use medical record numbers and codes assigned to individual prescribers within reports. It is also important not to inadvertently identify a practitioner. For example, if the results of an evaluation are reported by practitioner specialty (e.g., pediatrics, pediatric infectious disease, etc.) and there are only one or two practitioners in certain subspecialties, you have in essence identified the practitioner for the small subspecialty area.

Ultimately, practitioner-specific reports should be generated in most cases, because JCAHO requires that information related to medication use be considered in the reappointment/recredentialing of medical staff. Following peer review, the practitioner name may be revealed only to those responsible for the reappointment/recredentialing functions. Medical department chairpersons usually carry out this function. An example of a practitioner-specific report appears in Appendix 15–5.

Data Analysis

The multidisciplinary oversight group should conduct the analysis of results. Reports should compare actual performance with expectations defined by the standards (or thresholds or control limits) established and approved prior to data collection. Performance not meeting standards (or threshold or control limits) may be considered opportunities for improvement. Alternatively, the oversight group may determine that the standards were too rigorous, that unforeseen exceptions were encountered, and/or that actual performance falls within current acceptable standards of practice. Specific corrective actions should be recommended for all identified opportunities for improvement (e.g., for all criteria statements for which the standard of performance was not met). The need for and nature of follow-up should also be assessed based on the frequency, prevalence, and/or severity of the issue. For example, if an evaluation of the management of pneumonia identified no issues with drug selection, but did identify an unacceptable delay in time to first dose of antibiotic (e.g., greater than 2 hours after admission), the follow-up evaluation could focus on the time to first dose and not assess antibiotic selection. Furthermore, if this issue was identified in patients admitted to a particular unit, then the follow-up could focus on assessing and documenting improvement in only that unit.

Often, a multidisciplinary group does not perform the actual data analysis. In this situation, the findings and actions must be reviewed and approved by the appropriate multidisciplinary group prior to initiation of any corrective action or distribution of the results.

Computer software programs (e.g., relational databases and spreadsheets) can be very helpful in collecting data, managing data, and reporting results.[33,62-64] Palm top units, bar code technology, proprietary software products, and computer systems used within the organization's clinical departments can be employed as tools to assist in patient identification, data collection and analysis, and documentation.[62-65]

The report to the oversight group should contain the rationale for the topic selection, team members involved in the evaluation, a description of the patient population evaluated, any selection criteria used, a copy of the criteria/indicators, discussion of the results, identification of likely causes for opportunities identified, and recommendations for corrective action and follow-up evaluation. An example is provided in Appendix 15–6. In most settings, delineation of results on a practitioner-specific basis is not appropriate at this level. The exception would be if the practice of only a small subset of practitioners consistently fell outside the criteria. In this situation, some sort of code (e.g., physician A or physician 28) should be used instead of an actual name.

Interventions and Corrective Actions

The key to quality improvement is improving the process and ultimately the results, not blaming an individual or group of individuals. Steps to improve performance or avoid similar outcomes in the future fall into three categories: educational interventions, restrictive interventions, and process changes. *Educational interventions* are most appropriate when knowledge deficits contribute to performance outside the criteria. They are most effective when they are directed personally, take place soon after the problem occurs, the educator is a peer or superior of the person being educated, and when the education is well supported in the literature or by practice standards.[66] One-on-one or group discussion of results, letters, newsletters, computerized order entry educational screens, protocols, or guidelines and presentation via quality improvement channels are examples of educational approaches.[67,68] Generally, educational interventions incorporated into ongoing processes (e.g., education screens in computer order entry systems) are more effective while one-time efforts (e.g., newsletters) may not have a sustained effect. In most situations, educational interventions are the most palatable.[69]

Restrictive approaches may involve special ordering procedures, compliance with guidelines for use, consultation with a specialty service, or formulary restrictions. The impact of restrictive interventions often reverses when the restrictions are removed.[70] Restrictive interventions are perhaps most effective when used to establish appropriate practice patterns when an agent is first made available for use within the organization (see Chap. 14).

Process changes incorporate the correction into routine practice. This approach may involve changes in policy or procedures, implementation of new services, acquisition of new equipment, changes in staffing, or generation of regular notifications, etc., when practice does not appear to meet standards.

Follow-Up

Follow-up evaluation should occur within a reasonable time frame after completion of the initial evaluation and completion of the corrective action. Follow-up is designed to assess the effectiveness of the intervention. The same criteria, standards, and sample should be used for the follow-up assessment as in the initial evaluation. Exceptions to this rule should be made if there was a problem with the initial criteria, standards, and sample; the standard of practice changes in the interim; or there is an opportunity to focus on a subset of the original data elements or patient population. For example, if issues were only found in the administration component of the use of a medication (and not in the prescribing, dispensing, or monitoring components) or only in a specific age group, follow-up evaluation could focus on these issues or populations rather than repeating the broader assessment performed initially.

DUE has been criticized as being heavy handed, non–patient focused, and for not addressing the issue of accountability for provision of care based on a unique body of knowledge.[3] If the approach termed MUE is utilized in its true spirit, many of these challenges are addressed. MUE is a truly multidisciplinary, process-oriented approach to evaluate the quality of medication use. The process goes beyond numbers and percentages to identify opportunities for improvement and, more importantly, to improve the quality of care.

Quality in Drug Information

Quality standards for drug information practice have not been established to date and quality assessment techniques used in drug information practice vary greatly among practice sites.[71-74] Several studies have found inconsistencies in the quality of drug information practice and have called for increased emphasis on quality and the development of practice standards.[75-77] Most drug information services conduct some form of quality assessment based on the scope of service provided by that center and preestablished levels of acceptable performance. Quality assessment is usually conducted on the responses provided to drug information requests, medical literature search and evaluation processes, availability, accuracy and timeliness of drug information resources, and the quality of materials produced by the drug information center staff (e.g., monographs, newsletters, continuing education programs). Although some quality assessment processes are conducted concurrently, most assessments are done retrospectively often by randomly sampling of drug information requests, monographs, and so forth. Furthermore, assessments may be performed via peer review or may be performed by the director of the service. Currently, no standards have been developed for this process.

Assessment of the quality of responses to drug information inquiries may include components such as timeliness, completeness and appropriateness of response, and the method of communication of the response. Additionally, aspects such as documentation of search terms, references used, and the availability of appropriate background or patient-specific information may also be assessed. This assessment may be carried out internally based on standards of practice at the site. This usually offers the advantage of peer review by practitioners skilled in these functions. Another method is to poll those using the service about the quality of service and response received. This approach is hampered because consumers of the response are rarely able to assess the quality or appropriateness of the search strategy utilized to formulate the response they received in lieu of performing the search themselves or being present while the search is performed. An example assessment tool appears in Appendix 15–7. Questions that are often asked in the process of assessing drug information responses include:

- Is the response correct and appropriate to the situation presented?
- Is the response provided promptly?
- Does the response completely address the question posed?
- Is the response communicated appropriately?
- Are search terms and references appropriately documented?
- Is the response clear, concise, and appropriate for the clinical situation?
- If follow-up was appropriate, was it provided?

The search process itself can be assessed by evaluation of the appropriate depth and breath of resources used, the timeliness of the resources accessed, and the search strategy. This process can also assess documentation issues, the application of literature evaluation skills to the information, and resources used by the practitioner completing the search.

Drug information practitioners are often responsible for assessing and recommending drug information resources available within the organization. These resources may include printed references such as handbooks, textbooks, or educational materials, or electronic resources such as large search engines or Internet web sites. This process should assess whether the appropriate information resources are available based on the scope of care provided and expertise of the practitioners and whether the resources contain accurate and timely information that can be applied in clinical situations. Available primary, secondary, and tertiary resources should be evaluated based on established standards. The explosion of medical information on the Internet has created new challenges in evaluating drug and medical information resources (see Chap. 5). Because there are currently no regulations of content of Internet sites, caution must be used when referencing these resources to support clinical decision making. With the number of web sites expanding faster than most practitioners can assess their content and editorial policies (if any), it has become increasingly difficult for drug information practitioners to stay abreast of those sites that offer legitimate and validated information compared to those offering only conjecture and opinion. Information obtained from other sources including manufacturer's drug information services should also be assessed.

A final component of quality relates to material produced by the drug information service. This includes newsletters, drug monographs, and guidelines developed by the service. Most measures of quality relate to the accuracy, timeliness, and clinical applicability of such documents. Unfortunately, more time is often spent assessing quality of grammar and writing style than is often devoted to clinical content and interpretation. Chapters 6 and 7 provide further information on assessing the quality of the material itself.

Conclusion

The focus of quality in health care has increased significantly in the past decade and has become a major initiative among governmental agencies and accreditation organizations. Within organizations, the emphasis has shifted from departmental efforts to multidisciplinary efforts related to key processes reflecting the move to continuous quality improvement. Within this context, the role of the pharmacist in quality improvement functions related to the medication use process has expanded. A practical working knowledge of total quality management principles is essential for pharmacists to contribute to and lead initiatives to improve patient care.

Study Questions

1. Describe the differences between TQM and quality assurance.

2. List at least four statistical tools used in TQM to identify barriers to quality and to improve processes.

3. Describe the role of the pharmacist in TQM programs.

4. As asked by JCAHO, what two questions define the "Dimensions of Performance"?

5. Give two examples of clinical measures that might be used to meet ORYX requirements.

6. List two specific drug measures included in the HEDIS 2000 quality measures.

7. Compare and contrast DRR, DUR, and MUE based on current definitions.

8. Compare and contrast retrospective, concurrent, and prospective data collection in terms of timing relative to the provision of care, personnel requirements, and accessibility of important information.

9. Give one example of each of the following: educational intervention, restrictive intervention, and process intervention.

10. List three criteria or indicators that could be used to assess the use of a problematic medication within your practice.

11. Give one example of how each of the following could be used at your practice site to assist in a quality improvement effort: a flowchart, a Pareto chart, and a control chart.

REFERENCES

1. Goldstone J. The role of quality assurance versus continuous quality improvement. J Vasc Surg 1998;28(2):378–80.
2. Decker MD. The application of continuous quality improvement to healthcare. Infect Control Hosp Epidemiol 1992;13(4):226–9.

3. Enright SM, Flagstad MS. Quality and outcome: pharmacy's professional imperative. Am J Hosp Pharm 1991;48:1908–11.

4. Zellmer WA. Symposium: opportunity for pharmacy leadership in integrated health care systems. Am J Health-Syst Pharm 1996;53(4):3S–4S

5. Costello RB, ed. The American Heritage College Dictionary. Boston: Houghton, Mifflin Company; 1997.

6. Jablonski JR. Implementing TQM. Competing in the nineties through total quality management. 2nd ed. Albuquerque: Technical Management Consortium, Inc.; 1992.

7. Decker MD. Continuous quality improvement. Infect Control Hosp Epidemiol 1992;13(2):165–9.

8. Chambers DW. TQM: The essential concepts. J Am Coll Dent 1998;65(2):6–13.

9. Dorodny VS. Quality and caring: A fad or a religion? Hosp Pharm 1997;32(3):316, 320, 325–6.

10. Relman AS. Assessment and accountability. The third revolution in medical care. N Engl J Med 1988;319(18):1220–2.

11. Chassin MR. Quality improvement nearing the 21st century: Prospects and perils. Am J Med Qual 1996;11(1):S4–7.

12. Cohen MR. Cooperative approaches to medication error management. Top Hosp Pharm Manage 1991;11(1):53–65.

13. Tremblay J. Creating an appropriate climate for drug use review. Am J Hosp Pharm 1981;38(2):212–15.

14. O'Malley C. Quality measurement for health systems: Accreditation and report cards. Am J Health-Syst Pharm 1997;54:1528–35.

15. Ente BH. The Joint Commission's agenda for change. Curr Concept Hosp Pharm Manage 1989; Summer:7–14.

16. Joint Commission on the Accreditation of Healthcare Organizations. Accreditation Manual for Hospitals. Chicago: Joint Commission on Accreditation of Healthcare Organizations; 1999.

17. Joint Commission of the Accreditation of Health Care Organizations. Approach to use of performance measurement data in the accreditation process during 2000–2001. 1999:[1 screen] Available from: URL: http://www.jcaho.org/.

18. Joint Commission to require performance data. Am J Health-Syst Pharm 1997;54:743.

19. Andrusko-Furphy KT. Oryx and performance measurement in home care. Am J Health-Syst Pharm 1998;55:2299–2301.

20. Kazandjian VA, Lawthers J, Cernak CM, Pipesh FC. Relating outcomes to care: The Maryland Hospital Association's Quality Indicator Project (QI Project®). Joint Comm J Qual Improvement 1993;19(11):530–8.

21. Himmelstein DU, Woolhandler S, Hellander I, Wolfe SM. Quality of care in investor-owned vs. not-for-profit HMOs. JAMA 1999;282(2):159–63.

22. National Committee for Quality Assurance. 2000:[1 screen]. Available from: URL: http://www.ncqa.org/.

23. Cortterell CC. Pharmacy and the proposed quality measures for managed care plans. Am J Health-Syst Pharm 1996;53:2619–22.

24. Spoeri RK, Ullman R. Measuring and reporting managed care performance: Lessons learned and new initiatives. Ann Intern Med 1997;127(8 part 2):726–32.

25. Managed care shows moderate gains, reluctance to share performance data in 1998, says NCQA. Am J Health-Syst Pharm 1998;55:2351–2.

26. Spragins EE. What are they hiding? HMOs are getting more secretive about quality. Newsweek 1999;133(9):74.

27. Omnibus Budget Reconciliation Act of 1987. Section 843.60, Level A requirement; Pharmacy services. 54 FR1989:5359–69.

28. Omnibus Budget Reconciliation Act of 1990. Section 1903(I)10(B)(g) Drug Use Review and (A) Prospective Drug Review.

29. Navarro RP. DUR applications in managed care. Medical Interface 1995;8(3):67–8.

30. Briesacher D, DuChane J. Drug utilization review in the managed care environment. Medical Interface 1995;8(3):72–8.

31. Feinberg JL. Meeting the mandate for quality assurance through drug-use evaluation. Consult Pharm 1991;6:611–20.

32. Stolar MH. Drug use review: Operational definitions. Am J Hosp Pharm 1978;35:76–8.

33. ASHP guidelines on medication-use evaluation. American Society of Health System Pharmacists. Am J Health-Syst Pharm 1996;53(16):1953–5.

34. Nadzam DM. Development of medication-use indicators by the Joint Commission on Accreditation of Healthcare Organizations. Am J Hosp Pharm 1991;48:1925–30.

35. Cousins DD. Medication Use: A systems approach to reducing errors. Chicago: Joint Commission on Accreditation of Healthcare Organizations; 1998.

36. DHEW Task force on prescription drugs: final report. Washington: U.S. Department of Health, Education, and Welfare; 1969.

37. Gutshall EL, Davidson HE, Ninno SD, editors. Medication usage evaluation: Primer, third edition. Norfolk: Insight Therapeutics, LLC; 1999.

38. Todd MW, Keith TD, Foster MT. Development and implementation of a comprehensive, criteria-based drug-use review program. Am J Hosp Pharm 1987;44:529–35.

39. New accreditation process model for 1994 and beyond. Am J Hosp Pharm 1993;50:1111–2, 1121.

40. Flagstad MS, Williams RB. Assuming responsibility for improving quality. Am J Hosp Pharm 1991;48:1898.

41. Terry AK, Draugalis JR, Bootman JL. Drug-use evaluation programs in short-term-care general hospitals. Am J Hosp Pharm 1993;50:940–4.

42. ASHP guidelines on the pharmacist's role in drug use evaluation. Am J Hosp Pharm 1988;45:385–6.

43. The Joint Commission on Accreditation of Hospitals. 1990 AMH. Accreditation Manual for Hospitals. Chicago: Joint Commission on Accreditation of Hospitals; 1989.

44. Covington TR, Alexander VL. Drug use evaluation: The fundamentals. 1991. Indianapolis: Eli Lilly & Co.

45. Schaff RL, Schumock GT, Nadzam DM. Development of the Joint Commission's indicators for monitoring the medication use system. Hosp Pharm 1991;26:326–9, 350.

46. Bernstein SJ, Hilborne LH. Clinical indicators: The road to quality care? J Qual Improvement. 1993:19(11):501–9.

47. American Society of Consultant Pharmacists. Drug Regimen Review: A Process Guide For Pharmacists. 2nd ed. Arlington: American Society of Consultant Pharmacists; 1992.

48. Angaran DM. Selecting, developing, and evaluating indicators. Am J Hosp Pharm 1991;48: 1931–7.

49. Beers MH, Ouslander JG, Rollingher I, Reuben DB, Brooks J, Beck JC. Explicit criteria for determining inappropriate medication use in nursing home residents. Arch Intern Med 1991; 151:1825–32.

50. Criteria for drug use evaluation. Volume 1. Bethesda: American Society of Hospital Pharmacists; 1989.

51. Criteria for drug use evaluation. Volume 2. Bethesda: American Society of Hospital Pharmacists; 1990.

52. Criteria for drug use evaluation. Volume 3. Bethesda: American Society of Hospital Pharmacists; 1992.

53. Gutshall EL, Davidson HE, Ninno SD, editors. Drug usage evaluation: a screening criteria manual for use in concurrent drug usage evaluation. 2nd ed. Norfolk: Insight Therapeutics, LLC; 1999.

54. Knapp DA. Development of criteria for drug utilization review. Clin Pharmacol Ther 1991; 50(Part 2):600–3.

55. American Psychiatric Association. Manual of psychiatric quality assurance. A report of the American Psychiatric Association Committee on Quality Assurance. Washington, D.C.: American Psychiatric Association; 1992.

56. Model drug use review criteria. Year one of HCFA project, Model for developing strategies for outpatient drug use review. Baltimore: Center on Drugs and Public Policy, University of Maryland; 1991.

57. Screening criteria for outpatient drug use review. Final report of HCFA project, Model for developing methodological strategies for outpatient drug use review. Baltimore: Center on Drugs and Public Policy, University of Maryland; 1992.

58. Melby MJ. A mid-sized hospital's experience in indicator data collection. Am J Hosp Pharm 1991;48:1937–40.

59. Threshold vs. standards. QRC Advisor 1988;5(2).

60. Makela EH, Davis SK, Piveral K, Miller WA, Pleasants RA, Gadsden RH Sr, et al. Effect of data collection method on results of serum digoxin concentration audit. Am J Hosp Pharm 1988; 45:126–30.

61. What is an adequate sample? QRC Advisor 1985;1(Aug);4–5

62. Grasela TH, Walawander CA, Kennedy DL, Jolson HM. Capability of hospital computer systems in performing drug-use evaluations and adverse event monitoring. Am J Hosp Pharm 1993; 50:1889–95.

63. Zarowitz BJ, Petitta A, Mlynarek M, Touchette M, Peters M, Long P, et al. Bar-code technology applied to drug-use evaluation. Am J Hosp Pharm 1993;50:935–9.

64. Burnakis TG. Facilitating drug-use evaluation with spreadsheet software. Am J Hosp Pharm 1989;46:84–88.

65. Libby D, Grove C, Adams M. Collaborative use of informatics among hospitals to benchmark medication use processes. Joint Comm J Qual Improvement 1997;23:626–52.

66. Soumerai SB, McLaughlin TJ, Avorn J. Improving drug prescribing in primary care: A critical analysis of the experimental literature. Millbank Q 1989;67:268–317.

67. Avorn J, Soumeri SB, Taylor W. Reduction of incorrect antibiotic prescribing through a structured educational order form. Arch Intern Med 1991;151:1825–32.

68. Kowalsky SF, Echols RM, Peck F. Preprinted order sheet to enhance antibiotic prescribing and surveillance. Am J Hosp Pharm 1982;39:1528–9.

69. Pierson JF, Alexander MR, Kirking DM, Solomon DK. Physician's attitudes toward drug-use evaluation interventions. Am J Hosp Pharm 1990;47:388–90.

70. Himmelberg CJ, Pleasants RA, Weber DJ, Kessler JM, Samsa GP, Spivey JM, et al. Use of antimicrobial drugs in adults before and after removal of a restriction policy. Am J Hosp Pharm 1991;48:1220–7.

71. Restino MS, Knodel LC. Drug information quality assurance program used to appraise students' performance. Am J Hosp Pharm 1992;49(6):1425–9.

72. Wheeler-Usher DH, Hermann FF, Wanke LA. Problems encountered in using written criteria to assess drug information responses. Am J Hosp Pharm 1990;47(4):795–7.

73. Moody ML, Revising a drug information center quality assurance program to conform to Joint Commission standards. Am J Hosp Pharm 1990;47(4):792–4.

74. Smith CH, Sylvia LM. External quality assurance committee for drug information services. Am J Hosp Pharm 1990;47(4):787–91.

75. Halbert MR, Kelly WN, Miller DE. Drug Information Centers: Lack of generic equivalence. Drug Intell Clin Pharm 1977;11:728–35.

76. Beaird SL, Coley RM, Blunt JR. Assessing the accuracy of drug information responses from drug information centers. Ann Pharmacother 1994;28(6):707–11.

77. Calis KA, Anderson DW, Auth DA, Mays DA, Turcasso NM, Meyer CC, et al. Quality of pharmacotherapy consultations provided by drug information centers in the United States. Pharmacotherapy 2000;20:830–6.

16

Chapter Sixteen

Medication Misadventures: Adverse Drug Reactions and Medication Errors

Philip J. Gregory • Karen L. Kier

Objectives

After completing this chapter, the reader will be able to:

- Define medication misadventures, adverse drug events, adverse drug reactions, and medication errors.
- Classify adverse drug reactions based on type and severity.
- Explain methods for determining probability and causality of an adverse drug reaction.
- Identify reporting systems for adverse drug reactions.
- Identify steps to develop an adverse drug reaction reporting program.
- Classify medication errors based on type and severity.
- Differentiate between slips and mistakes as they pertain to medication errors.
- Describe factors affecting cognitive function that lead to medication errors.
- Identify reporting systems for medication errors.
- Identify strategies health care practitioners and health systems can implement to reduce medication errors.

Pharmacists play a pivotal role in the medication use process. Throughout this process there is potential for unexpected adverse events, including errors in prescribing, dispensing, and administering medications, idiosyncratic reactions, and other adverse effects. These events can all be described as medication misadventures.[1] Pharmacists should understand the potential for various medication misadventures and be prepared to recognize and prevent such occurrences when possible.

The terminology surrounding medication misadventures is often confusing. *Medication misadventure* is a very broad term, referring to any iatrogenic hazard or incident associated with medications. All adverse drug events (ADEs), adverse drug reactions (ADRs), and medication errors fall under the umbrella of medication misadventures. An *ADE* is the next broadest term and refers to any injury caused by a medicine. An ADE refers to all ADRs, including allergic or idiosyncratic reactions, as well as medication errors that result in harm being done to a patient.[1-5] ADRs and medication errors are the most specific terms. *ADRs* refer to any unexpected, unintended, undesired, or excessive response to a medicine. A medication error is any preventable event that has the potential to lead to inappropriate medication use or patient harm.[1] Figure 16–1 shows one way of graphically classifying these terms.

Medication misadventures are a worldwide problem that have become an issue of national priority in the United States.[2-4] The economic burden of these events is staggering. Estimates suggest that costs of ADEs may range from $30 billion to more than $130 billion per year in the United States.[5-7] These costs may exceed the total costs of diabetes or cardiovascular care.[6] Up to 28% of these events are thought to be preventable.[5]

Several agencies and professional organizations across the country contribute efforts to minimize these events. Some of the key organizations include the Food and Drug Administration (FDA), the Joint Commission on Accreditation of Healthcare Organizations (JCAHO), the World Health Organization (WHO), the Institute for Safe Medication Practices (ISMP), the United States Pharmacopoeia (USP), and the American Society of Health-System Pharmacists (ASHP). Despite the numerous organizations

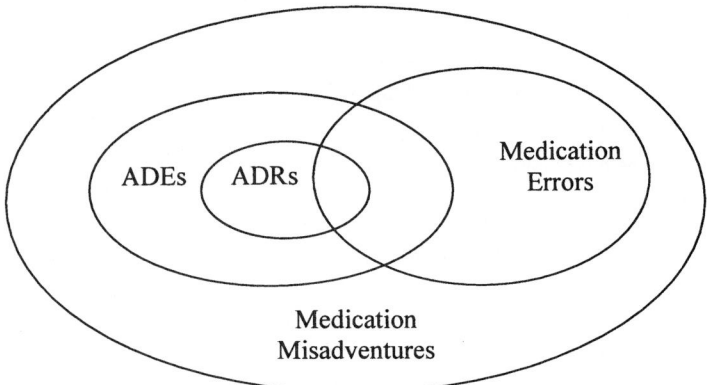

Figure 16–1. Relationship Among Medication Misadventures, Adverse Drug Events, Medication Errors, and Adverse Drug Reactions. Adapted from *American Society of Health-System Pharmacists. Suggested definitions and relationships among medication mis-adventures, medication errors, adverse drug events, and adverse drug reactions. Am J Health-Syst Pharm 1998;55:165–6.*

involved, efforts to minimize medication misadventures depend heavily on individual health care practitioners, including pharmacists, physicians, and nurses, to take measures to minimize and report events. For example, multiple studies have highlighted the tremendous impact individual pharmacists can have on minimizing medication misadventures.[8,9] In one study published in the *Journal of the American Medical Association,* pharmacists participating in hospital rounds in an intensive care unit decreased prescribing errors by 66% and saved an estimated $270,000 per year.[9]

This chapter focuses on ADRs and medication errors, highlighting pertinent definitions, classifications, reporting systems, and methods to minimize such events.

Adverse Drug Reactions

ADRs are frequent consequences of medication administration. All medications, including the excipients of a product, are capable of producing adverse effects.[10] ADRs are estimated to account for 8% to 15% of all hospital admissions, lead to an increase in morbidity and mortality, and result in an annual cost of $5 to $7 billion to the health care system.[6,11] Approximately 20% of the ambulatory population receiving medications suffers from ADRs.[12] These outpatient events do not always result in hospitalization. The incidence of ADRs for patients in the hospital has been reported to be as high as 28%. Health care professionals agree that these percentages are somewhat conservative because many ADRs go undetected, unreported, and untreated.[12] One reason for these low percentages is many patients and health care professionals are not always adequately informed about medications and their potential for adverse events. Many countries, including the United States, have developed systems to encourage the reporting of adverse events. In addition, JCAHO requires hospitals to have a mechanism in place to monitor ADRs. Many hospitals have developed extensive programs that provide a foundation for the monitoring of adverse reactions, including a warning system to prevent further problems. The sharing of information about ADRs between health care practitioners and groups is vital to the success of these programs. In addition, the networking of ADR information can help in providing a useful database to use for recognition or prevention of future ADRs

DEFINITIONS

One of the first steps in establishing an ADR program is to define what the institution or facility categorizes as ADRs. There are many definitions for ADRs that have been described in the literature. Institutions, as well as clinicians, have used different definitions depending on their practice needs.

WHO defines an ADR as "any noxious or unintended response to a drug that occurs at doses usually used for prophylaxis, diagnosis, or therapy of disease or for the modification of psychological function."[13]

The FDA definition of an ADR is

> any adverse event associated with the use of a drug in humans, whether or not considered drug related, including the following: adverse event occurring in the course of the use of a drug product in professional practice; an adverse event occurring from drug overdose, whether accidental or intentional; an adverse event occurring from drug abuse; an adverse event occurring from drug withdrawal; and any significant failure of expected pharmacologic action.[13]

This definition is fairly broad and includes overdose situations as well as areas involving abuse.

The FDA goes on to define an unexpected drug reaction, which is what they would like to have reported, as

> one that is not listed in the current labeling for the drug as having been reported or associated with the use of the drug. This includes an ADR that may be symptomatically or pathophysiologically related to an ADR listed in the labeling, but may differ from the labeled ADR because of greater severity or specificity (e.g., abnormal liver function vs. hepatic necrosis). An ADR may also be due to a drug interaction, defined as a pharmacologic response that cannot be explained by the action of a simple drug, but is due to two or more drugs acting simultaneously.[13]

The use of "unexpected" in the language does limit the number of ADRs that the FDA would like health care professionals to report. This definition focuses on reporting the unusual, uncommon, or newly identified ADRs. Although the common or usual ADRs are relevant and important, they do not provide the FDA with additional information.

Karch and Lasagna,[14] two prominent researchers in the area of ADRs, define a drug, an adverse event, and a patient drug exposure as

> Drug: a chemical substance or product available for an intended diagnostic, prophylactic or therapeutic purpose.
>
> Adverse Drug Reaction: any response to a drug which is noxious and unintended and which occurs at doses used in man for prophylaxis, diagnosis or therapy, excluding ther-

apeutic failures. (As stated by the WHO, this definition excludes intentional and accidental poisoning as well as drug abuse situations.)

Patient–Drug Exposure: a single patient receiving at least one dose of a given drug.

Many hospital programs use this definition because it excludes accidental poisonings as well as problems with drugs of abuse.

CAUSALITY AND PROBABILITY OF ADVERSE DRUG REACTIONS

One of the difficulties in defining an ADR is determining causality. Cause and effect is difficult to prove, in general, and ADRs are no exception. Many publications have dealt with this problem by developing definitions, algorithms, and questionnaires that try to determine the probability of a reaction. To date, none of these attempts have been able to prove actual causality. These tools, however, are used to determine the probability that a particular drug caused an adverse event and are described below

These algorithms and definitions use several key concepts.[15] Dechallenge and rechallenge are often discussed. *Dechallenge* occurs when the drug is discontinued and the patient is then monitored to determine whether the ADR abates or decreases in intensity. *Rechallenge* occurs when the drug is discontinued and, after the ADR abates, the drug is readministered in an attempt to elicit the response again. Dechallenge and rechallenge are effective means for establishing a strong case that the drug was responsible for the ADR. Unfortunately in clinical practice, a rechallenge may not be practical and may actually cause further harm to the patient. Patients who suffer a serious ADR may not be thrilled about experiencing the reaction again in the name of science! A rechallenge may not always be practical, but a dechallenge may be essential.

Another important factor to consider is the temporal relationship between the drug and the event. Does the time frame for development of the ADR make sense? If there is literature on the ADR, does it describe a temporal relationship between the drug and the event? Medical literature and package inserts can be helpful in noting if a drug has been known to cause a certain type of reaction in a certain time frame in the past. Unfortunately, for rare or new ADRs, the literature is not likely to be helpful, but this does not discount the fact that a reaction may have occurred.

Naranjo and associates[15] developed the following definitions to assist in determining the probability of an ADR.

Definite ADR is a reaction which: (1) follows a reasonable temporal sequence from administration of the drug, or in which the drug level has been established in body fluids or tissue; (2) follows a known response pattern to the suspected drug; and (3) is confirmed by dechallenge; and (4) could not be reasonably explained by the known characteristics of the patient's clinical state.

Conditional ADR is a reaction which: (1) follows a reasonable temporal sequence from administration of the drug; (2) does not follow a known response pattern to the suspected drug; and (3) could not be reasonably explained by the known characteristics of the patient's clinical state.

Doubtful ADR is any reaction which does not meet the criteria above.

Several algorithms have been published that try to incorporate information about an ADR into a more scientific form. These algorithms determine the likelihood that the drug was responsible for the reaction and establish a rational and scientific approach to what previously required strictly clinical judgment. All of the algorithms are time consuming and the results can vary according to the interpretation of multiple observers. In 1979, Kramer and co-workers[16] published a questionnaire composed of 56 yes or no questions (Appendix 16–1). This questionnaire includes sections about the patient's previous experience with the drug or related drugs, alternative etiologies, timing of events, drug concentrations, dechallenge, and rechallenge. Responses to each question are given a weighted value and these values are totaled. The total value then belongs to one of four categories: unlikely, possible, probable, or definite. One of the problems with this method is that clinicians can disagree on the weighted values because the user must make subjective judgments for some of the questions. Hutchinson and colleagues[17] evaluated the reproducibility and validity of the Kramer questionnaire. The authors concluded that although the questionnaire was cumbersome to use, the method described by Kramer was superior to clinical judgment alone. Another problem inherent with this questionnaire is that an unexpected ADR may not score well because of lack of literature or previous experience with the ADR. If the reaction is not universally accepted or in the most recent edition of the *Physicians' Desk Reference,* the reaction would score a zero in this section. Overall, however, the questionnaire provides professionals with the opportunity to use a standardized tool.

Naranjo and colleagues developed an alternative algorithm (Appendix 16–2). This algorithm has 10 questions. The questions involve the following areas: the temporal relationship, the pattern of response, dechallenge or administration of an antagonist, rechallenge, alternative causes, placebo response, drug level in the body fluids or tissue, dose–response relationship, previous patient experience with the drug, and confirmation by any other objective evidence. The answer to each question is then assigned a score. The score is then totaled and placed into a category from definite to doubtful. The Naranjo algorithm also places emphasis on rechallenge and dechallenge, which may pose some problems in evaluating ADRs using this method. In the initial published report of this algorithm, Naranjo and colleagues[15] tested the reproducibility and validity of the algorithm. Like the study by Kramer and associates,[16] this algorithm was found to be a valid means of assessing ADRs.

In 1982, Jones and co-workers[18] published an algorithm that allows health care practitioners to answer a series of yes or no questions to determine if a true ADR occurred (Appendix 16–3). This type of format is similar to other published algorithms. The Jones algorithm is shorter and quicker to complete compared to Kramer's questionnaire.

All of the algorithms possess a certain degree of observer variability. However, all can be used to help determine whether an adverse event was precipitated by a certain drug or drug-drug combination. Michel and Knodel[19] compared the three algorithms by Kramer, Jones, and Naranjo. The study found that the Naranjo algorithm was simpler and less time consuming, and compared favorably to the 56 questions asked by Kramer. The study found a higher correlation between the Naranjo algorithm and the Kramer questionnaire. Although there was agreement between the Naranjo and Jones algorithms, the correlation was not as high as that seen between the Naranjo and Kramer algorithms. The authors stated that more data was needed to support the use of the algorithm developed by Jones.

A Bayesian approach to assessing adverse reactions has also been developed by Lane.[20] Using the Bayesian approach, relevant information is collected and a quantitative measure of the odds that a particular drug caused a particular event is calculated. The Bayesian approach has the potential to be an outstanding tool for predicting populations that may be at higher risk for ADRs. The method needs further study, including determining whether the approach is applicable to the hospital environment. The reader is referred to this reference for further insight into the Bayesian approach.

CLASSIFICATION

Definitions and algorithms have also been used to classify the probability and severity of ADRs. Classification systems such as those developed by Naranjo, Kramer, and Jones have used the definite, probable, possible, and unlikely categories to establish probability of ADRs. Other classification systems ranked the severity of ADRs from minor to severe.

One such classification system was developed by Lasagna and Karch, and classifies severity of ADRs into minor, moderate, severe, and lethal as defined below.[18]

- *Minor:* no antidote, therapy or prolongation of hospitalization is required.
- *Moderate:* requires a change in drug therapy, specific treatment, or an increase in hospitalization by at least 1 day.
- *Severe:* potentially life threatening, causing permanent damage or requiring intensive medical care.
- *Lethal:* directly or indirectly contributes to the death of the patient.

The FDA classifies an ADR as serious when it results in death, is life threatening, causes or prolongs hospitalization, causes a significant persistent disability, results in a congenital anomaly, or requires intervention to prevent permanent damage.[21]

When developing an ADR monitoring program, these various systems can be used to determine probability (cause and effect) and severity of ADRs and help describe and quantify data.

MECHANISM OF ADVERSE DRUG REACTIONS

Karch and Lasagna also described various mechanisms for adverse drug reactions.[14] These mechanisms are related to the pharmacologic or pharmacodynamic aspects of drugs and can be used to classify the type of reaction that occurs.

- *Idiosyncrasy:* an uncharacteristic response of a patient to a drug, usually not occurring on administration.
- *Hypersensitivity:* a reaction, not explained by the pharmacologic effects of the drug, caused by altered reactivity of the patient and generally considered to be an allergic manifestation.
- *Intolerance:* a characteristic pharmacologic effect of a drug produced by an unusually small dose, so that the usual dose tends to induce a massive overaction.
- *Drug interaction:* an unusual pharmacologic response that could not be explained by the action of a single drug, but was caused by two or more drugs.
- *Pharmacologic:* a known, inherent pharmacologic effect of a drug, directly related to dose.

When implementing an ADR program, these classifications can help health care practitioners to organize and present data. Potential causative drugs involved in ADRs can be listed allowing trends to be followed over time. These trends can be used to change prescribing habits or alert the institution to potential problems. In addition, the data may also suggest the severity of reactions that are occurring and which medications cause the most severe reactions.

REPORTING

Well-designed programs that monitor ADRs, as well as network information to the medical community, are essential. Gerald A. Faich, MD, Director, Office of Epidemiology and Biostatistics, Center for Drugs and Biologics, for the FDA stated that "ADR surveillance serves primarily to provide early signals about possible problems." He further states, "neither industry nor the FDA should consider its scientific job complete when a new drug is approved."[22] Faich is explaining the importance of postmarketing surveillance and the need to continually monitor drugs and report any adverse consequences. Postmarketing ADR reporting has been responsible for changes in prescribing as well as withdrawal of various drugs from the market.

FDA REPORTING

Due to the limited size of studies required for approval of a new drug entity, the FDA relies on postmarketing information to establish a better understanding of adverse events. Historically, some drugs have been approved by the FDA only to be withdrawn from the market due to postmarketing adverse events. Pharmaceutical companies are required by the FDA to submit quarterly reports of all ADRs for the first 3 years that a drug is on the market as part of the postmarketing surveillance system.

The FDA was required to have a Spontaneous Reporting System (SRS) with the passage of the Kefauver–Harris Amendment of 1962 (due to limited numbers of study subjects, rare adverse effects could otherwise be missed). This program allows for an inexpensive monitoring system of ADRs for all drugs marketed in the United States.[23] The problem in the past has been the lack of reporting by the medical community. In a study of community based physicians, only 57% were aware of the voluntary system of reporting.[24] In the past, the FDA utilized Form 1639 to allow anyone to report an adverse event through the SRS. However, in June 1993, the FDA switched to a new program called MedWatch: The FDA Medical Products Reporting Program. With this new program, the FDA receives reports via mailings, phone calls, faxes, and the Internet. Between June 1993 and September 30, 1993, the FDA received 1717 voluntary reports from pharmacists, physicians, nurses, risk managers, dentists, and other health and non-health professionals. Pharmacists gave 53% of the reports. Of the 1717 reports, 65% were ADEs and 3% were ADRs to biologics. To report a problem to the FDA, consumers and health care professionals can call 1-800-FDA-1088, fax a report to 1-800-FDA-0178, or send via the Internet from <<www.fda.gov/medwatch>>. In addition, the MedWatch Form, also known as FDA Form 3500, can be completed and mailed to the FDA[25] (Appendix 16–4). A unit of the FDA called the Central Triage Unit receives voluntary reports. This unit screens the reports and forwards them to the appropriate FDA program within 24 hours of receiving the report. In addition, they mail a letter to the sender acknowledging the report's receipt. The report becomes part of a database used by the agency to identify signals or warnings that would require further study or regulatory action. Like the previous FDA program, MedWatch is still interested in *serious* adverse events, which they describe as death, life-threatening events, hospitalization, disability, congenital anomaly, or requiring intervention to prevent permanent impairment or damage. The MedWatch program asks people to report an event even if they are not certain that the product was the cause.[25]

The MedWatch program does not overcome lack of reporting due to a voluntary system. It is important to note that pharmaceutical manufacturers are required to report all adverse events to the FDA, whereas, individual health care practitioners only do so voluntarily. Various explanations can account for the failure of practitioners to participate in the FDA program. Hoffman[26] best describes the lack of ADR reporting by physicians as follows:

1. "Failure to detect the reaction due to a low level of suspicion.
2. Fear of potential legal implications.
3. Lack of training about drug therapy.
4. Uncertainty about whether the drug causes the reaction.
5. Lack of clear responsibility for reporting.
6. Paper work and time involved.
7. No financial incentive to report.
8. Unaware of reporting procedure or little understanding of it.
9. Lack of readily available reporting forms.
10. Desire to publish the report.
11. Fear that a useful drug will be removed from the market or given a bad name.
12. Complacency and lethargy.
13. Guilty feelings because of patient harm.
14. Reaction not worth reporting."

Other explanations for the lack of reporting are that medical record personnel, who might be used to categorize and report data, are not familiar with ADRs and/or their method of documentation. Therefore, the pharmacist can provide a valuable service by participating in the MedWatch program.

JCAHO AND ASHP GUIDELINES

The JCAHO requires that hospitals have an ADR reporting program. The programs are generally a function of the Pharmacy and Therapeutics (P&T) Committee and the department of pharmacy. The JCAHO encourages the reporting of serious ADRs to the FDA. Furthermore, JCAHO requires intense analysis of significant ADEs to determine the cause of the event and pursue a remedy to prevent further occurrence.

ASHP also encourages pharmacists to take an active role in monitoring adverse events. ASHP has published very specific guidelines as part of its practice standards. The ADR standards can be found on the Internet at <<http://www.ashp.org/bestpractices/ medmis/guide/adverse.pdf>>.[27]

IMPLEMENTING A PROGRAM

Prior to implementing an ADR program, the health care facility must educate its staff on the importance and significance of the program. The pharmacy department is in an excellent position to provide this education because of its involvement in the P&T Committee, pharmacokinetic dosing, drug utilization evaluation (DUE), and drug distribution. The pharmacy department can be an excellent resource for developing an ADR program, as well as providing data about ADRs to the P&T Committee.

The JCAHO and the ASHP standards can be used as a basis for starting an ADR monitoring program. In addition to the standards, the pharmacy and medical literature are abundant with examples of successful programs, some of which will be reviewed in this chapter. Guidelines for starting a program include the following.

1. Develop definitions and classifications for ADRs that work for the institution. The definitions and classifications in this chapter provide a good starting point for discussion.
2. Assign responsibility for the ADR program within the pharmacy and throughout other key departments. A multidisciplinary approach is an essential factor.
3. Develop a program with approval from the pharmacy department, medical staff, nursing department, as well as other appropriate areas within the facility. Cooperation is essential in initiation of a successful program.
4. Promote awareness of the program.
5. Promote the awareness of ADRs and the importance of reporting such events.
6. Develop policies and procedures for handling ADRs being sent to the FDA. Indicate who is responsible for sending them.
7. Establish mechanisms for screening ADRs. These mechanisms should include retrospective reviews, concurrent monitoring, as well as prospective planning for high-risk groups. It is worthwhile to educate pharmacists to check for ADRs when they see orders for certain "indicator drugs" that are often used in treating an ADR (Table 16-1), orders to discontinue or "Hold" drugs, and orders to decrease the dose or frequency of a drug.[28] Also, electronic screening methods to check for laboratory tests that are indicative of ADRs (e.g., drug levels, *Clostridium difficile* toxin assays, elevated serum potassium, low white blood cell counts) can be helpful.[29]
8. Develop forms for data collection and reporting or other mechanisms for reporting (some institutions use computer reporting, as well as hotline phone numbers).
9. Establish procedures for evaluating ADRs.
10. Routinely review ADRs for trends.
11. Monitor ADRs continuously and concurrently.

TABLE 16–1. ADR "INDICATOR DRUGS"

- Antidiarrheal agents
- Atropine (except preoperatively)
- Dextrose 50% (IV push)
- Diphenhydramine (except at bedtime)
- Epinephrine (IV push)
- Flumazenil
- Naloxone
- Potassium supplement (diuretic or digoxin patients)
- Protamine
- Sodium polystyrene sulfonate (patients on potassium sparing diuretics or ACE inhibitors)
- Topical steroids
- Vitamin K

12. Develop preventive interventions.
13. Report all findings to P&T Committee.
14. Develop strategies for decreasing the incidence of ADRs (depending on the opportunities presented by the ADRs reported). *Please note* this vital step has basically been ignored in the literature; however, for an ADR program to be part of the quality assurance process, it must be included, wherever possible.

There are numerous examples of successful ADR programs that have been published over the past several years, some of which will be covered below. The reader is encouraged to review the literature to evaluate published programs. In addition, colleagues are often willing to share information about their established programs. Reviewing existing programs can provide insight into what works and what may pose problems. The following examples are meant to be informative about the literature, but are by no means reflective of the full body of published ADR programs.

Meriter Hospital, a 500-bed community teaching institution, located in Madison, Wisconsin, reevaluated its ADR program in September of 1990.[30] The institution used the WHO definition of ADRs and identified an event as "a change or discontinuation of the drug therapy, treatment of the ADR, prolongation of hospital stay, and/or mortality." JCAHO guidelines and FDA reporting forms were also used. A communication pathway to monitor their ADRs, along with retrospective, concurrent and prospective drug monitoring was instituted. A retrospective review was performed if the drug information pharmacists noticed any unusual occurrence or trends on monthly reports generated by medical records. The ADRs were identified by coding in the medical record. The concurrent process employed an ADR alert card initiated by either a pharmacist or a utilization review nurse. The pink alert card was filled out for a suspected ADR. Information was obtained that included name, room number, drug, reaction, and reporter's name. This provided the necessary data to identify the causative agent and allowed pharmacy to intervene if necessary. The pharmacy was responsible for prospectively monitoring for allergies, drug–drug interactions, drug–food interactions, and any duplications of therapy.

After implementation of the program, awareness and reporting by the institution's staff significantly increased. The number of reports went from 11 in 1990 to 277 in 1992. Approximately 30% of the total responses were significant enough to forward to the FDA. The program also impacted patient care. Documentation of allergies prompted prospective changes to drug therapy. The ADR program has also become a screen for the DUE program. Likewise, the program improved channels of communication among the pharmacists, as well as throughout the hospital.

The pharmacy updated other departments in the hospital with a newsletter that increased awareness and produced valuable feedback. The program had a positive benefit on patient outcomes, new protocols were established for their DUE program, and new guidelines were set for medication administration.

Another example of a successful adverse drug reaction reporting program was documented in Warren, Michigan, at Macomb Hospital Center.[31] This program was the direct result of an inspection by the JCAHO. An expert on ADRs gave a presentation to a variety of hospital departments and employees. This resulted in increased reporting of ADRs, primarily contrast media reactions. The pharmacy intervened and, with help from the radiology department, developed an ADR program. The cardiac catheterization laboratory was due to open in October of 1989. Following the lead of the radiology department, the ADR forms were modified and used for all inpatients. The forms were placed on the patients' room doors to increase visibility of the program. After another visit from JCAHO, reporting for the institution was still low. A DUE specialist was hired to implement a working ADR and DUE program. Incentives such as discounts in the hospital cafeteria for the first person reporting ADRs helped involve all employees. Specialty services, cardiac and intensive care, psychiatry, and others soon followed suit with each department beginning to report ADRs. The patients' records all had stickers placed on them to increase physician awareness and to ensure allergies were being updated regularly. All staff pharmacists' job descriptions were altered to include ADRs as part of their responsibilities and a merit-based system was added as an incentive to report ADRs.

The Macomb hospital program received favorable reports from the Michigan Department of Public Health and increased its ADR reports from a baseline of 59 to 872 in 1991. In their program, only severe reactions were forwarded to the FDA. The hospital is still updating and improving its program with follow-up procedures, improvements in data collecting, and management of data. The hospital has not only benefited from meeting JCAHO standards, but has shown an improvement in drug usage as well. An unexpected benefit from this program has been increased clinical knowledge of the staff pharmacists and improvement in its literature evaluation and drug information skills.

One of the most impressive ADR programs to date was reported by the Cedars–Sinai Medical Center.[28] While the institution had tried various methods, including ICD-9 codes and a checkbox on the physician's discharge form, their best success resulted from training the utilization review nurses to monitor for ADRs. These nurses reviewed every patient chart at least every 3 days as a routine function of their jobs, and were therefore in a good position to monitor for ADRs. A simple ADR form was developed that the nurses completed and returned to pharmacy for review and collation into a computer database. All severe ADRs were reported to the FDA. The program resulted in ADRs being reported for 4% of hospital admissions. Although its program is certainly not catching 100% of all ADRs, its reporting rate is higher than many institutions.

TECHNOLOGY

Information systems and high-end technology may play an important role in monitoring, identifying, and minimizing ADRs. Information systems are available that can identify and alert practitioners to potential ADRs and detect potential drug–drug interactions that may contribute to ADRs. One system was developed at Brigham and Women's Hospital to detect potential ADRs. The system was programmed to detect a combination of patient-specific factors and medications that may indicate a patient who has the potential to experience an ADR. For example, patients taking medications that require renal function–based dosing who have elevated serum creatinine may be flagged as patients at risk for development of an ADR. Various other screening rules were also programmed. This system was compared to voluntary stimulated reporting and retrospective chart review. The system detected more ADRs than spontaneous reports, but fewer than chart review. Interestingly, the errors detected by the computer system were different than those detected by chart review, indicating that a combination of ADR and ADE detection systems may provide the best results. As expected, using the computer system saved work time, requiring five times fewer person-hours than the chart review method.[32]

In another study, a similar ADE detection system identified potential ADEs in 64 of every 1000 admissions. The prescribing physician did not recognize 44% of the ADEs detected by the system.[33] Computer systems that detect clinically significant drug–drug interactions may also be relevant for reducing ADRs. Although software is readily available for this purpose, one survey indicates that only slightly more than half of the hospitals are using drug interaction software integrated with their drug distribution system. Despite this finding, most pharmacists believe that drug interaction software does or would increase their ability to detect clinically significant drug–drug interactions that may contribute to ADRs.[34]

The health care industry is lagging behind other industries in the implementation of high-end technology information systems.[35] Health care organizations will likely be required to invest in that technology to significantly improve the quality of care and stay competitive in the health care market.[32,35]

Pharmacists can play a vital role in developing, maintaining, and promoting ADR monitoring programs These programs can provide valuable information about ADRs within the institution, as well as provide information that can be forwarded to the FDA. ADR monitoring programs have been developed that impact positively on patient care. ADR programs have been shown to improve communication channels, as well as provide additional education on adverse events. An ADR program should have a multidisciplinary approach and provide a mechanism to impact the quality of patient care. Although the examples concentrated on hospital practice, the concepts are applicable to any practice area and all pharmacists should be involved in adverse drug reaction reporting to improve both knowledge about drugs and individual patient care.

Medication Errors

Patients depend on health systems and health professionals to help them stay healthy. As a result, frequently patients receive drug therapy with the notion that these medications will help them lead a more healthy life. In fact, the initiation of drug therapy is the most common medical treatment received by patients.[36] In virtually all cases, patients and their health care providers understand that when medications are given, there are some known and some unknown risks. Many patients may experience expected side effects. However, patients also experience significant unexpected drug-related morbidity and mortality. These events may occur in up to 6.5% of hospitalized patients.[8] As many as 19% of disabling medical injuries are caused by ADEs, 45% of which are related to medication errors.[2] Errors in the medication use process, including errors in medication prescribing, dispensing, administering, and monitoring, are responsible for 14% of drug-related deaths.[37] In the early 1980s, an average of one medication error per patient per day was reported.[38] A review of medication error–related deaths from 1983 to 1993 has shown an increase from 2876 deaths in 1983 to 7391 deaths in 1993, a 2.57-fold overall increase. Medication error–related deaths in outpatients had an 8.48-fold increase and in inpatients there was a 2.37-fold increase during the same period.[4]

"First do no harm" is a common adage very familiar to most health care practitioners. It is the responsibility of all health professionals and health systems to maintain this adage and contribute to the minimization of medication errors. Because the medication use process is complex and involves multiple individuals representing several health professions and some nonprofessionals, communication and teamwork among the various professions are a necessity. Because society perceives pharmacists to be responsible for the safe and effective use of drugs,[37] however, the pharmacy profession needs to take a prominent role in the maximization of safe medicine use as a core responsibility of pharmaceutical care.[39]

DEFINITIONS

In general terms, "an error is a failure to perform an intended action that was appropriate given the circumstances."[40] The pharmacy and medical community have taken this rather simple general definition and applied the language of the professions to define what precisely constitutes an error in a medical environment within the scheme of medication misadventures and ADEs. The National Coordinating Council for Medication Error Reporting and Prevention (NCC MERP), an organization composed of 19 national organizations and individual members, including the FDA, American Medical Association (AMA), American Pharmaceutical Association (APhA), USP, and several others (Table 16–2), has developed a detailed definition of what constitutes a medication error.

> Any preventable event that may cause or lead to inappropriate medication use or patient harm while the medication is in the control of the health care professional, patient, or consumer. Such events may be related to professional practice, health care products, procedures, and systems, including prescribing; order communication; product labeling,

TABLE 16–2. NATIONAL COORDINATING COUNCIL FOR MEDICATION ERROR REPORTING AND PREVENTION MEMBER ORGANIZATIONS

- American Association of Retired Persons
- American Health Care Association
- American Hospital Association
- American Medical Association
- American Nurses Association
- American Pharmaceutical Association
- American Society of Health-System Pharmacists
- American Society for Healthcare Risk Management
- Department of Veterans Affairs
- Generic Pharmaceutical Industry Association
- Institute for Safe Medication Practices
- Joint Commission on the Accreditation of Healthcare Organizations
- National Association of Boards of Pharmacy
- National Council of State Boards of Nursing
- Pharmaceutical Research and Manufacturers of America and U.S. Pharmacopoeia
- U.S. Food and Drug Administration
- U.S. Pharmacopoeia

packaging, and nomenclature; compounding; dispensing; distribution; administration; education; monitoring; and use.[1]

As mentioned, medication errors fall within the broad category of medication misadventures. In cases where the medication error results in injury to a patient, that error also falls into the medication misadventure subcategory of ADEs (see Fig. 16–1).[1]

Based on the NCC MERP definition, an error may occur as a result of not adequately counseling or educating a patient on proper use of medication. When, for example, a patient inappropriately uses a metered-dose inhaler for asthma and fails to receive the full amount of the medication, a medication error has occurred. The error may be secondary to a lack of education or may have occurred despite adequate counseling and education. Independent of the cause, based on the above definition, a medication error did occur.

Based on the above definition, medication errors also occur when a prescriber writes an incorrect dose on a prescription pad. Even if the prescriber is called by a dispensing pharmacist to clarify and change the order and the patient eventually receives an appropriately dosed medication, an error did occur in the process. An adverse outcome does not necessarily have to occur to classify an event as a medication error.[40]

The "five rights" is a commonly used, but less precise, method of evaluating medication errors. Each medication dose that is administered must comply with these five rights to be free of error: (1) right patient, (2) right drug, (3) right dose, (4) right time, and (5) right route. The five rights are a tool to assist health care professionals at every step in the medication use process to minimize the occurrence of errors.[41] Each professional, when prescribing, dispensing, or administering, should clarify that the five rights are in order before furthering the process of medication use. The five rights also provide an easy and understandable way to identify when medication errors occur. Whenever the five rights are not met, a medication error has occurred. However, when using this very simplified method of looking at medication errors, many of the more common errors, such as dose omissions, may be missed.

The precise definitions for medication errors may vary among institutions. The general principles will be similar, but there may be differences in what qualifies as a reportable error. For example, at one institution it may be determined that an error has occurred when a dose is not received by a patient within 15 minutes of the scheduled time. At another institution, there may be more flexibility, with errors reported only if medication is not administered until more than 30 minutes beyond the scheduled time. Also, some institutions may not report errors that do not affect the patient. For example, institutions may not report an inappropriately written prescription if that error is caught by a pharmacist or nurse before the medication reaches the patient. Instead, a pharmacist or nurse may report it as a professional intervention. Although, according to the NNC MERP definition, it would technically count as an error.

CLASSIFICATION

Defining medication errors is important. It is necessary to develop definitions so that organizations and institutions can identify and track errors. After medication errors have been identified, it is also important to classify the errors. Classification helps to determine where errors are occurring and the severity of the errors, and assists with development of measures to improve the medication use process and minimize the occurrence of such errors.

Medication errors can be classified in a variety of ways. Some medication error reporting systems focus on the type of error. For example, organizations might be interested in whether the error was a dispensing, administering, or prescribing error. Other systems may be more interested in the outcome of the error. These systems focus on what effect, if any, the error had on a patient. For example, organizations may want to know if an extended hospital stay was necessary as a result of the error or if a patient died or suffered a disabling injury. Medication errors may also be subclassified. For example, errors may be further classified based on the profession committing the error or the particular drug involved in the error. Each of these systems will be described in more detail in the following sections.

Error Type

Probably the most common way to classify errors is to identify them by type. This classification focuses on whether an error was related to dispensing, administering, prescribing, or patient compliance. ASHP has provided definitions for various types of errors in 11 categories.[38,42]

1. *Prescribing error:* Errors in this category are fairly broad, but generally focus on inappropriate drug selection, dose, dosage form, or route of administration. Examples may include ordering duplicate therapies for a single indication, prescribing a dose that is too high or too low for a particular patient, writing a prescription illegibly, prescribing an inappropriate dosage interval, or ordering a drug to which the patient is allergic.[38]

   In one study, the most common type of prescribing error (56.1%) was related to an inappropriate dose (either too high or too low). The second most common prescribing error was related to prescribing an agent to which the patient was allergic (14.4%). Prescribing inappropriate dosage forms was the third most common error (11.2%).[36] Other relatively common prescribing errors have included failing to monitor for side effects and serum drug levels, prescribing an inappropriate medication for a particular indication, and inappropriate duration of therapy.[43]

2. *Omission error:* An omission error occurs when a patient does not receive a scheduled dose of medication. This is considered to be the second most common error in the medication use process, behind wrong time errors.[44]

3. *Wrong time error:* What constitutes a wrong time error may vary considerably among institutions. In general, this type of error occurs when a dose is not administered in accordance with a predetermined administration interval. Most institutions realize that it is often impossible to be totally accurate with the administration interval and typically 15 to 30 minutes outside that interval is acceptable. Institutions must establish a policy to indicate what exactly constitutes an error in this category.

4. *Unauthorized drug error:* This type of error occurs when patients receive a drug that was not authorized by an appropriate prescriber. This might include giving the wrong patient a medication.

5. *Improper dose error:* This type of error is different from that which occurs when a prescriber orders an inappropriate dose of a medication. In this situation, the dose given is inconsistent with what was prescribed, assuming the prescribed dose was appropriate. If a prescriber orders an inappropriate dose and then the dose is changed by a clinical pharmacist to an appropriate dose, an "improper dose error" did not occur; however, a prescribing error did occur. This kind of error may occur when a dose is miscalculated or determined based on improper units or measured improperly.

6. *Wrong dosage form error:* This error is also different from the type described in the prescribing error section. This error occurs when a patient receives a dosage form different from that prescribed, assuming the appropriate dosage form was originally ordered.

7. *Wrong drug preparation error:* When medications require some type of preparation, such as reconstitution, this type of error may occur. These kinds of errors may also occur in the compounding of various intravenous admixtures and other products.

8. *Wrong administration technique:* These errors occur when a drug is given to a patient inappropriately. An example is when an intravenously administered agent is given at an excessive rate or when an agent meant for intramuscular administration is given intravenously.

9. *Deteriorated drug error:* This error occurs when drugs are administered that have expired or have deteriorated prematurely due to improper storage conditions.

10. *Monitoring error:* These errors occur when patients are not monitored appropriately either after they have received a drug or before they received a drug. For

example, if a patient is placed on warfarin therapy and adequate blood tests are not performed to assess the patient's response, resulting in a life-threatening hemorrhage, a monitoring error has occurred. Further, in a community pharmacy, if a pharmacist fails to review a patient's medication history prior to dispensing a medication, resulting in a significant drug–drug interaction, a monitoring error has occurred.

11. *Compliance error:* This type of error occurs when patients use medications inappropriately. Although it may seem that health care professionals have little responsibility here, proper patient education and follow-up may play a significant role in minimizing this type of error. This type of error may be a direct result of insufficient patient counseling from a dispensing pharmacist, a prescribing physician, or both.

These types of medication errors are not mutually exclusive. Multiple types of errors may occur during a single administration of a drug and a single adverse patient outcome may be the result of more than one type of error.[42]

Outcome or Severity

Although the classifications of errors frequently are based on type, most errors are also classified by the final result or outcome of an error. Even though errors may occur based on the types described above, there is not always an adverse outcome. It is important for institutions to monitor both the types of errors that occur and the outcomes associated with them. Most reporting systems request information regarding type and outcome of a medication error. Institutions may use information about outcomes to focus their error minimization efforts on the types of errors resulting in the most serious outcomes.

The NCC MERP has proposed a medication error index that serves to categorize errors based on the severity or outcome of the error. This index is divided into four main categories and nine subcategories as follows:[38,45]

1. No error
   Category A: Circumstances or events that have the capacity to cause error.
2. Error, no harm
   Category B: An error occurred, but the medication did not reach the patient.
   Category C: An error occurred that reached the patient, but did not cause the patient harm.
   Category D: An error occurred that resulted in the need for increased patient monitoring, but caused no patient harm.
3. Error, harm
   Category E: An error occurred that resulted in the need for treatment or intervention and caused temporary patient harm.

Category F: An error occurred that resulted in initial or prolonged hospitalization and caused temporary patient harm.

Category G: An error occurred that resulted in permanent patient harm.

Category H: An error occurred that resulted in a near-death event (e.g., anaphylaxis, cardiac arrest).

4. Error, death

Category I: An error occurred resulting in patient death.

Subclassifications

Errors may need to be classified based on the professional involved with the error and the particular drug involved in the error. For example, if a health system notices that most of its errors are prescribing errors, that system may want to implement some training programs for physicians or develop new policies to help minimize those errors. If it is found that a particular dispensing error is increasing, an institution may ask for a review of the pharmacy procedures associated with that particular error.

It has also been found that certain drugs or classes of drugs are more commonly involved in errors than other drugs. For example, in hospitals, intravenous drugs are involved in 70% of medication errors. Medication errors resulting in pharmacist malpractice cases most often involve the drugs warfarin, corticosteroids, hypoglycemic agents, digoxin, amoxicillin, and phenytoin. Physician malpractice cases most commonly involve antibiotics, corticosteroids, and narcotics.[43] In one study evaluating prescribing errors, the agents most commonly involved included antibiotics (34.1%), cardiovascular agents (15.9%), gastrointestinal agents (7%), narcotics (5.7%), other analgesics (4.9%), and hormonal agents (4.1%).[36]

The classification of errors serves an important role. Health systems need detailed information on the extent, types, and consequences of medication errors to appropriately allocate efforts and resources to reduce their occurrence.

PSYCHOLOGY OF MEDICATION ERRORS: WHY DO ERRORS OCCUR?

I presume you are mortal, and may err.

—Shirley, *The Lady of Pleasure,* 1635[40]

Being human, health care professionals of all types have a propensity to commit errors in every area of their professional lives, including the medication use process. To understand why errors occur, it is necessary to examine the medication use system and the vital components in that system, health care professionals.

According to Senders, "An error is a psychological event with psychological causes. . . ."[40] To better understand why health care professionals commit errors, we must look at the cognitive processes that occur at the time of the error. However, even the best understanding of the psychology of errors will not likely eliminate the problem entirely. Humans will most likely commit errors at an unacceptable rate despite our best efforts to understand and remedy their occurrence. With this in mind, it is necessary to develop systems of medication use that account for human error and have processes in place to identify and correct human error before medications reach patients.

At a very basic level, Dr. James Reason suggests that there are two broad types of errors committed: slips and mistakes. *Slips* generally occur when the professional's attention is diverted from the activity at hand, resulting in an inadvertent error such as typing the wrong name on a label. A *mistake* occurs when an error is committed in problem solving due to inadequate knowledge or inappropriate information. For example, this is likely to occur when a seasoned practitioner makes therapeutic decisions based on personal experience rather than overwhelming research evidence.[38]

Davis[46,47] also suggests a broad categorization of causes of errors: (1) performance lapses, (2) lack of knowledge, and (3) lack or failure of safety systems. Davis's definitions parallel Reason's in that performance lapses could also be called slips and lack of knowledge falls into the mistakes category. Lack or failure of safety systems will be discussed in more detail in another section.

Personal and environmental factors are thought to interact to influence cognitive function that may lead to slips. There are several factors specific to the professional involved and their working environment that may contribute to their committal of an error. Grasha and O'Neill[48] have outlined some of the factors that may affect cognitive processes, resulting in lapses of performance.

1. *Excessive task demand:* Many dispensing pharmacists attribute their errors to this situation, complaining that their workload is so heavy and they are overloaded with tasks, making it difficult to work error free. In one survey, 68% of pharmacists rated "work overload" as a major contributing factor to the committal of dispensing errors.[49] Most pharmacists and experts in medication errors agree that work overload may be the most significant factor contributing to medication errors.[43,49]

2. *Personal characteristics:* Personal factors such as age, sensory deficits, or state of health may contribute to performance lapses. Personal levels of stress or fatigue may also have an impact. Someone who is bored at work may also be more error prone.

3. *Extra-organizational factors:* Factors such as similar product names or packaging from pharmaceutical companies may have an extensive impact on the committal of errors with particular drugs. In one study, look-alike or sound-alike drugs were involved in 37% of medication errors.[50] As an example, this issue is currently being addressed for the sound-alike drugs celecoxib (Celebrex), fosphenytoin (Cerebyx), and citalopram (Celexa). Complex insurance plans are also extra-organizational factors that may serve to complicate the medication use

process and contribute to slips. The profession of pharmacy has been referred to as the most heavily regulated of all professions. Legal mandates for policing illegal prescriptions and other regulatory requirements are also good examples of extra-organizational factors.

4. *Work environment:* Poor working conditions may influence the rate of error committal. Poor illumination and high noise levels have been shown to affect the dispensing error rate in pharmacies.[48] Other factors in this category may include high ambient temperatures and frequent interruptions from the telephone or patients.

5. *Intra-organizational factors:* In the era of managed care, there is a significant emphasis on the bottom line. Policies and procedures demanding high output or mandating long working hours may significantly affect cognition and the ability to prevent error occurrence.

6. *Interpersonal factors:* Conflicts among co-workers or with patients may distract professionals from the tasks at hand and contribute to error committal. General interruptions from people may also fall into this category.

Some factors that may contribute to cognitive lapses and the committal of medication errors may fall into more than one of these categories. Furthermore, factors from multiple categories may occur simultaneously to contribute to error committal.

Health care professionals have indicated that other factors may also contribute to medication errors. Some of those factors are as follows.

1. *Lack of communication:* This factor may also fall under interpersonal factors listed above. Failure to communicate among fellow employees or among health care professionals has frequently been named as contributing to medication error. For example, an error may be more likely to occur if a pharmacist chooses not to clarify unclear physician orders. Poor physician handwriting and verbal orders are also significant factors.[44]

2. *Failure to comply with policy:* This is a common factor in dispensing and administering drugs. In one survey, 42% to 46% of pharmacists said that failing to check drugs before dispensing was a significant factor in dispensing errors.[49] Noncompliance with policy has also been associated with drug administration errors. Often nurses develop specific personal routines for administration of certain agents, which they perceive to be an improvement in the medication administration process, despite contrary policy.[44]

3. *Lack of knowledge:* This is a frequently cited factor in the committal of medication errors. Mistakes rather than slips are typically committed as a result of inadequate knowledge. Placing inexperienced recent graduates in positions where they cannot interact with more experienced practitioners may increase medication errors. Nonspecialists covering a service that is normally staffed by a spe-

cialist may also lead to errors.[47] Nurses untrained in pharmacology may be more unlikely to recognize potential inconsistencies in disease state and medication usage and doses, resulting in the possibility of increased medication errors reaching the patient.[44]

4. *Lack of patient counseling:* It has been said that the last safety check prior to dispensing medication should be counseling the patient. Talking to the patient allows the pharmacist to correlate the medication and dose with the patient's condition and helps the pharmacist to detect any errors that may have occurred in the medication use process. In one study, 89% of errors committed in a community pharmacy were detected during patient counseling.[43] However, errors may occur not only from lack of counseling, but also from providing incorrect information during patient counseling.[51] Providing incorrect information may also fall in the *lack of knowledge* category.

There are a variety of intrapersonal, interpersonal, and environmental factors that may contribute to errors in the medication use process. The examples provided above are a partial list of contributory factors at the level of the health care practitioner. These factors influence the occurrence of slips or performance lapses and mistakes committed by individuals. They do not address failure of a system or failure of a safety net as a whole process. The medication use process involves multiple health care professionals, non-professional staff, patients, and multiple physical environments. The safety net should work with all professionals and in all environments and may consist of multiple checks by individuals of other people's work, computer systems that screen for errors, barcode scanning systems, quality assurance measures, extra-organizational measures (e.g., to minimize ordering medications from companies with similar packaging), and multiple other systems. To adequately address the causes of errors, failures in the system must also be addressed. Although it is important to address the problem of individuals committing errors (e.g., increasing training, enforcing policy), adequately developed safety systems should be in place to significantly minimize the number of errors reaching patients. When errors do occur, it is necessary to address the event in the context of failure of the system or safety net.[52]

MEDICATION ERROR REPORTING

To err is human; to forgive is against company policy.

—John Senders, 1978[40]

Reporting medication errors, particularly severe or life-threatening errors, may have adverse consequences for both the individuals and the organization involved. Health care professionals have lost their jobs and been sued as a result of medication errors. As a result, health care professionals and health systems are reluctant to open themselves up to adverse outcomes associated with reporting medication errors.[43] As an example, in one hospital, there were only 36 incident reports regarding medication errors over a yearlong reporting period. At the same institution, an observational study revealed that as many as 51,200 errors were likely to have actually occurred during that same reporting period.[38] In New York, a pharmacist had his license suspended after committing a single dispensing error that resulted in brain damage in a patient. In Nevada, a pharmacy was fined 2 weeks net profit for understaffing that resulted in dispensing errors.[43] A medical center in New Jersey was successfully sued for $12 million and fined by the state board of pharmacy after a medication error killed an infant.[53] In Colorado, three nurses were indicted on charges of criminal negligence after a medication administration error killed an infant.[54] In the current environment, the disincentives for error reporting seem to outweigh the incentives.[55]

The case in Colorado is particularly disheartening for experts in the field of medication misadventures. It demonstrates an example of a system failure that resulted in punishment of individual health care professionals. In this case, a 1-day-old baby was prescribed long-acting penicillin because its mother had acquired an infection. The medication was erroneously administered intravenously to the infant instead of intramuscularly, resulting in death of the infant. It was also found that a pharmacist had actually dispensed 10 times the appropriate dose. Cases similar to this one have been reported in the literature and had even occurred at that same institution as reported a few weeks before this particular incident. Although this case is saddening and disturbing, there was clearly a serious malfunctioning of the medication use process at this institution that allowed two serious errors to go unrecognized. District attorneys in Colorado pressed criminal charges against the nurses involved that could result in 3 to 5 years' imprisonment. The exact cause of this error is unknown, but it points to a lack of availability of clear and relevant drug information. It is also an example of blaming individuals for errors that are obviously the result of system breakdown.[54]

Despite the negative actions taken against individuals and organizations that commit medication errors, reporting errors is an absolute necessity for at least three reasons. First, to improve current medication use systems, the circumstances under which errors occur must be understood. Without adequate reporting, institutional and national self-evaluation would be impossible. Second, taking a proactive role in identifying errors and using that information to improve medication use systems may actually protect organizations from negligence claims. When errors are not reported, it may be interpreted as concealment.[43] In one study conducted at a Veterans Affairs Medical Center, it was shown that an institutional policy to immediately report medical errors to patients and their families and offer compensation resulted in liability payments among the lowest of 35 similar Veterans Affairs Medical Centers.[56] Finally, voluntary error reporting is necessary to avoid being placed on "accreditation watch" by JCAHO. If JCAHO discovers that a serious error occurred at an accredited organization that was not previously reported, JCAHO will perform an immediate on-site survey and place the organization on accreditation watch. The JCAHO has recently made voluntary reporting appear less risky for organizations and individuals in an effort to increase medication error reporting. Under a relatively new policy, when an error occurs and is reported, the institution is now given an opportunity to investigate and implement corrective measures on its own. Previously, JCAHO would immediately launch its own investigation and place the organization on accreditation watch. JCAHO has also acknowledged that firing professionals involved with an error is not a proper response or consistent with quality improvement principles.[3] This new approach has already resulted in increased reporting in 1998.[53] Time will tell if professionals and organizations continue to take this opportunity to conduct vigorous internal review to implement and improve systems to minimize medication errors.[55]

Institutional Reporting

Individual institutions must develop a reporting system specific to their institution, designed to meet their specific needs. There are at least four methods for collecting reports of medication errors.[38,43] These methods may be used alone or in combination.

1. *Anonymous self-reports:* In this system, anyone detecting or committing an error can report it without associating their name with the error. It is essentially risk free for the reporter and therefore it may increase the likelihood of having an error reported. Despite this theoretical advantage, there is still underreporting, particularly in cases that do not result in patient harm.[38]
2. *Incident reports:* This type of self-reporting system is the most commonly used. In this system, errors are written up as legal reports and are often used to satisfy JCAHO requirements. In this system, errors are highly underreported.[38]
3. *Critical-incident technique:* Although not really a reporting system, this technique uses observations and interviews of professionals involved in medication errors to analyze and identify weaknesses in the system. This method uses errors reported by other systems in an attempt to provide solutions to existing medication use problems.[38]
4. *Disguised observation:* Instead of relying on individuals to report errors, this method places an observer among health care professionals to watch for the occurrence of errors. The purpose of the observation is unknown by the professionals. Errors are then recorded and reported. This method is more reliable than self-reporting, but is time consuming and expensive.[38]

National Reporting

Reporting within specific institutions is important to maintain the safety of that institution's patients as well as to maintain the institution's accreditation status. In an effort to share institutional experiences to avoid the same errors being repeated at several institutions, national reporting systems have evolved. There is a great deal of controversy regarding legal concerns and reporting errors outside of respective institutions. It is thought by some in the legal community that reporting errors in any way may expose institutions to less legal protection.[3,43] Despite the objections of some in the legal community, national reporting must be done to share information among practitioners and institutions in an effort to increase the safety of patients. Several systems are available for this purpose.

1. *MedWatch:* This program was developed by the FDA Medical Products Reporting Program for the purpose of monitoring clinically significant adverse drug events and problems with medical products. MedWatch monitors quality, performance, and safety of medical products, devices, and medications. This program contributes to surveillance of medication errors that may be associated with product labeling and names.[38] The MedWatch program does not monitor reports of medication errors not specifically associated with a problematic product. Medication errors associated with strictly human error are not reported to MedWatch. Significant reports may result in distribution of e-mail and "Dear Doctor" alerts to health care professionals. These announcements can be viewed on the Internet at <<http://www.fda.gov/medwatch/safety.htm>>. Health care professionals and consumers can report adverse drug events and product problems by completing a MedWatch form (see Appendix 16–4) and mailing it to the FDA, by calling 1-800-FDA-1088, or reporting on-line at <<http://www.fda.gov/medwatch>>.

2. *USP-ISMP Medication Errors Reporting Program (MERP):* This system is a collaboration between USP and ISMP. Errors can be reported anonymously 24 hours a day by calling 1-800-23-ERROR. Report forms (Appendix 16–5) can also be mailed or submitted online at <<http://www.usp.org/>>. Reported errors are reviewed by USP and forwarded to the manufacturer and the FDA.[38,49]

3. *MedMARx:* This system was developed by USP and is the only service that requires payment of a fee for use. However, this service provides much more than an anonymous method of reporting errors. This service allows subscribing organizations to report and monitor organization-specific errors online. Furthermore, organizations can compare their error rates with other subscribing organizations of similar type. The program also allows organizations to perform root cause analysis as required by JCAHO when errors occur that result in patient

harm.[57] More information regarding MedMARx can be found at <<http://www.usp.org/>>.

At the institutional, organizational, or national level, medication error reporting systems generally require that a form be completed that describes the error, how it was treated, and its outcome. To standardize information associated with medication error reporting, the NCC MERP has developed a taxonomy for medication errors that may be applied in reporting and analyzing medication errors. This taxonomy ensures use of standard language and structure of information reported. Use of this taxonomy may help organizations develop reporting systems and analyze their specific medication errors. This 17-page document can be viewed and printed at <<http://www.nccmerp.org/taxo0514.pdf>>.

ERROR PREVENTION

The ultimate purpose for defining, classifying, analyzing, and reporting medication errors is to enable individuals and organizations to implement better systems that prevent medication errors. ASHP has identified a multitude of risk factors associated with the occurrence of medication errors as outlined below.[42]

- Work shift—more errors occur during the day shift
- Inexperienced or inadequately trained staff
- Medical services with special needs (e.g., pediatrics, oncology, etc.)
- Higher number of medications per patient
- Environmental factors such as high levels of noise, poor lighting, and frequent interruptions
- High workload for staff
- Poor communication among health care providers
- Dosage form—more errors with injectable drugs
- Drug category—more errors with certain classes of drugs (e.g., antibiotics)
- Type of drug distribution systems—unit dose system is associated with fewer errors; high levels of floor stock are associated with increased errors
- Improper drug storage
- Calculations—increased errors with increased complexity and frequency of amount of calculations required
- Poor handwriting
- Verbal orders
- Lack of effective policies and procedures
- Poorly functioning oversight committees

Although this is not necessarily a comprehensive list, prevention strategies that successfully address these risk factors may be successful at minimizing the occurrence of medication errors. In the remainder of this section, some strategies for reducing medication errors will be described.

PRACTITIONER STRATEGIES

Individual health care practitioners play an integral role in the medication use process and must be familiar with factors that may contribute to medication errors. Although individuals are merely one part of a medication use system, each must take some responsibility for ensuring that their individual practices are consistent with the goal of reducing medication errors. Practitioners that recognize the potential for errors in various situations and implement personal practice habits to minimize errors can have a significant impact on error reduction. The following is a look at some things individual practitioners can do to minimize medication errors.

1. *Patient communication:* As discussed, interaction with the patient may significantly reduce medication errors. A pharmacist who counsels patients before handing out the medication is more likely to catch a dispensing error.[58] Similarly, nurses may minimize errors that reach a patient by asking the patient about allergies and describing the medication to the patient just prior to administration. Physicians may similarly contribute to better medication use by counseling a patient more thoroughly when writing the prescription.[42] When the pharmacist also counsels, there will be reinforcement of the information. Also, if the directions are different from the pharmacist compared to the physician, that may indicate that an error was committed somewhere in the medication use process.[58]

2. *Intra-professional communication:* In addition to communicating with patients, health care professionals need to improve communication among themselves. Illegible writing, extensive verbal medication orders, and a "Lone Ranger" approach to practice has no place in a health system devoted to reducing medication errors. When a medication order is unclear, it is a necessity to clarify that order before the medication use process continues. Poor prescription writing is commonly cited as a cause for medication errors. Abbreviations should be avoided. Lack of knowledge about the proper use of drugs is also frequently cited as a cause of prescribing errors.[8,59] Prescribers should ensure proper use of medications by consulting with pharmacists, other physicians, or the medical literature.[42]

3. *Education and training:* Lack of knowledge among all health care practitioners is commonly associated with medication errors. Health care professionals should

stay abreast of current medical literature.[42] In the health care environment the phrase "in my clinical experience . . ." is often used. Undoubtedly experience counts for a lot, but past experiences are no substitute for a thorough understanding of current medical literature.

4. *Reporting:* Health care professionals should recognize the necessity of medication error reporting. To enable other organizations and professionals to avoid the mistakes of others, reporting must be carried out consistently and routinely.

HEALTH-SYSTEM STRATEGIES

The medication error literature emphasizes the importance of health system involvement in minimizing medication errors. It is not good enough for health systems to tell their employees to be more careful or to try to minimize errors. The medication use process involves multiple professional and nonprofessional staff that are prone to errors. Health systems must recognize that even the most highly trained and proficient practitioners will commit errors as a result of being human. In addition to individual responsibility, health systems must ensure that they provide the tools needed by all parties involved to help prevent medication errors. A medication error that reaches a patient is not the result of error committed by a single person, but a flaw in the medication use process. The following identifies some of the things health systems can do to help minimize medication errors.

1. *Environmental factors:* As discussed, there are numerous work place factors that may contribute to performance lapses and medication errors. Low lighting, high levels of noise, high temperatures, and stressful work environments are examples. Health systems should ensure that their facilities do not contribute to the commission of errors.[42]

2. *Policy:* Health systems should implement policies supportive of the effort to minimize medication errors. For example, policies that support the employment of adequate personnel for staffing and supervision should be implemented. There is a direct correlation with high workloads and inadequate staffing and medication errors.[44] Policies that demand multiple checks prior to dispensing or administering medication should also be implemented. Unit dose drug distribution systems are preferred.[37] Policies that limit floor stock and do not allow nonpharmacists to dispense medications should be implemented. Health systems must define medication errors and their classifications, and implement policies for monitoring and correcting such errors. Policies for medication error reporting should minimize risk to reporters of error and allow for the development of a system that supports improvement of the system rather than punishment of employees.[42]

3. *Failure mode and effect analysis:* This is a system of identifying potential errors and adverse outcomes before they occur. It has been adapted from the aerospace industry and can be applied to the medication use process. With the use of failure mode and effect analysis, health systems should be able to design and implement medication use processes that have a significantly lower incidence of medication error.[60]

4. *Drug and patient information:* Lack of information has been frequently cited as a cause of medication errors, particularly prescribing errors. Health systems should ensure that all health care providers have ready access to necessary patient-specific information and general drug information. Health systems may implement technology that allows viewing of a patient chart over a computer terminal or provides electronic medical references. Health systems may establish a drug information center where pharmacists are readily available to answer drug therapy questions. Considerable success has also been found in reducing medication errors when a knowledgeable pharmacist participates on medical rounds.[9]

5. *Training:* It is important for health care professionals to stay up to date regarding drug therapy. Health systems should contribute to this effort by supporting educational programs for their employees.[42]

6. *Technology:* The health care industry seems to be behind other industries in the area of informatics.[35] To significantly improve quality of care and minimize medication errors, health systems need to make a substantial investment in information technology. According to Arthur Caplan, "You've got a 19th-century Charles Dickens's system in an era of high technology,"[9] referring to the use of information technology in health care. Health care practitioners need to have ready access to medical and drug information, patient data, and an automated medication order system. The lack of drug and patient information, as described, has been associated with a large number of prescribing errors. Implementation of automated medication orders, also known as physician order entry, would minimize many problems with illegible writing and abbreviations and would save time for pharmacists and physicians.[61] Furthermore, physician order entry has been shown to significantly reduce the number of serious medication errors.[62] Other types of technology that may minimize errors include automated dispensing equipment and software that screens for drug–drug interactions and proper dosing.[63,64]

7. *Reporting:* Health systems should implement nonpunitive systems for medication error reporting. Accurate error monitoring will help organizations implement successful medication use processes that minimize adverse outcomes associated with medication errors.

An editorial appearing in the *American Journal of Health-System Pharmacy* encourages institutions to recognize the role that pharmacists play in minimizing errors.[65] Adequate staffing by qualified pharmacists who actively participate in all aspects of the medication use process, including prescribing, dispensing, and administering, has been shown to significantly decrease medication errors.[9] Institutions are urged to use pharmacists to their full potential, by more actively employing pharmacists in clinical settings where they can collaborate with other health care professionals, so that they may strengthen efforts to reduce medication errors. ASHP has published guidelines that describe specific methods for the individual practitioner (prescriber, pharmacist, nurse) and for organizations to consider for minimization of medication errors. These guidelines can be viewed and printed at the following Internet address: <<www.ashp.org/bestpractices/medmis/guide/preventing.pdf>>.

National Priority

Medication error prevention may be more important now than ever before for health systems. The Health Care Financing Administration (HCFA) has initiated new quality of care measures to ensure that health systems participating in the Medicare and Medicaid programs are minimizing medication errors. The new conditions of participation are now less focused on procedures and more focused on outcomes. Citing modern drug information systems and drug packaging as significant tools to reduce medication errors, HCFA expects health systems to document a medication error rate of 2% or less.[66]

In 1998, the Institute of Medicine (IOM) formed the Quality of Health Care in America Committee that was charged with developing a strategy to improve quality in health care. In their published report, "To Err is Human: Building a Safer Health System," the committee highlights what is currently known about the extent of medical errors, what contributes to medical errors, and recommendations to minimize errors and improve the quality of health care in the United States. The report can be found in full-text on the Internet at <<http://books.nap.edu/html/to_err_is_human/>>. The Committee's recommendations include the following.[4]

1. *Creation of a Center for Patient Safety.* This center would fall within the control of the Agency for Health Care Policy and Research (AHCPR) and would be responsible for setting national goals for patient safety, tracking progress toward those goals, and reporting progress to the President of the United States and Congress. The Center would also contribute to better understanding of errors in health care and identify methods for preventing errors by funding research activities and information dissemination programs.

2. *Development of a national mandatory reporting system.* This system would initially focus on hospital mandatory reporting of deaths and serious harm secondary to medical error to state governments. State governments would then share information with other states as coordinated by the Center for Patient Safety. Eventually, other institutional settings, including ambulatory care settings, would also have the same requirements. Furthermore, standards would be developed for reporting, including uniform reporting nomenclature and taxonomy.

3. *Encouragement of voluntary reporting systems.* The Center for Patient Safety would encourage increased participation in voluntary reporting programs and fund pilot projects for reporting systems.

4. *Extend peer review protection to information about medical errors used to improve organizational quality and safety.* The Committee suggests that the United States Congress ensure confidentiality in cases of medical error that do not result in serious harm to a patient by enacting specific legislation to protect that information. This will create an environment conducive to increasing reporting of certain kinds of errors that will help organizations fix flaws in their systems.

5. *Performance standards for health care organizations should focus more on patient safety.* The Committee suggests that licensing and accreditation standards should eventually be implemented that require patient safety programs as a minimum standard. Purchasers of health care (i.e., insurance companies) should then provide incentives for demonstration of continuous improvement in patient safety.

6. *Performance standards for health care professionals should focus more on patient safety.* Health care professional licensing bodies (e.g., state boards of pharmacy) should begin to require periodic reexamination to ensure competence and understanding of safety practices. Licensing or credentialing bodies should develop ways to identify practitioners that are unsafe. Professional organizations should develop and offer training to health care professionals and disseminate informative publications regarding patient safety. Safety issues should also be incorporated into practice guidelines. Professionals and professional organizations should collaborate on issues of patient safety.

7. *The FDA should focus more attention on the safe use of drugs.* The committee suggests that the FDA should develop standards for drug packaging and labeling to minimize medication errors associated with labeling and sound-alike drugs. The FDA, pharmaceutical industry, and health care professionals should work together to identify and remedy safety issues associated with problematic labeling and naming.

8. *Health care organizations and professionals should make continually improved patient safety a serious pursuit with defined executive responsibility.* Patient safety programs should be developed with well-described and understood standards

and a nonpunitive system for reporting and analyzing errors. Interdisciplinary team training programs should be completed.

9. *Health care organizations should implement medication safety practices proven to reduce errors.* All health care organizations should implement programs for improving safety of the medication use process based on published recommendations shown to reduce medication errors.

The recommendations of the committee are broad and do not address many of the finer points that health care organizations must deal with to implement an environment safer for patients. However, the recommendations provide a map to improved patient safety for organizations to pursue. The committee suggests reevaluation of the same issues again in 5 years to assess progress toward improved patient safety and decreased medical error.

Conclusion

Medication misadventures are a serious problem in the U.S. health care system. Recognition of the problem is an important first step in developing strategies to minimize their occurrence. Reporting of medication misadventures is an absolute necessity to gauge our progress and direct our efforts.

Pharmacists have the responsibility of ensuring the safe and effective use of medications. Although other health care providers and health care systems must significantly contribute to this effort, pharmacists, as champions of the medication use process, must take a leading role. Several studies have already demonstrated the tremendous benefit pharmacists can provide to patients through reduction of medication misadventures. As a mandate of pharmaceutical care, pharmacists need to continue to contribute to improving patient care by actively pursuing improvements in the medication use process.

Study Questions

1. Describe the relationship of medication misadventures, adverse drug events, adverse drug reactions, and medication errors.

2. Define adverse drug reaction.

3. Describe the JCAHO requirements for adverse drug reaction reporting.

4. List 10 reasons physicians may not report adverse drug reactions.

5. Describe a successful adverse drug reaction program.

6. Explain how technology might improve adverse drug reaction programs.

7. Explain the "five rights."

8. Who is responsible for minimizing medication errors?

9. Why should pharmacists take a leading role in minimizing adverse drug events?

10. Identify three national medication error reporting programs.

11. Explain why it is important to analyze the medication use process when errors occur rather than blaming individuals.

12. Describe strategies practitioners and health systems can use to minimize medication errors.

REFERENCES

1. American Society of Health-System Pharmacists. Suggested definitions and relationships among medication misadventures, medication errors, adverse drug events, and adverse drug reactions. Am J Health-Syst Pharm 1998;55:165–6.

2. Rich DS. A process for interpreting data on adverse drug events: Determining optimal target levels. Clin Ther 1998;20(suppl C).

3. Rich DS. The Joint Commission's revised sentinel event policy on medication errors. Hosp Pharm 1998;33:881–5.

4. Institute of Medicine. To err is human: Building a safer health system. Washington, D.C.: National Academy Press; 1999.

5. White TJ, Arakelian A, Rho JP. Counting the costs of drug-related adverse events. Pharmacoeconomics 1999;15:445–58.

6. Classen DC, Pestotnik SL, Evans S, Loyd JF, Burke JP. Adverse drug events in hospitalized patients. JAMA 1997;277:301–6.

7. Bates DW, Spell N, Cullen DJ, Burdick E, Laird N, Petersen LA, et al. The costs of adverse drug events in hospitalized patients. JAMA 1997;277:307–11.

8. Lesar TS, Briceland L, Stein DS. Factors related to errors in medication prescribing. JAMA 1997;277:312–17.

9. Leape LL, Cullen DJ, Clapp M, Burdick E, Demonaco HJ, Erickson JI, et al. Pharmacist participation on physician rounds and adverse drug events in the intensive care unit. JAMA 1999; 282:267–70.

10. Wong YL. Adverse effect of pharmaceutical recipients in drug therapy. Ann Acad Med 1993; 22:99–102.

11. Swanson KM, Landry JP, Anderson RP. Pharmacy-coordinated, multidisciplinary adverse drug reaction program. Top Hosp Pharm Manage 1992;12:49–59.

12. Fincham JE. An overview of adverse drug reactions. Am Pharm 1991;NS31:435–41.

13. Lamy PP. Adverse drug effects. Clin Ger Med 1990;6:293–307.

14. Karch FE, Lasagna L. Toward the operational identification of adverse drug reactions. Clin Pharmacol Ther 1977;21:247–54.

15. Naranjo CA, Busto U, Sellers EM, Sandor P, Ruiz I, Roberts EA, et al. A method of estimating the probability of adverse drug reactions. Clin Pharmacol Ther 1981;30:239–45.

16. Kramer MS, Leventhal JM, Hutchinson TA, Feinstein AR. An algorithm for the operational assessment of adverse drug reactions: I. Background, description, and instructions for use. JAMA 1979;242:623–32.

17. Hutchinson TA, Leventhal JM, Kramer MS, Karch FE, Lipman AG, Feinstein AR. An algorithm for the operational assessment of adverse drug reactions: II. Demonstration of reproducibility and validity. JAMA 1979;242:633–8.

18. Jones JK. Adverse drug reactions in the community health setting: Approaches to recognizing, counseling, and reporting. Fam Comm Health 1982;5(2):58–67.

19. Michel DJ, Knodel LC. Comparison of three algorithms used to evaluate adverse drug reactions. Am J Hosp Pharm 1986;43:1709–14.

20. Lane DA. The Bayesian approach to causality assessment: An introduction. Drug Info J 1986; 20:455–61.

21. What is a serious adverse event? [cited 2000 Feb 28]:[1 screen]. Available from: URL: http://www.fda.gov/medwatch/report/desk/advevnt.htm.

22. Faich GA, Dreis M, Tomita D. National adverse drug reaction surveillance: 1986 Arch Intern Med 1988;148:785–7.

23. Stang PE, Fox JL. Adverse drug events and the Freedom of Information Act: An apple in Eden. Ann Pharmacother 1992;26:238–43.

24. Rogers AS, Israel E, Smith CR, Levine D, McBean AM, Valente C, et al. Physician knowledge, attitudes, and behaviour related to reporting adverse drug events. Arch Intern Med 1988;148: 1596–1600.

25. MedWatch: The FDA Medical Products Reporting Program. FDA Med Bull 1993;23:insert.

26. Hoffman RP. Adverse drug reaction reporting—problems and solutions. J Mich Pharm 1989;27: 400–3, 407–8.

27. ASHP guidelines on adverse drug reaction monitoring and reporting. Am J Hosp Pharm 1989; 46:336–7.

28. Saltiel E, Johnson E, Shane R. A team approach to adverse drug reaction surveillance: Success at a tertiary care hospital. Hosp Form 1995;30:226–32.

29. Classen DC, Pestotnik SL, Evans RS, Burke JP. Computerized surveillance of adverse drug events in hospital patients. JAMA 1991;266:2847–51.

30. Saine DR. A successful community hospital program for monitoring adverse drug reactions. Top Hosp Pharm Manage 1992;12:19–30.

31. Burkhardt ME, Ripepe SD. Reporting adverse drug reactions is everyone's business: An adverse drug reaction reporting program that works. Top Hosp Pharm Manage 1992;12:31–9.

32. Jha AK, Kuperman GJ, Teich JM, Leape L, Shea B, Rittenberg E, et al. Identifying adverse drug events: Development of a computer-based monitor and comparison with chart review and stimulated voluntary report. JAMIA 1998;5:305–14.

33. Raschke RA, Gollihare B, Wunderlich TA, Guidry JR, Leibowitz AI, Peirce JC, et al. A computer alert system to prevent injury from adverse drug events. JAMA 1998;280:1317–20.

34. Dalton M, Chambers G, Halvachs F. Implementing an effective drug interaction reporting program. Hosp Pharm 1999;34:31–42.

35. Felkey BG. Health system informatics. Am J Health-Syst Pharm 1997;54:274–80.

36. Lesar TS, Lomaestro BM, Pohl H. Medication-prescribing errors in a teaching hospital: A 9-year experience. Arch Intern Med 1997;157:1569–76.

37. Kelly WN. Pharmacy contributions to adverse medication events. ASHP Online 1999 [cited 1999 Sept 8]:[1 screen]. Available from: URL: http://www.ashp.org/public/proad/mederror/pkel.html.

38. Coleman IC. Medication errors: Picking up the pieces. Drug Topics 1999;143:83–92.

39. Chenier GE, Vogel DP. Medication error prevention guidelines. Pharm Pract News 1999;May: 25–8.

40. Senders JW. Theory and analysis of typical errors in a medical setting. Hosp Pharm 1993; 28:505–8.

41. Institute for Safe Medication Practices. The "five rights." 1999 August 17 [cited 1999 Sept]: [1 screen]. Available from: URL: http://www.ismp.org/MSAarticles/FiveRights.html.

42. American Society of Hospital Pharmacists. ASHP guidelines on preventing medication errors in hospitals. Am J Hosp Pharm 1993;50:305–14.

43. Abood RR. Errors in pharmacy practice. US Pharm 1996;21:122–32.

44. Pepper GA. Errors in drug administration by nurses. ASHP Online 1999. [cited 1999 Sept 8]:[1 screen]. Available from: URL: http://www.ashp.org/public/proad/mederror/pep.html.

45. Dunn EB, Wolfe JJ. Medication error classification and avoidance. Hosp Pharm 1997;32:860–5.

46. Davis NM. Performance lapses as a cause of medication errors. Hosp Pharm 1996;31:1524–5.

47. Davis NM. Lack of knowledge as a cause of medication errors. Hosp Pharm 1997;32:16–25.

48. Grasha AF, O'Neill M. Cognitive processes in medication errors. US Pharm 1996;21:96–109.

49. Ukens C. Breaking the trust: Exclusive survey of dispensing errors. Drug Top 1992;136: 58–69.

50. DeMichele D. Preventing medication errors. US Pharm 1995;20:69–75.

51. Fitzgerald WL, Wilson DB. Medication errors: Lessons in law. Drug Top 1998;142:84–93.

52. Davis NM. Lack or failure of the safety net as a cause of medication errors. Hosp Pharm 1997;32:143–4.

53. Glut of medication errors focuses pharmacists on event reporting. Drug Utilization Rev 1998; December:201–6.

54. Cohen MR. ISMP medication error report analysis: The mistake of blaming people and not the process. Hosp Pharm 1997;32:1106–11.

55. Leape LL, Woods DD, Hatlie MJ, Kizer KW, Schroeder SA, Lundberg GD. Promoting patient safety by preventing medical error. JAMA 1998;280:1444–7.

56. Landis NT. Disclosure of errors may have financial benefit. Am J Health-Syst Pharm 2000; 57:312.

57. Cousins DD. Developing a uniform reporting system for preventable adverse drug events. Clin Ther 1998;20:C45–C58.

58. Proulx SM. Medication errors. US Pharm 1997;22:73.

59. Jones EH, Speerhas R. How physicians can prevent medication errors: Practical strategies. Clev Clin J Med 1997;64:355–9.

60. McNally KM, Page MA, Sunderland B. Failure-mode and effects analysis in improving a drug distribution system. Am J Health-Syst Pharm 1997;54:171–7.

61. Davis NM, Cohen MR. Computer generated prescription orders. Am Pharm 1995;NS35(9):10.

62. Bates DW, Leape LL, Cullen DJ, Laird N, Petersen LA, Teich JM, et al. Effect of computerized physician order entry and a team intervention on prevention of serious medication errors. JAMA 1998;280:1311–16.

63. Neuenschwander M. Limiting or increasing opportunities for errors with dispensing automation. Hosp Pharm 1996;31:1102–6.

64. McMullin ST, Reichley RM, Kahn MG, Dunagan WC, Bailey TC. Automated system for indentifying potential dosage problems at a large university hospital. Am J Health-Syst Pharm 1997; 54:545–9.

65. Sellers JA. Too many errors, not enough pharmacists. Am J Health-Syst Pharm 2000;57:337.

66. Wechsler J. Federal agencies seek to reduce drug errors, improve information on adverse events. Formulary 1998;33:161–2.

17

Chapter Seventeen

Investigational Drugs

Bambi Grilley

Objectives

After completing this chapter, the reader will be able to:

- List the major legislative acts that led to our current system of drug evaluation, approval, and regulation.
- List all of the requirements (as specified by the Office of Human Research Protections [OHRP]) for an institutional review board (IRB).
- Prepare appropriate pharmacy reviews of protocols for use by the IRB or other review committees when they evaluate new protocols.
- List the steps in the drug approval process.
- Recognize the difference between a treatment investigational new drug (IND), an emergency IND, and an individual investigator IND.
- Define orphan drug status and list the advantages of classifying a drug as an orphan drug.
- Provide pharmacy support for clinical research including (but not limited to):
  - ordering drug supplies for ongoing clinical trials.
  - maintaining drug accountability records as required by the FDA.
  - preparing drug and protocol data sheets for use by health care personnel in the hospital.
  - preparing pharmacy budgets for sponsored clinical research.
  - aiding study sponsors in designing and conducting clinical trials in their institution.
  - assisting investigators in initiating and conducting clinical trials (including emergency use INDs).

It is estimated that $231 million is spent to get a new drug product to market in the United States. For every 4000 products synthesized in the lab, only 5 will ever be tested in humans and only one of those will ever reach the market.[1] Currently, more than 9000 registered drug products and their dosage forms are available in the American marketplace. The Food and Drug Administration (FDA) is the federal agency that decides which drug products are marketed in this country. On average, the FDA approves two new molecular entities (NMEs) each month. Since 1940, more than 1000 NMEs have been approved in the United States.[2] It is very important that the clinical trials upon which the FDA will base their decisions be both scientifically accurate and complete. Pharmacists can play an important role in ensuring that the clinical trials conducted at their institutions meet the goals set forth by the study sponsor, the local investigator, and ultimately the FDA.

In some institutions, a pharmacist will be hired specifically to handle investigational drugs. More frequently, however, this role falls to a specified staff pharmacist or the drug information pharmacist. To successfully manage investigational drugs, the pharmacist must be a bookkeeper, inventory control manager, and most importantly an information disseminator. Before proceeding, it is necessary to define a number of terms that will be used in this chapter.

Definitions

- *Clinical investigation:* Any experiment in which a drug is administered or dispensed to one or more human subjects. An experiment is any use of a drug (except for the use of a marketed drug) in the course of medical practice. Although there are many other definitions, this is the FDA's definition and would seem the appropriate one to use given the nature of this topic. Please note that the FDA does not regulate the practice of medicine and prescribers are (as far as the agency is concerned) free to use any marketed drug for "off-label use."
- *Clinical safety officer* (*CSO*): Also known as the regulatory management officer (RMO). This will be the sponsor's FDA contact person. Generally the CSO/RMO assigned to a drug's Investigational New Drug (IND) application will also be assigned to the New Drug Application (NDA).
- *Control group:* The group of test animals or humans that receive a placebo (a dosage that does not contain active medicine) or active (a dosage that does contain active medicine) treatment. For most preclinical and clinical trials, the FDA will require that this group receive placebo (commonly referred to as the placebo control). However, some studies may have an "active" control, which generally consists of an available (standard of care) treatment modality. An active control

may, with the concurrence of the FDA, be used in studies where it would be considered unethical to use a placebo. A historical control is one in which a group of previous patients is compared to a "matched" set of patients receiving the new therapy. A historical control might be used in cases where the disease is consistently fatal (i.e., AIDS).

- *Contract research organization* (*CRO*): An individual or organization that assumes one or more of the obligations of the sponsor through an independent contractual agreement.
- *Drug master file* (*CMC-DMF*): References on file with the FDA that contain information regarding the drug. There are five different types of DMFs. The one most commonly used when filing an IND is the CMC-DMF, which contains information regarding the chemistry, manufacturing, and controls (CMC) of the drug.
- *Drug product:* The final dosage form prepared from the drug substance.
- *Drug substance:* Bulk compound from which the drug product is prepared.
- *Food and Drug Administration* (*FDA*): The agency of the U.S. government that is responsible for ensuring the safety and efficacy of all drugs on the market.
- *Institutional Review Board* (*IRB*): A committee of reviewers that evaluates the ethical implications of a clinical study protocol.
- *Investigational New Drug:* A drug, antibiotic, or biological that is used in a clinical investigation. The label of an investigational drug must bear the statement: "Caution: New Drug—Limited by Federal (or United States) law to investigational use."
- *Investigational New Drug Application* (*IND*): A submission to the FDA containing chemical information, preclinical data, and a detailed description of the planned clinical trials. Thirty days after submission of this document to the FDA by the sponsor, clinical trials may be initiated in humans (unless the FDA places a clinical hold). When the FDA allows the studies to proceed, this document allows unapproved drugs to be shipped in interstate commerce.
- *Investigator:* The individual responsible for initiating the clinical trial at the study site. This individual must treat the patients, assure that the protocol is followed, evaluate responses and adverse reactions, assure proper conduct of the study, and solve problems as they arise.
- *New Drug Application* (*NDA*): The application to the FDA requesting approval to market a new drug for human use. The NDA contains data supporting the safety and efficacy of the drug for its intended use.
- *Sponsor:* An organization (or individual) who takes responsibility for and initiates a clinical investigation. The sponsor may be an individual or pharmaceutical com-

pany, government agency, academic institution, private organization, or other organization.

- *Sponsor-investigator:* An individual who both initiates and conducts a clinical investigation (i.e., submits the IND and directly supervises administration of the drug as well as other investigator responsibilities).
- *Subject:* An individual who participates in a clinical investigation (either as the recipient of the investigational drug or as a member of the control group).[3]

History of Drug Development Regulation in the United States

For more than a century after the Declaration of Independence, drug products were not regulated in this country. Available drugs were often ineffective, but some were addictive, toxic, or even lethal. During this same period, doctors were not licensed and nearly anyone could practice medicine. The public was, for the most part, responsible for using common sense when evaluating which products they would use.

The evolution of drug regulations in this country is a study in human tragedy. Crises have instigated the development of many of the laws regulating drug development, preparation, and distribution.

The first federal law developed to deal with drug quality and safety was the Import Drug Act of 1848. This law was passed after it was discovered that American troops involved in the Mexican War had been supplied with substandard imported drugs. The act provided for the inspection, detention, and destruction or re-export of imported drug shipments that failed to meet prescribed standards.

The Pure Food and Drugs Act was passed in 1906. This law required that drugs not be mislabeled or adulterated and stated that they must meet recognized standards for strength and purity. Mislabeling in this context only referred to the identity or composition of drugs (not false therapeutic claims). False therapeutic claims were prohibited with the passing of the Sherley Amendment in 1912.

In 1937 the drug sulfanilamide was released. This drug showed promise as an anti-infective agent and was prepared as an oral liquid. The vehicle used for this preparation was diethylene glycol (a sweet-tasting solvent similar to ethylene glycol, which was used as an automobile antifreeze). A total of 107 people died after taking this preparation. Within 1 year of this tragedy, the Food, Drug and Cosmetic Act of 1938 was enacted. This law required that the safety of drugs, when used in accordance with the labeled instructions, be proven through testing before they could be marketed. It was in this law that the submission of an NDA to the FDA was first described. The NDA was required to list the drug's intended uses and provide scientific evidence that the drug was safe. If after 60 days the FDA had not responded to the manufacturer regarding the NDA, the manufacturer was free to proceed with marketing of the product.

In 1951 the Durham–Humphrey Amendment was passed. This law divided pharmaceuticals into two distinct classes:

1. Over-the-counter (OTC) medications that could be safely self-administered.
2. Prescription (Rx) medications that had potentially dangerous side effects and therefore required expert medical supervision.

This law required the following statement be added to the labels for all prescription medications: "Caution: Federal Law prohibits dispensing without a prescription."

In 1962 another drug tragedy occurred that resulted in additional regulations. In that year, an inordinate number of pregnant women in Western Europe gave birth to children with severe deformities. These deformities were related to the use of the drug thalidomide. Although U.S. consumers were not directly affected by this tragedy (because thalidomide had not been released in the U.S. market), it was a compelling reason for the legislature to develop stronger laws regarding the testing of new drug products. The Kefauver–Harris Drug Amendment was passed the same year. This law specified that the manufacturer had to demonstrate proof of efficacy, as well as safety, prior to marketing any new drug. Additionally, this law required that drug manufacturers operate in conformity with current good manufacturing practices (CGMP). Finally, it stated that the FDA had to formally approve an NDA before the drug could be marketed.[4]

There are numerous other laws and regulations that affect drug products in the United States, but those mentioned above provide the legal foundation for the current regulation of drug products in this country. Based on these laws, the FDA has assumed a large role in assessing the safety and efficacy of drug products prior to their distribution in the United States.

As stated, the goal of the FDA is to provide American consumers with safe and effective therapy. Extensive debate regarding the need to reform the FDA has been ongoing in the United States for years. Critics of the FDA claim the approval process for drugs in this country is too costly and time consuming.[5] Interestingly, a comparison of the drug approval times between the United States, the United Kingdom, Germany, and Japan, reveals that the United Kingdom and United States have similar patterns of drug availability. Additionally, the United States outpaces both Germany and Japan in the approval of "global" drugs (those drugs that are important enough to ultimately be approved in more than one of the four countries mentioned above). Nevertheless, the FDA and the federal government have initiated reforms designed to address criticism.[6]

Recent reform acts include the Prescription Drug User Fee Act of 1992 (PDUFA) and the Food and Drug Administration Modernization Act of 1997 (FDAMA). PDUFA redefined the time frames for NDA reviews and established revenues to fund the increased demands created by the new time frames. The FDAMA, which reauthorized PDUFA, was much broader in scope and impacted not only the drug approval process, but also other aspects of the practices of pharmacy and medicine. Finally, the FDA has undertaken many information technology initiatives to facilitate the regulatory review process. Included in these initiatives is the development of systems allowing for electronic submission, management, and review of regulatory information. Other attempts by the FDA to increase availability of investigational drugs and to expedite the drug approval process will be discussed later in this chapter.

Increasingly, drug companies are involved in global drug development. Historically, the regulatory requirements for drug approval varied from country to country, resulting in a significant amount of time and money being spent to receive multiple approvals. For this reason, the International Conference on Harmonization (ICH) has brought together officials from Europe, the United States, and Japan to develop common guidelines for ensuring the quality, safety, and efficacy of drugs. The FDA has been very involved in the development of the ICH guidelines.[7] The ultimate goal of these guidelines is to provide pharmaceutical firms a method to ensure simultaneous submission and rapid regulatory approval in the world's major markets. This would minimize duplication of effort, improve efficiency, and increase the quality and consistency of medical treatments available to patients worldwide.

For gene therapy products, review and approval by the National Institutes of Health Office of Biotechnology Activities (NIH/OBA) are required in addition to review and approval by the FDA. Submission requirements are similar to those mandated by the FDA (covered later in this chapter). The review process for gene therapy products is a separate topic that will not be further addressed in this chapter.

In addition to the regulatory review of investigational drugs by the FDA, research protocols are also reviewed for ethical appropriateness by IRBs. The formalized process for protecting human subjects began with the Nuremberg Code. This code was used to judge the human experimentation conducted by the Nazis around the middle of the twentieth century. The Nuremberg Code states that "the voluntary consent of the human subjects is absolutely essential."[8] The code goes on to specify that the subject must have the capacity to consent, must be free from coercion, and must comprehend the risks and benefits involved in the research.[8] The Declaration of Helsinki reemphasized the above points and distinguished between therapeutic and nontherapeutic research. This document was first developed in 1964 and was revised in 1975 and again in 1989.[9]

The National Institutes for Health (NIH), as part of the Department of Health and Human Services (DHHS), used these two documents to develop its own policies for the Protection of Human Subjects in 1966. These policies were raised to regulatory status in 1974 and established the IRB as a mechanism through which human subjects would be protected. The Belmont Report, released in 1978, further delineates the basic ethical principles underlying medical research on human subjects.[10] Title 45 Part 46 of the Code of Federal Regulations (CFR), which was released in 1981, was designed to make uniform the protection of human subjects in all federal agencies.[11] Title 21 Part 50 (approved in 1980) of the CFR sets forth guidelines for appropriate informed consent and Title 21 Part 56 (approved in 1981) of the CFR sets forth guidelines for the IRB.[12,13] Copies of these regulations are available from the federal government upon request.

These two documents are used by the FDA and the DHHS to evaluate the ethical conduct of clinical trials in the United States. Further information regarding the role of the IRB will be presented later in this chapter.

The Drug Approval Process

The first step in the drug approval process is preclinical testing. This testing is either in vitro or in animals. Before filing an IND, the sponsor must have developed a pharmacologic profile of the drug, determine its acute toxicity in at least two species of animals, and conducted short-term toxicity studies (2 weeks to 3 months). Chronic toxicity studies in animals can coincide with the use of the drug in clinical trials in humans (although they must be initiated at least 13 weeks in advance). The preclinical chronic toxicity studies must be of at least the same duration as any planned clinical trial (i.e., a 6-month study in humans requires at least 6 months of preclinical data).[1,4]

After the preclinical testing is completed, the sponsor will file an IND with the FDA. The IND is the application by the study sponsor to the FDA to begin clinical trials in humans. Most often, the sponsor is usually a pharmaceutical company, but occasionally an individual investigator will file an IND and serve as a sponsor-investigator. The investigator IND is submitted when a physician plans to use an approved drug for a new indication (i.e., one that is outside the package labeling) or on occasion, for an unapproved product or for an NME. The IND requirements for the sponsor-investigator are the same as those for any other sponsor. For that reason, no differentiation will be made in the following discussion of the drug approval process.

The IND can be filed after the study sponsor has identified the pharmacologic profile of the drug and has results from both acute and short-term toxicity studies in animals. An IND is not required if the drug to be studied is marketed in the United States and all of the following requirements are met.

1. The study is not to be reported to the FDA in support of a new indication.
2. The study does not involve a different dose, route, or patient population that increases the risk to patients.
3. IRB approval and informed consent are secured.
4. The study will not be used to promote the drug's effectiveness for a new indication.

In situations where it is unclear whether an IND is required or not, a call to the FDA may be beneficial. If an IND is required, the application needs to contain the following information.

1. *Cover sheet:* Form 1571 (see Appendix 17–1). This form identifies the sponsor, documents that the sponsor agrees to follow appropriate regulations, and identifies any involved CRO. This is a legal document.
2. *Table of contents*
3. *Introductory statement:* States the name, structure, pharmacologic class, dosage form, and all active ingredients in the investigational drug; the objectives and planned duration of the investigation should be stated here.
4. *General investigational plan:* Describes the rationale, indications, and general approach for evaluating the drug, the types of trials to be conducted, the projected number of patients that will be treated, and any potential safety concerns; the purpose of this section is to give FDA reviewers a general overview of the plan to study the drug.
5. *Investigator's brochure:* An information packet containing all available information on the drug including its formula, pharmacologic and toxicologic effects, pharmacokinetics, and any information regarding the safety and risks associated with the drug; it is important that this brochure be kept current and comprehensive; therefore, it should be amended as necessary. The investigator's brochure may be used by the investigator or other health care professionals as a reference during the conduct of the research study.
6. *Clinical protocol* (*note:* in general, phase I protocols are allowed to be less detailed than phase II and phase III protocols).

   - *Objectives and purpose:* a description of the purpose of the trial (a typical phase I objective would be to determine the maximum tolerated dose of the investigational drug, whereas a typical phase III objective would be to compare the safety and efficacy of the investigational drug to placebo or standard therapy).

   - *Investigator data:* provides qualifications and demographic data of the investigators involved in the clinical trial (may be presented on form 1572 [see Appendix 17–2]).

- *Patient selection:* describes the characteristics of patients that are eligible for enrollment in the trial (and states factors that would exclude the patient).

- *Study design:* describes how the study will be completed; if the study is to be randomized, this will be described here (with a description of the alternate therapy).

- *Dose determination:* describes the dose (with possible adjustments) and route of administration of the investigational drug; if retreatment or maintenance therapy of patients is allowed, it will be detailed in this section.

- *Observations:* describes how the objectives stated earlier in the protocol are to be assessed.

- *Clinical procedures:* describes all laboratory tests or clinical procedures that will be used to monitor the effects of the drug in the patient; the collection of this data is intended to minimize the risk to the patients.

- *IRB approval for protocol:* documentation of this approval is not required as part of the IND application process; however, form 1571 does state that an IRB will review and approve each study in the proposed clinical investigation before allowing initiation of those studies.

7. *Chemistry, manufacturing, and control data*
   - *Drug substance:* describes the drug substance including its name, biological, physical, and chemical characteristics; the address of the manufacturer; the method of synthesis or preparation; and the analytical methods used to assure purity, identity, and the substance's stability.

   - *Drug product:* describes the drug product including all of its components; the address of the manufacturer; the analytical methods used to ensure identity, quality, purity, and strength of the product; and the product's stability.

   - *Composition, manufacture, and control of any placebo used in the trial:* the FDA does not require that the placebo be identical to the investigational drug; however, it wants to ensure that the lack of similarity does not jeopardize the trial.

   - *Labeling:* copies of all labels (drug substance, product, and packages).

   - *Environmental assessment:* presents a claim for categorical exclusion from the requirement for an environmental assessment (a statement that the amount of waste expected to reach the environment may reasonably be expected to be nontoxic).

8. *Pharmacology and toxicology data*
   - *Pharmacology and drug disposition:* describes the pharmacology, mechanism of action, absorption, distribution, metabolism, and excretion of the drug in animals and in vitro.

   - *Toxicology:* describes the toxicology in animals and in vitro.

   - A statement that all nonclinical laboratories involved in the research adhered to Good Laboratory Practice (GLP) regulations.

9. *Previous human experience:* summary of human experiences, which includes data from the United States and, where applicable, foreign markets. Known safety and efficacy data should be presented (especially if the drug was withdrawn from foreign markets for reasons of safety or efficacy).

10. *Additional information:* other information that would help the reviewer evaluate the proposed clinical trial should be included here. For example, if a drug has the potential for abuse, data on the drug's dependence and abuse potential should be discussed in this section.[3]

The Letter of Authorization (LOA) to Cross-reference a Drug Master File (referred to in item 9 on page 1 of form 1571) is required when the investigational product (or some component of the investigational product) being used in the research is being supplied by a manufacturer other than the study sponsor. The original holder of the IND/NDA prepares the LOA. An LOA is frequently required when two companies are working together toward development of a product.[14]

The IND should be amended as necessary. There are four types of documents that may be used to amend the IND. They are as follows:

1. *Protocol amendments:* submitted when a sponsor wants to change a previously submitted protocol or add a new study protocol to an existing IND.
2. *Information amendments:* submitted when information becomes available that would not be presented using a protocol amendment, IND safety report, or annual report (example: new chemistry data).
3. *IND safety reports:* reports clinical and animal adverse reactions; reporting requirements depend on the nature, severity, and frequency of the experience. The following definitions are used to help evaluate adverse reactions.
   a. *Serious adverse drug experience:* Any adverse drug experience occurring at any dose that results in any of the following outcomes: death, a life-threatening adverse drug experience, inpatient hospitalization or prolongation of existing hospitalization, a persistent or significant disability/incapacity, or a congenital anomaly/birth defect. Important medical events that may not result in death, be

life threatening, or require hospitalization may be considered a serious adverse drug experience when, based on appropriate medical judgment, they may jeopardize the patient or subject and may require medical or surgical intervention to prevent one of the outcomes listed in this definition.

b. *Unexpected adverse drug experience:* Any adverse drug experience that is not listed in the current labeling for the drug product. This includes events that may be symptomatically and pathophysiologically related to an event listed in the labeling, but differs from the event because of greater severity or specificity.

For serious and unexpected, fatal, or life-threatening adverse reactions associated with the use of the drug, the sponsor is required to notify the FDA by telephone or fax within 7 calendar days after the sponsor receives the information. The sponsor must also submit a written report within 15 calendar days. For clinical and nonclinical adverse events that are both serious and unexpected, the sponsor must notify the FDA in writing within 15 calendar days. The written reports should describe the current adverse event and identify all previously filed safety reports concerning similar adverse events. The written report may be submitted as a narrative or as form 3500A.[15]

4. *Annual reports:* submitted within 60 days of the annual effective date of an IND; it should describe the progress of the investigation including information on the individual studies, summary information of the IND (summary of adverse experiences, IND safety reports, preclinical studies completed in the last year), relevant developments in foreign markets, and changes in the investigators brochure.

Each submission to a specific IND is required to be numbered sequentially (starting with 000). A total of three sets (the original and two copies) of all submissions to an IND file (whether a new IND or revisions to an existing IND) are sent to the FDA.[3]

Once submitted to the FDA, the IND will be forwarded to one of nine divisions for review (each division handles different therapeutic categories). These divisions are based on the therapeutic group of the drug.[4] The FDA has 30 days after receipt of an IND to respond to the sponsor. The sponsor may begin clinical trials if there is no response from the FDA within 30 days. The FDA delays initiation of a new study or discontinues an ongoing study by issuing a clinical hold. Clinical holds are most often used when the FDA identifies an issue (through initial review or through later submissions) that the agency feels poses a significant risk to the subjects. After this issue has been satisfactorily resolved, the clinical hold can be removed and the investigations can be initiated or resumed.

There are four phases of clinical trials. Clinical studies generally begin cautiously. As experience with the agent grows, the dose and duration of exposure to the agent may also increase. The number of patients treated at each phase of study and the duration of the studies can vary significantly depending on statistical considerations, the prevalence of patients affected by the disease, and the importance of the new drug. However, some general guidelines regarding the four phases of clinical testing are presented below.

A *phase I trial* is the first use of the agent in humans. As such, these studies are usually initiated with cautious (low) doses and in small numbers of subjects. Doses may be increased as safety is established. A phase I study will usually treat 20 to 80 patients and last an average of 6 months to 1 year. The purpose of a phase I trial is to determine the safety and toxicity of the agent. Frequently these trials include a pharmacokinetic portion. These trials assist in identifying the preferred route of administration and a safe dosage range. When possible, these trials are initiated in normal, healthy volunteers. This allows for evaluation of the effect of the drug on a subject who does not have any preexisting conditions. In situations in which this is not practical (such as oncology drugs, in which the drug itself can be highly toxic) these drugs are usually reserved for patients who have exhausted all conventional options.

A *phase II trial* is one in which the drug is used in a small number of subjects who suffer from the disease or condition that the drug is proposed to treat. The purpose of a phase II trial is to evaluate the efficacy of the agent. Data from the phase I trial, in vitro testing, and animal testing may be used to identify which group of patients is most likely to benefit from therapy with this agent. Phase II trials usually treat between 100 and 200 patients and will average about 2 years in duration.

Phase III trials build on the experience gained during the phase II trials. The purpose of a phase III study is to further define the efficacy and safety of the agent. Frequently, in phase III studies, the new agent is compared to current therapy. These trials are usually multicenter studies, generally treat from 600 to 1000 patients, and usually last about 3 years. Some of the phase III trials will be "pivotal" studies and will serve as the basis for the NDA for a drug's marketing approval.

After phase III trials have been completed, the sponsor will submit an NDA to the FDA requesting approval of the drug for marketing. The FDA requires the completion of two well-designed, controlled clinical trials prior to submission to the FDA. However, the sponsor will include information gathered from all of the clinical trials to show that the drug is safe and effective and to describe the pharmacology and pharmacokinetics of the drug. The NDA will include all preclinical data, clinical data, manufacturing methods, product quality assurance, relevant foreign clinical testing (or marketing experience), and all published reports of experience with the drug (whether sponsored by the company or not). A proposed package insert will be supplied as well.[3]

The NDA will be distributed to the appropriate FDA drug review divisions. This is one of the same divisions described earlier in this chapter in the section discussing the IND evaluation process. As noted, these divisions are based on the therapeutic group of the drug. The same reviewer may be assigned to review the IND and the NDA.[4]

The speed at which the NDA will be processed is to some extent determined by the classification the drug receives during its initial review. Each drug is rated with a number–letter designation that evaluates two separate aspects of the drug. The number portion of the rating is associated with the uniqueness of the drug product (ranging from 1 for an NME to 7 for a drug that has already been marketed but without an approved NDA). The letter portion of the rating is associated with the therapeutic potential of the drug product. The P (priority review) designation is given to drugs that represent a therapeutic advance with respect to available therapy, whereas an S (standard review) is given to drugs that have little or no therapeutic gain over previously available drugs).[16] A detailed description of these different codes can be found in Tables 14–3 thru 14–6.

During the review process, the FDA may utilize one of its 15 prescription drug advisory committees to help review the NDA. These committees are composed of experts. They provide the agency with independent, nonbinding advice and recommendations regarding the NDA.[4] After completing its review, the FDA issues an NDA with an "action letter" (stating the NDA is either "approved," "approvable," or "not approvable"). When an approval letter is sent the drug is considered "approved" as of the date of the letter (this rarely occurs with an original NDA). When an "approvable" letter is sent it means that the application "substantially meets the requirements for marketing approval and the agency believes that it can approve the application if specific additional information or material is submitted or specific conditions are agreed to by the applicant."[17] The sponsor has 10 days to respond to the "approvable" letter (although an extension is usually granted if requested within the 10-day period). A "not approvable" letter is sent when the FDA believes the NDA is insufficient for approval. The letter will describe the deficiencies in the application. Once again the sponsor has 10 days to respond to the letter. The sponsor can amend the NDA, withdraw the NDA, or request a hearing with the FDA to clarify whether grounds exist for denying approval of the application.[17]

After the drug has been approved, phase IV trials may be initiated. These trials are also referred to as postmarketing studies. They are conducted for the approved indication, but may evaluate different doses, the effects of extended therapy, or the drug's safety in patient populations that were not represented in premarketing clinical trials. These phase IV trials may be requested by the FDA or they may be initiated by the sponsor in an attempt to gather more data on the safety and efficacy of the drug or to identify a competitive advantage of the drug over other available therapies.[1,18]

The average time from initial synthesis of an agent to approval of an NDA is approximately 100 months.[1] On average, the NDA review process (from submission to approval) takes 2 years (range of 2 months to 7 years).[1] For diseases (such as AIDS and cancer) where these investigational drugs may be the only therapy available, this time delay can be a significant factor. The FDA has developed procedures to expedite the drug development and review process and has established methods for providing promising experimental drugs to desperately ill patients.

The treatment IND is one way the FDA has allowed for increased accessibility of experimental drugs for desperately ill patients. For a drug to qualify for use under a treatment IND it must meet the following criteria:

1. The drug must be intended to treat a serious or immediately life-threatening disease.
2. There must be no satisfactory alternative therapy for the patient.
3. The drug must be under investigation in controlled clinical trials.
4. The sponsor must be actively pursuing FDA approval of the drug.

There are two different categories of treatment IND: immediately life-threatening conditions and serious conditions. The FDA defines immediately life-threatening conditions as those where death is likely to occur within a matter of months. In this situation, the FDA would allow treatment with the drug earlier than phase III, but not earlier than phase II. Serious conditions are defined as those in which the disease causes major irreversible morbidity (such as Alzheimer's disease). For use in treating serious conditions, the drug must meet tougher requirements for safety and efficacy. As a result, treatment INDs for serious illnesses are more likely to be granted during phase III trials or after all clinical trials have been completed. Provisions of the treatment IND regulations permit charging for the investigational drug under certain conditions. The amount the sponsor may charge for the investigational drug cannot exceed the amount necessary to recover costs associated with drug production, development, and distribution. Both drug sponsors and individual investigators are eligible to request FDA approval of a treatment IND. The drug sponsor may do so via submission of a treatment protocol, which states how and why the drug will be used. If the drug sponsor will not establish a treatment protocol and an investigator feels access to the drug is necessary, the investigator may submit a treatment IND for the drug, assuming the drug is available. The treatment IND that the investigator submits should contain all of the components of a treatment protocol as well as information about the investigator and a description of the steps taken by the investigator to obtain the drug under a treatment protocol from the drug sponsor.

The parallel track is a way the FDA has allowed for increased accessibility of experimental drugs specifically for AIDS patients. Using this mechanism, drugs may be made available after completion of phase I studies to patients who are ineligible for enrollment in the clinical trials and are unable to benefit from current therapies. Regular controlled studies for safety and efficacy are still essential and the sponsors are required to monitor the impact of the parallel track on enrollment in ongoing clinical trials.

The most recent effort to improve access to potentially beneficial products is known as the Oncology Initiative. This policy was designed to address the needs of oncology patients. This initiative allows for

1. accelerating drug approval by using surrogate end points to approve oncology drugs. A surrogate end point of a clinical trial is "a laboratory measurement or a physical sign used as a substitute for a clinically meaningful endpoint that measures directly how a patient feels, functions, or survives. Changes induced by a therapy on a surrogate endpoint are expected to reflect changes in a clinically meaningful endpoint."[19]
2. treating patients in the United States with drugs approved in other countries via expanded access protocols.
3. expanding the number of consumer members on the advisory committees.
4. reducing the number of INDs required to conduct studies of marketed oncology drugs.

There has been much interest in this program and it has shown promising results.[4]

Emergency use INDs are another way that the FDA allows access to investigational drugs for desperately ill patients. The emergency use IND allows shipment of a drug by the sponsor prior to the submission of an IND. This type of IND can only be used to treat individual patients with life-threatening diseases where all other options have been exhausted. The FDA must authorize the emergency use IND; however, IRB approval is not required.

The FDA has also attempted to expedite the review process for new drugs. One such initiative is the accelerated drug approval program. This program can be utilized if the drug is intended for the treatment of a serious or life-threatening condition and it demonstrates the potential to address unmet medication needs for the condition. The application would then be evaluated by weighing the risk/benefit relationship of the severity of the disease and alternatives to the new product. These products could be approved based on surrogate end points or on clinical end points other than survival or irreversible morbidity if the product can provide a meaningful therapeutic benefit to patients. In some cases, this approval could be given as early as post–phase II studies. Two pivotal phase II studies would be required before the NDA could be submitted. In these situations, the FDA can apply restrictions to the marketing and distribution of such products and significant postmarketing studies (phase IV) will be required because they would provide information regarding larger and more diverse patient populations than may be seen in the earlier phases of study.

Finally, the FDA has attempted to improve the drug development and approval process by initiating a program of meeting with study sponsors to discuss and review the preclinical and clinical studies that will be necessary for drug development and approval. The purpose of these meetings is to help the sponsor minimize wasteful expenditures of time and money while still meeting the scientific objectives necessary for drug approval. For products designed to treat desperately ill patients, these meetings can occur prior to submission of the initial IND and at the end of phase I studies. Additionally, the FDA will meet with the sponsor of any IND at the end of Phase II studies and prior to submission of the NDA.[3,20,21]

The Institutional Review Board

The IRB is a committee of at least five members formed to review proposed clinical trials and the progress of such studies to ensure that the rights and welfare of human subjects are protected. The IRB must contain at least one member who has specialized in a scientific area (usually this will be a physician) and at least one board member who has a specialty in a nonscientific area such as law, ethics, or religion. Additionally, the IRB must contain at least one individual who is not affiliated with the institution where the research is being conducted. Membership of the IRB varies between institutions. Common members of IRBs include physicians, pharmacists, nurses, lawyers, clergy, and lay persons. The IRB is also responsible for ensuring that the proposed clinical trial is not in conflict with the institution's research policies or philosophy. The IRB and the study sponsor will have little if any direct contact. The primary investigator generally acts as the liaison between these two parties. The IRB should evaluate the research proposal to ensure that the following requirements are met.

- The risks to subjects are minimal.
- The expected risk/anticipated benefit ratio must be reasonable.
- Equitable subject selection is used.
- Informed consent must be received from each participant (or his or her representative).
- Informed consent must be documented in writing.
- Data must be monitored to ensure subject safety.
- Patient confidentiality must be maintained.
- If appropriate, additional safeguards against coercion must be included in studies that include vulnerable subjects (children, prisoners, pregnant women, mentally disabled people, or economically or educationally disadvantaged persons).

A notable exception to the requirements for written informed consent, as described above, has been provided for research done in emergency circumstances. In these situations, the IRB will evaluate the research to ensure that it meets the strictly limited conditions outlined by the DHHS. Additionally, the investigator must provide the communities in which the research will be conducted with information on the research and its risks and expected benefits.[22]

The IRB must, at a minimum, perform annual reviews of all ongoing clinical trials and evaluate adverse experiences to ensure that the criteria listed above continue to be met.

The IRB must maintain documentation of all IRB activities including copies of all research proposals reviewed, minutes of IRB meetings, records of continuing review activities, copies of all correspondence between the IRB and the investigators, a list of IRB members, written procedures of the IRB, and statements of significant new findings provided to subjects. This documentation should be retained for at least 3 years. Records that pertain to research should be retained for 3 years after the research is completed.[23]

Some institutions divide their review of proposed clinical research into two separate processes. One of these is the review of the protocol for scientific worth (scientific review), and the other is the review of the protocol for ethical considerations (IRB review). Recently, the role of the IRB and the effectiveness of the informed consent process have been questioned.[24] Federal officials and the regulatory agencies are considering reform of this process. Information regarding the role the pharmacist can assume in these reviews will be presented later in the chapter.

The Orphan Drug Act

The Orphan Drug Act was passed in 1983. This act provides incentives for manufacturers to develop orphan drugs. An *orphan drug* is one used for the treatment of a rare disease (affecting fewer than 200,000 people in the United States) or one that will not generate enough revenue to justify the costs of research and development. The Orphan Drug Act is administered by the FDA's Office of Orphan Products Development. The orphan drug designation provides the following incentives.

- *Tax incentives:* The sponsor is eligible to receive a 50% tax credit for money spent on research and development of an orphan drug; unfortunately, this is only beneficial to profitable companies as this credit cannot take the form of a tax refund.
- *Protocol assistance:* If a sponsor can show that a drug will be used for a rare disease, the FDA will provide assistance developing the preclinical and clinical plan for the product.
- *Grants and contracts:* The FDA budget may allot up to $12 million annually for grants and contracts to be used in developing orphan drugs.

- *Marketing exclusivity:* The first sponsor to obtain marketing approval for a designated orphan drug is allowed 7 years of marketing exclusivity for that indication, but identical versions of the same product marketed by another manufacturer may be approved for other indications.

The Orphan Drug Act does not provide advantages for the drug approval process. Sponsors seeking approval for drugs that will be designated as orphan drugs must still provide the same safety and efficacy data as all other drugs evaluated by the FDA. Exceptions to the rules governing the number of patients that should be treated in the clinical trials may be made based on the scarcity of patients with the condition. Additionally, because in many cases there are no alternative therapies for the disease, the drug may be given a high review priority during the NDA process.[4,16,25,26]

Role of the Pharmacist

The pharmacist can play a vital role in the clinical research process by

- being the primary investigator (PI) on a study.
- reporting adverse events.
- preparing the IND.
- serving on the IRB and, where applicable, on the Scientific Review Committee.
- providing financial evaluations of investigational protocols.
- disseminating information regarding both the protocol and the investigational drug to other health care personnel.
- maintaining drug accountability records.
- ordering, maintaining, and, when necessary, returning drug supplies for ongoing clinical trials.
- randomizing and, when necessary, blinding drug supplies for a clinical trial.

The pharmacist can serve as the PI on clinical research studies. The type of study for which a pharmacist is PI varies based on the expertise and experience of the pharmacist. Common types of studies for which pharmacists serve as PIs include pharmacoeconomic and pharmacology/pharmacokinetic studies. For some of these trials, a physician must be a co-investigator.

The pharmacist can assist the investigator by reporting adverse events that occur during clinical trials to the FDA. A discussion of the types of adverse events and the applicable reporting requirements was presented in the IND section of this chapter. Further information about the concept of adverse drug reaction reporting, including identification and classification of adverse events can be found in the adverse drug reaction section of Chap. 16.

The pharmacist can assist in preparing the IND by following the guidelines presented earlier in this chapter.

The pharmacist should be a voting member of the IRB and as such may have some control over clinical trials initiated at the institution. More important, however, is the role the pharmacist may have in the scientific review of the protocol, whether this occurs as part of the scientific review board review or as part of the IRB review. When reviewing a protocol for scientific purposes, the pharmacist should verify that the protocol contains the following information.

1. The name and synonyms of the study drug.
2. The chemical structure of the study drug.
3. The mechanism of action of the study drug.
4. The dosage range of the study drug (with appropriate rationale).
5. Animal toxicologic and pharmacologic information (when available, any known human toxicologic and pharmacologic information should also be presented).
6. How the drug will be supplied (dosage form and size).
7. The preparation guidelines for the drug (including stability and compatibility information when appropriate).
8. The storage requirements of the drug (both before and, when appropriate, after preparation).
9. The route of administration (and, if applicable, the rate of administration).

In addition, the pharmacist should confirm that any toxicities specified in the protocol are detailed for the patient in the informed consent of the protocol.

The pharmacist should also review the protocol for other potential problems (such as incompatibilities and inappropriate infusion devices). Frequently, nursing does not have an opportunity to review protocols prior to initiation and it falls to the pharmacist to ensure that the drug can be given as specified in the protocol. For complex protocols, it may be best to request secondary reviews by other specialists such as the nurses who will be giving the doses or the pharmacists who will be preparing the doses. The pharmacist can review the protocol for clinical and scientific issues appropriate to his or her knowledge level and experience. Those pharmacists with research experience or a strong clinical background may, and probably should, comment on the study design or scientific merit of a particular protocol.

With the central role of financial considerations in today's research environment, pharmacists can also provide valuable insight into the costs associated with clinical research. Traditionally, the study sponsors would provide the investigational drug free of charge to the hospital (and to the patient) and the patient (or the third-party payer) would be responsible for paying for all other charges associated with therapy. Increasingly, third-party payers are reluctant to pay for investigational therapy. This leaves the patient, and subsequently the hospital, in a financially risky situation. A significant portion of costs associated with clinical research is pharmacy related (either supportive care medications or infusion devices, solutions, etc., that are used to administer the investigational drug). If during the review process the pharmacist can provide the investigator and the scientific review board with information regarding the potential cost of the research (at least as it relates to pharmacy charges), both the investigator and the review board can make a more educated decision regarding appropriation of resources for research purposes. When preparing an economic review of a protocol the pharmacist should pay specific attention to the following items.

1. Can the therapy be converted from inpatient to outpatient?
2. Can the method of infusion or the infusion device be changed to one that is more cost effective?
3. Does the treatment plan call for administration of compatible medications that could be mixed in the same container?
4. Is the supportive care adequate and not excessive (this is especially important with high-cost drugs such as antiemetics and growth factors)?
5. Does the protocol have a high risk of reimbursement denial? This can be evaluated by reviewing the package insert, *American Hospital Formulary Service Drug Information, US Pharmacopeia—Drug Information (USP-DI),* and for oncology products, *Association of Community Cancer Centers Compendia-Based Drug Bulletin.* Other factors in reimbursement risk include the cost of the drug and the supportive care or tests associated with the drug. If the protocol does have a high risk of reimbursement denial, can free drug supplies offset part or all of this risk?

See Appendix 17–3 for an economic review template that can be used to evaluate this information.

The pharmacist can assist in disseminating information regarding both the protocol and the investigational drug by preparing data sheets that may be used by pharmacy and nursing personnel (and in some situations by physicians who may be unfamiliar with the research). This information can be distributed using various methods including paper, the hospital mainframe, and the Intranet. The drug data sheet should include the following elements.

- Drug name (synonyms)
- Therapeutic classification
- Pharmaceutical data
- Stability and storage data
- Dose preparation guidelines (where applicable)

- Usual dosage range
- Route of administration
- Known side effects and toxicities
- Mechanism of action
- Status (phase of study)
- Study chairperson
- Date effective (and dates of revision)
- References

The protocol data sheet should include the following elements.

- Protocol number (as assigned by the institution)
- Protocol title
- Drug name(s) (synonym[s])
- Protocol description
  1. Objectives
  2. Study design
     a. Registration requirements
     b. Primary location of patients
     c. Type of study
  3. Treatment course (including retreatment criteria)
- Availability
  1. Supplier
  2. Status
  3. How supplied
- Storage, stability, and compatibility
  1. Intact drug
  2. Prepared drug (for injectables this should include both reconstitution and dilution guidelines)
- Dosage range
- Dose preparation guidelines
- Administration guidelines
- Special notes
- Primary investigator
- Research nurse

The primary investigator and study sponsor should approve both the drug data sheet and the protocol data sheet before dissemination. This will help eliminate any potential errors and may reduce the liability the pharmacist assumes in preparing and distributing these documents. The pharmacist should assume primary responsibility for ordering and maintaining adequate drug supplies for conducting the clinical trial. All investigational drugs should be stored in the pharmacy. Usually, ordering can be done via telephone; however, sometimes study sponsors require written drug orders. If the drug under investigation is a controlled substance, a written order will definitely be required. Shipment and receipt of the drug can vary from 1 day to several weeks (or sometimes months for very specialized drug products). The pharmacist must be sufficiently knowledgeable regarding the rate of patient enrollment in the protocol and subsequent drug usage to ensure that the institution does not run out of drug. The pharmacist should also assume responsibility for returning unused drug supplies at the completion of the study. The sponsor may authorize on-site destruction of unused supplies provided this will not increase the risk to humans (or provide a risk to the environment). Many study sponsors will attempt to have the pharmacist save and return all used drug supplies as well. This is not a FDA requirement and for safety and space reasons should be discouraged.

Another role the pharmacist should assume is maintaining drug accountability records. These records can be maintained manually or on a computer. The records must document all drug shipments, returns, and dispensing to patients. At a minimum, these records should document:

- the date of the transaction.
- the patient initials and an identifying number.
- the dose.
- the number of vials of drug used or received.
- the lot number of the drug (if multiple lot numbers were used, each one should be documented).
- the initials of the individual who performed the transaction.

The National Cancer Institute (NCI) has prepared a sample drug accountability form that may be used as a guide (see Appendix 17–4).[27]

Computer systems that will maintain drug accountability records are available commercially. Both personal computer (PC) based and mainframe-based systems exist. A PC-based system allows the user greater flexibility. Some of these systems will also provide drug labels, drug and protocol information, summaries of investigational drug dispensing (useful in the preparation of productivity reports), and even monthly billing summaries to be used for posting charges to the study budget. Two PC-based systems that are currently on the market are IDRx (available through Cygnus Systems*) and PharmAsyst (available through HealthCare Consulting Associates[†]). Obviously, the development of a personalized system that meets the specific needs of the institution or

---

*Ben Bluml, Cygnus Systems Development, Inc., 2505 N.W. Bent Tree Circle, Lee's Summit, MO 64084.
[†] Randall Marler, Health Care Consulting Associates, 918 Sam Hill, Irving, Texas 75062.

pharmacy is ideal. However, this can be costly, laborious, and time consuming. If a personalized system is developed, it is important to remember that the system must be able to maintain the integrity of the records and that a clear audit trail needs to be maintained. Ultimately, the decision to computerize drug accountability records and the selection of which system to use, is one that the pharmacist should make only after evaluating the needs of the institution/pharmacy and the available budget.[28-31]

Drug accountability records and drug supplies may be inspected at any time by the sponsor. The frequency of these inspections may vary according to the wishes of the sponsor. They may be monthly, quarterly, or annually. The FDA also has the right to inspect these records. The investigational drug pharmacist should play a key role in providing drug accountability information to either the FDA or the sponsor during an audit. If proper records are not being maintained, the sponsor or the FDA may discontinue the investigator's participation in the clinical investigation.

After the clinical trial is complete, records must be maintained at the study site for the following time periods:

- Two years after approval of the NDA *or*
- Two years after the FDA received notification that the investigation was discontinued.[3]

The pharmacist should also assume primary responsibility for randomizing and, where appropriate, blinding clinical trials. These two activities assist the sponsor in reducing or eliminating the bias of the clinical trial. A randomized study is one in which patients are "randomly" assigned (similar to flipping a coin) to different therapies. Usually the assignment is done using a computer-generated randomization list; however, a manual list may be used as well. The randomization groups may include a number of different therapy options (e.g., a study may have four different treatment arms with an equal number of patients assigned to each arm). The number of patients assigned to the different groups may vary as well (e.g., a study may have two different treatment regimens where patients will be assigned in a 2:1 ratio to the first treatment option). The investigator should not be aware which arm the patient has been assigned to before randomization. Therefore, the involvement of a third party (such as the pharmacist) is important. A blinded study is one in which, after the patient has been randomized, the drug is masked so that at least one of the involved parties (e.g., physician, nurse, patient, or pharmacist) is not aware of what the patient is to receive. In a single-blind study the only individual who is not aware of what the patient is receiving is the patient himself. In a double-blind study neither the nurse, doctor, or patient is aware of what the patient is receiving. The role of a pharmacist in a double-blind study is crucial, and sloppy work in this area destroys a clinical investigation. A triple-blind study is one in which the drug arrives at the pharmacy already blinded. In this scenario, the patient, nurse, doctor, and pharmacist are not aware of what drug the patient is to receive. Although this may seem simpler than a double-blind study, it is equally difficult because each patient has his or her own supply of medication and it is important that the supplies be dispensed appropriately. In a triple-blind study, the sponsor supplies the investigator with a mechanism for removing the blind from the patient (in case of emergency). It is critical that the pharmacist keep the master list. The protocol should state who has access to the master list and under what conditions this access should occur. If the FDA discovers that the investigator had access to this list, the study will be considered invalid.

Pharmacists should be willing and able to request reimbursement for the services they provide. Funds for these services are usually negotiated directly with the study sponsor before initiation of the protocol. The majority of pharmacies charge a base fee for each protocol initiated at its institution (these fees generally range from $50 to $3000 per protocol). This base fee may be fixed or it may vary based on the size of the patient population or the number of doses to be prepared. Some institutions also charge an annual renewal fee for ongoing clinical trials (ranging from $40 to $750). Most pharmacies will charge a separate fee for randomizing and blinding a clinical trial. This fee can be a one-time (per study) fee or it can be a per-patient fee (one time fees range from $25 to $300 while per-patient fees range from $1 to $50). Some hospitals also charge a monthly fee for drug storage and inventory (ranging from $10 to $50 per month). This fee varies based on the amount of space and type of storage (freezer, room temperature, or refrigerator) required. The pharmacist can also charge a professional fee for services that exceed the standard services provided for in the base fee (range of $20 to $70 per hour). Examples of services that should be charged for separately include monitoring of patients, completing case report forms, and completing sponsor specific drug accountability records. These services are usually charged for using an hourly fee.[32]

Conclusion

Assisting in the implementation and conduct of clinical trials can be a satisfying role for the pharmacist. The laws governing these trials can be complex, but they are understandable once the pharmacist has taken the time to study them. The pharmacist can and should play an integral role in the conduct of clinical trials at their institution.

Helpful Web sites
- NIH/Office of Biotechnology Activities (OBA): <<http://www.nih.gov/od/oba>>
- FDA: <<http://www.fda.gov>>
- FDA forms: <<http://forms.psc.gov/forms/FDA/fda.html>>

- Archives of the Federal Register: <<http://www.access.gpo.gov/su_docs/aces/aces140.html>>
- Code of Federal Regulations: <<http://www.access.gpo.gov/nara/cfr/index.html>>
- ICH: <<http://www.pharmweb.net/pwmirror/pw9/ifpma/ich1.html>>
- NIH/OHRP: <<http://ohrp.osophs.dhhs.gov/polasur.htm>>
- CenterWatch: <<http://www.centerwatch.com>>

Study Questions

1. What are the steps in the drug approval process?

2. What type of information is contained in the investigator's brochure?

3. What type of information is gathered in a phase I, phase II, phase III, and phase IV trial? Why is this relevant to the drug approval process?

4. What is the purpose of the institutional review board?

5. What incentives does the Orphan Drug Act provide to the manufacturers? Does this accelerate the drug approval process?

6. What role does the pharmacist play in the clinical research process?

REFERENCES

1. Molecule to market: The drug development process. Continuing education brochure distributed by Glaxo; 1992.
2. Manasse HR. Toward defining and applying a higher standard of quality medication use in the United States. Am J Hosp Pharm 1995;52:374–9.
3. Investigational New Drug Application, Title 21, Code of Federal Regulations, Part 312. Washington, DC: US Government Printing Office via GPO Access, revised as of April 1, 1998.
4. Mathieu M. New drug development: a regulatory overview. 4th ed. Cambridge (MA): PAREXEL International Corporation; 1997.
5. Bruderle TP. Reforming the Food and Drug Administration: legislative solution or self-improvement? Am J Health-Syst Pharm 1996;53:2083–90.
6. Kessler DA, Hass AE, Feidin KL, Lumpkin, M, Temple, R. Approval of new drugs in the United States. JAMA 1996;276:1826–31.
7. Reynolds, T. European drug agency promises quicker approvals. JNCI 1995;87:1050–1.
8. The Nuremberg Code. Trials of War Criminals before the Nuremberg Military Tribunals under Control Council Law No. 10, Vol. 2, pp. 181–182. Washington, DC: US Government Printing Office; 1949.

9. World Medical Association: Declaration of Helsinki. Washington, DC: US Government Printing Office; September 1989.

10. The Belmont Report: Ethical Principles and Guidelines for the Protection of Human Subjects of Research. Washington, DC: US Government Printing Office; April 18, 1979.

11. Protection of Human Subjects. Title 45, Code of Federal Regulations, Part 46. Washington, DC: US Government Printing Office; 1991.

12. Protection of Human Subjects. Title 21, Code of Federal Regulations, Part 50. Washington, DC: US Government Printing Office via GPO Access; revised as of April 1, 1998.

13. Institutional Review Boards, Title 21, Code of Federal Regulations, Part 56. Washington, DC: US Government Printing Office via GPO Access; revised as of April 1, 1998.

14. CDER: Food and Drug Administration. Guideline for Drug Master Files. Washington, DC: US Government Printing Office; September 1989.

15. Records and reports concerning adverse drug experiences on marketed prescription drugs for human use without approved new drug applications. Title 21 Code of Federal Regulations Part 310, Section 305. Washington, DC: U.S. Government Printing Office; effective April 6, 1998.

16. CDER: Food and Drug Administration. Drug Classification and Priority Review Policy. Staff manual Guide CDER 4820.3. Washington, DC: US Government Printing Office; January 22, 1992.

17. Applications for FDA Approval to market a new drug or an antibiotic, Title 21, Code of Federal Regulations, Part 314. Washington, DC: US Government Printing Office via GPO Access; revised April 1, 1998.

18. Bready BB. Conducting clinical trials in oncology. Cancer Bull 1990;42:411–15.

19. Temple RJ. A regulatory authority's opinion about surrogate endpoints. In: Nimmo WS, Tucker GT, editors. Clinical measurement in drug evaluation. New York: Wiley; 1995.

20. How FDA Expedites Evaluation of Drugs for AIDS and Other Life-Threatening Illnesses. Wellcome Programs in Pharmacy. January 1993.

21. Food and Drug Administration Modernization Act of 1997 (Senate bill S-830). Washington, DC: US Government Printing Office via GPO Access; November 21, 1997.

22. Protection of Human Subjects; Informed Consent and Waiver of Informed Consent Requirements in Certain Emergency Research; Final Rules. Federal Register 1996;51:498–51, 533.

23. Protecting Human Research Subjects: Institutional Review Board Guidebook. Washington, DC: US Government Printing Office; 1993.

24. Davis R. 1998. U.S.: Human medical tests lack oversight. USA Today 1998 June 8;Sect.A:1, 19–20.

25. Orphan Drugs, Title 21, Code of Federal Regulations, Part 316. Washington, DC: US Government Printing Office via GPO Access; revised April 1, 1998.

26. CDER: Food and Drug Administration. Frequently Asked Questions Concerning the OOPD Grant Program. Washington, DC. US Government Printing Office via GPO Access; updated November 9, 1998.

27. Investigator's Handbook: A Manual for Participants in Clinical Trials of Investigational Agents Sponsored by the Division of Cancer Treatment, National Cancer Institute. Bethesda (MD): National Cancer Institute; 1986.

28. Burnham NL, Elcombe SA, Skorlinski CR, Kosanke L, Kovach JS. Computer program for handling investigational oncology drugs. Am J Hosp Pharm 1989;46:1821–4.

29. Grilley BJ, Trissel LA, Bluml BM. Design and implementation of an electronic investigational drug accountability system. Am J Hosp Pharm 1991;48:2816.

30. Lakamp JE, Lunik MC, Wilson AL, Armbruster CJ. Using a hospital mainframe computer for pharmacy investigational drug study management. Top Hosp Pharm Manage 1993;13:37–46.

31. Iteen SE, Ceppaglia J. Investigational drug information through a hospitalwide computer system. Am J Hosp Pharm 1992;49:2746–8.

32. Rockwell, K. Pharmacy-based investigational drug services: A national survey. Top Hosp Pharm Manage 1993;13:1–15.

Appendices

2–1

Appendix 2–1

Drug Information Response Quality Assurance Evaluation Form

Drug Information Service
Department of Pharmacy Services, MCVH
Quality Assurance Review

Month under review_____   Date of request_____
Primary responder_____   DIS staff supervisor_____

	Satisfactory	Unsatisfactory	N/A	Comment
Requestor's demographic data was complete	___	___	___	___
Background information inquiry was thorough	___	___	___	___
. . . was appropriate	___	___	___	___
Search question was clearly noted	___	___	___	___
. . . was succinct	___	___	___	___
Search strategy and reference selection were relevant	___	___	___	___
. . . were comprehensive	___	___	___	___
Literature and information retrieved were				
. . . evaluated	___	___	___	___
. . . interpreted	___	___	___	___
. . . documented	___	___	___	___
Conclusions were appropriate per				
. . . data collected	___	___	___	___
. . . data assimilation	___	___	___	___
Oral or verbal response was				
. . . accurate	___	___	___	___
. . . complete	___	___	___	___
. . . succinct	___	___	___	___
. . . provided in a timely manner	___	___	___	___
Follow-up communication				
. . . was clearly documented	___	___	___	___
. . . showed appropriate reaction	___	___	___	___

	Excellent		Acceptable		Unacceptable
Summary (circle 1):	5	4	3	2	1

Recommendations:_____
Reviewer's initials:____

Appendix 2-2

Drug Information Request/Response Form

REQUEST/RESPONSE FORM   DATE__/__/__
Drug Information Service—Department of Pharmacy Services   TIME__:__
Medical College of Virginia Hospitals   (use military time)

DEMOGRAPHIC DATA:
Requestor_____ Dept/Affiliation_____
Phone/Pager_____ Location/City_____
MCV-VCU____   Profession: Physician____   Nurse____   PA/NP___Student____
NON-MCV____   Pharmacist____   Dentist____   Other_____

Initial Question:_____
BACKGROUND INFORMATION (age, sex, weight, disease states, medications, lab values, allergies, etc.)

ULTIMATE QUESTION: _____
                              Receiver_____   Respond by_____
Classification: (check only one category)
__Availability (strength,   __Drug Interactions (drug, lab,   __Dosage/Regimen
   manufacturer, formul.)   disease, food)   Recommendations
__Identification   __Pharmaceutics (compounding,   __Adverse Effects
__General Product Information   formulations)   __Poisoning/Toxicology
__Laws/Policy & Procedure/P & T   __Pharmacokinetics (ADME/   __Teratogenicity/Genetic
__Cost   levels/HD, PD, HPI)   Effects
__Foreign/Investigational   __Therapy Eval./Drug   __Lactation/Infant Risks
__Compatibility/Stability/   of Choice   __Other:_____
   Administration (rate/method)
__Referral: __ Clinical Pharmacokinetics __Poison Control __Nutrition Support __Library
__Other:_____
SEARCH STRATEGY: (Indicate resource and utility [+ or –]; record specific data on back)

FINDINGS/EVALUATION (see back):
RESPONSE:

Responder/Supervisor_____/_____ Written Response:__Y__N Date__/__/__
Time:__:__   Time Spent: <5__ 5–30__ 30–60__ >60__

__Quality Assurance __Statistics __Projects __Pharmacy Trend Written Reference Search____
Verbal Reference Search_____   Drug Information Service Consult_____

FOLLOW-UP INFORMATION (also note attempts to contact, messages left):

2–3

Standard Questions for Obtaining Background Information from Requestors

GENERAL

Regardless of the type or classification of the question, the following information should be obtained.

1. Requestor's name
2. Requestor's location and/or page number
3. Requestor's affiliation (institution or practice), if a health care professional
4. Requestor's frame of reference (i.e., title, profession/occupation, rank)
5. Resources the requestor has already consulted
6. If the request is patient specific or academic
7. Patient's diagnosis and other medications
8. Urgency of the request (negotiate time of response)

SPECIFIC*

The following questions should be asked when appropriate for calls of the following classes.

Availability of Dosage Forms
1. What is the dosage form desired?
2. What administration routes are feasible with this patient?
3. Is this patient alert and oriented.
4. Does the patient have a water or sodium restriction?
5. What other special factors regarding drug administration should be considered?

---

*Specific questions for only selected types of requests presented; other questions would be appropriate for other types of requests.

Identification of Product

1. What is the generic or trade name of the product?
2. Who is the manufacturer? What is the country of origin?
3. What is the suspected use of this product?
4. Under what circumstances was this product found? Who found the product?
5. What is the dosage form, color markings, size, etc.?
6. What was your source of information? Was it reliable?

General Product Information

1. Why is there a particular concern for this product?
2. Is written patient information required?
3. What type of information do you need?
4. Is this for an inpatient, outpatient, or private patient?

Foreign Drug Identification

1. What is the drug's generic name, trade name, manufacturer, and/or country of origin?
2. What is the dosage form, markings, color, strength, or size?
3. What is the suspected use of the drug? How often is the patient taking it? What is the patient's response to the drug? Is the patient male or female?
4. If the medication was found, what were the circumstances/conditions at the time of discovery?
5. Is the patient just visiting or is he or she planning on staying?

Investigational Drug Information

1. Why do you need this information? Is the patient in need of the drug or currently enrolled in a protocol?
2. If a drug is to be identified, what is the dosage form, markings, color, strength, or size of the product?
3. Why was the patient receiving the drug? What is the response when the patient was on the drug? What are the patient's pathologic conditions?
4. If a drug is desired what approved or accepted therapies have been tried? Was therapy maximized before discontinued?

Method and Rate of Administration

1. What dosage form or preparation is being used (if multiple salts available)?
2. What is the dose ordered? Is the drug a one-time dose or standing order?
3. What is the clinical status of the patient? Could the patient tolerate a fluid push of XX mL? Is the patient fluid or sodium restricted? Does the patient have CHF or edema?
4. What possible delivery routes are available?
5. What other drugs is the patient receiving currently? Are any by the same route?

Incompatibility and Stability

1. What are the routes for the patient's medications?
2. What are the doses (in mg), concentrations, and volumes for all pertinent medications?
3. What are the infusion times/rates expected or desired?
4. What is the base solution or diluent used?
5. Was the product stored in a refrigerator or at room temperature? For how long?
6. Was the product exposed to sunlight? For how long?
7. Was the product frozen? For how long?
8. When was the product compounded/prepared?

Drug Interactions

1. What event(s) suggest that an interaction occurred? Please describe.
2. For the drugs in question, what are the doses, volumes, concentrations, rates of administration, administration schedules, and length of therapies?
3. What is the temporal relationship between the drugs in question?
4. Has the patient received this combination or a similar combination in the past?
5. Other than the drugs in question, what other drugs is the patient receiving currently? When were these started?

Drug-Laboratory Test Interference

1. What event(s) suggest an interaction occurred? Please describe.
2. For the drug in question, what is the dose, volume, concentration, rate of administration, administration schedule, and length of therapy?
3. What is the temporal relationship between drug administration and laboratory test sampling?
4. What other drugs is the patient receiving?
5. Has clinical chemistry (or the appropriate laboratory) been contacted? Are they aware of any know interference similar to this event?
6. Was this one isolated test or a trend in results?

Pharmacokinetics

1. What is the generic name, dose, and route of the drug?
2. What is the patient's age, sex, height, and weight?
3. What is the disease being treated and the severity of the illness?
4. What is the patient's hepatic and renal function?
5. What other medications is the patient receiving?
6. What physiologic conditions exist (e.g., pneumonia, severe burns, or obesity)?
7. What are the patient's dietary and ethanol habits?

Serum or Urine Therapeutic Levels

1. Is the patient currently receiving the drug? Have samples already been drawn? At what time?
2. What is the disease or underlying pathology being treated? If infectious in nature, what is the organism suspected/cultured?
3. If not stated in the question, what was the source of the sample (blood, urine, saliva; venous or arterial blood)?
4. What was the timing of the samples relative to drug administration? Over what period of time was the drug administered and by what route?
5. What were the previous concentrations for this patient? Was the patient receiving the same dose then?
6. How long has the patient received the drug? Is the patient at steady state?

Therapy Evaluation/Drug of Choice

1. What medications, including doses and routes of administration, is the patient receiving?
2. What is the patient's pathology(ies) and disease(s) severity?
3. What are the patient's specifics: age, weight, height, gender, organ function/ dysfunction?
4. Has the patient received the drug previously? Was response similar?
5. Has the patient been compliant?
6. What alternative therapies has the patient received? Was therapy maximized for each of these before discontinuation? What other therapies are being considered?
7. What monitoring parameters have been followed (serum concentrations/levels, clinical status, other clinical laboratory results, objective measurements, and subjective assessment).
8. What is the patient's name and location?

Dosage Recommendations (Normal and Compromised)

1. What disease is being treated? What is the extent/severity of the illness?
2. What are the drugs (all) being prescribed? Has the patient been receiving any to date?
3. Does the patient have any insufficiency of the renal, hepatic, or cardiac system(s)?
4. For drugs with renal elimination, what are the serum creatinine/creatinine clearance, BUN, and/or urine output? Is the patient receiving peritoneal dialysis or hemodialysis?
5. For drugs with hepatic elimination, what are the liver function tests, bilirubin (direct and indirect), and/or albumin?

6. For drugs with serum level monitoring utility, characterize the most recent levels relative to dose.
7. Are these laboratory values recent? Is the patient's condition stable?
8. Does this patient have a known factor that could affect drug metabolism (ethnic background such as Oriental, or acetylator status)?

Adverse Effects
1. What is the name, dosage, and route for all drugs currently and recently prescribed?
2. What are the patient specifics (age, sex, height, weight, organ dysfunction, and indication for drug use)?
3. What is the temporal relationship with the drug?
4. Has the patient experienced this adverse relationship (or a similar event) with this drug (or similar agent) previously?
5. Was the suspected drug ever administered before? Why was it discontinued then?
6. What were the events/findings that characterize this adverse drug reaction (ADR) (include onset and duration)?
7. Has any intervention been initiated at this time?
8. Does the patient have any food intolerance?
9. Is there a family history for this ADR and/or drug allergy?

Toxicology Information
1. What is your name, relationship to the victim, and telephone number?
2. What are the patient specifics (age, sex, height, weight, organ dysfunction, and indication for drug use)?
3. Is this a suspected ingestion or exposure?
4. What product is suspected to have been ingested? What is the strength of the product and the possible quantity ingested (e.g., how much was in the bottle)?
5. How long ago did the ingestion occur?
6. How much is on the victim or surrounding floor?
7. How much was removed from the victim's hands and mouth? Was the ingestion in the same room where the product was stored?
8. What has been done for the patient already? Has the Poison Control Center or ER been called?
9. Do you have syrup of ipecac available? Do you know how to give it properly?
10. What is the patient's condition (sensorium, heart rate, respiratory rate, temperature, skin color/turgor, pupils, sweating/salivation, etc.)?
11. Does the patient have any known illnesses or organ dysfunction?

Teratogenicity

1. What is the drug the patient received and what was the dose? What was the duration of therapy?
2. Is the patient pregnant or planning to become pregnant?
3. When during pregnancy was the exposure (trimester or weeks)?
4. What are the patient specifics (age, height, weight, sex)?
5. What is the source of the case information?
6. Was the patient compliant?
7. For what indication was the drug being prescribed?

Drugs in Breast Milk

1. What drug did the patient receive and what was the dose? What was the duration of therapy?
2. How long has the infant been breast feeding?
3. Has the infant ever received nonmaternal nutrition? Is bottle feeding a plausible alternative?
4. What is the frequency of the breast feeds? What is the milk volume?
5. How old is the infant?
6. Does the mother have hepatic or renal insufficiency?
7. What was the indication for prescribing the drug? Was this initial or alternate therapy?
8. Has the mother breast fed previously while on the drug?

2-4

Appendix 2-4

Drug Information Request—An Example Completed Form

REQUEST/RESPONSE FORM
Drug Information Service—Department of Pharmacy Services
Medical College of Virginia Hospitals

DATE_/_/_
TIME_:_
(use military time)

DEMOGRAPHIC DATA:
Requestor <u>Dr. Kolinski</u>
Phone/Pager <u>555-1234</u>
MCV-VCU __   Profession <u>XX</u>Physician
NON-MCV __   __Pharmacist

Dept/Affiliation <u>Dermatology</u>
Location/City <u>MCV</u>
__Nurse   __PA/NP   __Student
__Dentist   __Other_____

Initial Question: <u>How do I get thalidomide?</u>
BACKGROUND INFORMATION (age, sex, weight, disease states, medications, lab values, allergies, etc.)
male, 67-year-old patient with Behcet's disease × 5 years
disease is progressing, destroying most of palate
has heard thalidomide may be useful (recommendation from Louisiana)
pt has received steroids, dapsone, colchicine, chlorambucil
other patient background obtained and WNL
MD, a dermatologist, has also heard of possibly using cyclosporine

ULTIMATE QUESTION: <u>What are (third line) therapeutic recommendations for this patient?</u>
                          Receiver_____   Respond by_____
Classification: (check only one category)
__Availability (strength,   __Drug Interactions (drug, lab,   __Dosage/Regimen
  manufacturer, formul.)   disease, food)   Recommendations
__Identification   __Pharmaceutics (compounding,   __Adverse Effects
__General Product Information   formulations)   __Poisoning/Toxicology
__Laws/Policy & Procedure/P & T   __Pharmacokinetics (ADME/   __Teratogenicity/Genetic
__Cost   levels/HD, PD, HPI)   Effects
__Foreign/Investigational   <u>X</u>Therapy Eval./Drug   __Lactation/Infant Risks
__Compatibility/Stability/   of Choice   __Other:_____
  Administration(rate/method)

__Referral: __ Clinical Pharmacokinetics __Poison Control __Nutrition Support __Library __Other:____
SEARCH STRATEGY: (Indicate resource and utility [+ or –]; record specific data on back)

This would start with general (tertiary) references, and proceed through secondary references to the primary literature.

FINDINGS/EVALUATION (see back): (On back [not shown])
RESPONSE:
Recommend cyclosporine before thalidomide, considering response rates and commercial availability . . .
Responder/Supervisor____/____ Written Response:__Y__N Date_/_/_
Time:__:__ Time Spent:__ <5__ 5–30__ 30–60__ >60

| __Quality Assurance __Statistics __Projects __Pharmacy Trend Written Reference Search_____ |
| Verbal Reference Search_____   Drug Information Service Consult_____ |

FOLLOW-UP INFORMATION: (also note attempts to contact, messages left)

557

Appendix 4–1

Useful Resources for Commonly Requested Drug Information

Type of Inquiry	Tertiary Resources	Secondary Resources
Adverse events	ClinAlert 2000,* Meyler's Side Effects of Drugs,* Textbook of Adverse Drug Reactions* AHFS Drug Information, Clinical Pharmacology, DRUGDEX, Drug Facts and Comparisons, Drug Information Handbook, Handbook of Clinical Drug Data, Martindale: The Complete Drug Reference, Physicians' Desk Reference, Mosby's GenRx, STAT!-Ref, USPDI Volume 1	Reactions Weekly,* ClinAlert* Embase, Index Medicus, International Pharmaceutical Abstracts, Iowa Drug Information System, MEDLINE
Alcohol-free/sugar-free products	American Drug Index,* Red Book,* Drug Facts and Comparisons* DRUGDEX, Handbook of Non-Prescription Drugs	—
Bioequivalency ratings	Approved Bioequivalence Codes,* USPDI Volume 3,* Mosby's GenRx,* PDR Generics*	Lexis-Nexis*
Chemical data (molecular weight, solubility, pKa, etc.)	Merck Index,* Remington's,* Martindale's: The Complete Drug Reference*	International Pharmaceutical Abstracts*
Cost	Red Book,* Mosby's GenRx* PDR Generics, Price Chek PC, Facts and Comparisons (Cost Index)	Lexis-Nexis,* Pharmacoeconomics,* InPharma, International Pharmaceutical Abstracts
Disease state information	Cecil Textbook of Medicine,* Harrison's Principles of Internal Medicine,* The Merck Manual,* Scientific American Medicine,* STAT!-Ref* Applied Therapeutics, Clinical Pharmacy and Therapeutics, Conn's Current Therapy, Current Medical Diagnosis and Treatment, Non-Prescription Drug Therapy, Pharmacotherapy, Handbook of Non-prescription Drugs	Index Medicus,* Iowa Drug Information System,* MEDLINE,* Lexis-Nexis,* Embase, InPharma, International Pharmaceutical Abstracts, Journal Watch

*Indicates resources particularly useful for locating information on the specified subject.

Type of Inquiry	Tertiary Resources	Secondary Resources
Dosage guidelines (general)	*AHFS Drug Information,* DRUGDEX,* Drug Facts and Comparisons,* Physicians' Desk Reference,* Mosby's GenRx,* STAT!-Ref,* USPDI Volume 1* Clinical Pharmacology, Drug Information Handbook, Handbook of Clinical Drug Data, Martindale: The Complete Drug Reference, Handbook of Nonprescription Drugs, Physicians' Desk Reference for Non-Prescription Drugs, PDR Generics Applied Therapeutics, Clinical Pharmacy and Therapeutics, Conn's Current Therapy, Pharmacotherapy*	*Index Medicus,* InPharma,* International Pharmaceutical Abstracts,* Iowa Drug Information System,* MEDLINE,* Lexis-Nexis** *Embase*
Dosage guidelines (geriatrics)	*Geriatric Dosage Handbook,* Geriatric Pharmacology* Drug Prescribing in Renal Failure,* AHFS Drug Information, DRUGDEX, Drug Facts and Comparisons, Drug Information Handbook, Handbook of Clinical Drug Data, Physicians' Desk Reference, Physicians' GenRx, STAT!-Ref, USPDI Volume 1, Applied Therapeutics, Clinical Pharmacy and Therapeutics, Conn's Current Therapy, Pharmacotherapy*	*Embase, Index Medicus, InPharma, International Pharmaceutical Abstracts, Iowa Drug Information System, MEDLINE, Lexis-Nexis*
Dosage guidelines (hepatic failure)	*Geriatric Dosage Handbook,* Merck Manual of Geriatrics,* AHFS Drug Information, DRUGDEX Drug Facts and Comparisons, Drug Information Handbook, Handbook of Clinical Drug Data, Physicians' Desk Reference, Mosby's GenRx, STAT!-Ref, USPDI Volume 1, Applied Therapeutics, Textbook of Therapeutic, Conn's Current Therapy, Pharmacotherapy*	*Embase, Index Medicus, InPharma, International Pharmaceutical Abstracts, Iowa Drug Information System, MEDLINE, Lexis-Nexis*
Dosage guidelines (pediatrics)	*Harriet Lane Handbook,* Pediatric Dosage Handbook,* Problems in Pediatric Drug Therapy,* Drug Information Handbook,* AHFS Drug Information, DRUGDEX, Drug Facts and Comparisons, Handbook of Clinical Drug Data, Physicians' Desk Reference, Mosby's GenRx, STAT!-Ref, USPDI Volume 1, Applied Therapeutics, Textbook of Therapeutics, Conn's Current Therapy, Pharmacotherapy*	*Paediatrics Today** *Embase, Index Medicus, InPharma, International Pharmaceutical Abstracts, Iowa Drug Information System, MEDLINE, Lexis-Nexis*

*Indicates resources particularly useful for locating information on the specified subject.

Type of Inquiry	Tertiary Resources	Secondary Resources
Dosage guidelines (renal failure)	*Geriatric Dosage Handbook,* Drug Prescribing in Renal Failure,* Dosing Guidelines for Adults,* Pocket Reference to Renal Dialysis,* Scientific American Medicine,* Drug Information Handbook,* DRUGDEX,** *AHFS Drug Information, Drug Facts and Comparisons, Handbook of Clinical Drug Data, Physicians' Desk Reference, Mosby's GenRx, STAT!-Ref, USPDI Volume 1, Applied Therapeutics, Textbook of Therapeutics, Conn's Current Therapy, Pharmacotherapy*	*Embase, Index Medicus, InPharma, International Pharmaceutical Abstracts, Iowa Drug Information System, MEDLINE, Lexis-Nexis*
Drug administration	*AHFS Drug Information,* DRUGDEX,* Drug Information Handbook** *Clinical Pharmacology, Drug Facts and Comparisons, Handbook of Clinical Drug Data, Martindale: The Complete Drug Reference, Physicians' Desk Reference, Mosby's GenRx, PDR Generics, STAT!-Ref, USPDI Volume 1*	*Embase, Index Medicus, International Pharmaceutical Abstracts, Iowa Drug Information System, MEDLINE, STAT!-Ref, Lexis-Nexis*
Drug information centers	*Red Book**	
Drug interactions	*Drug Interaction Facts,* Drug Interactions and Updates,* Drug-REAX,* Evaluation of Drug Interactions** *MediSpan Drug Therapy Screening System,* Clinical Reference Library, AHFS Drug Information, Clinical Pharmacology, DRUGDEX, Drug Facts and Comparisons, Drug Information Handbook, Handbook of Clinical Drug Data, Martindale: The Complete Drug Reference, Physicians' Desk Reference, Mosby's GenRx, STAT!-Ref USPDI Volume 1*	*ClinAlert,* Reactions,* International Pharmaceutical Abstracts** *Embase, Index Medicus, Iowa Drug Information System, MEDLINE, Lexis-Nexis*
Drug use in pregnancy and lactation	*Drugs in Pregnancy and Lactation,* Reprorisk,* DRUGDEX** *AHFS Drug Information, Drug Facts and Comparisons, Drug Information Handbook, Handbook of Clinical Drug Data, Physicians' Desk Reference, Mosby's GenRx, STAT!-Ref, USPDI Volume 1, PDR Generics*	*Reactions,* Lexis-Nexis** *Embase, Index Medicus, Iowa Drug Information System, MEDLINE, International Pharmaceutical Abstracts*
Extemporaneous compounding	*Extemporaneous Ophthalmic Preparations,* Stability of Compounded Formulations,** *Handbook of Extemporaneous Compounding,**	*International Pharmaceutical Abstracts,* Iowa Drug Information System** *MEDLINE, Embase, Index Medicus*

*Indicates resources particularly useful for locating information on the specified subject.

Type of Inquiry	Tertiary Resources	Secondary Resources
	Pediatric Formulations, * Remington's Pharmaceutical Sciences, * AHFS Drug Information, DRUGDEX	
Herbal and homeopathic medications	A Clinical Guide to Chinese Herbs and Formulae, * The Honest Herbal, * Information Sourcebook of Herbal Medicine, * PDR Herbal, * Natural Medicines Comprehensive Database, * Professional's Handbook of Complementary and Alternative Medicine, * Review of Natural Products, * POISINDEX, * Martindale: The Complete Drug Reference, * Commission E Monographs, * PDR for Herbal Medicine, * Therapeutic Use of Phytochemicals *	International Pharmaceutical Abstracts, * Iowa Drug Information System, * Reactions, * ClinAlert, * Lexis-Nexis, * Embase, Index Medicus, MEDLINE
Identification (domestic products)	Herbs of Choice, F-D-C Tan Sheets	
	American Drug Index, * POISINDEX, * Drug Facts and Comparisons * Red Book, Clinical Pharmacology,	Embase, Index Medicus, InPharma, International Pharmaceutical Abstracts, Iowa Drug Information System, MEDLINE, Lexis-Nexis
	USP Dictionary of USAN & International Names, AHFS Drug Information, DRUGDEX, Drug Information Handbook, Handbook of Clinical Drug Data, Physicians' Desk Reference, Mosby's GenRx, USPDI Volume 1, Handbook of Nonprescription Drugs, Physicians' Desk Reference for Non-Prescription Drugs, STAT!-Ref, PDR Generics	
Identification (foreign products)	British National Formulary, * Diccionario de Especialidades Farmaceuticas, * European Drug Index, * Index Nominum, * Martindale: The Complete Drug Reference *	Embase, * InPharma, * International Pharmaceutical Abstracts * Index Medicus, Iowa Drug Information System, MEDLINE, Lexis-Nexis
Identification (imprint code)	IDENTIDEX, * PDR, * PDR Generics, * Mosby's GenRx, * Ident-A-Drug Reference, * Clinical Reference Library	—
Identification (street drug)	IDENTIDEX, * POISINDEX *	—
Indications (approved only)	Physicians' Desk Reference, * Mosby's GenRx, * PDR Generics *	Lexis-Nexis *
Indications (approved and unapproved)	AHFS Drug Information, * DRUGDEX, * Martindale: The Complete Drug Reference, * PDR Generics * Clinical Pharmacology, Drug Facts and Comparisons, Drug Information Handbook, Handbook of Clinical Drug Data, STAT!-Ref, USPDI Volume 1	Embase, * Index Medicus, * InPharma, * Iowa Drug Information System, * MEDLINE, * International Pharmaceutical Abstracts, * Lexis-Nexis *

*Indicates resources particularly useful for locating information on the specified subject.

Type of Inquiry	Tertiary Resources	Secondary Resources
Investigational drugs	DRUGDEX,* Martindale: The Complete Drug Reference,* USP Dictionary of Drug Names,* Handbook of Clinical Drug Data, Drug Facts and Comparisons	Embase,* Index Medicus,* InPharma,* Iowa Drug Information System,* MEDLINE,* International Pharmaceutical Abstracts,* Lexis-Nexis
Laboratory tests	Clinical Guide to Laboratory Tests,* Laboratory Test Handbook,* Laboratory Tests and Diagnostic Procedures,* STAT!-Ref*	Embase,* Index Medicus,* MEDLINE*
		Reactions, Lexis-Nexis, Iowa Drug Information Services, International Pharmaceutical Abstracts
	Cecil Textbook of Medicine, Harrison's Principles of Internal Medicine, The Merck Manual, Scientific American Medicine	
Manufacturer information (foreign)	European Drug Index,* Index Nominum,* Martindale: The Complete Drug Reference,* Merck Index,* other foreign pharmacopeias	—
Manufacturer information (domestic)	American Drug Index,* Red Book,* POISINDEX,*Drug Facts and Comparisons,* Physicians' Desk Reference,* Mosby's GenRx,* PDR Generics, USP Dictionary	—
Over-the-counter drugs	Handbook of Nonprescription Drugs,* Nonprescription Drug Therapy,* Nonprescription Products: Formulations and Features,* Physicians' Desk Reference for Non-Prescription Drugs,* Drug Facts and Comparisons, DRUGDEX, POISINDEX, USPDI Volume 1	Lexis-Nexis*
		Embase, Index Medicus, InPharma, International Pharmaceutical Abstracts, Iowa Drug Information System, MEDLINE
Patient counseling	Aftercare,* Medication Teaching Manual,* Patient Counseling Handbook,* Patient Drug Facts,* USPDI Volume 2*	Lexis-Nexis*
	AHFS Drug Information, DRUGDEX, Drug Facts and Comparisons, Drug Information Handbook, Handbook of Clinical Drug Data, Physicians' Desk Reference, Physicians GenRx, Dr. Schueler's Home Medical Advisor	
Pharmaceutical calculations	Remington's Pharmaceutical Sciences*	—
	Redbook, Handbook of Clinical Drug Data, A Practical Guide to Contemporary Pharmacy Practice	
Pharmaceutical organizations (state and national)	Red Book*	—
Pharmacy law	Pharmacy Law Digest,* Individual state law books	Lexis-Nexis,* International Pharmaceutical Abstracts*
Physical assessment	Physical Assessment: A Guide for Evaluating Drug Therapy*	—

*Indicates resources particularly useful for locating information on the specified subject.

Type of Inquiry	Tertiary Resources	Secondary Resources
Pharmacokinetics	*Applied Pharmacokinetics: Principles of Therapeutic Drug Monitoring,* * *Basic Clinical Pharmacokinetics,* * *Handbook of Basic Pharmaceutics* * *AHFS Drug Information, DRUGDEX, Drug Facts and Comparisons, Drug Information Handbook, Handbook of Clinical Drug Data, Martindale: The Complete Drug Reference, Physicians' Desk Reference, Mosby's GenRx, USPDI Volume 1, PDR Generics*	*International Pharmaceutical Abstracts* * *Embase, Index Medicus, Iowa Drug Information System, MEDLINE, InPharma*
Pharmacology	*Goodman and Gilman's Pharmacologic Basis of Therapeutics,* * *Human Pharmacology: Molecular to Clinical,* * *Principles of Pharmacology, Basic Concepts & Clinical Applications* * *AHFS Drug Information, DRUGDEX, Drug Facts and Comparisons, Drug Information Handbook, Handbook of Clinical Drug Data, Martindale: The Complete Drug Reference, Physicians' Desk Reference, Physicians GenRx, STAT!-Ref, USPDI Volume 1*	*Iowa Drug Information System,* * *Embase, Index Medicus, MEDLINE, InPharma, International Pharmaceutical Abstracts*
Poison control centers	*Red Book,* * *Mosby's GenRx,* * *Poisoning & Toxicology Handbook,* * *PDR Generics* *	
Stability/compatibility	*Guide to Parenteral Admixtures,* * *Handbook on Injectable Drugs* * *AHFS Drug Information, DRUGDEX, STAT!-Ref*	*International Pharmaceutical Abstracts* * *Index Medicus, Iowa Drug Information System, MEDLINE*
Toxicology/poisoning	*Clinical Management of Poisoning and Drug Overdose,* * *Ellenhorn's Medical Toxicology,* * *POISINDEX,* * *Poisoning & Toxicology Handbook,* * *Principles of Clinical Toxicology,* * *Goldfrank's Toxicologic Emergencies* * *AHFS Drug Information, DRUGDEX, Drug Facts and Comparisons, Drug Information Handbook, Handbook of Clinical Drug Data, Physicians' Desk Reference, Physicians GenRx, USPDI Volume 1*	*Reactions* * *Embase, Index Medicus, International Pharmaceutical Abstracts, Iowa Drug Information System, MEDLINE*
Veterinary	*The Merck Veterinary Manual,* * *Small Animal Medicine Therapeutics,* * *Veterinary Drug Handbook,* * *Veterinary Drug Therapy,* * *Veterinary Pharmaceuticals and Biologicals (VPB),* * *DRUGDEX, POISINDEX, USP-DI Vol. 1*	*Biosis, Embase, MEDLINE*

*Indicates resources particularly useful for locating information on the specified subject.

5–1

Appendix 5–1

Alternative Medicine Web Addresses

Important note: The quality of the information in these web sites is open to interpretation. They are listed to provide the user a way to find out what is being claimed by various proponents of alternative medicine.

Web sites often move or change. The information provided was accurate at the time of writing.

Name of Site	Web URL
About.com Alternative Medicine	http://www.about.com/health/altmedicine
The Alexander Technique	http://www.life.uiuc.edu/jeff/alextech.html
Algy's Herb Page	http://www.algy.com/herb/index.html
Alternative Medicine Center	http://www.healthy.net/clinic/therapy
Alternative Health—The Directory of Natural Medicine Homepages	http://members.aol.com/altamed/inter.htm
Alternative Medicine Associations, Trade Groups, etc.	http://www.healthy.net/associations
Alternative Medicine Digest	http://www.alternativemedicine.com
Alternative Medicine Homepage	http://www.pitt.edu/~cbw/altm.html
American Association of Naturopathic Physicians	http://www.naturopathic.org
American Botanical Council	http://www.herbalgram.org
American College for Advancement in Medicine	http://www.acam.org
American Herbal Pharmacopoeia	http://www.herbal-ahp.org
American Herbal Product Association	http://www.ahpa.org
American Holistic Health Association	http://www.healthy.net/ahha
American Nutraceutical Association	http://www.americanutra.com
American Whole Health, Inc.	http://www.americanwholehealth.com
A Modern Herbal (hypertext version of a 1931 book)	http://www.botanical.com/botanical/mgmh/mgmh.html
Ask Dr. Weil	http://cgi.pathfinder.com/drweil
Association of Natural Medicine Pharmacists	http://www.anmp.org
Association of Teachers of Preventive Medicine	http://www.atpm.org
Ayurvedic Foundations	http://www.ayur.com
The Backrubs FAQ	http://www.ii.uib.no/~kjartan/backrubfaq/index.html
Botanical.com	http://www.botanical.com
Cathay Herbal Laboratories (traditional Chinese medicine) Traditional Chinese Medicine Library & Search Engine	http://www.cathayherbal.com http://www.cathayherbal.com/library/index.htm
Center for Empirical Medicine	http://www.empiricaltherapies.com

Name of Site	Web URL
The Chiropractic Page	http://www.mbnet.mb.ca/~jwiens/chiro.html
CHIRO-WEB	http://pages.prodigy.com/CT/doc/doc.html
Combined Health Information Database (CHID) (U.S. government)	http://chid.nih.gov
Complementary Medicine References, General	http://www.forthrt.com/~chronicl/archiv.htm
Cyberbotanica	http://biotech.icmb.utexas.edu/botany
Datadiwan (Germany)	http://www.datadiwan.de/neuigkeiten/index_e.htm
Dietary Supplements—An Advertising Guide for Industry (FTC)	http://www.ftc.gov/bcp/conline/pubs/buspubs/dietsupp.htm
Dr. Bower's Complementary and Alternative Home Page	http://www.people.virginia.edu/~pjb3s/Complementary_Practices.html
Dr. Duke's Phytochemical and Ethnobotanical Databases	http://www.ars-grin.gov/duke
eNutrition	http://www.enutrition.com
FDA's Special Nutritionals' Adverse Event Monitoring	http://vm.cfsan.fda.gov/~dms/aems.html
foodandlife.com	http://www.foodandlife.com
Gifts of Health	http://users.ox.ac.uk/~gree0179
GlycoScience	http://www.glycoscience.com/glycoscience
Healthcare Reality Check—science-based information on alternative and complementary medicine	http://www.hcrc.org
Health-n-Energy	http://www.health-n-energy.com
healthshop.com	http://www.healthshop.com
Health World Online	http://www.healthy.net
Healthy World Herbal Medicine Center	http://www.healthy.net/clinic/therapy/herbal/index.asp
Health World Homeopathy Center	http://www.healthy.net/clinic/therapy/homeopat/
Health World Naturopathy Medicine Center	http://www.naturopathy.com
Herbal Pharmacy	http://www.herbalpharmacy.com
HerbMed	http://www.amfoundation.org/herbmed.htm
Herb Research Foundation	http://www.herbs.org
HerbWeb	http://www.herbweb.com
Holistic Healing Web Page	http://www.holisticmed.com
Holistic.com	http://www.holistic.com
Holisticmedicine.com	http://www.holisticmedicine.com
Home of Reflexology	http://www.reflexology.org
Homeopathic Educational Services	http://www.homeopathic.com
Homeopathy Home Page	http://www.homeopathyhome.com
IBISMedical.com (Integrative Medicine and Natural Health)	http://www.ibismedical.com
International Bibliographic Information on Dietary Supplements (IBIDS) (NIH)	http://odp.od.nih.gov/ods/databases/ibids.html
LifePlus Nutrition	http://www.lifeplusnutrition.com
The Massage Therapy Homepage	http://www.massagetherapyhomepage.com
Medherb.com	http://www.medherb.com
MEDMarket.com	http://www.medmarket.com/alternative.com
MotherNature.com	http://www.mothernature.com
Museum of Questionable Medical Devices	http://www.mtn.org/~quack/index.htm
National Center for Complementary and Alternative Medicine (National Institutes of Health)	http://nccam.nih.gov

Name of Site	Web URL
Complementary and Alternative Citation Medicine Citation Index	http://nccam.nih.gov/nccam/resources/cam-ci
National Center for Homeopathy	http://www.homeopathic.org
National Institutes of Health Office of Dietary Supplements	http://odp.od.nih.gov/ods/default.html
International Bibliographic Information on Dietary Supplements	http://odp.od.nih.gov/ods/databases/ibids.html
Natural and Alternative Medicine Home Page	http://www.geocities.com/HotSprings/4353
Natural Health and Longevity Resource Center	http://www.all-natural.com
Natural Medicine Online	http://www.nat-med.com/index.htm
Natural Products Industry Center (NPI Center)	http://www.npicenter.com
The Natural Pharmacist	http://www.tnp.com
Nature's Resource (company)	http://www.vitamin.com/brands/naturesresource/about.html
New York Access to Health (NOAH) Alternative (Complementary) Medicine	http://www.noah.cuny.edu/alternative/alternative.html
Nurses Portal Alternative Health	http://www.wholenurse.com/alternative.htm
OneMedicine	http://www.onemedicine.com
OnHealth.com	http://www.onhealth.com
Osteopathic Medicine International WWW Resource Website	http://www.rscom.com/osteo
Prevention Magazine	http://www.healthyideas.com
Rosenthal Center for Complementary and Alternative Medicine	http://cpmcnet.columbia.edu/dept/rosenthal
Royal Botanic Gardens Kew, Scientific Research Programmes	http://www.rbgkew.org.uk
Shiatsu—Therapeutic Art of Japan	http://www.doubleclickd.com/shiatsu.html
Snowbound Herbals	http://www.sbherbals.com
Southwest School of Botanical Medicine	http://chili.rt66.com/hrbmoore/HOMEPAGE/HomePage.html
Specialty Enzymes and Biochemicals Company	http://www.4enzymes.com
SupplementWatch.com	http://www.supplementwatch.com
Twinlab	http://www.twinlab.com
vitacost.com	http://www.vitacost.com
VitaminShoppe.com	http://www.vitaminshoppe.com
WholeHealthMD.com	http://www.wholehealthmd.com
Yahoo! Alternative Medicine	http://dir.yahoo.com/health/alternative_medicine
Zinc Acetate Lozenges	http://www.coldcure.com

5-2

Appendix 5-2

Associations' and Organizations' Web Addresses

Important note: Web sites often move or change. The information provided was accurate at the time of writing.

Organization	Web URL
Academy of Managed Care Pharmacy	http://www.amcp.org
AdvaMed (Advanced Medical Technology Association)	http://www.himanet.com
Agency for Healthcare Research and Qualtiy (AHRQ)	http://www.ahrq.gov
Alabama Pharmacy Association	http://www.aparx.org
Alaska Pharmaceutical Association	http://www.alaska.net/~akphrmcy
Alternative and Conventional Medicine Association	http://www.healthy.net/associations
Alzheimer's Association	http://www.alz.org
American Academy of Allergy, Asthma & Immunology (Allergy and Asthma Disease Management Center)	http://www.aadmc.org
American Association of Colleges of Pharmacy	http://www.aacp.org
American Association of Pharmaceutical Scientists (AAPS Online)	http://www.aaps.org
American Association of Pharmacy Technicians, Inc.	http://www.pharmacytechnician.com
American Cancer Society	http://www.cancer.org
American College of Apothecaries Research and Education Resource Center	http://www.acaresourcecenter.org
American College of Clinical Pharmacy	http://www.accp.com
American Council on Pharmaceutical Education (ACPE)	http://www.acpe-accredit.org
American Diabetes Association	http://www.diabetes.org
American Geriatrics Society	http://www.americangeriatrics.org
American Heart Association	http://www.americanheart.org
American Hospital Association	http://www.aha.org
AHA Quality Initiatives	http://www.aha.org/quality
American Lung Association	http://www.lungusa.org
American Medical Association	http://www.ama-assn.org
American Medical Informatics Association	http://www.amia.org
American Nutraceutical Association	http://www.americanutra.com

Organization	Web URL
American Pain Society	http://www.ampainsoc.org
American Pharmaceutical Association (APhA)	http://www.aphanet.org
American Psychiatric Association	http://www.psych.org
American Public Health Association (APHA)	http://www.apha.org
American Society for Automation in Pharmacy (ASAP)	http://www.asapnet.org
American Society of Consultant Pharmacists (ASCP)	http://www.ascp.com
American Society for Healthcare Risk Management	http://www.ashrm.org
American Society of Health-Systems Pharmacists	http://www.ashp.org
American Society for Parenteral & Enteral Nutrition (ASPEN)	http://www.clinnutr.org
American Society for Pharmacy Law	http://www.aspl.org
American Telemedicine Association	http://www.atmeda.org
American Thoracic Society	http://www.thoracic.org
Arkansas Pharmacists Association	http://www.arpharmacists.org
Association of Natural Medicine Pharmacists	http://www.anmp.org
Board of Pharmaceutical Specialties (BPS)	http://www.bpsweb.org
California Pharmacists Association	http://www.cpha.com
California Society of Health-System Pharmacists	http://www.cshp.org
Canadian Lung Association	http://www.lung.ca
Canadian Society for Pharmaceutical Sciences	http://www.ualberta.ca/~csps
Canadian Wholesale Drug Association	http://www.cwda.com
Center for the Study of Autism	http://www.autism.org
Chain Drug Marketing Association (CDMA)	http://www.chaindrug.com
Colorado Pharmacists	http://www.coloradopharmacy.org
Consumer Coalition for Quality Health Care	http://www.consumers.org
Consumer Healthcare Products Association	http://www.ndmaininfo.org
Cosmetic, Toiletry, and Fragrance Association (CTFA)	http://www.ctfa.org
Cystic Fibrosis Foundation	http://www.cff.org
Delaware Pharmacists Society	http://www.depharmacy.org/Index.htm
Drug Information Association	http://www.diahome.org
Drug, Chemical and Allied Trades Association (DCAT)	http://www.dcat.org
Florida Pharmacy Association	http://www.pharmview.com
Florida Society of Health-System Pharmacists	http://www.fshp.org
Food and Drug Law Institute (FDLI)	http://www.fdli.org
Foundation for Accountability (FACCT)	http://www.facct.org
Generic Access.com	http://www.genericaccess.com
Generic Pharmaceutical Industry Association (GPIA)	http://www.gpia.org
Georgia Pharmacy Association	http://www.gpha.org
Georgia Society of Health System Pharmacists	http://www.gshp.org
Gerontological Society of America	http://www.geron.org
Hawaii Pharmacists Association	http://www.helix.com/helix/assoc/assn_pharm/hpha/hpha.htm
Healthcare Leadership Council	http://www.hlc.org
Health Insurance Association of America (HIAA)	http://www.hiaa.org
Illinois Council of Health-System Pharmacists	http://www.ichpnet.org
Immunization Action Coalition	http://www.immunize.org
Indiana Pharmacists Alliance	http://www.indianapharmacists.org

Organization	Web URL
International Medical Informatics Association	http://www.imia.org
Institute for Safe Medication Practices	http://www.ismp.org
International Pharmaceutical Federation (FIP)	http://www.fip.nl
International Society for Pharmacoeconomic and Outcomes Research (ISPOR)	http://www.ispor.org
Iowa Pharmacists Association	http://www.iowapharmacists.org
Joint Commission on Accreditation of Healthcare Organizations	http://www.jcaho.org
Joint Healthcare Information Technology Alliance	http://www.jhita.org
Juvenile Diabetes Foundation International	http://www.jdf.org
Kentucky Society of Health-System Pharmacists	http://www.kshp.org
Louisiana Pharmacists Association	http://www.lpha.com
Louisiana Society of Health-System Pharmacists	http://www.louisianapharmacists.org
Lymphoma Research Foundation of America	http://www.lymphoma.org
Maine Society of Health-System Pharmacists	http://www.meshp.org
Maryland Pharmacists Association	http://www.erols.com/mpha
Maryland Society of Health-System Pharmacists	http://www.mshp.org
Massachusetts Pharmacists Association	http://www.channel1.com/users/mpha
Medical Lobby for Appropriate Marketing (MaLAM)	http://www.camtech.net.au/malam
Michigan Pharmacists Association	http://www.mipharm.com
Minnesota Pharmacists Association	http://www.mpha.org
Minnesota Society of Health-System Pharmacists	http://www.mnshp.org
Missouri Pharmacy Association	http://www.morx.com
Montana Society of Health-System Pharmacists	http://www.umt.edu/mshp
National Association of Boards of Pharmacy (NABP)	http://www.nabp.net
National Association of Chain Drug Stores	http://www.nacds.org
National Association for Healthcare Quality	http://www.nahq.org/index.htm
National Association of Pharmaceutical Manufacturers	http://www.napmnet.org
National Association of Pharmacy Regulatory Authorities (NAPRA) (Canada)	http://www.napra.org
National Childhood Cancer Foundation	http://www.nccf.org
National Coalition for Adult Immunization	http://www.nfid.org/ncai
National Committee for Quality Assurance (NCQA)	http://www.ncqa.org
National Community Pharmacy Association (NCPA) (formerly NARD)	http://www.ncpanet.org
National Coordinating Council for Medication Error Reporting and Prevention	http://www.nccmerp.org
National Council on the Aging	http://www.ncoa.org
National Council on Patient Information and Education (NCPIE)	http://www.talkaboutrx.org
National Council for Prescription Drug Programs	http://www.ncpdp.org

Organization	Web URL
National Council of State Pharmacy Association Executives (NCSPAE)	http://www.ncspae.org
National Depressive and Manic-Depressive Association	http://www.ndmda.org
National Foundation for Infectious Diseases	http://www.nfid.org
National Foundation for Depressive Illness, Inc.	http://www.depression.org
National Mental Health Association	http://www.nmha.org
National Osteoporosis Foundation	http://www.nof.org
National Organization for Rare Disorders (NORD)	http://www.rarediseases.org
National Ovarian Cancer Coalition	http://www.ovarian.org
National Pediculosis Association	http://www.headlice.org
National Pharmaceutical Alliance	http://www.n-p-a.org
National Pharmaceutical Association (NPhA)	http://www.helix.com/helix/assoc/assn_pharm/npha/npha_home.htm
National Wholesale Druggists' Association (NWDA)	http://www.nwda.org
Nebraska Pharmacists Association	http://npa.creighton.edu
Nebraska Society of Health-Systems Pharmacists	http://nshp.creighton.edu
New Jersey Pharmacists Association	http://www.njpha.com
New Mexico Pharmaceutical Association	http://www.nm-pharmacy.com
New Mexico Society of Health-System Pharmacists	http://www.nmshp.org
New York State Council of Health-System Pharmacists	http://www.nyschp.org
North American Association of Central Cancer Registries	http://www.naaccr.org
North Carolina Association of Pharmacists	http://www.ncpharmacists.org
North Dakota Pharmaceutical Association	http://www.nodakpharmacy.com
Ohio Pharmacists Association	http://www.ohiopharmacists.org
Ohio Society of Health-System Pharmacists	http://www.ohioshp.org
Oklahoma Pharmacists Association	http://www.opha.com
Oklahoma Society of Health-System Pharmacists	http://www.oshp.net
Oregon Society of Health-System Pharmacists	http://www.oshp.org
Osteoporosis Society of Canada	http://www.osteoporosis.ca
Ovarian Cancer National Alliance	http://www.ovariancancer.org
Parenteral Drug Association	http://www.pda.org
Pediatric Pharmacy Advocacy Group	http://www.ppag.org
Pennsylvania Pharmacists Association	http://www.papharmacists.com
Pennsylvania Society of Health-System Pharmacists	http://www.pshp.org
Pharmaceutical Care Management Association	http://www.pcmanet.org
Pharmaceutical Society of New Zealand	http://www.psnz.org.nz
Pharmaceutical Research and Manufacturers of America (PhRMA)	http://www.phrma.org
Pharmacists Society of the State of New York	http://www.pssny.org
Pharmacy Society of Wisconsin	http://www.pswi.org
Pharmacy Technician Certification Board	http://www.ptcb.org
Rhode Island Society of Health-System Pharmacists	http://www.rishp.org

Organization	Web URL
Society of Competitive Intelligence Professionals	http://www.scip.org
Society for Medical Decision Making	http://www.gwu.edu/~smdm
Texas Pharmacy Association	http://www.txpharmacy.com
Texas Society of Health-System Pharmacists	http://www.tshp.org
U.S. Pharmacopeia (USP)	http://www.usp.org
Utah Society of Health-System Pharmacists	http://www.ushp.org
Virginia Pharmacists Association	http://pharmacy.su.edu/vpha
Virginia Society of Health-System Pharmacists	http://www.vshp.org
Washington Metropolitan Society of Health-System Pharmacists	http://www.his.com/~quinnj
Washington State Pharmacists Association	http://www.pharmcare.org
Washington State Society of Health-System Pharmacists	http://www.wsshp.org
West Virginia Society of Health-System Pharmacists	http://www.wvshp.org
World Health Organization	http://www.who.int
WHO Guide to Good Prescribing	http://www.geocities.com/HotSprings/3660/home.html
Wyoming Pharmacists Association	http://www.wpha.net

5-3

Boards of Pharmacy Web Addresses

Important note: Web sites often move or change. The information provided was accurate at the time of writing.

Name of Site	Web URL
United States	
Alabama	http://www.albop.com
Alaska	http://www.dced.state.ak.us/occ/ppha.htm
Arizona	http://www.pharmacy.state.az.us
Arkansas	http://www.state.ar.us/asbp
California	http://www.pharmacy.ca.gov
Colorado	http://www.dora.state.co.us/Pharmacy
Connecticut	http://www.ctdrugcontrol.com
Florida	http://www.doh.state.fl.us/mqa/pharmacy/pshome.htm
Georgia	http://www.sos.state.ga.us/ebd-pharmacy
Idaho	http://www.state.id.us/bop
Illinois	http://www.dpr.state.il.us
Indiana	http://www.state.in.us/hpb/isbp
Iowa	http://www.idph.state.ia.us/pa/pl/pharmacy.htm
Kansas	http://www.ink.org/public/pharmacy
Louisiana	http://www.labp.com
Massachusetts	http://www.state.ma.us/reg/boards/ph
Michigan	http://www.cis.state.mi.us/bhser/home.htm
Minnesota	http://www.phcybrd.state.mn.us
Mississippi	http://www.mbp.state.ms.us
Missouri	http://www.ecodev.state.mo.us/pr/pharmacy
Montana	http://www.com.state.mt.us/License/POL/pol_boards/pha_board/board_page.htm
Nebraska	http://www.hhs.state.ne.us
Nevada	http://www.state.nv.us./pharmacy
New Hampshire	http://www.state.nh.us/pharmacy
New Jersey	http://www.state.nj.us/lps/ca/brief/pharm.htm
New Mexico	http://www.state.nm.us/pharmacy/index.html
New York	http://www.op.nysed.gov/pharm.htm
North Carolina	http://www.ncbop.org
Ohio	http://www.state.oh.us/pharmacy
Oklahoma	http://www.state.ok.us/~pharmacy
Oregon	http://www.pharmacy.state.or.us
Pennsylvania	http://www.dos.state.pa.us/bpoa/phabd.htm
South Carolina	http://www.llr.state.sc.us/bop.htm

Name of Site	Web URL
South Dakota	http://www.state.sd.us/dcr/pharmacy/pharm-ho.htm
Texas	http://www.tsbp.state.tx.us
Utah	http://www.commerce.state.ut.us/dopl/dopl1.htm
Vermont	http://170.222.200.71/pharmacists
Virginia	http://www.dhp.state.va.us/levelone/pharm.htm
Washington	http://www.doh.wa.gov/pharmacy
Canada	
Ontario	http://www.ocpharma.com
Quebec	http://www.opq.org/eng/default.htm

5–4

Appendix 5–4

Drug Information/Informatics Centers Web Addresses

Important note: Web sites often move or change. The information provided was accurate at the time of writing.

Name of Site	Web URL
AAPCC Directory of Poison Control Centers	http://www.nlu.edu/~pharmacy/aapcclst.html
Arizona Poison and Drug Information Center	http://www.pharm.arizona.edu/centers/poison_center/index.html
Coy C. Carpenter Library Drug Information Service Center (Wake Forest University)	http://www.bgsm.edu/library/disc.html
Creighton University Drug Informatics	http://druginfo.creighton.edu
Glasgow (Scotland) Area Drug Information Center	http://www.digri.demon.co.uk
Grafic Health Drug Information Service	http://www.gerrygraf.com
Idaho Drug Information Service	http://rx.isu.edu/services_contracts/idis
Iowa Drug Information Network	http://idin.idis.uiowa.edu
Louisiana Drug and Poison Information Center	http://rxweb.nlu.edu/ldpic
Marshall University Drug Information Service	http://musom.marshall.edu/CHH/DrugInfo/home.htm
Ohio Northern University Drug Information Center	http://www.onu.edu/pharmacy/DrugInfo
University of Chicago Hospitals Drug Information Service	http://dacc.bsd.uchicago.edu/drug/dis.html
University of Colorado Health Sciences Center Drug Information Center	http://www.coloradohealthnet.org/pharmacology/pharm_about.html
University of Florida Drug Information and Pharmacy Resource Center (DIPRC)	http://www.health.ufl.edu/professional/diprc.html
University of Kansas Drug Information Center	http://www2.kumc.edu/druginfo
University of Kansas Radiopharmaceutical Drug Information Center	http://www2.kumc.edu/druginfo/radio.html
University of Kentucky Drug Information Center	http://www.mc.uky.edu/pharmacy/DIC
University of Maryland Drug Information Center	http://www.pharmacy.ab.umd.edu/~umdi/umdi.html
University of the Pacific Drug Information Center	http://jarl.cs.uop.edu/pharmacy/info/uopdruginfo.html

5–5

Appendix 5–5

Evidence-Based Medicine/Outcomes/ Clinical Practice Guidelines Web Addresses

Important note: Web sites often move or change. The information provided was accurate at the time of writing.

Name of Site	Web URL
Agency for Healthcare Research and Quality (AHRQ)	http://www.ahrq.gov
Agency for Healthcare Research and Quality Guidelines	http://www.ahrq.gov/clinic
Agency for Quality in Medicine (Germany)	http://www.leitlinien.de/aezqengl.htm
Alberta Medical Association Clinical Practice Guidelines	http://www.amda.ab.ca/cpg/index.html
American Academy of Pediatrics	http://www.aap.org/policy/pprgtoc.html
American Association of Clinical Endocrinologists Guidelines	http://www.aace.com/clinguideindex.htm
American College of Cardiology/American Heart Association Clinical Guidelines	http://www.acc.org/clinical/guidelines/index.html
American College of Gastroenterology Guidelines	http://www.acg.gi.org
American College of Rheumatology Clinical Guidelines	http://www.rheumatology.org
American Society of Anesthesiologists Clinical Guidelines	http://www.asahq.org/practice/homepage.html
Australian Clinical Guidelines	http://www.nbcc.org.au/pages/info/resource/ nbccpubs/nbccpubs.htm#gui
Canadian Coordinating Office for Health Technology Assessment	http://www.ccohta.ca
Canadian Medical Association Clinical Practice Guidelines	http://www.cma.ca/cpgs/index.asp
Center for the Evaluative Clinical Sciences at Dartmouth	http://www.dartmouth.edu/dms/cecs
Center for Health Policy, Law and Management (Duke University)	http://www.hpolicy.duke.edu
Centre for Evidence-Based Medicine (Great Britain)	http://cebm.jr2.ox.ac.uk
Cholesterol Clinical Guidelines	http://dsg.harvard.edu/public/guidelines/ cholesterol/chlintun.html
Clearing House for Health Outcomes	http://www.leeds.ac.uk/nuffield/infoservices/ UKCH/find.html
Cochrane Collaboration (McMaster University)	http://hiru.mcmaster.ca/COCHRANE
The Cochrane Library	http://www.update-software.com/cochrane/ cochrane-frame.html

Name of Site	Web URL
Combined Health Information Database (CHID) (U.S.government)	http://chid.nih.gov
CPG Infobase (Canadian Medical Association)	http://www.cma.ca/cpgs/index.htm
European Clearing Houses on Health Outcomes (ECHHO)	http://www.leeds.ac.uk/nuffield/infoservices/ECHHO
Evidence-Based Medicine (definition)	http://cebm.jr2.ox.ac.uk/ebmisisnt.html
Evidence-Based Medicine (journal)	http://www.acponline.org/journals/ebm/pubinfo.htm
Evidence Based Medicine Tool Kit (University of Alberta, Canada)	http://www.med.ualberta.ca/ebm/ebm.htm
Guideline (United Kingdom)	http://www.ihs.ox.ac.uk/guidelines
Health Care Libraries Unit	http://libsun1.jr2.ox.ac.uk
Health Information Research Unit (McMaster University, Canada)	http://hiru.mcmaster.ca
Henry Ford Health System Center for Health Services Research	http://www.hfhs-cce.org
Institutes of Health Sciences (Oxford)	http://www.ihs.ox.ac.uk
International Society for Pharmacoeconomic and Outcomes Research (ISPOR)	http://www.ispor.org
JAMA Asthma Information Center	http://www.ama-assn.org/special/asthma
Medical Journal of Australia Clinical Guidelines	http://www.mja.com.au/public/guides/guides.html
National Guideline Clearinghouse	http://www.guideline.gov
New Zealand Guidelines Group	http://www.nzgg.org.nz/index.efm
NHS R&D Strategy in Eastern Region	http://www.rdd-phru.com.ac.uk/nhserdd
Office of Health Policy and Clinical Outcomes Thomas Jefferson University Hospital/ Jefferson Health System	http://jeffline.tju.edu/CWIS/OHP/solutions.html
ORION: Outcomes Research Information On-line	http://www.healthoutcomesresearch.com
Pediatric Clinical Guidelines (Loyola University)	http://www.meddean.luc.edu/lumen/DeptWebs/peds/clinguid.htm
Pediatric Current Practice Parameters (American Academy of Pediatrics)	http://www.aap.org/policy/paramtoc.html
Pediatric Evidence-Based Medicine (University of Washington)	http://depts.washington.edu/pelebm
Primary Care Clinical Practice Guidelines (UCSF)	http://medicine.ucsf.edu/resources/guidelines
PRISE (Oxford)	http://libsun1.jr2.ox.ac.uk/prise
Queen's University at Kingston Clinical Practice Guidelines Index	http://post.queensu.ca/~bhc/gim/cpgs.html
ScHARR Introduction to Evidence-Based Practice on the Internet	http://www.shef.ac.uk/~scharr/ir/netting.html
Stratis Health	http://www.stratishealth.org
TALARIA Hypermedia Clinical Practice Guidelines for Cancer Pain	http://www.talaria.org
Therapeutics Initiative	http://www.ti.ubc.ca
Virtual Hospital Clinical Practice Guidelines	http://vh.radiology.uiowa.edu/Providers/ClinGuide/CGType.html
WHO Guide to Good Prescribing	http://www.geocities.com/HotSprings/3660/home.html

5–6

Appendix 5–6

General and Specialty Medicine Site Web Addresses

Important note: Web sites often move or change. The information provided was accurate at the time of writing.

Name of Site	Web URL
General Medicine Sites	
Achoo	http://www.achoo.com
AMEDEO The Medical Literature Guide	http://amedeo.com
BioSpace.com	http://www.biospace.com
Disease Management Forum	http://www.sapien.net/dm/index.htm
Doctor's Guide Global Editor	http://www.pslgroup.com/docguide.htm
DoctorNet.com	http://www.doctornet.com
DoctorPage (find a physician)	http://www.doctorpage.com
Health Communication Network	http://www.hcn.net.au
Health-Center.com	http://www.health-center.com
HealthWorld Online (includes free MEDLINE)	http://www.healthy.net
MedConnect	http://www.medconnect.com
Mediconsult	http://www.mediconsult.com
Specialty Medical Sites	
AEROSPACE MEDICINE	
Space Environmental Health Database	http://www.envmed.rochester.edu/htbin/ nasaindex
ALLERGY	
Allerdays	http://www.allerdays.com
Allergy and Asthma Disease Management Center (American Academy of Allergy, Asthma & Immunology)	http://www.aadmc.org
AUTISM	
Center for the Study of Autism	http://www.autism.org
CARDIOLOGY	
Cardiology Compass	http://www.cardiologycompass.com
DERMATOLOGY	
Dermatology Department (University of Iowa)	http://tray.dermatology.uiowa.edu/home.html
Dermatology Department (Waikato Hospital, New Zealand)	http://www.dermnet.org.nz/index.html

Name of Site	Web URL
Electronic Textbook of Dermatology	http://telemedicine.org/stamford.htm
Skin Cancer and Benign Tumor Image Atlas	http://www.meddean.luc.edu/lumen/MedEd/medicine/dermatology/content.htm

GASTROENTEROLOGY

GERD Information Resource Center (sponsored by Astra/Zeneca)	http://www.gerd.com

HIV/AIDS

Aegis (claims to be the world's largest HIV/AIDS web site)	http://www.aegis.com
AIDS Clinical Trials Information Service	http://www.actis.org
AIDS Knowledge Base (online version of The Textbook on HIV Disease from UCSF)	http://hivinsite.ucsf.edu/akb
Aidsmap	http://www.aidsmap.com
Aids.org	http://www.aids.org
CDC National Prevention Information Network	http://www.cdcnpin.org
Center for AIDS Prevention Studies (CAPS)	http://www.caps.ucsf.edu
Critical Path AIDS Project	http://www.critpath.org
Food and Drug Administration HIV/AIDS Activities	http://www.fda.gov/oashi/aids/hiv.html
Global HIV/AIDS and STD (sexually transmitted diseases) Surveillance	http://www.who.int/emc-hiv
HIV InfoWeb	http://www.infoweb.org
HIV Insite	http://hivinsite.ucsf.edu
HIV Medication Guide (Canada)	http://www.jag.on.ca/hiv
HIV AIDS Treatment Information Service (ATIS)	http://www.hivatis.org
JAMA's HIV/AIDS Information Center	http://www.ama-assn.org/special/hiv
Johns Hopkins AIDS Service	http://www.hopkins-aids.edu
Medscape HIV/AIDS	http://www.medscape.com/Home/Topics/AIDS/AIDS.html
National Institute on Allergy and Infectious Diseases	http://www.niaid.nih.gov/research/Daids.htm
National Library of Medicine AIDS Publications	http://sis.nlm.nih.gov/aidswww.htm
Positive Health AIDS Program at San Francisco General Hospital	http://sfghaids.ucsf.edu

INFECTIOUS DISEASE

All the Virology on the WWW	http://www.tulane.edu/~dmsander/garryfavweb.html
FluNet (international epidemiologic data on influenza)	http://oms2.b3e.jussieu.fr/flunet
Glossary of Microbiology	http://www.hardlink.com/~tsute/glossary/index.html
HepNet: The Hepatitis Information Network (Canada)	http://www.hepnet.com
Pediatric Infectious Diseases	http://www.pedid.uthscsa.edu
ProMed (Program for Monitoring Emerging Diseases, Federation of American Scientists)	http://www.sun00781.dn.net/promed
Resistance Web (Bacterial Antibiotic Resistance)	http://resistanceweb.mfhs.edu

MISCELLANEOUS

Doc's Diving Medicine Home Page	http://weber.u.washington.edu/~ekay
GeneMed Network (gene therapy)	http://genemed.org
Medications, Drugs, and Diving	http://www.gulftel.com/~scubadoc/drugsdiv.htm
PainLink	http://www.edc.org/PainLink

ONCOLOGY

Association of Cancer Online Resources, Inc.	http://www.medinfo.org

Name of Site	Web URL
Cancer Europe	http://www.cancereurope.org
Cancer Information Network	http://www.cancernetwork.com
Cancer News on the Net	http://www.cancernews.com
Carcinogenic Potency Project	http://potency.berkeley.edu/cpdb.html
Medicine Online (oncology information)	http://www.meds.com
North American Association of Central Cancer Registries	http://www.naaccr.org
OncoLink (oncology information) includes video	http://www.oncolink.upenn.edu
Ovarian Cancer Research Notebook	http://www.slip.net/~mcdavis/ovarian.html

OPHTHALMOLOGY

EyeMax	http://www.eyemax.com

PEDIATRICS

KidsMeds	http://www.kidsmeds.com

PSYCHIATRY/PSYCHOLOGY

Internet Mental Health	http://www.mentalhealth.com

SUBSTANCE ABUSE

National Substance Abuse Web Index	http://nsawi.health.org/compass

TERATOGENICITY

Clinical Teratology Web	http://depts.washington.edu/~terisweb
Reprotox	http://www.reprotox.org

TOXICOLOGY

Integrated Risk Information System (IRIS)	http://www.epa.gov/iris
Karolinska Institute (Sweden) Toxicology Information	http://www.mic.ki.se/Diseases/c21.613.html
Poisons Information Database (Singapore)	http://valentine.mip.nus.edu.sg/PID
Tox.it (Italy)	http://www.tox.it/emerindex.htm
United Nations Environment Programme (UNEP) Chemicals	http://irptc.unep.ch/irptc

5–7

Appendix 5–7

Government Web Addresses

Important note: Web sites often move or change. The information provided was accurate at the time of writing.

Government Bureau	Web URL
Agency for Toxic Substances and Disease Registry (ATSDR)	http://www.atsdr.cdc.gov/atsdrhome.html
Canadian Coordinating Office for Health Technology Assessment	http://www.ccohta.ca
cancerTrials (National Cancer Institute)	http://cancertrials.nci.nih.gov
Centers for Disease Control and Prevention	http://www.cdc.gov
Centers for Disease Control Search Engine	http://www.cdc.gov/search.htm
CDC National Prevention Information Network	http://www.cdcnpin.org
Code of Federal Regulations	http://www.access.gpo.gov/nara/cfr/index.html
Combined Health Information Database (CHID) (U.S. government)	http://chid.nih.gov
Department of Health and Human Services	http://www.os.dhhs.gov
Department of Veterans' Affairs—Pharmacy Benefit Management Strategic Health Group	http://www.vapbm.org/PBM/menu.htm
Department of Veterans' Affairs—Treatment Guidelines	http://www.vapbm.org/PBM/treatment.htm
Department of Veterans' Affairs—Drug Class Reviews	http://www.vapbm.org/PBM/reviews.htm
Department of Veterans' Affairs—National Formulary	http://www.vapbm.org/PBM/natform.htm
Department of Veterans' Affairs—Criteria for Use of Selected Drugs	http://www.vapbm.org/PBM/criteria.htm
Department of Veterans' Affairs—Drug and Pharmaceutical Prices	http://www.vapbm.org/PBM/prices.htm
Drug Enforcement Administration (DEA)	http://www.usdoj.gov/dea
Eudra Portal (European Agency) for the Evaluation of Medicinal Products	http://eudraportal.eudra.org
Federal Register Archives	http://www.access.gpo.gov/su_docs/aces/aces140.html
Federal Web Locator	http://www.infoctr.edu/fwl
FedWorld.gov	http://www.fedworld.gov
Food and Drug Administration	http://www.fda.gov
Drug Information	http://www.fda.gov/cder/drug.htm
HIV/AIDS Activities	http://www.fda.gov/oashi/aids/hiv.html
NDA Information—approvals	http://www.fda.gov/cder/da/da.htm
GPO access on the web	http://thorplus.lib.purdue.edu/gpo

Government Bureau	Web URL
GrantsNet (Department of Health and Human Services)	http://www.os.dhhs.gov/progorg/grantsnet/index.html
HealthCanada Online	http://www.hc-sc.gc.ca/english
HealthFax (Australian Immunisation Guidelines)	http://www.healthfax.org.au/control.htm
Healthfinder (patient oriented site)	http://www.healthfinder.gov
Health Information (NIH)	http://www.nih.gov/health
HIV/AIDS Treatment Information Service (U.S. government site with official recommendations)	http://www.hivatis.org
Medicare	http://www.medicare.gov
MedWatch Program (FDA)	http://www.fda.gov/medwatch
National Cancer Institute—CancerNet	http://cancernet.nci.nih.gov
PDQ (NCI's Comprehensive Cancer Database)	http://cancernet.nci.nih.gov/pdqfull.htm
National Center for Biotechnology Information	http://www.ncbi.nlm.nih.gov
National Center for Complementary and Alternative Medicine (National Institutes of Health)	http://nccam.nih.gov
National Center for Health Statistics	http://www.cdc.gov/nchs
National Center for Infectious Diseases	http://www.cdc.gov/ncidod/index.htm
National Health Care Anti-Fraud Association (NHCAA)	http://www.nhcaa.org
National Health Information Center	http://nhic-nt.health.org
National Heart, Lung, and Blood Institute	http://www.nhlbi.nih.gov/nhlbi/nhlbi.htm
National Institute on Aging	http://www.nih.gov/nia
National Institute on Allergy and Infectious Diseases (home page)	http://www.niaid.nih.gov
National Institute on Allergy and Infectious Diseases (AIDS Information)	http://www.niaid.nih.gov/research/Daids.htm
National Institute of Arthritis and Musculoskeletal and Skin Diseases (NIAMS)	http://www.nih.gov/niams
National Institute of Diabetes and Digestive and Kidney Diseases	http://www.niddk.nih.gov
National Institute on Drug Abuse	http://www.nida.nih.gov/NIDAHomel.html
National Institute of Mental Health	http://www.nimh.nih.gov
National Institutes of Health Grants and Funding Opportunities	http://www.nih.gov/grants
National Library of Medicine	http://www.nlm.nih.gov
PubMed Central	http://www.pubmedcentral.nih.gov
National Substance Abuse Web	http://nsawi.health.org/compass
National Technical Information Service (NTIS)	http://www.ntis.gov
National Vaccine Injury Compensation Program (VICP)	http://www.hrsa.dhhs.gov/bhpr/vicp/index.htm
Office of Dietary Supplements	http://odp.od.nih.gov/ods
Office of Rare Diseases	http://rarediseases.info.nih.gov/ord
Occupational Safety and Health Administration	http://www.osha.gov
Practice of Pharmacy Compounding (FDA site)	http://www.fda.gov/cder/pharmcomp/default.htm
South African Package Inserts	http://home.intekom.com/pharm
Substance Abuse and Mental Health Services Administration (SAMHSA)	http://www.samhsa.gov
USGovsearch (Search Engine for US Government)	http://usgovsearch.northernlight.com
U.S. State Department Travel Warnings and Consular Information Sheets	http://travel.state.gov/travel_warnings.html

5-8

Appendix 5–8

Miscellaneous Web Addresses

Important note: Web sites often move or change. The information provided was accurate at the time of writing.

Name of Site	Web URL
American Hospital Directory (hospital statistics)	http://www.ahd.com
Bioethics.net	http://www.med.upenn.edu/bioethics/index.shtml
California Internet Formulary Reference (compilation of HMO drug formularies sponsored by The Citizens for the Right to Know)	http://ca.mcodrugs.com
DoseCalc OnLine (oncology dosing calculation program)	http://www.meds.com/DChome.html
Drug Testing Services (information on drug testing, including law and procedures)	http://www.drugscreenlab.com
Food Allergy Network (FAN)	http://www.foodallergy.org
Guide to Locating Health Statistics (University of Pittsburgh)	http://www.hsls.pitt.edu/intres/guides/statcbw.html
Health Hippo (policy and regulatory information)	http://hippo.findlaw.com
Health Law	http://www.ljx.com/practice/health/index.html
Helix	http://www.helix.com
Kashrut.com (Kosher information)	http://www.kashrut.com
Knowledge Pharm.com	http://knowledgepharm.com
Maggot Therapy Project	http://www.ucihs.uci.edu/path/sherman/home_pg.htm
MedErrors	http://www.mederrors.com
Medical College of Wisconsin and Froedtert Memorial Lutheran Hospital Drug Formulary	http://www.intmed.mcw.edu/drug.html
MedNet Quality Improvement Connections	http://www.sermed.com/quality.htm
Mental Health Infosource	http://www.mhsource.com
National Reference Center for Bioethics Literature	http://adminweb.georgetown.edu/nrcbl
Needy Meds (Pharmaceutical Manufacturer's Drug Assistance Programs)	http://www.needymeds.com
On-line Dictionary of Street Drug Slang	http://www.drugs.indiana.edu/slang/home.html
pharmacistplacement.com	http://www.pharmacistplacement.com
Pharmacy Week (job listings)	http://www.pweek.com
Pharmajobs	http://www.pharmajobs.com
PharmInfoNet	http://www.pharminfo.com
Pharmulary	http://www.pharmulary.com
PharmWeb	http://www.pharmweb.net

Name of Site	Web URL
Practice of Pharmacy Compounding (FDA site)	http://www.fda.gov/cder/pharmcomp/default.htm
RxList	http://www.rxlist.com
RxMed (References for Family Physicians—including medication information)	http://www.rxmed.com
Symbios, Inc. (Pharmaceutical and Biotechnology Job Search)	http://www.symbiosinc.com
Uniform Requirement for Manuscripts Submitted to Biomedical Journals (5/2000)	http://icmje.org/index.html
The Virtual Clinical Pharmacologist (Anticoagulation Consultation Service)	http://www.clinpharmacologist.bigstep.com
Virtual Hospital (University of Iowa)	http://www.vh.org
Virtual Library Pharmacy	http://www.pharmacy.org
Virtual Drugstore (Canadian)	http://www.virtualdrugstore.com
WebMD	http://www.webmd.com/
World Wide Drugs	http://community.net/~neils/new.html

Appendix 5–9

News Web Addresses

Important note: Web sites often move or change. The information provided was accurate at the time of writing.

Name of Site	Web URL
ABC News	http://abcnews.go.com
Associate Press Wire Service	http://www.wire.ap.org
CBS News	http://www.cbs.com/navbar/news.html
CBSHealthWatch by Medscape	http://CBS.HealthWatch.com
CNN	http://www.cnn.com
CNN Health	http://www.cnn.com/HEALTH
HotBot News	http://www.newbot.com
MSNBC	http://www.msnbc.com
News Rounds	http://www.newsrounds.com
New York Times	http://www.nytimes.com
The Paperboy (newspapers from many locations)	http://www.thepaperboy.com
pharmscope.com	http://www.pharmscope.com
PR Newswire	http://www.prnewswire.com
ReutersHealth	http://www.reutershealth.com
RxTV (video information for patients) (requires RealVideo player)	http://www.rxtv.com
WorldNewsTV (English-language TV-type broadcasts from various countries)	http://www.foreigntv.com/worldnews/index.html
48 Hours Health and Medical News	http://www.48hours.net

5–10

Appendix 5–10

Patient Education Web Addresses

Important note: Web sites often move or change. The information provided was accurate at the time of writing.

Name of Site	Web URL
Allergy, Asthma & Immunology Online	http://allergy.mcg.edu
allHealth.com	http://www.allhealth.com
AMA Health Insight	http://www.ama-assn.org/consumer.htm
American Psychological Association Help Center	http://helping.apa.org
AmericasDoctor.com	http://www.americasdoctor.com
California Formulary Internet Reference (compilation of HMO drug formularies sponsored by The Citizens for the Right to Know)	http://ca.mcodrugs.com
Cancer Care, Inc.	http://www.cancercare.org
Complete Home Medical Guide (Columbia University)	http://cpmcnet.columbia.edu/texts/ guide/all.html
CyberPharmacy.com	http://www.cyberpharmacy.com
Depression.com	http://www.depression.com
Diabetes Action Research and Education Foundation (DAREF)	http://www.daref.org
Diabetes Education and Research Center	http://www.libertynet.org/diabetes
Diabetes Prevention Program	http://www.preventdiabetes.com
Doctor's Page	doctorspage.net
Dr.Koop.com	http://www.drkoop.com
Drug Digest	http://www.drugdigest.org
familydoctor.org (American Academy of Family Physicians)	http://familydoctor.org
Group Health Cooperative of Puget Sound	http://www.ghc.org/
HealthAnswers.com (English and Spanish)	http://www.healthanswers.com
Healthcare Reality Check—science-based information on alternative and complementary medicine	http://www.hcrc.org
Health-Center.com	http://www.healthguide.com
HealthCentral (Dr. Dean Edell)	http://www.healthcentral.com/home/ home.html
HealthGate	http://www.healthgate.com
The Health Gazette	http://www.freenet.tlh.fl.us/healthgazette
Health Scout	http://www.healthscout.com
Healthtouch Online	http://www.healthtouch.com/level1/hi_toc.htm
Heart Information Network	http://www.heartinfo.org
HeartPoint	http://www.heartpoint.com

Name of Site	Web URL
Hepatitis Education Project (HEP)	http://www.scn.org/health/hepatitis
Imaginis.net	http://www.imaginis.net
Informed Patient Decision Group	http://www.ohsu.edu/bicc-ipdg
InteliHealth	http://www.intelihealth.com
Lifeclinic.com	http://www.lifeclinic.com
Louisiana State University Patient Education Materials	http://lib-sh.lsumc.edu:80/fammed/ pted/pted.html
Managing Your Diabetes	http://diabetes.lilly.com/
Mayo Clinic Health Oasis	http://www.mayohealth.org
MedicineNet	http://www.medicinenet.com
MSN Health	http://health.msn.com
Multimedia Medical Reference Library	http://www.med-library.com/medlibrary
National Institutes of Health—Health Information	http://www.nih.gov/health
NetWellness	http://www.netwellness.org
New York Online Access to Health (NOAH)	http://www.noah.cuny.edu
OnHealth	http://www.onhealth.com
Pain.com	http:/www.pain.com
PDR Family Guide Encyclopedia of Medical Care	http://home.cyberave.com/~hsquare/ medcare2.htm
Prevention (part of women.com)	http://www.prevention.com
Project Inform (HIV/AIDS information)	http://www.projinf.org
The Prostate Cancer InfoLink (sponsored by Comed Communications, Inc.)	http://comed.com/Prostate/index.html
Prostateinfo.com (sponsored by AstraZeneca)	http://www.prostateinfo.com
Protocare	http://www.quickcare.org
RxTV (video information for patients) (requires RealVideo player)	http://www.rxtv.com
thehealthchannel.com	http://www.thehealthchannel.com
thriveonline	http://www.thriveonline.com
Viagra (Pfizer Site)	http://www.viagra.com
Viagra Talk	http://www.bigv.com
Virtual Hospital—Information for Patients	http://vh.radiology.uiowa.edu/Patients/ Patients.html
Virtual Medical Center Mediconsult	http://www.mediconsult.com
VTMEDNET	http://www.vtmednet.org/diner/home.htm
WebMD	http://www.webmd.com
Wellness Web, The Patient's Network	http://www.wellweb.com
YourHealth.com	http://www.yourhealth.com

5-11

Appendix 5-11

Pharmaceutical Manufacturer Web Addresses

Important note: Web sites often move or change. The information provided was accurate at the time of writing.

Name of Site	Web URL
3M Pharmaceuticals	http://www.mmm.com/pharma
3M Worldwide	http://www.3m.com
Abbott Laboratories	http://www.abbott.com
AGI (Applied Genetics Inc.) Dermatics	http://www.agiderm.com
Agouron Pharmaceuticals, Inc.	http://www.agouron.com
Alcon Laboratories, Inc.	http://www.alconlabs.com
Allergan Online	http://www.allergan.com
Alliance Pharmaceutical Corporation	http://www.allp.com
Allscripts, Inc.	http://www.allscripts.com
Almirall	http://www.intercom.es/almirall/eng/21alm.html
Alpharma	http://www.alpharma.com
Alza Corporation	http://www.alza.com
American Home Products Corporation	http://www.ahp.com/
Amgen, Inc.	http://www.amgen.com
Amrad Corporation Limited (Australia)	http://www.amrad.com.au
Amstelfarma (Netherlands)	http://www.amstelfarma.nl
Amylin Pharmaceuticals	http://www.amylin.com
Andrx Corporation	http://www.andrx.com
Anesta Corp.	http://www.anesta.com
Apothecon	http://www.apothecon.com
Ariad Pharmaceuticals, Inc.	http://www.ariad.com
Aronex Pharmaceuticals, Inc.	http://www.aronex.com
ASAC Pharmaceutical International AIE (Spain)	http://asac.net
Ascent Pediatrics, Inc.	http://www.ascentpediatrics.com
Asta Medica (Brazil)	http://www.astamedica.com.br
AstraZeneca	http://www.astrazeneca.com
Aurobindo Pharma Ltd.	http://www.aurobindo.com
Aventis	http://www.aventispharma-us.com
Aventis Behring	http://www.aventisbehring.com
Azupharma GmbH	http://www.azupharma.de
Barr Laboratories	http://www.barrlabs.com
Bausch & Lomb Pharmaceuticals, Inc.	http://www.bausch.com
Bausch & Lomb Surgical	http://www.blsurgical.com
Baxter Healthcare Corporation	http://www.baxter.com
Bayer	http://www.bayer.com

Name of Site	Web URL
Bayer Diagnostics	http://www.bayerdiag.com
Becton Dickinson and Company	http://www.bd.com
Berlix (Betaseron site)	http://www.betaseron.com
Berlix (Fludara site)	http://www.fludara.com
Berna Products	http://www.bernaproducts.com
Bertek Pharmaceuticals, Inc.	http://www.bertek.com
Beutlich Pharmaceuticals	http://www.beutlich.com
Biogen	http://www.biogen.com
Biorex	http://www.biorex.hu
Blaine Pharmaceuticals	http://www.blainepharma.com
Boehringer Ingelheim	http://www.boehringer-ingelheim.com
Bradley Pharmaceuticals, Inc.	http://www.bradpharm.com
Bristol-Meyers Squibb Company	http://www.bms.com
Britannia Pharmaceuticals Limited (United Kingdom)	http://www.britannia-pharm.co.uk
Caraco Pharmaceutical Laboratories, Ltd.	http://www.caraco.com
Cathay Herbal Laboratories (traditional Chinese medicine)	http://www.cathayherbal.com
CCL Pharmaceuticals (Pakistan)	http://www.cclpharma.com
Centocor	http://www.centocor.com
Cephalon	http://www.cephalon.com
Cheshire Pharmaceutical Systems	http://www.cpsrx.com
Chiron	http://www.chiron.com
Chugai Pharma Europe Ltd.	http://www.chugai.co.uk
Ciba Vision Ophthalmics	http://www.cvo-us.com
Colgate-Palmolive Company	http://www.colgate.com
Connetics Corporation	http://www.connective.com
Contract Pharmacal Corporation	http://www.contractpharmacal.com
CP Pharmaceuticals (United Kingdom)	http://cppharma.co.uk
Cytogen	http://www.cytogen.com
Dakryon Pharmaceuticals	http://www.he.net/~dakryon
Daniel Pharmaceuticals	http://www.soloxine.com
Darya-Varia Group	http://www.darya-varia.com
Datex-Ohmeda	http://www.datex-ohmeda.com
DepoTech	http://www.depotech.com
Dermik Laboratories, Inc.	http://www.dermik.com
Dey	http://www.deyinc.com
Dimethaid Research, Inc. (Canada)	http://www.dimethaid.com
Dista (see Eli Lilly & Co.)	http://www.dista.com
Dupont Pharmaceuticals Company	http://www.dupontmerck.com
Dura Pharmaceuticals, Inc.	http://www.durapharm.com
Duramed Pharmaceuticals, Inc.	http://www.duramed.com
Efroze Chemical Industries (Pvt.) Ltd. (Pakistan)	http://www.efroze.com
Eli Lilly & Co.	http://www.lilly.com
ELPEN Pharmaceuticals (Greece)	http://www.elpen.gr
Endo Pharmaceuticals, Inc.	http://www.endoinc.com
Enzon, Inc.	http://www.enzon.com
Esteve Group (Spain)	http://www.esteve.com/
ETHEX Corp.	http://www.ethex.com
Everett Laboratories Inc.	http://www.everettlabs.com
Faulding	http://www.faulding.com.au
Fischer Pharmaceuticals	http://www.dr-fischer.com
Forest Pharmaceuticals, Inc.	http://www.forestpharm.com
Forum (Holdings) Ltd. (United Kingdom)	http://www.forum.co.uk

Name of Site	Web URL
Fougera	http://www.fougera.com
Fujisawa Healthcare, Inc.	http://www.fujisawausa.com
G&W Laboratories Inc.	http://www.gwlabs.com
Galderma S.A. (Infoderm)	http://www.galderma.com
Gebauer Company	http://www.gebauerco.com
Genaissance Pharmaceuticals	http://www.genaissance.com
Genetech, Inc.	http://www.gene.com
Genetics Institute	http://www.genetics.com
Genome Therapeutics	http://www.cric.com
Genzyme	http://www.genzyme.com
Geron Corporation	http://www.geron.com
Gilead Sciences	http://www.gilead.com
Glades Pharmaceuticals	http://www.glades.com
Glaxo Wellcome	http://www.glaxowellcome.com
G.C. Hanford Mfg. Co.	http://www.hanford.com
Helix Biopharma Corp.	http://www.helixbio.com
Hemosol Inc. (Canada)	http://www.hemosol.com
Henry Schein Inc.	http://www.henryschein.com
Horizon Diagnostics, Inc.	http://horizondiagnostics.com
Hovid Sdn Bhd—Malaysia	http://www.hovid.com
Institut Biochimique SA (IBSA) (Switzerland)	http://www.ibsa.ch
ICI Pharmaceuticals	http://www.icipharms.com
ICN Biomedicals	http://www.icnbiomed.com
ICN Pharmaceuticals, Inc.	http://www.icnpharm.com
Immune Response Corporation	http://www.imnr.com
Immunex	http://www.immunex.com
ImmunoScience, Inc.	http://www.immunoscience.com
Incara Pharmaceuticals	http://www.incara.com
Incyte Pharmaceuticals, Inc.	http://www.incyte.com
Inhale Therapeutics Systems	http://www.inhale.com
Introgen Therapeutics, Inc.	http://www.introgen.com
Isis Pharmaceuticals	http://www.isip.com
ivpcare	http://www.ivpcare.com
Janssen-Cilag	http://www.janssen-cilag.com
Jenapharm (Denmark)	http://www.jenapharm.de
Johnson & Johnson	http://www.jnj.com
Jones Pharma Inc.	http://www.jmedpharma.com
Kiel Pharmaceuticals	http://www.kielpharm.com
King Pharmaceutical	http://www.kingpharm.com
KONSYL Pharmaceuticals, Inc.	http://www.konsyl.com
Laboratorios Rubio, SA	http://www.laboratoriosrubio.com
Lacer (Spain)	http://www.lacer.es
Lannett Co., Inc.	http://www.lannett.com
Leo Pharmaceutical Products Ltd.	http://www.leo-pharma.com
Mallinckrodt	http://www.mkg.com
McNeil (see Ortho-McNeil)	
Tylenol web site	http://www.tylenol.com
Medco Research, Inc.	http://www.medcores.com
medicis	http://www.medicis.com
MedImmune, Inc.	http://www.medimmune.com
Menarini Group (Spain)	http://www.menarini.es
Merck & Co., Inc.	http://www.merck.com
Meridian Medical Technologies, Inc.	http://www.meridianmeds.com
Merz Inc.	http://www.merzusa.com

Name of Site	Web URL
Mikart Inc.	http://www.mikart.com
Mochida Pharmaceutical Co. Ltd. (Japan)	http://www.mochida.co.jp
Monarch Pharmaceuticals, Inc.	http://www.monarchpharm.com
Monsanto Company	http://www.monsanto.com
Moore Medical Corp.	http://www.mooremedical.com
MOVA Laboratories Inc.	http://www.movalabs.com
Mylan Laboratories, Inc.	http://www.mylan.com
Nabi	http://www.nabi.com
Nagase Pharmaceuticals	http://www.nagase.com/Pharmaceuticals.html
North American Vaccine	http://www.nava.com
Nova Factor, Inc	http://www.novafactor.com
Novartis	http://www.novartis.com/index.html
Novo Nordisk A/S	http://www.novo.dk
Nycomed Amersham (United Kingdom)	http://www.amersham.co.uk
Octamer Inc.	http://www.octamer.com
Ocular Pharmaceuticals	http://www.eyedoc.com/profpharm.html
Oculex Pharmaceuticals	http://oculex.com
Ohmeda Medical	http://www.ohmedamedical.com
Organon	http://www.organon.com
Ortho Biotech (Procrit site)	http://www.procrit.com
Ortho-McNeil	http://www.ortho-mcneil.com
Otsuka Pharmaceutical Co., Ltd. (Japan)	http://www.otsuka.co.jp
Paddock Laboratories, Inc.	http://www.paddocklabs.com
Parkedale Pharmaceuticals, Inc.	http://www.kingpharm.com/parkedale/aboutUs/index.shtml
Parnell Pharmaceuticals	http://www.parnellpharm.com
PathoGenesis Corporation	http://www.pathogenesis.com
PDRx Pharmaceuticals, Inc.	http://www.pdrx.com
Pedinol Pharmacal, Inc.	http://www.pedinol.com
Penwest Pharmaceuticals Co.	http://www.penw.com
Peptech Limited	http://www.peptech.com
Perrigo Company	http://www.perrigo.com
Pfizer	http://www.pfizer.com
Viagra	http://www.viagra.com
Pharmaceutical Specialties, Inc.	http://www.psico.com
Pharmacia and Upjohn	http://www.pnu.com
Pharmacyclics	http://www.pcyc.com
Pharma Pac	http://www.pharmapac.com
PowderJect Pharmaceuticals PLC	http://www.powderject.com
Protein Design Labs	http://www.pdl.com
Provalis	http://www.provalis.com
Procter & Gamble	http://www.pg.com
Ribozyme Pharmaceuticals Incorporated	http://www.rpi.com
Roche	http://www.roche.com
Roxane Laboratories, Inc.	http://www.roxane.com
R&D Laboratories (kidney disease information)	http://www.rndlabs.com
Sai Pharmaceutical Works	http://www.saipharma.com
Sankyo Co., Ltd. (Japan)	http://www.sankyo.co.jp
Sanochemia Pharmazeutika AG (Germany)	http://www.sanochemia.at
Savage Laboratories	http://www.savagelabs.com
Scandipharm	http://www.scandipharm.com
Schein Pharmaceutical	http://www.schein-rx.com
Schering-Plough	http://www.sch-plough.com

Name of Site	Web URL
Schwarz Pharma	http://www.schwarzpharma.com
Searle	http://www.searle.com
Serono, Inc.	http://www.seronousa.com
SHS International	http://www.shsweb.co.uk
North American Office	http://www.shsna.com
Shire Pharmaceuticals Group plc	http://www.shiregroup.com
SICOR Corporation, Inc.	http://www.gensiaicor.com
Sigma-Aldrich	http://www.sigma-aldrich.com
Sigma-Tau	http://www.sigmatau.com
SkyePharma PLC	http://www.SkyePharma.com
SmithKline Beecham	http://www.sb.com
Solka Laboratories, Inc. (Nicaragua)	http://www.ibw.com.ni/~solka/solk_ing.html
Solvay	http://www.solvay.com
Sonus Pharmaceuticals	http://www.sonuspharma.com
SP Pharmaceuticals, LLC	http://www.sppharma.com
Storz Ophthalmics	http://www.expovision.com/storz/default.htm
SuperGen	http://www.supergen.com
Superior Pharmaceutical Co.	http://www.superiorpharm.com
Synthon (The Netherlands)	http://www.synthon.nl
Takeda Pharma GmbH (Denmark)	http://www.takeda.de
Takeda Pharmaceuticals America, Inc.	http://www.takedapharm.com
Tanox, Inc.	http://www.tanox.com
Taro Pharmaceutical U.S.A., Inc.	http://www.taropharma.com
Technilab (Canada)	http://www.technilab.ca
Telluride Pharmaceutical Corporation	http://www.tellpharm.com
Teva Pharmaceuticals USA	http://www.tevapharmusa.com
Texas Biotechnology Corporation	http://www.tbc.com
Tianjia Central Pharm (China)	http://www.ipine.com
Upjohn	See Pharmacia and Upjohn
Valentis	http://www.valentis.com
Value in Pharmaceuticals (VIP)	http://www.vippharm.com
VectorPharma	http://www.vectorpharma.com
Vertex Pharmaceuticals, Inc.	http://www.vpharm.com
Viscount Pharma Inc.	http://www.viscountpharma.com
Vital Helpsys PVT, Ltd.	http://www.angelfire.com/biz/vitaldrugs
Watson Pharmaceuticals, Inc.	http://www.watsonpharm.com
Westwood-Squibb	http://www.westwood-squibb.com
Wyeth Ayerst	See American Home Products
Xoma	http://www.xoma.com
Zila, Inc.	http://www.zila.com

Appendix 5–12

Pharmacies Web Addresses

Important note: Web sites often move or change. The information provided was accurate at the time of writing.

Name of Site	Web URL
Allegro Medical.com	http://www.allegromedical.com
Click Pharmacy	http://www.clickpharmacy.com
CornerDrugstore.com	http://www.cornerdrugstore.com
Corner Drugstore Specialties	http://www.cornerdrug.com
CVS (WebMD) Pharmacy	http://www.cvs.com
Drug Emporium.com	http://www.drugemporium.com
drugstore.com	http://www.drugstore.com/
Eckerd	http://www.eckerd.com
ExpressScripts.com	http://www.express-scripts.com
Good Neighbor Pharmacy	http://www.mygnp.com
HealthQuick.com	http://www.healthquick.com
J&D International Pharmacy	http://www.jdpharmacy.com
Longs Drugs	http://www.longs.com
MedicalEdge.com	http://www.medicaledge.com
Medicine Shoppe Pharmacies	http://www.medshoppe.com
Mediconsult	http://www.mediconsult.com
merckmedco.com	http://www.merck-medco.com
millenium-rx.com	http://www.millennium-rx.com
more.com	http://www.more.com
nevoca.com (prescription verification system)	http://www.nevoca.com
Other smaller pharmacies or pharmacy chains	http://dir.yahoo.com/Business_and_economy/ shopping_and_services/health/pharmacies
PharmaSays.com	http://www.pharmasays.com
PlanetRx.com	http://www.planetrx.com
PrescriptionRx (connections with non-US pharmacies)	http://www.prescriptionrx.com
Rite Aid	http://www.riteaid.com
GNC and Rite Aid	http://www.gnc.riteaid.com
Rx.com	http://www.rx.com
Strictly Pharmacy	http://www.strictlypharmacy.com
Valu-Rite (McKesson)	http://www.valu-rite.com
Virtual Drugstore (Canadian)	http://www.virtualdrugstore.com
Virtual Pharmacy (Dr. Koop's/Rite Aid)	http://www.drkoop.com/hcr/drugstore
Walgreens	http://www.walgreens.com

5-13

Appendix 5-13

Pharmacoeconomics Web Addresses

Important note: Web sites often move or change. The information provided was accurate at the time of writing.

Name of Site	Web URL
Canadian Coordinating Office of Health Technology Assessment	http://www.ccohta.ca
Cochrane Collaboration Home Page	http://hiru.mcmaster.ca/cochrane
Department of Defense Pharmacoeconomic Center	http://www.pec.ha.osd.mil
HealthEconomics.com	http://www.healtheconomics.com
Institute of Health Economics	http://www.ipe.ab.ca
International Society for Pharmacoeconomics and Outcomes Research	http://www.ispor.org
Department of Pharmaceutical Economics and Policy (University of Southern California School of Pharmacy)	http://www.usc.edu/go/pharmecon

Appendix 5–14

Publication Web Addresses

Important note: Web sites often move or change. The information provided was accurate at the time of writing.

Name of Site	Web URL
AMA Publications (e.g., JAMA)	http://pubs.ama-assn.org/scipub.htm
American Druggist	http://www.americandruggist.com
American Journal of Health-System Pharmacy	http://www.ashp.org/public/pubs/ajhp
Antimicrobial Use Guidelines (University of Wisconsin)	http://www.medsch.wisc.edu/clinsci/amcg/amcg.html
Archives of Neurology	http://archneur.ama-assn.org/
BioMedNet	http://www.bmn.com
Biotech Life Science Dictionary	http://biotech.icmb.utexas.edu/search/dict-search/html
Bloodline (oncology/hematology information)	http://www.bloodline.net
British Medical Journal	http://www.bmj.com
Bulletin of Experimental Treatments for AIDS (BETA)	http://www.sfaf.org/beta
Cadmus Dynamic Diagrams	http://www.dynamicdiagrams.com/Home.htm
Canadian Immunization Guide	http://www.hc-sc.gc.ca/hpb/lcdc/publicat/immguide/index.html
Clinical Drug Investigation	http://www.medscape.com/adis/CDI/public/journal.CDI.html
Clinical Pharmacology	http://cp.gsm.com
computertalk.com	http://www.computertalk.com
CyberStacks (Iowa State University)—a virtual library card catalog	http://www.public.iastate.edu/~CYBERSTACKS
Dermatology Times	http://164.109.17.92
Dietary Supplements—An Advertising Guide for Industry (FTC)	http://www.ftc.gov/bcp/conline/pubs/buspubs/dietsupp.htm
Drug Topics.com	http://www.dt.pdr.net/dt/index.htm
DynaMed (Dynamic Medical Information System)	http://www.dynamicmedical.com
Econtent	http://www.ecmag.net
Electronic Orange Book (FDA Approved Drug Products with Therapeutic Equivalence Evaluations)	http://www.fda.gov/cder/ob/default.htm
Electronic Textbook of Dermatology	http://telemedicine.org/stamford.htm
Emedicine (electronic textbooks)	http://www.emedicine.com
Dermatology	http://www.emedicine.com/derm/index.shtml
Emergency Medicine	http://www.emedicine.com/emerg/index.shtml
Medicine, Ob-Gyn, Psychiatry, and Surgery	http://www.emedicine.com/med/index.shtml

Name of Site	Web URL
Neurology	http://www.emedicine.com/neuro/index.shtml
Ophthalmology	http://www.emedicine.com/oph/index.shtml
Otolaryngology and Facial Plastic Surgery	http://www.emedicine.com/ent/index.shtml
Pediatrics	http://www.emedicine.com/ped/index.shtml
Plastic Surgery	http://www.emedicine.com/plastic/index.shtml
Emerging Infectious Diseases	http://www.cdc.gov/ncidod/eid/index.htm
Ethics Manual (Annals of Internal Medicine position paper)	http://www.acponline.org/journals/annals/01apr98/ethicman.htm
Evidence Based Medicine	http://www.acponline.org/journals/ebm/pastiss.htm
Federal Register	http://www.access.gpo.gov/su_docs/aces/aces140.html
First DataBank	http://www.firstdatabank.com
Formulary	http://164.109.17.89
Galen II (University of California at San Francisco)—(publication metasite)	http://galen.library.ucsf.edu
Gastroenterology	http://www.gastrojournal.org
Geri.com	http://164.109.17.91
Glossary of Microbiology	http://www.hardlink.com/~tsute/glossary/index.html
Gold Standard Multimedia	http://www.gsm.com
Handbook of Parenteral Drug Administration (Australia)	http://www.ozemail.com.au/~jamesbc
Health and Medical Informatics Digest	http://144.92.205.41/hmid/home/htm
Healthcare Intelligence Network (subscriptions to multiple publications)	http://www.hin.com
Healthcare Informatics	http://www.healthcare-informatics.com
HerbalGram (Journal of the American Botanical Council and the Herb Research Foundation)	http://www.herbalgram.org/herbalgram/index.html
Hypertension Dialysis Clinical Nephrology (electronic journal)	http://www.hdcn.com
Immunisation Handbook (New Zealand)	http://210.48.125.104/moh.nsf/49ba80c00757b8804c256673001d47d0/d011b7afeff395084c256671000d75f8
Immunization Gateway	http://www.immunofacts.com
Indiana University Ruth Lilly Medical Library (list of journal sites)	http://www.medlib.iupui.edu/techserv/ejournals.html
Infectious Disease News	http://www.slackinc.com/general/idn/idnhome.htm
InfoLink (University of Wisconsin Medical School)	http://www.medsch.wisc.edu/infolink/pubs/medjs.html
Infomed Drug Guide	http://www.infomed.org/100drugs/index.html
The Informatics Review (e-journal)	http://www.informatics-review.com
Integrated Medical Curriculum (includes Clinical Pharmacology)	http://www.imc.gsm.com
Iowa Drug Information Service	http://lime.weeg.uiowa.edu/~idis
Journal Club on the Web	http://www.journalclub.org/index.html
Journal of the American Medical Association	http://jama.ama-assn.org
Journal of the American Medical Informatics Association	http://www.jamia.org
Journal of Cost and Quality	http://www.cost-quality.com
Journal of Clinical Outcomes Management	http://www.turner-white.com/cgi-bin/rbox/jmein2.cgi
Journal of Information Technology in Medicine	http://www.j-itm.com

Name of Site	Web URL
Journal of Medical Internet Research	http://www.jmir.org/index.htm
Journal of Managed Care Pharmacy	http://www.amcp.org/public/pubs/journal
Journal of the National Cancer Institute	http://www.jnci.oupjournals.org
Journal of Pharmacy and Pharmaceutical Sciences (Canadian Society for Pharmaceutical Sciences)	http://www.ualberta.ca/~csps/Journal/JPPS.htm
Managed Care Interface	http://www.medicomint.com
ManagedHealthcare	http://164.109.17.94
Martindale's Health Sciences Guide	http://www-sci.lib.uci.edu/~martindale/Pharmacy.html
Material Safety Data Sheets (guide from the University of Kentucky)	http://www.ilpi.com/msds/index.html
McGill Journal of Medicine	http://www.mjm.mcgill.ca
Medical Computing Today	http://www.medicalcomputingtoday.com
Medical Journal of Australia	http://www.mja.com.au/index.html
MedWebLit (multiple medical journals)	http://www.webmedlit.silverplatter.com/index.html
Merriam-Webster's Medical Desk Dictionary	http://www.medscape.com/home/partners/MWebster/about.MWebster.html
Modern Medicine	http://164.109.17.96
Multimedia Healthcare/Freedom LLC	http://www.mmhc.com
Multimedia Medical Reference Library	http://www.mmrl.com/medlibrary
Nature (abstracts)	http://www.nature.com
netLibrary	http://www.netlibrary.com
New England Journal of Medicine	http://www.nejm.org
New Jour (List of new journals and newsletters available on the Internet)	http://gort.ucsd.edu/newjour
Online	http://www.onlineinc.com/onlinemag/index.html
PDQ (NCI's Comprehensive Cancer Database)	http://cancernet.nci.nih.gov/pdqfall.htm
PDR Family Guide Encyclopedia of Medical Care	http://www.healthsquare.com/medcare2.htm
PDR Family Guide to Drugs and Medicine	http://www.healthsquare.com/drugmain.htm
PDR Family Guide to Women's Health	http://www.healthsquare.com/fgwh01.html
PDR net (charge for PDR)	http://www.pdr.net
Pediatric Critical Care Medicine	http://pedsccm.wustl.edu
Pediatrics	http://www.pediatrics.org
Pharmaceutical Information Network	http://pharminfo.com
Pharmacotherapy	http://www.accp.com/pharmacotherapy.html
Pharmacy and Therapeutics	http://www.pharmacyandtherapeutic.com
Pharmacy Times	http://www.pharmacytimes.com
Pharmacy Week (job listings)	http://www.pweek.com
The Physician and Sportsmedicine Online (electronic journal)	http://www.physsportsmed.com
Postgraduate Medicine Online	http://www.postgradmed.com
Power-Pak C.E. (continuing education for pharmacists)	http://www.powerpak.com
Project Gutenberg (downloadable free books, mostly classics)	http://www.gutenberg.net
PubMed Net Central (National Library of Medicine)	http://www.pubmedcentral.nih.gov
Psychiatric Times	http://www.mhsource.com/psychiatrictimes.html
PubMed (National Center for Biotechnology Information)	http://biomednet.com
Science Direct	http://www.sciencedirect.com
Science Magazine	http://www.sciencemag.org
South African Package Inserts	http://home.intekom.com/pharm
Spellex Development (medical spelling checker)	http://www.spellex.com/speller.htm

Name of Site	Web URL
Swiss Medical Weekly	http://www.smw.ch
Telemedicine Today	http://www.telemedtoday.com
U.S. Pharmacist	http://www.uspharmacist.com
Virtual Drugstore (Canada)	http://www.virtualdrugstore.com
WebMedLit (Medical Journal Web Metasite)	http://www.webmedlit.com

Appendix 5–15

Publication Search Engine Web Addresses

Important note: Web sites often move or change. The information provided was accurate at the time of writing.

Name of Site	Web URL
Medline Journals with Links to Publisher Web Sites	http://www.ncbi.nlm.nih.gov/PubMed/fulltext.html
medsite ISI journal tracker	http://www.journaltracker.com
PubList.com (Internet Directory of Publications)	http://www.publist.com
PubMed Journal Database Browser	http://www4.ncbi.nlm.nih.gov/PubMed/ jbrowser.html
WebMed Lit (sponsored by SilverPlatter)	http://webmedlit.silverplatter.com
Yahoo! Health and Medical Journals	http://dir.yahoo.com/health/medicine/journals

5–16

Appendix 5–16

Quality Assurance Web Addresses

Important note: Web sites often move or change. The information provided was accurate at the time of writing.

Name of Site	Web URL
AHA Quality Initiative	http://www.aha.org/quality
American Society for Healthcare Risk Management	http://www.ashrm.org
Consumer Coalition for Quality Health Care	http://www.consumers.org
Foundation for Accountability (FACCT)	http://www.facct.org
Healthcare Quality Resources at Quality.org	http://www.quality.org/html/hc-res.html
Institute for Safe Medication Practices	http://www.ismp.org/ISMP
Joint Commission on Accreditation of Healthcare Organizations	http://www.jcaho.org
Journal of Cost and Quality	http://www.cost-quality.com
MedNet Quality Improvement Connections	http://www.sermed.com/quality.htm
National Committee for Quality Assurance (NCQA)	http://www.ncqa.org
National Coordinating Council for Medication Error Reporting and Prevention	http://www.nccmerp.org
Picker Institute	http://www.picker.org
Quality Indicator Project	http://www.qiproject.org
Quality Measurement Advisory Service	http://www.qmas.org
Simcoe County Mental Health Education MHCP CQI Links Page (links to CQI information) (Canadian)	http://www.mhcva.on.ca/CQI/cqilinks.htm

5-17

Appendix 5-17

Research Web Addresses

Important note: Web sites often move or change. The information provided was accurate at the time of writing.

Name of Site	Web URL
AIDS Clinical Trial Information Service (ACTIS)	http://www.actis.org
Alberta Clinical Trials Resources (Canada)	http://www.med.ualberta.ca/clinical
BioMedNet	http://www.biomednet.com/db/biomedlink
Breast Cancer Clinical Trials Matching System	http://research.bmn.com
cancerTrials (National Cancer Institute)	http://cancertrials.nci.nih.gov
CenterWatch Clinical Trials Listing Service	http://www.CenterWatch.com
Clinical Trials and Noteworthy Treatments for Brain Tumors	http://www.virtualtrials.com
Code of Federal Regulations	http://www.access.gpo.gov/nara/cfr/index.html
Current Controlled Trials	http://www.controlled-trials.com
Cystic Fibrosis Foundation Clinical Trials	http://www.cff.org/clinical.htm
Drug Study Central (Formerly MedTrial)	http://www.drugstudycentral.com
Federal Register Archives	http://www.access.gpo.gov/su_docs/aces/aces140.html
Food and Drug Administration	http://www.fda.gov
Food and Drug Administration Forms	http://forms.psc.gov/forms/FDA/fda.htm
Foundation Center	http://fdncenter.org
GrantsNet	http://www.os.dhhs.gov/progorg/grantsnet/index.html
International Conference on Harmonisation	http://www.pharmweb.net/pwmirror/pw9/ifpma/ich1.html
JAMA's HIV/AIDS Information Center	http://www.ama-assn.org/special/hiv
Medical Study Register (Germany)	http://medweb.uni-muenster.de/msr
National Cancer Institute's PDQ Cancer Clinical Trials Listing	http://cancernet.nci.nih.gov/pdqfull.html
National Institutes of Health Grants and Funding Opportunities	http://grants.nih.gov/grants
NIH Office of Biotechnology Activities	http://www.nih.gov/od/oba
NIH Office for Human Research Practices	http://ohrp.osophs.dhhs.gov/polasur.htm
New York Eye & Ear Infirmary (NYEEI)—Clinical Trials	http://www.nyee.edu/research/research.htm
OncoLink (clinical trials information)	http://www.oncolink.com/clinical_trials
Pew Charitable Trusts	http://www.pewtrusts.com
Rare Diseases Clinical Research Database (NIH)	http://rarediseases.info.nih.gov/ord/wwwprot/index.shtml

Name of Site	Web URL
Recombinant Capital Clinical Trials Database	http://www.recap.com/mainweb.nsf/HTML/clinical+frame?OpenDocument
Robert Wood Johnson Foundation	http://www.rwjf.org/main.html
Swiss Academy of Medical Sciences Documentation Service	http://www.sams.ch
University of Connecticut Health Center Division of Rheumatic Diseases—Clinical Trials	http://www2.uchc.edu/~rheum/pag11.html

5–18

Appendix 5–18

Search Engine Web Addresses

Important note: Web sites often move or change. The information provided was accurate at the time of writing.

Search Engine Name	Web URL
Medicine/Pharmacy	
About.com (formerly Mining Co.) Guide to Pharmacology	http://pharmacology.about.com/health/pharmacology
Achoo	http://www.achoo.com
BONES: Biomedically Oriented Navigator of Electronic Services	http://bones.med.ohio-state.edu/bones/bones.html
Citeline.com	http://www.citeline.com
CliniWeb International	http://www.ohsu.edu/cliniweb
Drug InfoNet	http://www.druginfonet.com
Hardin MP	http://www.lib.uiowa.edu/hardin-mdinform.html
HealthFinder (patient-oriented site)	http://www.healthfinder.gov
HealthGate (includes free MEDLINE)	http://www.healthgate.com
Infomine	http://www.infomine.com
MDchoice.com	http://www.mdchoice.com
MedBot	http://www-med.stanford.edu/medworld/medbot/reference.html
MedExplorer	http://www.medexplorer.com
MedHunt (Health on the Net Foundation) (includes free MEDLINE)	http://www.hon.ch
Medical Matrix (various medically related web sites)	http://www.medmatrix.org
Medinex Systems	http://www.medinex.com
Mednav.com	http://mednav.com
MedNets (a collection of medical search engines, grouped by specialty)	http://www.internets.com/mednets/smedlink.htm
MedScout	http://www.medscout.com
Medical World Search	http://www.mwsearch.com
MedWeb @ Emory University	http://www.medweb.emory.edu/MedWeb
MedWeb Plus	http://www.medwebplus.com
Multimedia Medical Reference Library	http://www.med-library.com
Organising Medical Networked Information (OMNI)	http://omni.ac.uk
PEDINFO (pediatric information)	http://www.pedinfo.org
Stayhealthy.com	http://www.stayhealthy.com/
Virtual Library Pharmacy	http://www.pharmacy.org

Search Engine Name	Web URL
General Search Engines	
About.com (formerly Mining Co.)	http://home.about.com
Alta Vista	http://www.altavista.digital.com
AOL.com	http://searchaol.com
CyberStacks (Iowa State University)—a virtual library card catalog	http://www.public.iastate.edu/~CYBERSTACKS
Direct Hit (rates sites depending on how much time users spend at those sites)	http://www.directhit.com
Excite	http://www.excite.com
Fast Search (Claims to be worlds biggest and fastest search engine)	http://www.ussc.alltheweb.com
galaxy	http://www.einet.net
Go.com	http://www.go.com
GoGettem	http://www.gogettem.com
Google	http://www.google.com
HotBot (Lycos Network)	http://hotbot.Lycos.com
LookSmart	http://www.looksmart.com
Lycos	http://www.lycos.com
NetGuide (cmpnet)	http://www.netguide.com
Northern Light	http://www.northernlight.com
WebCrawler	http://www.webcrawler.com
Yahoo	http://www.yahoo.com
Multiple Web Search Engine Sites (Metasearch Engines)	
All4one Search Machine	http://www.all4one.com
Ask Jeeves!	http://www.askjeeves.com
The BigHub.com	http://www.thebighub.com
C4 Total Search Technology	http://www.4.c4.com
Debriefing	http://www.debriefing.com
Dogpile	http://www.dogpile.com
FinderSeeker	http://www.finderseeker.com
Go2Net	http://www.go2net.com
Highway 61	http://www.highway61.com
HuskySearch	http://huskysearch.cs.washington.edu
inFind	http://www.infind.com
Mamma (The Mother of All Search Engines)	http://www.mamma.com
metacrawler	http://www.metacrawler.com
MetaGopher	http://www.metagopher.com
OneSeek.com	http://www.oneseek.com
ProFusion.com	http://www.profusion.com
Search.com	http://www.search.com
Spaniel Search	http://www.searchspaniel.com
Starting Point	http:http://www.stpt.com
Verio Metasearch	http://search.verio.net

5–19

Appendix 5–19

Address and Phone Number Search Engine Web Addresses

Important note: Web sites often move or change. The information provided was accurate at the time of writing.

Search Engine Name	Web URL
AnyWho	http://www.anywho.com
BigBook (Yellow Pages)	http://www.bigbook.com
Bigfoot	http://www.bigfoot.com
BigYellow	http://www.bigyellow.com
DoctorPage (find a physician)	http://www.doctorpage.com
Excite Education	http://www.excite.com/education/reference/people_finders
Hospital Select	http://www.hospitalselect.com
HotBot White Pages	http://www.hotbot.com/partners/people.asp
HotBot Yellow Pages	http://www.hotbot.com/partners/business.asp
InfoSpace	http://www.infospace.com
LocateADoc.com	http://www.locateadoc.com
Switchboard.com	http://www.switchboard.com
WhoWhere	http://www.whowhere.lycos.com
WorldPages.com	http://www.worldpages.com
Yahoo! People Search	http://www.people.yahoo.com

5–20

Appendix 5–20

Image Search Engine Web Addresses

Important note: Web sites often move or change. The information provided was accurate at the time of writing.

Search Engine Name	Web URL
Alta Vista Image Search	http://www.altavista.com/cgi-bin/ query?pg-q&stype-simage
Amazing Picture Machine	http://www.ncrtec.org/picture.htm
Lycos Multimedia	http://multimedia.lycos.com/picturethis
Medical Indexed Visuals	http://www.indexedvisuals.com
Medical Legal Art	http://www.medical-legal.com
Web Places Clip Art Searcher	http://webplaces.com/search
WebSeek Image and Video Search	http://disney.ctr.columbia.edu/webseek
Yahoo Image Surfer	http://ipix.yahoo.com

5–21

Appendix 5–21

Search Engine Information Web Addresses

Important note: Web sites often move or change. The information provided was accurate at the time of writing.

Search Engine Name	Web URL
Beaucoup (listing of 800+ search engines, with Links)	http://www.beaucoup.com/engbig.html
Discern Online (quality criteria for consumer health information)	http://www.discern.org.uk
Encyclopedia Britanica Online Guide	http://www.ebig.com
Internet Resources	http://library.berkeley.edu/TeachingLib/Guides/Internet
Megasite Project	http://www.lib.umich.edu/megasite/toc.html
MetaSearch Engines (general information)	http://www.lib.berkeley.edu/TeachingLib/Guides/Internet/MetaSearch.html
Search Engine Watch	http://www.searchenginewatch.com
SeekHelp.com	http://www.seekhelp.com

ACKNOWLEDGMENT

Meghan J. Malone is acknowledged for her assistance in preparing the appendices for Chapter 5.

6-1

Evaluation Questions for Assessing Clinical Research Reports

OVERALL ASSESSMENT

- Was the article published in a reputable, peer-reviewed journal?
- Were the investigators qualified to conduct the study?
- Did the authors contribute substantially to the research effort?
- Did the research site have appropriate resources and patients for the study?
- Was study funding obtained from an unbiased source?

TITLE/ABSTRACT

- Was the title of the article unbiased?
- Did the abstract provide a clear overview of the purpose, methods, results, and conclusions of the study?

INTRODUCTION

- Did the authors provide sufficient background information to demonstrate that the study was important and ethical?
- Were study objectives clearly explained?
- Were planned subgroup or covariate analyses indicated?
- Were the research and null hypotheses stated?
- Was the study approved by an institutional review board (IRB)?
- Was the study ethical?

METHODS

- Was an appropriate study design used?
- Did the inclusion and exclusion criteria represent an appropriate patient population for the study?

- Was sample size large enough to detect a statistically significant difference between treatment groups?
- Was the study sample representative of the patient population to which the study results were intended to be generalized?
- Was the study controlled? Were the controls appropriate?
- Were outcome variables relevant, clearly defined, objective, and clinically and biologically significant? Was methodology used to measure outcome variables described in detail? Were outcome variables measured at appropriate time intervals?
- Was the study randomized using an appropriate method? After randomization, were demographics for the treatment and control groups similar?
- Were subjects, investigators, outcome assessors, and data entry personnel blinded? Were these individuals unable to determine whether treatment or control was administered before the blind was broken?
- Were data collected appropriately?
- Was patient compliance with the study medication measured?
- Were patient and investigator compliance with the study protocol monitored?
- Were appropriate statistics used to analyze data?

RESULTS

- Were dates for study initiation and completion of the study provided? Is the study current and relevant?
- Were numbers of patients screened, enrolled, administered study treatment, completing, and withdrawing from the study reported? Were reasons for study withdrawal described?
- Were demographics for treatment and control subjects similar at baseline?
- Were data presented in a clear and understandable format? Were data for both efficacy and safety of the treatment clearly reported?
- Was an intent-to-treat analysis conducted?
- Were exact p-values or confidence intervals reported?
- Was study power calculated?
- Could a Type I or Type II error have occurred?
- Were study results valid?
- Can study results be generalized to patients in clinical practice?
- Were the results both statistically and clinically significant?

CONCLUSIONS/DISCUSSION

- Did the authors compare their study results to those of a systematic review of all previously published data?

- Were study conclusions consistent with the results and did they relate to the study conclusion?
- Did the study results support the conclusions?

REFERENCES

- Is current literature well represented?

7–1

Questions to Consider for Critique of Primary Literature Documents

TRUE EXPERIMENT

- Refer to Chap. 6

N-OF-1 TRIAL

- Was assignment of active and control treatment to study periods randomized?
- Was the study blinded?
- Were multiple observation periods used?
- Were study endpoints clearly defined?

STABILITY STUDY

- Were study methodologies and test conditions clearly defined?
- Were validated assays used?
- Were assays validated using time-zero measurements and an adequate number of test samples taken?

BIOEQUIVALENCY STUDY

- Did the protocol define the characteristics of the subjects?
- Were confounding factors (e.g., smoking, alcohol use) identified and controlled?
- Was a crossover design used?
- Was the study randomized and blinded?

PROGRAMMATIC RESEARCH

- Were one of two options used for subject comparison: (1) comparison of subjects to those not using the program or service, (2) comparison of subjects before or after initiation of the program or service?

- Was the program or service clearly defined?
- Did the authors specify from whose perspective (e.g., patient, provider, physician, third-party payer) the study was undertaken?
- If costs were analyzed, were all costs associated with provision of the program or service included in the analysis?
- Were clinically important outcome parameters used to assess the effectiveness of the program or service?

FOLLOW-UP (COHORT) STUDY

- Were exposed and unexposed subjects similar in terms of demographic characteristics and susceptibility to disease states?
- Were subjects randomized to exposure or nonexposure, if possible?
- Were inclusion and exclusion criteria described in detail?
- Was the research question clearly stated?
- Were the same efforts to measure outcomes made in each group?
- Were 95% confidence intervals calculated?
- Were follow-up rates the same for the exposed and unexposed groups?

CASE-CONTROL STUDY

- Was predisposition of disease similar in cases and controls except for exposure to the risk factor?
- Were cases and controls matched?
- Was exposure to the risk factor similar to that which would occur in the general population?
- Did cases and controls undergo similar diagnostic evaluations?
- Were investigators who assessed patients or collected data blinded to the status of the subject as a case or control?
- Did the investigators compare cases with several different control groups?
- Were 95% confidence intervals calculated?

CROSS-SECTIONAL STUDY

- Did investigators ensure accuracy in data collection?
- If a survey or questionnaire was used, was it validated?
- Were the inclusion and exclusion criteria clearly defined and stated?
- Was selection of cases clearly described?

CASE STUDY OR CASE SERIES

- Did the authors recognize the preliminary nature of the results (i.e., recommendations for clinical application of the results should be guarded)?

SURVEY STUDY

- Was the survey instrument valid and reliable? Was a pretest or pilot test conducted on the survey instrument?
- Was the sample size large enough to detect a difference between groups?
- Was the survey objective and carefully planned?
- Were data quantifiable?
- Was the sample representative of the target population?
- Was response rate high enough to reflect results that would be expected of the target population?
- Did the investigators determine whether nonresponders differed from responders?

POSTMARKETING SURVEILLANCE STUDY

- Was a large enough sample studied to reflect current uses of and side effects associated with the new drug therapy?
- Were appropriate methods used to measure clearly defined endpoints?

NONSYSTEMATIC REVIEWS (NARRATIVE REVIEWS)

- Was an extensive search for available studies undertaken?
- Did the authors use a variety of resources to identify studies for inclusion in the review article?
- Was the review article focused on a clearly defined patient population?
- Did the studies included in the review article use valid research methods?
- Did the author examine reasons for differences in study results and conclusions?
- Were outcomes of the studies clinically important?
- Did the author consider benefits and risks of the drug therapy?

SYSTEMATIC REVIEWS (QUALITATIVE OR QUANTITATIVE)

- Did the authors clearly define the research question?
- Was the review article focused on a clearly defined patient population?
- Was an extensive search for available studies undertaken?
- Did the authors consider using results from both published and unpublished studies in the analysis?
- Did the authors clearly define criteria for study inclusion in the analysis?
- Did the authors list studies that were included in and excluded from the analysis?
- Did the authors provide details concerning methodologies of studies used in the analysis?

- Were tests of homogeneity performed and results reported?
- Were those who selected studies for inclusion in the analysis blinded to the names of the original authors, place of publication of the study, and final study results?
- If a meta-analysis, were appropriate statistical tests used and the probability of type I and type II errors considered?
- If a meta-analysis, were 95% confidence intervals calculated?
- If a meta-analysis, were sensitivity analyses conducted?
- Was the source of funding provided and could it be a source of bias in the results?

PRACTICE GUIDELINES

- Is there an explicit description of the procedures used to identify, select, and combine evidence?
- Are the recommendations valid?
- Are the guidelines regularly reviewed and updated to incorporate new evidence as it becomes available?
- Was the guideline peer-reviewed?
- Can the recommendations be generalized to a larger population?
- Was the source of funding for the development of the guideline provided and could it bias the conclusions?
- If another group of experts were to independently develop a guideline on the same clinical situation, would the recommendations be the same (are the recommendations reliable)?

PHARMACOECONOMIC ANALYSIS

- Readers are referred to Chap. 8 for a discussion of the evaluation of these types of trials.

QUALITY-OF-LIFE STUDIES

- Did the study design simulate clinical practice?
- Were aspects of the patients' lives that patients consider important measured?
- Are the results biased by the presence of training effect?
- If it is a multicenter trial, did all of the sites evaluate QOL?
- Is the QOL instrument used valid for examining the specific disease in question?

11-1

Appendix 11–1

Question Example

DRUG INFORMATICS CENTER

St. Anywhere Hospital

Name of Inquirer:	Dr. Meghan Malone	Date: XX/XX/XX
Address	2184 Fall St. Seneca Falls, NY 13148	Time Received: XX:XX am/pm
		Time Required: 5 hours
		Nature of Request: Therapeutics
Telephone Number:	(315)555-1212	Type of Inquirer: MD

Question

A young, adult male patient recently arrived from Japan and presented to the physician sparse medical records indicating he is suffering from tsutsugamushi disease. Because of the language difficulties, not much is known about the patient, other than he is taking drug X for the illness. Physical exam reveals a patient in some discomfort with elevated temperature, swollen lymph glands, and red rash. All other findings appear to be normal. (*Note:* the person answering this question obtained as much background as possible about the patient.) The physician has little information on the disease and would like to know if that drug X is the most appropriate treatment.

Answer

Tsutsugamushi disease is an acute infectious disease seen in harvesters of hemp in Japan.[1] It is caused by *Rickettsia tsutsugamushi.* Common symptoms of the disease include fever, painful swelling of the lymph glands, a small black scab in the genital region, neck or axilla, and large dark-red papules. The disease is known by a number of other names, including akamushi disease, flood fever, inundation fever, island disease, Japanese river fever, and scrub typhus.[2-4] (*Note:* background information presented.) The standard treatment of the disease includes either drug X or drug Y, although there are several other less effective treatments.[5-7] In the remainder of this paper, a comparison of the two major drugs will be presented. (*Note:* clear objective for paper is presented.)

A thorough search of the available literature was conducted. Unfortunately, there were few textbooks available on this disease. A search of MEDLINE (1966 to present) and Embase's *Drugs and Pharmacology* (1980 to present) produced a number of articles that were obtained and are reviewed below. (*Note:* This documents the type of search and acts as a lead-in to the remainder of the body of the paper.)

Smith and Jones[8] performed a double-blind, randomized comparison of the effects of drug X and drug Y in patients with tsutsugamushi fever. Patients were required to be between 18 and 70 years old, and could not have any concurrent infection or disorder that would affect the immune response to the disease (e.g., neutropenia, AIDS). Twenty patients received 10 mg of drug X three times a day for 15 days. Eighteen patients received 250 mg of drug Y twice a day for 10 days. The two groups were comparable, except that the patients receiving drug X were an average of 5 years younger ($p < .05$). Drug X was shown to produce a cure, both in terms of symptoms and cultures in 85% of patients, whereas drug Y only produced a cure in 55.5% of patients. The difference was statistically significant ($p < .01\%$). No significant adverse effects were seen in either group. Although it appears that drug X was the better agent, it should be noted that drug Y was given in its minimally effective dose, and may have performed better in a somewhat higher or longer regimen. (*Note:* evaluative comments made about article.)

(*Note:* Other articles would be described at this point.)

Based on the literature found, it appears that drug Y is generally accepted as the better agent, except in those patients with several renal insufficiency. Because this patient does not appear to be suffering from that problem, it is recommended that he receive a 3-week course of drug Y in a dose of 500 mg three times a day. Renal function should be monitored weekly. The patient should receive an additional week of therapy, if the symptoms have not been gone for the final week of therapy. (*Note:* this patient's situation was specifically addressed, rather than just presenting a general conclusion.)

Signature: _____ Date: March 20, 2000

       Sandy Q. Pharmacist, PharmD

References

(Present references here.)

11-2

Appendix 11–2

Abstracts

Abstracts are a synopsis (usually of 250 words or less) of the most important aspect of an article. They should be clear, concise, and complete enough for readers to have a reasonable understanding of the important portions of the article.[1] Since they are the most commonly read part of an article, they must be accurate and avoid the three most common errors: differences in information presented in the abstract and in the body of the article, information given in the abstract that was not presented in the article, and conclusions presented in the abstract that are not supported by information in the abstract.[2-4]

There are basically three types of abstracts that are seen in the literature. The first two (descriptive and informational) are somewhat traditional; however, they do not convey as much information as structured abstracts. Structured abstracts were originally designed to convey more information, and have only been in use since the 1980s. The type of abstract to be used depends on the type of information and the requirements of the particular place the work is being submitted or used.

In addition to writing an abstract, some journals ask that indexing terms be submitted. Whenever possible, Medical Subject Headings (MeSH) from the National Library of Medicine should be used for the indexing terms. Each of the abstracts will be discussed in more detail in the following sections.

DESCRIPTIVE ABSTRACTS

A descriptive abstract, as its name implies, simply describes the information found in an article. Few specific details are given and it would mostly be used in a review article. An example of this type of abstract is as follows:

> Lists of references that should be available, depending on location of the drug information service, are presented. These lists are specific to community, hospital, long-term care facility, and academic sites. Included are general references, indexing and abstracting services, and journals. Specialty references that would be useful in specific circumstances

are also presented. In addition, the equipment necessary to access the computerized resources is shown for the individual references.

INFORMATIONAL ABSTRACTS

Informational abstracts concisely summarize the factual information presented in a study. This type of abstract is more applicable to clinical studies.

Key points to include in an informational abstract include:

- Study design (e.g., double blind, cross-over)
- Purpose
- Number of patients
- Dosages
- Results
- Conclusions

An example of this type of abstract is as follows:

A double-blind, randomized comparison of the effects of drug X and drug Y was performed in patients with tsutsugamushi fever, in order to determine whether either drug was superior in efficacy or safety. Twenty patients received 10 mg of drug X three times a day for 15 days. Eighteen patients received 250 mg of drug Y twice a day for 10 days. The two groups were comparable, except that the patients receiving drug X were an average of 5 years younger ($p < .05\%$). Drug X was shown to produce a cure, both in terms of symptoms and cultures in 85% of patients, whereas drug Y only produced a cure in 55.5% of patients. The difference was statistically significant ($p < .01\%$). No significant adverse effects were seen in either group. Drug X was shown to be significantly better than drug Y in the treatment of tsutsugamushi fever.

STRUCTURED ABSTRACTS

Due to perceived deficiencies in abstracts,[5] including lack of sufficient information,[6] a new type of abstract was presented in 1987[7] and later updated in 1990.[8] This structured abstract was designed to present more information about clinical studies and possibly laboratory studies, as compared to the informational abstract presented earlier.[9,10] This type of abstract is not meant for case reports, studies of tissues or animals, opinion articles, and position papers.[8] Abstracts following this standard seem to be gaining in popularity and have been mandated by an influential group of journals (e.g., *New England Journal of Medicine*,[11] *Annals of Internal Medicine*,[8] *JAMA: Journal of the American Medical Association*,[9] *British Medical Journal*,[12] *Canadian Medical Association Journal*,[13] *Chest*[14]), sometimes in a somewhat modified form. Although the overall acceptance and approval of this format of abstract appears to be good, there are some who disapprove.[15-17] Also, there is at least some data suggesting that structured abstracts do not always contain as much information as they should, if the published rules are followed[18] and that they do not necessarily contain any more useful information than traditional abstracts.[19]

It is worth noting that articles with structured abstracts are indexed with a greater number of terms in MEDLINE, which may lead to ease of finding such articles on computer search.[20]

An abstract following this procedure would contain the following subheadings and information.

- *Objective*—The main objective and key secondary objectives.
- *Design*—The basic design of the study (e.g., randomized, double-blind, crossover, placebo-controlled) and duration of any follow-up.
- *Setting*—The location and level of clinical care available at that location (e.g., tertiary care hospital, ambulatory clinic).
- *Patients or other participants*—Description of the patients, including illnesses and key sociodemographic features and how they were selected for the study (including whether it was a random, volunteer, etc. sample); it should also include number of patients that refused to enroll in the study, proportion of the patients completing the study, and the number of patients withdrawn due to adverse effects.
- *Intervention(s)*—A brief description of any treatment(s) or intervention(s).
- *Main outcome measure(s)*—The main study outcome measurements, as planned before data collection was begun; if most of the article covers other material (e.g., data or hypotheses not planned to be observed before the study was started), that should be made clear.
- *Results*—The method(s) by which patients were assessed and the main results of the study, including any blinding. Statistical significance (particularly confidence intervals, odds ratios, numerators, and denominators) and levels of significance should be mentioned. Absolute, rather than relative, differences are presented (e.g., "adverse effects were seen in 5% of patients in group A and 10% of patients in group B," rather than "Group B had twice as many adverse effects"). Provide response rate in survey articles.
- *Conclusion(s)*—The key conclusion(s) directly supported by the evidence presented in the study and their clinical application(s). Should also include whether further study is necessary.

An example of this type of abstract is as follows:

Study Objective: To compare the safety and efficacy of drug X and drug Y in the treatment of tsutsugamushi fever.

Design: Randomized, double-blind trial.

Setting: Tertiary-care, military hospital located on Guam.

Patients: Sequential sample of 40 young (age 20 to 37), otherwise healthy male patients with tsutsugamushi fever. Patients randomly divided into two equal groups. Two patients were removed from the group receiving drug Y, due to transfer to U.S. mainland hospitals. The two groups were comparable, except that the patients receiving drug X were an average of 5 years younger ($p < .05\%$).

Interventions: Twenty patients received 10 mg of drug X three times a day for 15 days. Eighteen patients received 250 mg of drug Y twice a day for 10 days.

Main Outcome Measures: Physician and patients' global assessment of disease activity; five point scale from 0 (no symptoms) to 5 (severe disability). Presence or absence of organism on laboratory specimens.

Results: Drug X was shown to produce a cure, both in terms of symptoms and cultures in 85% of patients, whereas drug Y only produced a cure in 55.5% of patients. The difference was statistically significant ($p < .01\%$). No significant adverse effects were seen in either group.

Conclusions: Drug X was shown to produce significantly higher cure rates than drug Y in the treatment of tsutsugamushi fever, with no difference in adverse effects. Additional trials at different doses and lengths of therapy should be performed.

A method to prepare a structured abstract for a review article differs from the first example.[21] This method would only be applicable in specific situations, where a number of similar studies were evaluated together. It would not be useful in a situation where a number of dissimilar articles dealing with the same topic were discussed (e.g., a review of all therapies for a particular disease). Such an abstract would consist of the following items:

- *Purpose*—The main objective of the review article, including information about the population tested, how they were tested, and the outcome.
- *Data sources*—A brief summary of data sources and the time periods covered.
- *Study selection*—The number of studies covered in the article and how they were selected for inclusion.
- *Data extraction*—A description of the guidelines for abstracting data and how those guidelines were applied.
- *Data synthesis*—The main results of the review and the method to obtain the results are outlined.

- *Conclusions*—Important conclusions, including applications and need for further study.

An example of this type of abstract would be as follows:

Purpose: To evaluate the effect of the antihistamine, drug X, on symptoms of allergy, as determined by physicians' and patients' global symptom assessment.

Data sources: Studies published from January 1980 to December 1998 were identified by computer searches of MEDLINE and Embase—*Drugs and Pharmacology* and hand searching of bibliographies of the articles identified via the computer search.

Study selection: Fifty-three studies evaluating the effects of drug X in the treatment of allergy were located.

Data extraction: Descriptive data regarding the population, dosing, effects, and adverse effects were assessed, along with the study's quality.

Results of data analysis: Subjective and objective measures of effectiveness demonstrated that drug X decreased or eliminated allergic symptoms approximately 80% of the time in a variety of patient types (e.g., seasonal allergic rhinitis, perennial allergic rhinitis, anaphylaxis). The only adverse effects seen were dryness of mucous membranes and sedation, seen in approximately 5% and 2% of patients, respectively.

Conclusions: Drug X is an effective agent for the treatment of allergic reactions. It has a low incidence of typical antihistamine adverse effects. Further studies should be performed to verify the effectiveness of Drug X in comparison to other drugs commonly used for anaphylaxis.

REFERENCES

1. Staub NC. On writing abstracts. Physiologist 1991;34:276–7.
2. Pitkin RM, Branagan MA. Can the accuracy of abstracts be improved by providing specific instructions? A randomized controlled trial. JAMA 1998;280:267–9.
3. Pitkin RM, Branagan MA, Burmeister LF. Accuracy of data in abstracts of published research articles. JAMA 1999;281:1110–11.
4. Winker MA. The need for concrete improvement in abstract quality. JAMA 1999;281:1129–30.
5. Huth EJ. Structured abstracts for papers reporting clinical trials. Ann Intern Med 1987;106: 626–7.
6. Narine L, Yee DS, Einarson TR, Ilersich AL. Quality of abstracts of original research articles in CMAJ in 1989. CMAJ 1991;144:449–53.
7. Ad Hoc Working Group for Critical Appraisal of the Medical Literature. A proposal for more informative abstracts of clinical articles. Ann Intern Med 1987;106:598–604.

8. Haynes RB, Mulrow CD, Huth EJ, Altman DG, Gardner MJ. More informative abstracts revisited. Ann Intern Med 1990;113:69–76.

9. Rennie D, Glass RM. Structuring abstracts to make them more informative. JAMA 1991;266:116–17.

10. Haynes RB. Dissent. More informative abstracts: current status and evaluation. J Clin Epidemiol 1993;46:595–7.

11. Relman AS. New "Information for Authors"—and readers. N Engl J Med 1990;323:56.

12. Lock S. Structure abstracts. Now required for all papers reporting clinical trials. Br Med J 1988;297:156.

13. Squires BP. Structured abstracts of original research and review articles. CMAJ 1990;143:619–22.

14. Soffer A. Abstracts of clinical investigations. A new and standardized format. Chest 1987;92:389–90.

15. Spitzer WO. Second thoughts. The structured sonnet. J Clin Epidemiol 1991;44:729.

16. Heller MB. Dissent. Structured abstracts: a modest dissent. J Clin Epidemiol 1991;44:739–40.

17. Heller MB. Structured abstracts. [letter] Ann Intern Med 1990;113:722.

18. Froom P, Froom J. Variance and Dissent. Presentation. Deficiencies in structured medical abstracts. J Clin Epidemiol 1993;46:591–4.

19. Scherer RW, Crawley B. Reporting of randomized clinical trial descriptors and use of structured abstracts. JAMA 1998;280:269–72.

20. Harbourt AM, Knecht LS, Humphreys BL. Structured abstracts in MEDLINE®, 1989–1991. Bull Med Libr Assoc 1995:83(2):190–5.

21. Mulrow CD, Thacker SB, Pugh JA. A proposal for more informative abstracts of review articles. Ann Intern Med 1988;108:613–15.

11-3

Bibliography

Although there seems to be a different method to prepare a bibliography for every English class ever given, there is fortunately a standardized method to prepare a bibliography in medical writing. This method is used by the National Library of Medicine and has been incorporated into the "Uniform Requirements for Manuscripts Submitted to Biomedical Journals"[1-3]; it has been used widely since the 1970s in both journals and other medical writing. This method will be presented here.

References in the bibliography are placed in the order they are first cited in the text of a document, and each reference is assigned a consecutive Arabic number. Those cited only in tables or figures are numbered according to the place the table or figure is identified in the text. References are not listed multiple times in the bibliography, if they are cited more than once in the text of the document. Instead, subsequent citations to the same reference use the original reference number. It should also be noted that *Ibid* is not used. The reference number in the text will be the Arabic number in parenthesis or, commonly, superscript. This number is often cited after the sentence that contains the fact being referenced. If there are several references used to prepare a specific sentence, they may be listed at the end of the sentence or throughout the sentence. Also, if the sentence is a lead-in to an abstract, the authors' names are commonly listed followed by the reference number. See the sentences below for examples.

- Drug X has been shown to cause green rash with purple spots.[2,3]
- Drug Y is useful in the treatment of hypertension,[4] congestive heart failure,[5] and arrhythmias.[6]
- Smith and Jones[7] studied the effects of . . .
- Brown et al.[9] treated . . . (please notice on this example, al. is followed by a period since it is an abbreviation, whereas et is a full Latin word, and there is no need for a comma after the first author's name)

It should be mentioned that citations are often not found in conclusions of documents. The conclusions are based on the information presented, and cited, earlier in the article.

Before getting into the method for listing references and examples, it should be mentioned that there are a number of general rules to be followed. They are as follows.

- Avoid using abstracts as references.
- Do not use unpublished observations or personal communications as references. In the latter case, it is proper to insert references to written, but not oral, communications in parentheses in the text.
- If reference is made to an article that has been accepted by a journal, but not yet published, the phrase *In press* should be inserted where the year, volume, and page numbers would normally be listed.
- If there are more than six authors, the first six should be listed, followed by the phrase *et al.*

JOURNAL ARTICLES

To cite a journal article, the following information should be given.

- Last name of author(s) and initials (each separated by commas, with a period at the end).
- Title of article (do not use quotation marks, capitalize only the initial word of sentences and proper nouns in English) (followed by a period).
- Title source (abbreviated as found in the list of journals in *Index Medicus*—see <<http://www.nlm.nih.gov/tsd/serials/lji.html>>).
- Year (followed by a semicolon). Month and day of month can be listed after the year, but is optional in journals that have continuous pagination throughout the volume.
- Volume number (listing the issue number in parenthesis is optional, but necessary in journals that do not have continuous page numbers for the entire volume) (followed by a colon).
- Page numbers (If continuous, use first and last pages separated by a hyphen. If separate pages, list the pages separated by a comma. If a combination of continuous and separate pages, use both (e.g., 18–29,33,40).

Example Citations

Standard Journal Article

Smythe M, Hoffman J, Kizy K, Dmuchowski C. Estimating creatinine clearance in elderly patients with low serum creatinine concentrations. Am J Hosp Pharm 1994;51:198–204.

Beck DE, Aceves-Blumenthal C, Carson R, Culley J, Dawson K, Hotchkiss G, et al. Factors contributing to volunteer practitioner-faculty vitality. Am J Pharm Ed 1993;57:305–12.

Organization as Author

Task Force on Specialty Recognition of Oncology Pharmacy Practice. Executive summary of petition requesting specialty recognition of oncology pharmacy practice. Am J Hosp Pharm 1994;51:219-24.

No Author Given

N.Y. court rules against Medicaid co-pay. Drug Topics 1994;138(3):6.

Article not in English

Antoni N. Zur kritjk der irrtümlich sogenannten sehnen- und periostreflexe. Acta Psychiatrica Neurologica 1932;VII:9-19.

Volume with Supplement

Nayler WG. Pharmacological aspects of calcium antagonism. Short term and long term benefits. Drugs 1993;46 Suppl 2:40-7.

Issue with Supplement

Graves NM. Pharmacokinetics and interactions of antiepileptic drugs. Am J Hosp Pharm 1993;50(Suppl 5):S23-S29.

Volume with Part

Katchen MS, Lyons TJ, Gillingham KK, Schlegel W. A case of left hypoglossal neurapraxia following G exposure in a centrifuge. Aviat Space Environ Med 1990;61(Pt 2):837-9.

Issue with Part

Dudley MN. Maximizing patient outcomes of antiinfective therapy. Pharmacotherapy 1993;13(2 Pt 2):29S-33S.

Issue with no Volume

Slaga TJ, Gimenez-Conti IB. An animal model for oral cancer. Monogr J Nat Cancer Instit 1992;(13):55-60.

No Issue or Volume

Payne R. Acute exacerbation of chronic cancer pain: basic assessment and treatments of breakthrough pain. Acute Pain Sympt Manage 1998:4-5.

Pagination in Roman Numerals

Koretz RL. Clinical nutrition. Gastroenterol Clin North Am 1998 June:27(2):xi-xiii.

Expressing Type of Article (as needed)

Goldwater SH, Chatelain F. Taking time to communicate [letter]. Am J Hosp Pharm 1994;51:232,234.

Talley CR. Reducing demand through preventive care [editorial]. Am J Hosp Pharm 1994;51:55.

Article Containing a Retraction

Brown MD. Retraction [retraction of Slutsky RA, Olson LK. In: Am Heart J 1984;108:543–7]. Am Heart J 1986;111:623.

Article Retracted

Slutsky RA, Olson LK. Intravascular and extravascular pulmonary fluid volumes during chronic experimental left ventricular dysfunction [retracted in: Am Heart J 1986;111:623]. Am Heart J 1984;108:543–7.

Article Containing Comment

Relman AS. An error corrected, a conclusion withdrawn, and a lesson learned [comment]. N Engl J Med 1990;323:1482–3. Comment on: N Engl J Med 1989;320:376–9.

Article Commented on

Pintor C, Loche S, Cella SG, Müller EE, Bauman G. A child with phenotypic Laron dwarfism and normal somatomedin levels [see comments]. N Engl J Med 1989;320:376–9. Comment in: N Engl J Med 1990;323:1482–3.

Article with Published Erratum

Reitz MS Jr, Juo HG, Oleske J, Hoxie J, Popovic M, Read-Connole E, et al. On the historical origins of HIV-1 (MN) and (RF) [letter] [published erratum appears in AIDS Res Hum Retroviruses 1992;8:1731]. AIDS Res Hum Retroviruses 1992;8:1539–41.

BOOKS

To cite a book, the following information should be given (Please note, previously published styles incorrectly had a comma instead of a semicolon after the publisher[1]):

- Last name of author(s) and initials (followed by a period)
- Title of book (followed by period)
- Edition, other than first (followed by period)
- Place of publication (city) (followed by colon)
- Name of publisher (followed by semicolon)
- Year of publication (followed by period)

Example Citations

Personal Author(s)

Albright RG. A basic guide to online information systems for health care professionals. Arlington: Information Resource Press; 1988.

Editor(s), Compiler as Author

Billups NF, Billups SM. American drug index. 42nd ed. St. Louis: Facts and Comparisons; 1998.

No Specific Editor(s), Compiler, or Author Identified

Drug facts and comparisons. 1999 edition. St. Louis: Facts and Comparisons; 1998.

Organization as Author and Publisher

United States Pharmacopeial Convention, Inc. USAN and the USP dictionary of drug names. Rockville: United States Pharmacopeial Convention, Inc.; 1993.

Chapters in a Book or Full Text Computer Reference

Theesen KA, Stimmel GL. Disorders of infancy and childhood. In: DiPiro JT, Talbert RL, Hayes PE, Yee GC, Matzke GR, Posey LM, editors. Pharmacotherapy. A pathophysiologic approach. 2nd ed. Norwalk (CT): Appleton & Lange; 1993. p. 953–61.

Thompson GA, Kayahara C, DRUGDEX® Editorial Staff. Cluster headache—drug therapy. In: Rumack BH, Bird PE, Gelman CR, Clouthier M, Hutchison T, editors. DRUGDEX Information System. Englewood: MICROMEDEX, Inc.; 1998.

Duffy JP, Tong TG. Iron. In: Rumack BH, McCrory MR, Smith RD, editors. POISINDEX Information System. Englewood: MICROMEDEX, Inc.; 1999.

Conference Proceedings

Allebeck P, Jansson B, editors. Ethics in medicine. Individual integrity versus demands of society. Karolinska Institute Novel Conference Series. Proceedings of the Third International Congress on Ethics in Medicine; 1989; Stockholm. New York: Raven Press; 1990.

Conference Paper

Keyserlingk E. Ethical guidelines and codes—can they be universally applicable in a multi-cultural world? In: Allebeck P, Jansson B, editors. Ethics in medicine. Individual integrity versus demands of society. Karolinska Institute Novel Conference Series. Proceedings of the Third International Congress on Ethics in Medicine; 1989; Stockholm. New York: Raven Press; 1990. p. 137–49.

Scientific or Technical Report

Cohon MS, Rice BS, Noble V. Information sources in pharmacy and pharmacology. Kalamazoo (MI): Upjohn; 1980 Jan.

Dissertation

Wellman CO. Pain perceptions and coping strategies of school-age children and their parents: a descriptive-correlational study [dissertation]. Omaha (NE): Creighton University; 1985.

Patent

Schwartz B, inventor. New England Medical Center Hospital, Inc., assignee. Method of and solution for treating glaucoma. U.S. patent 5,212,168. 1993 May 18.

OTHER MATERIAL

Examples

Newspaper Article

Fein EB. Rise in fetal tests prompts ethical debate. The New York Times 1994 Feb 5; Sect. A:1(col. 2).

Audiovisual Material

Universal precautions: AIDS and hepatitis B prevention for home health care [video-recording]. Garden Grove (CA): Medcom; 1992.

Computer File

A.D.A.M. animated dissection of anatomy for medicine [computer program]. Version 2.2. Windows version. Marietta (GA): A.D.A.M. Software, Inc.; 1993.

Dictionary

Stedman's medical dictionary. 25th ed. Baltimore: Williams & Wilkins; 1990. Asthenia. p. 144.

Electronic Material

Nemecz G. Evening primrose. US Pharmacist [serial online] 1998 Nov [cited 1998 Dec 10]:[1 screen]. Available from: URL: http://www.uspharmacist.com/NewLook/Docs/1998/Nov1998/EveningPrimrose.htm.

Marone G. Tacrolimus ointment for atopic dermatitis. N Engl J Med [serial online] 1998 Dec 10 [cited 1998 Dec 10];339(24):[1 screen]. Available from: URL: http://www.nejm.org/content/1998/0339/0024/1788.asp.

FDA Backs Drug to Fight Hepatitis B. Omaha World Herald [serial online] 1998 Dec 10 [cited 1998 Dec 10]:[1 screen]. Available from: URL: http://www.omaha.com/OWH/StoryView/1,1344,73566,00.html.

Please note: Although all of the above citations are for web sites, the format would be the same for ftp or gopher sites; only the Internet address would change. In keeping with the general prohibition to the use of personal communications, USENET News, listserver and e-mail formats will not be dealt with here. They should be dealt with as previously stated in this appendix.

Monograph in Electronic Format

Phenytoin [monograph on CD-ROM]. Reents S. Clinical pharmacology. Version 1.17. Windows version. Tampa (FL): Gold Standard Multimedia Inc.; 1998.

Package Insert

Package inserts are commonly cited in professional writing, however, the "Uniform Requirements" do not address the format to use. The following is a common format that is similar to those presented in this appendix.

Prilosec® (omeprazole) delayed-release capsules [product information]. Wayne, PA: Astra Merck, June 1998.

REFERENCES

1. International Committee of Medical Journal Editors. Uniform requirements for manuscripts submitted to biomedical journals. JAMA 1997;277:927–34.
2. International Committee of Medical Journal Editors. Uniform requirements for manuscripts submitted to biomedical journals. Med Educ 1999;33:66–78.
3. International Committee of Medical Journal Editors. Uniform requirements for manuscripts submitted to biomedical journals [cited 2000 Sept 20]:[30 screens]. Available from: URL: http://www.icmje.org

13-1

Sample Case Scenarios

Sample case scenarios describing ethical dilemmas that might arise for pharmacists who are providing drug information.

1. A pharmacist is contacted by a patient inquiring about a medication his physician has recently prescribed for him called Obecalp (Placebo spelled backwards).

   Factors that may change the ethical decision: A nurse calls for the information at the request of her friend.

2. A cancer patient picking up a prescription for morphine tablets inquires, "How many of these pills could kill you?"

   Factors that may change the ethical decision: A physician calls to ask about the lethal dose of a product that the pharmacist knows he has prescribed for a relative with a terminal illness.

3. A physician requests detailed dosing information from a recent publication describing how two specific agents (methotrexate and misoprostol) are dosed in combination to induce abortion.

   Factors that may change the ethical decision: A patient requests this information.

4. A layperson calls to ask a drug information pharmacist how long amphetamines will remain in the urine.

   Factors that may change the ethical decision:

   a. *A medical resident calls with the same question.*

   b. *The caller asks for the name of a chemical that is understood to interfere with tests for marijuana in the blood or urine.*

Notes:

1. Consider addressing the above dilemma both where the caller provides demographic data (name, address, telephone number and profession), and where he or she refuses to do so.

2. Refer to a discussion of this topic by Uretsky and colleagues.[16]

5. A layperson requests information on how to obtain a homeopathic medicine promoted to treat cancer.
   Factors that may change the ethical decision:
   a. *The product appears to be harmless.*
   b. *The product appears to have substantial risk for harm.*
   c. *The product will replace standard therapy, versus being used along with the prescribed regimen.*

   Note: Consider addressing the above dilemma where the client is from a culture (Mexican, Chinese) that tends to strongly value the use of various homeopathic remedies.

6. The pharmacist responsible for assessing a new diagnostic imaging product for the P&T Committee of the hospital is encouraged, by the pharmacy director, to recommend that the agent *not* be added to the Formulary based on its high cost, even though it appears to have improved efficacy and safety compared to alternate products.

7. A pharmacist working in the marketing branch of a drug manufacturing company is asked to develop a direct-to-consumer advertisement that has high potential to encourage inappropriate use of a specific medication.

8. A patient calls a local pharmacist to request information about a medication obtained from a mail-order prescription service.
   Factors that may change the ethical decision:
   a. *The patient is a former client who has recently switched to the mail-order company for services.*
   b. *The patient has not previously used the local pharmacist for services.*

9. While picking up a prescription, a patient requests detailed information about the medication, which she or he must begin immediately. Six other clients are waiting for service, and only 30 minutes remain before closing.
   Factors that may change the ethical decision: The patient asks about the use of a generic product promoted by the pharmacy chain; the pharmacist has reservations about its bioequivalence.

10. A parent calls to request identification of a medication belonging to her 15-year-old daughter (found in the youngster's drawer).
    Factors that may change the ethical decision:
    a. *The product is a contraceptive agent recently dispensed by the pharmacist to the child.*
    b. *The product is a nonprescription decongestant product that has had some use as a "street drug."*

13–2

Appendix 13–2

Code of Ethics for Pharmacists

AMERICAN PHARMACEUTICAL ASSOCIATION, 1994

Pharmacists are health professionals who assist individuals in making the best use of medications. This Code, prepared and supported by pharmacists, is intended to state publicly the principles that form the fundamental basis of the roles and responsibilities of pharmacists. These principles, based on moral obligations and virtues, are established to guide pharmacists in relationships with patients, health professionals, and society.

I. A **pharmacist** respects the covenantal relationship between the patient and pharmacist.

Considering the patient-pharmacist relationship as a covenant means that a pharmacist has moral obligations in response to the gift of trust received from society. In return for this gift, a pharmacist promises to help individuals achieve optimum benefit from their medications, to be committed to their welfare, and to maintain their trust.

II. A **pharmacist** promotes the good of every patient in a caring, compassionate, and confidential manner.

A pharmacist places concern for the well-being of the patient at the center of professional practice. In doing so, a pharmacist considers needs stated by the patient as well as those defined by health science. A pharmacist is dedicated to protecting the dignity of the patient. With a caring attitude and a compassionate spirit, a pharmacist focuses on serving the patient in a private and confidential manner.

III. A **pharmacist** respects the autonomy and dignity of each patient.

A pharmacist promotes the right of self-determination and recognizes individual self-worth by encouraging patients to participate in decisions about their health. A pharmacist communicates with patients in terms that are understand-

This code was approved by members of the American Pharmaceutical Association on October 27, 1994. Code of ethics adopted. Am Pharm 1994; NS34(11):72.

able. In all cases, a pharmacist respects personal and cultural differences among patients.

IV. A **pharmacist** acts with honesty and integrity in professional relationships.

A pharmacist has a duty to tell the truth and to act with conviction of conscience. A pharmacist avoids discriminatory practices, behavior or work conditions that impair professional judgment, and actions that compromise dedication to the best interests of patients.

V. A **pharmacist** maintains professional competence.

A pharmacist has a duty to maintain knowledge and abilities as new medications, devices, and technologies become available and as health information advances.

VI. A **pharmacist** respects the values and abilities of colleagues and other health professionals.

When appropriate, a pharmacist asks for the consultation of colleagues or other health professionals or refers the patient. A pharmacist acknowledges that colleagues and other health professionals may differ in the beliefs and values they apply to the care of the patient.

VII. A **pharmacist** serves individual, community, and societal needs.

The primary obligation of a pharmacist is to individual patients. However, the obligations of a pharmacist may at times extend beyond the individual to the community and society. In these situations, a pharmacist recognizes the responsibilities that accompany these obligations and acts accordingly.

VIII. A **pharmacist** seeks justice in the distribution of health resources.

When health resources are allocated, a pharmacist is fair and equitable, balancing the needs of patients and society.

Appendix 14–1

Format for Drug Monograph

INSTITUTION NAME HEADING

Generic name (can include other common, nonofficial names; e.g., TPA for alteplase)

Trade name (if more than one, indicate company that each is from)

Manufacturer(s) (or source of supply)—include web site address(es)

Classification (Note—other classifications, such as the VA class, can also be used)
- AHFS number and classification (if not in the book yet, see the list in the front of *American Hospital Formulary Service—Drug Information* book and determine the most appropriate classification)
- FDA classification (include specific FDA web site URL concerning approval)
- Status—prescription, nonprescription, and/or controlled substance schedule (if applicable)

Similar agents (A list of common treatments used for the same indication[s].)

Summary (Includes a short summary of advantages and disadvantages of the drug, particularly in relation to other drugs or treatments used for each major indication, and any other significant information.)

Recommendations (Indicate whether or not the drug should be added to the drug formulary of an institution, assuming they would have patients that would be treated for illnesses where this drug might be used. Also indicate specific formulary status for the drug [i.e., uncontrolled, monitored, restricted, conditional—see ASHP guidelines] and whether the drug will replace any other product that might already be on the formulary. In addition, any information on how the drug is to be placed in any clinical guidelines.)

Page one consists of the above information

Pharmacologic data
- Mechanism of action (usually brief)
- Bacterial spectrum (if applicable)

Therapeutic indications

- FDA-approved indications (see package insert)—clearly indicate which indications are FDA approved.
- Potential unlabeled uses (list only if they are considered to be acceptable medical practice, although it is allowable to mention others that are early in investigation with a statement that the drug should not be used for them or that they require more study)—clearly indicate they are not FDA approved.
- How the drug, and similar drugs, fit into clinical guidelines.
- Clinical comparison (abstract at least two studies; see Appendix 11–2 for more guidelines. Include human efficacy studies and, where available, studies comparing the product to standard therapy. *Note:* if there are other supportive studies for an indication, they can be covered briefly, if you desire, along with the major study covered in detail. Be sure to note any deficiencies in the studies.)

Bioavailability/pharmacokinetics (A table summarizing the following, in comparison to the "gold standard," can be very useful.)

- Absorption
- Distribution
- Metabolism
- Excretion

Dosage forms

- Forms and strengths (compare to other agents [consider a table], because new products often have a limited number of dosage forms/routes as compared to established products]. Purity and composition information should be included for herbal and alternative medications.)
- Explain any special information needed for preparation and storage, in comparison to other products. Sometimes a product will be so difficult to prepare or have such a limited shelf life after preparation that it is not worth stocking.

Dosage range

- Adults
- Children
- Elderly
- Renal or hepatic failure
- Special administration requirements

Known adverse effects/toxicities

- Frequency and type (a table comparing the drug to others can be a clear and concise way of expressing this information)

- Prevention of toxicity
- Risk and benefit data

Special Precautions (usually includes pregnancy and lactation)

Contraindications

Drug Interactions (a simple one or two sentence statement for each—usually separate various interactions into separate short paragraphs and compare to other drugs)
- Drug–drug
- Drug–food
- Drug–laboratory

Patient monitoring guidelines
- Include effectiveness, adverse effects, compliance, and other appropriate items

Patient information
- Name and description of the medication
- Dosage form
- Route of administration
- Duration of therapy
- Special directions and precautions
- Side effects
- Techniques for self-monitoring
- Proper storage
- Refill information
- What to do if dose missed

Cost Comparison (use AWP and institutional prices, and make sure there is a comparison with any similar products at equivalent doses—a pharmacoeconomic analysis [see Chap. 8] is the best method of comparing drugs in this section.)

Date presented to Pharmacy and Therapeutics Committee, and name and title of the person preparing the document.

References
- Follow guidelines as described in Appendix 11–3.

14-2

Example Drug Monograph

(*Note:* This example is based on fictional products and is condensed. It shows examples of most sections in a real drug monograph, but often does not go into all of the details [e.g., a table of adverse effects is seen, but only a couple items are listed, whereas a full drug monograph would list at least all common and/or serious reactions.])

St. Anywhere Medical Center
Pharmacy and Therapeutics Committee
Drug Evaluation Monograph

Generic Name: artiblood
Brand Name: MegaBlood
Manufacturer: MegaPharmics (http://www.megapharmics.com)
Classification: AHFS 16:00 blood derivatives
FDA classification: 1A (http://www.fda.gov/cder/foi/
appletter/2000/99999ta.pdf)
Status: prescription only

Similar agents fakered

Summary

Artiblood is a new perfluorocarbon that has many similarities to the only other product in its class, fakered. Both products have the ability to temporarily replace the oxygen-carrying function of red blood cells in patients in whom use of whole blood or packed red blood cells is impossible due to medical or religious reasons. In general, artiblood was found to be more efficacious than fakered; however, it also has been shown to produce a greater number of adverse effects. The adverse effects are mostly gastrointestinal in nature; however, the increased INR can be a problem in some patients. Artiblood is not metabolized in the body, whereas fakered is approximately 50% metabolized to inactive components. These differences are generally not clinically significant, because the dose of either product is unlikely to need adjustment. Fakered is available in several different volume bags, allowing the dose to be matched more closely to the anticipated patient need. Although the cost of fakered appears to be lower, a pharmacoeco-nomic analysis shows that artiblood would produce the greatest cost savings for the institution.

Recommendations

It is recommended that artiblood be added to the drug formulary for use restricted to those who cannot use natural blood replacement products because of religious reasons or because suitable blood types are not available.

Pharmacologic Data

Artiblood is a type of perfluorocarbon, similar to fakered. These products have the unique ability to freely bind with or give up oxygen, depending on the partial pressures of the gas where the product is located (i.e., in the lungs there is an abundance of oxygen, so the product adsorbs oxygen; in the tissues there is a relative deficiency of oxygen, so the product gives up the gas).[1,2] The products do not have direct immunologic properties, nor do they have the ability to aid in blood clotting, although there may be some effect on blood clotting (either interference by coating platelets or precipitation of the clotting pathway mechanism).[3]

In addition to oxygen-carrying capabilities, the products have some plasma volume expansion properties. Artiblood has a similar effect to Dextran 40,[1] whereas fakered's properties are relatively insignificant.[4] Maximum plasma volume expansion occurs within several minutes of administration and lasts for approximately 1 day in normal patients. This results in increased central venous pressure, cardiac output, stroke volume, blood pressure, urinary output, capillary perfusion, and pulse pressure. Microcirculation is improved.

Therapeutic Indications

Indications

Artiblood is FDA approved for the short-term replacement of the oxygen-carrying capabilities of blood in patients who cannot use normal whole blood.[1] In addition, the product has been used successfully in cardiac catheter procedures, although this use is not FDA approved.[5] There is some early research into the use of the product as a plasma expansion product, but there is not enough information to support this use.[6]

Fakered is approved only for use in cardiac catheterization,[2] although it is commonly used as a blood replacement product in patients who cannot or will not use whole blood products.[7]

Evidence-Based Clinical Guidelines

A search of the literature was performed to identify evidence-based clinical guidelines. This included MEDLINE, *Embase Drugs and Pharmacology,* the National Guideline Clearinghouse web site, the American College of Cardiology (ACC) web site, and approximately a dozen Internet search engines; however, no applicable guidelines were identified.

Clinical Studies

Max and Sugar[6] conducted a comparison trial of artiblood (500 mL/d administered once over 1 hour in 80 patients) and fakered (750 mL administered once over 90 minutes in 82 patients) in patients (18 to 80 years of age) suffering from massive blood loss (>1 L), who could not use whole blood due to religious beliefs (e.g., Jehovah's Witnesses). In the artiblood group, all patients were undergoing open-heart surgery, as were 78 of the patients in the fakered group. The remainder of the fakered group consisted of gunshot wound patients. Patients with renal insufficiency (creatinine clearance <50 mL/min) or diagnosed with liver dysfunction were eliminated from consideration. Both groups were similar, except that the artiblood group had more smokers, which may have had an affect on oxygen requirements. Withdrawals from the artiblood group were for the following reasons: death due to failure of heart–lung machine (1 patient), noncompliance with protocol (10 patients), worsening symptoms (3 patients), and side effects (1 patient—vomiting). The authors noted that protocol compliance problems were due to inappropriate staff education and were not related to the drug itself. In the fakered group, withdrawals were due to side effects (1 patient—diarrhea, 1 patient—nausea, 1 patient—abdominal cramps) and noncompliance with protocol (2 patients). The patients were assessed on the following items: oxygen and carbon dioxide content of the blood (samples drawn immediately before and after administration, and every 4 hours for 24 hours), coagulation profile of patient (drawn within 2 hours before and after administration), effect on normal blood chemistry profiles (SMA-20) (drawn within 2 hours before and after administration), and time to discontinuation of supplemental oxygen to the patient. Adverse effects were also noted. Results were analyzed using appropriate statistical methods. Artiblood was found to increase the oxygen-carrying capabilities of the blood in comparison to fakered ($p <$ .01), although fakered did significantly improve oxygen-carrying capabilities over baseline ($p <$ .05). While fakered had minimal effect on blood chemistry and coagulation profile, it was noted that INRs were increased in patients receiving artiblood ($p <$ .001). Other adverse effects, mostly gastrointestinal in nature, were more common with fakered, although the symptoms typically disappeared within 2 hours of administration. Other measured characteristics seemed similar between the two groups. The authors concluded that artiblood was the superior agent, due to increased oxygen-carrying capabilities. The authors downplayed adverse effects, although the affects on INRs do appear worrisome.

[Other studies would be covered here for all likely uses within an institution.]

Bioavailability/Pharmacokinetics[16–18]

Absorption
Absorption is not applicable, because these agents are administered by IV infusion.

Distribution
Artiblood is found in the blood stream, with little being distributed to the tissues. Approximately 5% of fakered is found in the liver, with the rest being in the bloodstream.

Metabolism

Artiblood is not metabolized in the body, whereas approximately 50% of fakered is broken down to inactive components and is excreted in the bile.

Elimination

Artiblood has a half-life of 5 to 15 hours. It is excreted unchanged in the urine. The longer half-life is seen in patients with renal insufficiency. Because the drug is usually given as a single dose, renal insufficiency does not pose a significant problem. Fakered has a half-life of 4 to 7 hours in normal patients. Significant renal or hepatic impairment may double the half-life.

Dosage Forms

Large-Volume Parenteral

- Artiblood—500 mL IV bags
- Fakered—500, 750, and 1000 mL IV bags

No other forms or strengths available.

Dosage Range

The normal dose of artiblood for blood replacement is 500 mL, which may be repeated once after 4 hours. Doses may be cut in half for patients weighing less than 50 kg. No dosage adjustments are necessary in renal or hepatic impairment. The product has not been tested in patients younger than 12 years of age and is not recommended in that population. No dosage adjustment is necessary in the elderly.[1]

Fakered is given in doses of 500 mL to 1 L, with a maximum daily dose of 1.5 L. The dose is adjusted based on clinical response of the patient. The product can be used in patients as young as 6 years of age; however, the initial dose is 250 mL.[2]

Known Adverse Effects/Toxicities

The two agents are compared in the following table.

Adverse Effect	Artiblood (% of patients)	Fakered (% of patients)
Gastrointestinal		
Nausea	20	7
. . .	. . .	. . .

Special Precautions

Neither drug has been studied long term; therefore, the effects are not known.

Both products are considered Pregnancy Category C. Tests in pregnant animals have shown adverse effects and no adequate, well-controlled studies have been conducted in humans. There is no information available on the excretion of the drug in human milk. Overall, when considering use in pregnant or lactating women, the physician must consider the benefits versus the risks.

Safety and effectiveness of artiblood in children have not been established, although fakered may be used in children at least 6 years old.

Contraindications

Both agents are contraindicated in patients with hypersensitivities to the drug or any component of the dosage form.

Drug Interactions

Drug–Drug Interactions

Heparin—Effects of heparin or low-molecular-weight heparins may be significantly increased by either artificial blood replacement agent, although the effect of artiblood tends to be greater. There is no effect on either artiblood or fakered, although heparin may improve circulation of the products to underperfused tissues.

[Other interactions for both drugs would be listed and compared.]

Drug–Food Interactions

None are known or expected, because these agents are given intravenously and do not undergo enterohepatic recirculation.

Drug–Laboratory Test Interactions

INR—INRs can be increased by both agents, although the effect is more noticeable with artiblood.

[Other interactions for both drugs would be listed and compared.]

Patient Monitoring Guidelines

Monitor patient for objective evidence of effectiveness (e.g., oxygen content of blood and clinical effects). Obtain baseline INR and normal chemistry values, and monitor regularly. Monitor for adverse effects.

Patient Information

In a patient receiving the product due to trauma, it is likely that he or she will not be able to be given information. In that case, provide the information to the next of kin or guardian. Inform patients that the product is an intravenous product that does not contain any blood products. The patient or family should know that he or she may receive this product once or more during the first day after surgery. The patient or family should be informed that the drug has few noticeable adverse effects other than some gastrointestinal upset; however, the physician or pharmacist should be consulted if anything unusual occurs. The patient or family should know that some blood tests will be regularly performed to exclude the possibility of adverse effects. The nurse will keep the drug refrigerated until approximately 30 minutes before infusion. Warnings about missed doses are irrelevant.

Cost Comparison

General Pricing Information

	AWP (per bag)	Daily Dose*	St. AMC (per bag)	Daily Dose*
Artiblood 500 mL	$2500	$2500	$2310	$2310
Fakered 500 mL	$1000	$1000	$800	$800
Fakered 750 mL	$1500	$1500	$1200	$1200
Fakered 1000 mL	$2000	$2000	$1600	$1600

*Assume used one bag of each strength.

Pharmacoeconomic Analysis

Problem Definition—The objective of this analysis is to determine which artificial blood product should be included on our drug formulary.

Perspective—This will be from the perspective of the institution.

Specific treatment alternatives and outcomes—There are two drugs to be compared, artiblood and fakered. It will be assumed that natural blood products are not an alternative, because the ability to use natural products would preclude consideration of the artificial products. The outcomes to be measured are hospital costs.

Pharmacoeconomic model—A cost–benefit analysis will be performed. A cost–utility analysis would be desirable, but insufficient information is available. *Note:* no published pharmacoeconomic analysis is available. The following is based on information obtained from the literature concerning efficacy, adverse effects, monitoring, and so on and uses St. AMC costs, because outside prices would be irrelevant.

	Cost per patient	Benefit-to-Cost Ratio	Net Benefit
Cost of artiblood (including administration, monitoring, adverse reactions, etc.)	$5120	$7430/$5120 = 1.45:1	$7430 − $5120 = $2310
Benefits of artiblood (money saved by early patient discharge from ICU)	$7430		
Cost of fakered (including administration, monitoring, adverse reactions, etc.)	$4000	$4500/$4000 = 1.125:1	$4500 − $4000 = $500
Benefits of fakered (money saved by early patient discharge from ICU)	$4500		

[*Note:* The above information is a summary of information, including averages, decision analysis, and sensitivity analysis that would be used in a pharmacoeconomic evaluation. Although the details could be presented here, that may be distracting and confusing to some readers; a decision must be made as to whether all of the details will be presented. See Chap. 8 for details on how to prepare a pharmacoeconomic analysis of a drug being evaluated by the P&T Committee.]

Presented by John Q. Doe, PharmD to the Pharmacy and Therapeutics Committee on February 30, 20XX.

References

[References would be listed in the order in which they are cited in the text—see Appendix 11–2.]

15–1

Appendix 15–1

Comparison of Quality Assurance and Total Quality Management in Health Care

Comparison	TQM Approach	QA Approach
Purpose	Improve quality of all services/products for all patients and customers	Improve quality of patient care
Scope	All systems and processes (clinical and nonclinical)	Clinical systems and processes
	Actions directed to improving processes	Actions directed toward improving people
Leadership	All clinical and nonclinical leadership	Physicians and clinical leadership
Aims	Continuous improvements if no problems are identified	Problem solving
	Focus on common causes of failed quality	Identify individuals whose performance or outcomes are outside expectations
Focus	Process improvement and people	Individuals (peer review)
	Improve performance of everyone	Training or elimination of unacceptable few
	Prevention and process design	Inspection
	Customers are everyone involved in the system	Customers are patients, professionals, and review organizations
Customers and requirements	Measures based on customers and professionals	Measures established by health professionals
Methods	Brainstorming	Audits
	Nominal group technique	Nominal group technique
	Force field analysis	Hypothesis testing
	Coaching/mentoring	
	Flowcharts	
	Pareto charts	
	Cause-and-effect diagrams	

	Run chart	
	Control chart	
	Histogram	
	Scatter diagram	
	Stratification	
	Quality function deployment	
People involved	Everyone	Quality assurance committee/staff
	Actions are decided by a team with no time constraints	Actions decided by committees appointed for a specified time period
Outcomes	Improves performance for everyone involved in the process	Improves individual performance
	Reduces threats	Creates defensiveness
	Promotes team effort and eliminates territoriality	
Continuing activities	Continual process improvement through monitoring	Monitors deviations and actions occur when deviations occur

15-2

Tools Used in Quality Improvement

FLOWCHARTS

Flowcharts illustrate the steps of a process and how the steps are related to each other. They can be used to describe the process, increase a team's knowledge of the entire process, identify weaknesses or breakdown points in the current process, or design a new process. An example of a flowchart outlining how adverse reactions might be addressed within an organization appears on the next page.

PARETO CHART

Pareto charts are vertical bar graphs with the data presented so that the bars are arranged from left to right on the horizontal axis in order of decreasing frequency. This arrangement helps to identify which problems to address in what order. By addressing the data represented in the tallest bars (e.g., the most frequently occurring problems or contributing factors), efforts can be focused on areas where the most gain can be realized. Pareto charts are commonly used to identify issues to address, delineate potential causes of a problem, and monitor improvements in processes. An example of a Pareto chart appears below. This example illustrates frequently occurring factors contributing

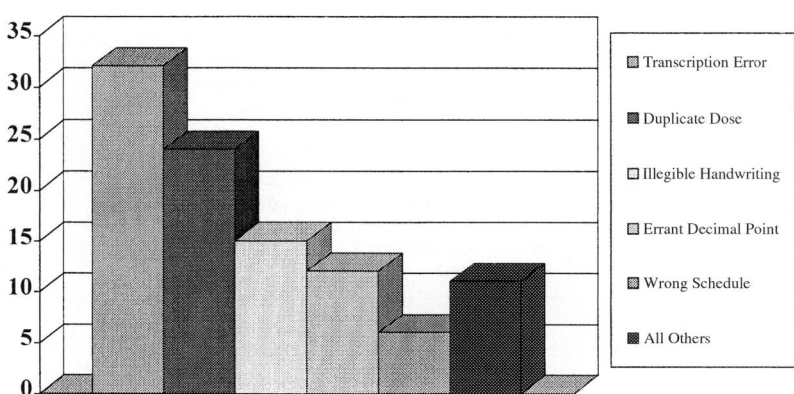

Flowchart: Suspected Adverse Drug Reactions

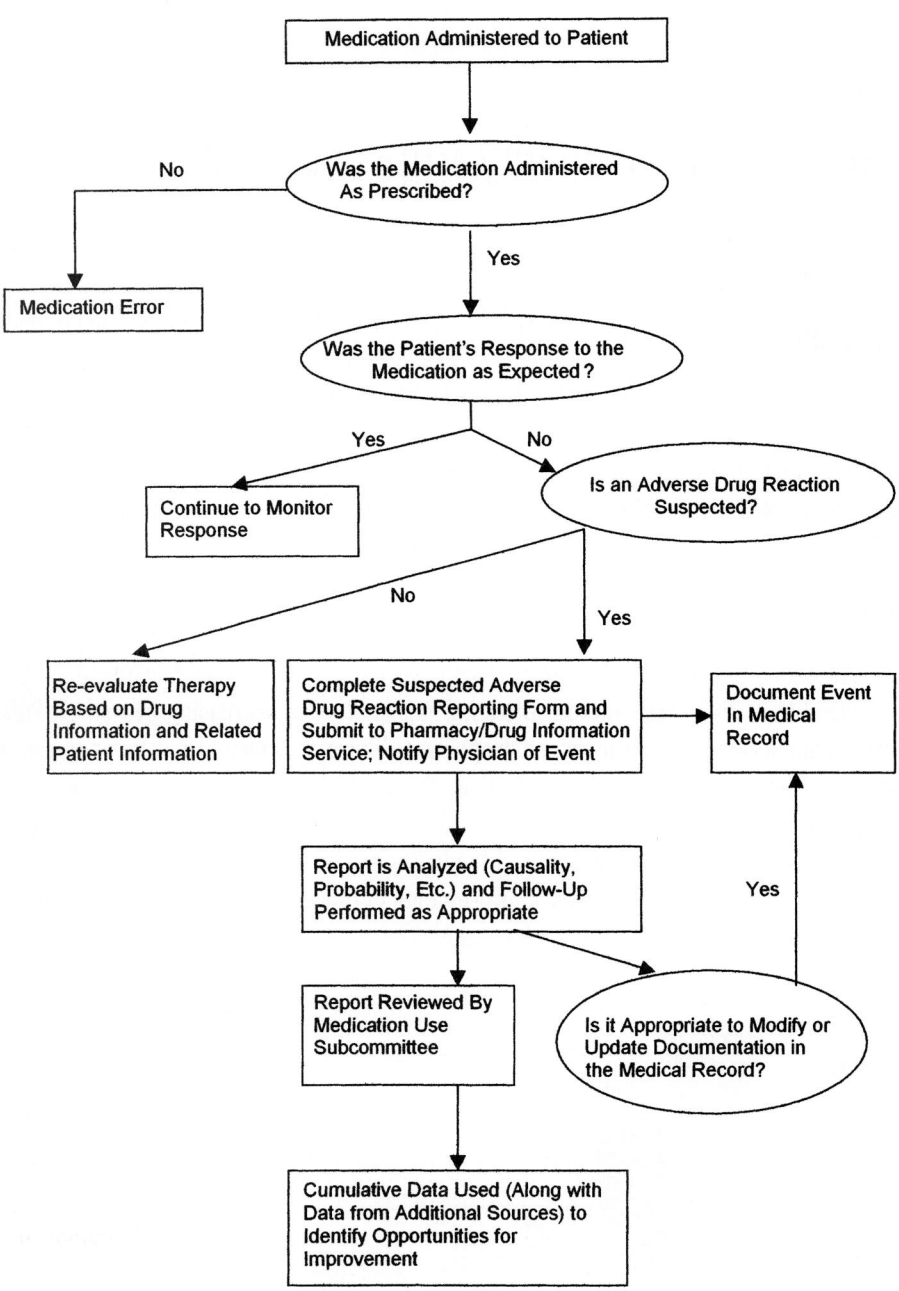

to improper dose medication errors. By focusing on transcription errors as a contributing factor on which to focus quality improvement efforts, the quality improvement team will generally gain more than by tackling the smaller bars.

FISHBONE OR CAUSE-AND-EFFECT DIAGRAM

Fishbone or cause-and-effect diagrams represent the relationship between an outcome (represented at the head of the fish) and the possible causes of the outcome (represented as the bones of the fish). The bones of the fish should represent causes and not symptoms of the issue. Fishbone diagrams are commonly used to identify components of a process to address, delineate potential causes of a problem, or identify practitioner groups that participate in producing an outcome and should be represented in the group addressing quality issues in the process(es). An example of a fishbone chart appears below.

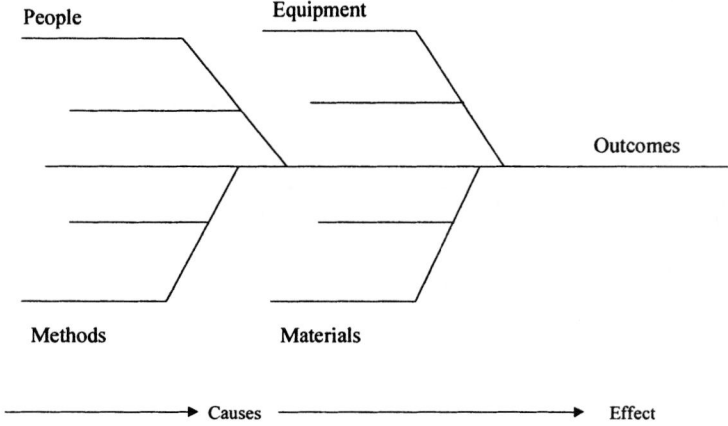

CONTROL CHARTS

Control charts are run charts or line graphs with defined allowable limits of variation. Data are plotted on the graph as they become available, with new data points connected to older data by a continuous line. The x-axis is usually a measure of time. The control limits help to identify which variations in data are important. Control limits are statistically determined based on average ranges and sample size. Fluctuation in data points above and below the average is expected and is referred to as "common variation" or "common cause" as long as they remain between the control limits. Data points above the upper control limit or below the lower control limit are referred to as "special variation" or "special cause." Special cause variation indicates that something different is going on outside the normal operation of the process. Also, a series of data points above or below average may indicate a trend in performance that may need to be addressed. As variability in a process is reduced by quality improvement efforts, control limits should be recalculated (and narrowed) based on ongoing data. An example of a control chart appears below. Calls from pharmacists to prescribers in response to questions or issues related to new medication orders are represented over a 6-month period. Data from the month of July indicate a significant increase in the number of calls made. A quality improvement team evaluating these data would then attempt to identify what contributed to this increase. A potential cause in many institutions might be the influx of new medical housestaff into the organization each July. One potential intervention to reduce this special cause is to improve the orientation of new practitioners to the medication use process within the organization.

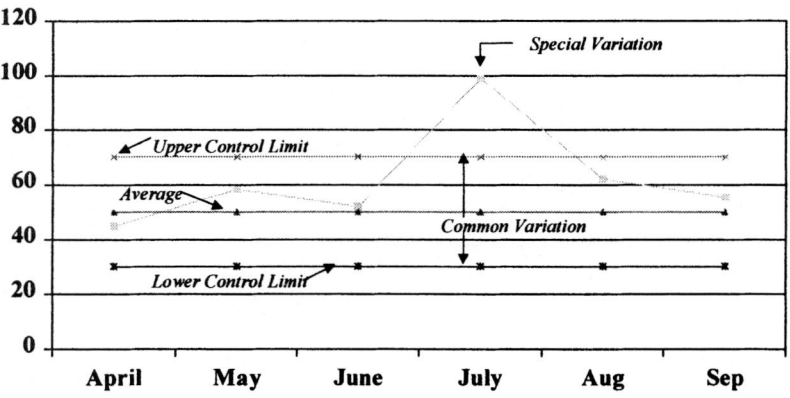

Appendix 15–3

Examples of Approaches to Quality Improvement

SMART PROBLEM SOLVING PROCESS

Statement: Written statement outlining problem or opportunity for improvement
Selection of problem
Definition of problem in measurable terms

Measurement: Collection of baseline data based on most influential factors
Determine what needs to be known about the problem
Develop data collection methods, compile data

Analysis: Analyze data and identify causes
Outline root causes of problems
Evaluate collected data to identify causes of specific outcomes

Remedy: Generate solutions and implement action
Identify action(s) needed to address root causes and implement

Test: Assess impact of corrective action(s)
Reassess (collect data) to determine if improvement has occurred

FOCUS-PDCA

Find a Process to Improve

Review of data, brainstorming a list of processes, and/or customer feedback can be used to identify processes in need of improvement.

Organize the Team

Team membership should include those who participate in the process and who are most familiar with its day to day function.

Clarify the Current Process

It is essential that team members understand how the process currently works. Flow-charts are useful tools to achieve this objective.

Understand the Current Process

Once the process is understood, causes of variation are identified. These could also be described as breakdowns of flaws in the process. Fishbone diagrams are useful tools to identify causes of variation.

This step also includes data collection on the process and more specifically, the variations identified. Check sheets, Pareto charts, histograms, and control charts are useful to display data.

Solution

Possible improvement solutions are then identified. Brainstorming and nominal group technique can be useful in this step.

Plan the Improvement

Plan who, what, when, where, and how solutions will be implemented. Also, determine what data will be needed to verify that the improvement has occurred.

Do the Improvement

Following appropriate coordination and training, implement the improvement solution.

Check the Results

Collect data to evaluate the effectiveness of the solution. These results should be compared to baseline data (obtained in the Understand the Current Process step). The same tools mentioned above can be useful in displaying this data.

Act on Results

If results were as expected, the new process should be standardized. If the results were not as expected, return to the Solution step to select an alternative solution and continue through the remaining steps. This cycle is repeated until the process improvement is achieved.

TEN-STEP PROCESS

1. Assign responsibility for monitoring and evaluation.
2. Delineate scope of care and service provided by the organization.
3. Identify important aspects of care and service provided by the organization.
4. Identify indicators, data sources, and collection methods to monitoring important aspects of care.
5. Establish means to trigger evaluation (e.g., trends or patterns of use, thresholds, etc.).
6. Collect and organize data.
7. Initiate evaluation of care (as indicated by triggers set in Step 5).
8. Take actions to improve care and service.
9. Assess the effectiveness of actions and maintain the improvement; document improvements in care.
10. Communicate results to relevant individuals and groups.

Appendix 15–4

Example of a Quality Improvement Activity Plan

The following components should be included in the presentation of a proposal.

1. A description of the aspect of care to be assessed including historical background if appropriate (e.g., if this is a follow-up to a previous evaluation).
2. A description of the group responsible for developing the criteria, indicators, guidelines, and so forth to be used in the evaluation.
3. The proposed criteria or indicators and performance expectations.
4. A summary of the data collection methods, case identification methods, time frame for data collection, and minimal cases to be evaluated.
5. The proposed reporting channels and frequency of reports.

EXAMPLE OF CRITERIA AND REQUEST FOR APPROVAL

Medication Use Evaluation Criteria

Antiemetic Use in the Prophylaxis of Chemotherapy-induced Nausea and Vomiting

Request for Approval by Medication Use Evaluation Committee

Purpose of evaluation: The purpose of this Medication Use Evaluation (MUE) is to evaluate the use of antiemetic therapy in the prevention of chemotherapy-induced nausea and vomiting. This agent was selected for evaluation based on its essential role in the management of this patient population, potential inappropriate use, and increased cost relative to other antiemetic agents. This class of medications has not been evaluated within the organization for at least 5 years.

Criteria: A multidisciplinary group including physicians, clinical nurse specialists, staff nurses from the oncology unit, and pharmacists developed the attached criteria. They are submitted to the MUE Committee for approval.

Data collection: Data will be collected on all patients with orders for this agent written throughout a period of approximately 30 days beginning in mid-January 2000. A minimum of 50 cases will be reviewed. Pharmacists and clinical nurse specialists will collect data concurrently from the medical record. Patients will be identified by means of the pharmacy information system.

Results: Results will be presented to this committee. Information will also be shared with the Cancer Care Committee and Hospital Quality Improvement Council. Prescriber-specific results will be confidentially provided to Medical Staff Support for use in the reappointment/recredentialing process.

MEDICATION USE EVALUATION CRITERIA

ANTIEMETIC USE IN THE PROPHYLAXIS OF CHEMOTHERAPY-INDUCED NAUSEA AND VOMITING

Name _____ RM _____ Age _____ Sex _____ WT _____ HT _____

Allergies _____ Service _____

Chemo/Dose/Date/Time _____ Attending MD: _____

Medication-Use Process Elements	Standard (%)	Exceptions
Prescribing		
A. Indication—Antiemetic (IV or PO)		
1. No other drug and nondrug causes of preexisting nausea and vomiting identified.	95	A2a) Pt receiving other less emetic cancer chemotherapy regimen and not responsive to other antiemetics. Chemo/Dose: Other antiemetic/Dose:
2. Prevention of acute nausea and vomiting during the first 24 hours following the initiation of highly or moderately highly emetogenic cancer chemotherapy regimens:	95	
a) Highly emetogenic (>90%): cisplatin, dacarbazine, mechlorethamine, streptozocin, cytarabine (>500 mg/m^2);		A2b) Pt has had significant documented adverse reactions to alternative antiemetics and is receiving a regimen with a lesser emetogenic potential.
b) Moderately high (60–90%): carmustine, lomustine, cyclophosphamide, dactinomycin, plicamycin, procarbazine, methotrexate (>200 mg/m^2) *or*		
3. Prevention of anticipatory nausea and vomiting associated with any chemotherapy regimen.		
Dispensing/administering		
A. Dosage—IV antiemetic		
1. 0.4 mg/kg infused over 15 min begun 30 min prior to initiation of chemotherapy regimen; then two additional doses given 4 and 8 hours after first dose of therapy *or*	95	Dosage reduced by 50% in patients with significant renal dysfunction (i.e., measured or estimated creatinine clearance <25 mL/min)
2. A single 85-mg dose infused over 15 min begun 30 min prior to initiation of chemotherapy regimen.		
B. Dosage—oral antiemetic		
1. 20 mg administered 30 min before chemotherapy is initiated, second dose 8 hours after first dose. Continue therapy bid for 1–2 days after completion of therapy.	95	
Monitoring		Preventive and/or responsive management:
Adverse Effects		
1. Headache	<15	• Identify other drug and nondrug causes.
2. Diarrhea	<15	• Provide supportive and symptomatic therapy.
3. Constipation	<10	
4. Sedation	<10	
Outcome measures		2) Medical contraindications:
1. Prevention of nausea and emesis.	95	a) to continuation of chemotherapy.
2. Cancer chemotherapy course not interrupted by nausea and vomiting.	95	b) patient expired.
		c) lost to follow-up.

654

15–5

Example Report—Prescriber-Specific Results

Prescriber-specific reports from MUE activities should be provided for use in the reappointment/recredentialing process. It is important that these reports contain sufficient information to facilitate peer review. A summary of all cases involving the prescriber should be included in the report including a brief description of cases in which criteria were not met. A mechanism to access the medical record (e.g., a medical record number) should be provided to allow chart review if needed.

PRESCRIBER-SPECIFIC INFORMATION FOR USE IN REAPPOINTMENT/RECREDENTIALING

Source: Medication Use Evaluation (MUE) Committee

Evaluation Topic: Antiemetic Medication Use Evaluation

Dates of Evaluation: January 2000

Data Enclosed:

    a. Summary of overall results reviewed by MUE Committee and actions taken by the Committee (see attached)
    b. Criteria used in evaluation (see attached, approved by MUE Committee prior to data collection)
    c. Prescriber-specific results (below)

1. Table outlining patient case number, medical record number, diagnosis, attending physician (by first letters of last name followed by ID #), and criteria not met (when applicable) for all patients managed by this attending during the evaluation period.
2. Any other prescriber-specific correspondence, and so on, from the Committee.

Results for Attending Physician #12345

Attending #	Case #	Medrec #	Diagnosis	Criteria Not Met
12345	43	54321	OVARIAN CA	
12345	44	43215	BREAST CA	Dosing
12345	55	32154	SMALL CELL CA/LIVER METS	Dosing
12345	58	15432	MET BREAST CA	Outcome
12345	59	53215	MET BREAST CA	
12345	71	42153	AML	Outcome
12345	121	15342	OVARIAN CA	

Summary of cases where dosing criteria not met
- Case #44 did not meet dosing criteria. Patient received 85 mg IV antiemetic on chemotherapy day 1 (cisplatinum and VP16) then 85 mg in 24 hours on day 2 (VP 16 only).
- Case #55 did not meet dosing criteria. Patient received 85 mg IV antiemetic on chemotherapy day 1 (cisplatinum and VP16) then 85 mg in 24 hours on day 2 (VP 16 only).

MUE Committee action taken (specific to this prescriber): letter written to prescriber (copy attached).

Summary of cases where outcome criteria not met
- Case #58 did not meet outcome criteria (i.e., prevention of nausea and vomiting). Patient experienced nausea/vomiting × 1 less than 24 h following antiemetic dose (85 mg IV × 1).
- Case #71 did not meet outcome criteria (i.e., prevention of nausea and vomiting). Patient received 85 mg IV antiemetic QD × 6 days. On sixth day had one episode nausea.

MUE Committee action taken (specific to this prescriber): none

Appendix 15–6

Example of MUE Results

MEDICATION USE EVALUATION

Summary of Overall Results

Antiemetic: January 2000

Background: This topic was selected based on high use, potential misuse, and high cost of these agents. Criteria for this evaluation were approved at the MUE Committee's December 1999 meeting. Please refer to attached criteria for additional information.

Total Patients Evaluated (All Indications for Use) = 52

Element	Standard	Results	Compliance
Prescribing			
Indication for use	95%	Overall results	
		Treatment/prevention of nausea/vomiting associated with chemotherapy	100% (52/52)
		Highly emetogenic chemotherapy	46/46
		Anticipatory N/V associated with chemotherapy	6/6
Dispensing/administering			
Dosing	95%	Overall results	71% (37/52)
		Highly emetogenic chemotherapy	31/46
		Anticipatory N/V associated with chemotherapy	6/6
Monitoring			
Adverse drug reaction(s)	≤10–25% (varies with ADR)	Overall results	4% (2/52)
		Headache: 1 patient	
		Constipation: 1 patient	

Outcome			
Prevention of nausea and emesis	95%	Overall results	92% (46/50)*
		Highly emetogenic chemotherapy	41/44
		Anticipatory N/V associated with chemotherapy	5/6
Chemotherapy course not interrupted	95%	Overall results (all indications)	100% (52/52)

*Includes only patients in whom outcome was documented. Outcome was not assessed in two patients who were discharged immediately following administration of chemotherapy.

Summary of Results

Prescribing: Criteria for indication for use were met in all cases.

Dispensing/Administering: Criteria for dosing were met in 37 of 52 cases with all cases involving anticipatory nausea and vomiting meeting criteria.

In 15 cases, patients receiving the antiemetic prior to highly emetogenic chemotherapy received doses not included in the approved criteria. Five of these patients received doses based on an investigational protocol. This dose is now under consideration by the FDA for approval and preliminary results (available only in abstract form) were recently presented at the American Society of Clinical Oncology meeting. Results with the new dosing regimen have been comparable to those with the currently approved doses.

In seven cases not meeting dosing criteria, patients received a single dose prior to chemotherapy consistent with the criteria. However, an additional dose was administered 24 hours after the first dose. Two prescribers wrote these orders.

Two cases did not meet dosing criteria because the dose was not adjusted based on renal dysfunction. In both cases, the estimated creatinine clearance was between 20 and 25 mL/min and nephrotoxic drugs were not being administered concurrently. In both cases, the estimated creatinine clearance increased to 30 mL/min or more by day 2 of the admission (probably due to rehydration of the patient). Neither patient experienced adverse effects.

One dose was not administered within the appropriate time frame. In this case, the antiemetic dose was administered just 5 minutes prior to the initiation of chemotherapy administration. The nurse administering the antiemetic documented its administration on the way to the patient's room. When she arrived, the patient was not in the room. The dose was administered after he was located, approximately 25 minutes later. The nurse did not correct the actual administration time until after a second nurse administered the chemotherapy.

Recommendations
1. Add new dosing regimen to dosing criteria.
2. Send letters to prescribers giving extra dose.
3. Renal dosing was not significantly outside guidelines. Mention findings in report to be published in quality improvement newsletter but do not take prescriber-specific action.
4. The dose administered late was reported via an incident report; no further action by this group is required at this time.

Monitoring: The rate of adverse drug reactions was less than that reported in the literature. This might be reflective of underreporting and underdocumenting of adverse drug events.

Recommendations
1. The Adverse Drug Event Task Force is currently implementing a new process to improve reporting and documentation. No specific action by this group is required at this time.

Outcome: Ninety-two percent of patients did not experience nausea or vomiting. Outcome was assessable in 50 patients; two patients were discharged immediately following the administration of chemotherapy.

The patient who received his antiemetic dose just 5 minutes prior to chemotherapy experienced moderate nausea and no vomiting. Otherwise, the occurrence of nausea and vomiting was not related to problems with administration or dosing.

Recommendations
1. 92% success rate is acceptable based on literature; no action is necessary.

General Recommendations

1. After approval, implement recommendations presented above.
2. Publish results in the *Quality Improvement Newsletter* following review by the Cancer Care Committee and the Quality Improvement Committee.
3. Perform a follow-up evaluation focusing on dosing issues.
4. Initiate planned assessment of this agent's use in post-operative nausea and vomiting as soon as possible.

Note to reader: An example of a prescriber-specific report for reappointment/recredentialing appears in Appendix 15–5.

Quality Evaluation—Response to Drug Information Request

Request # _____   Date of Request _____

Response by (circle one):   DI Staff   Resident   Student

Caller (circle type):   MD   RPh   Nurse   Other:

Assessment of Search and Response to Request

	Yes	No	NA	Standard %*
1. Is requestor's demographic information complete?				100%
2. Background information is:				
A. thorough				100%
B. appropriate to request				
3. Is the question clearly stated?				100%
4. Search Strategy/References				
A. Appropriate references were used				100%
B. Search was sufficiently comprehensive				
C. Is search strategy clearly documented				
5. Response				
A. was appropriate for the situation				
B. answered the question				100%
C. was provided in a timely manner				
D. was integrated with available patient data				
E. was supported by appropriate materials supplied to requestor				

6. If complete response could not be
   provided within time frame
   requested, was requestor advised as   100%
   to the status of their request and the
   anticipated delivery of the final
   response?

*If performance falls below 90% in any category during any month, the service director will coordinate an assessment of the process and report findings and actions taken to the Pharmacy Quality Improvement Council.

Comments:

Reviewed by: _____

16-1

Appendix 16–1

Kramer Questionnaire*

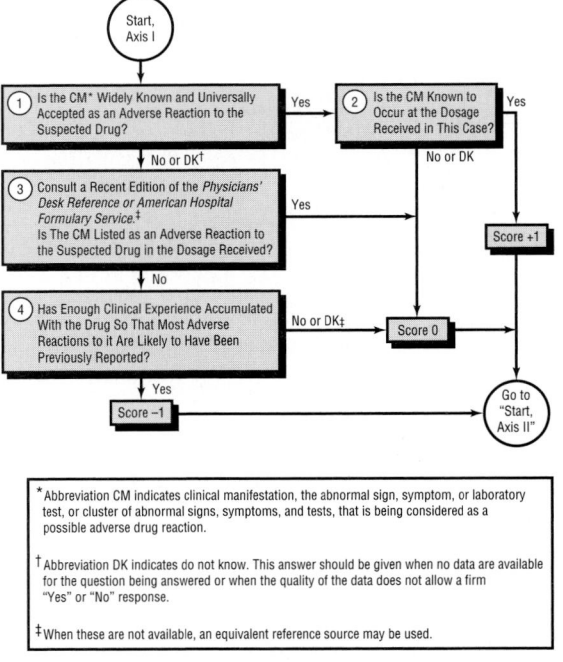

Figure 1. Axis I. Previous general experience with drug.

*Kramer MS, Leventhal JM, Hutchinson TA, Feinstein AR. An algorithm for the operational assessment of adverse drug reaction: I. background, descriptions, and instructions for use. JAMA 1979; 242(7):623–32.

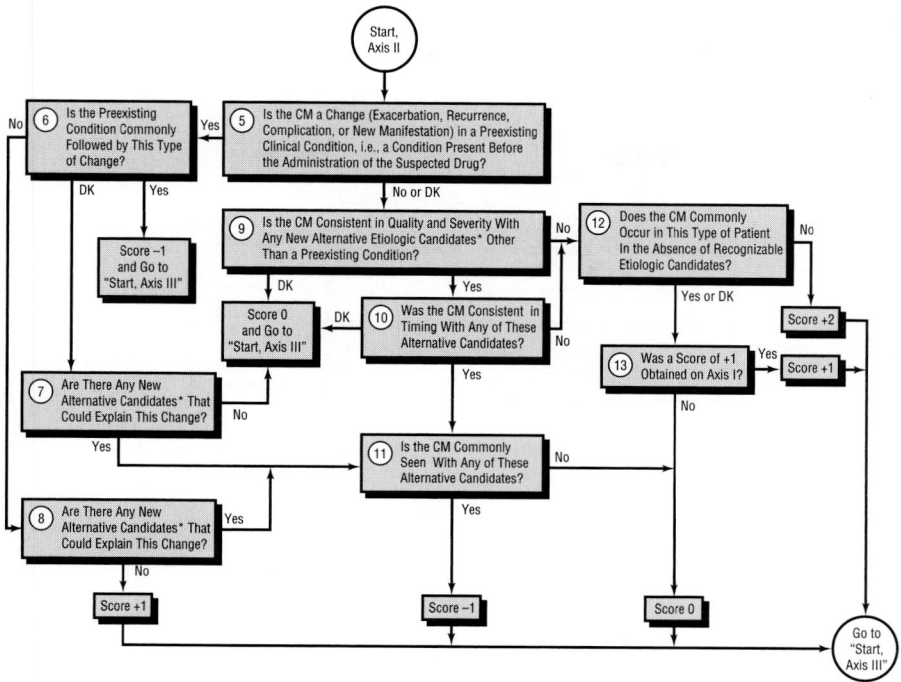

Figure 2. Axis II. Alternative etiologic candidates. For explanation of abbreviations, see Axis I.

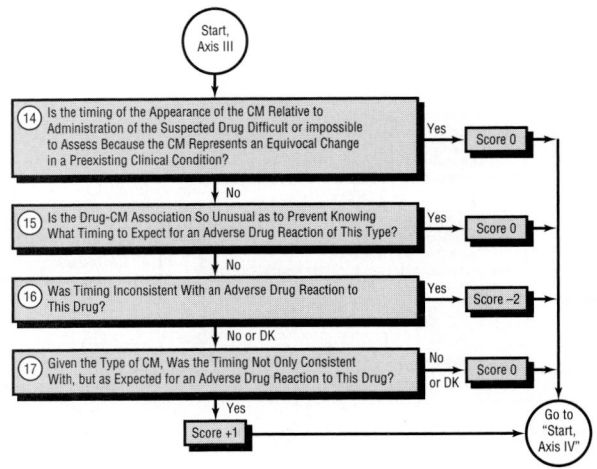

Figure 3. Axis III. Timing of events. For explanation of abbreviations, see Axis I.

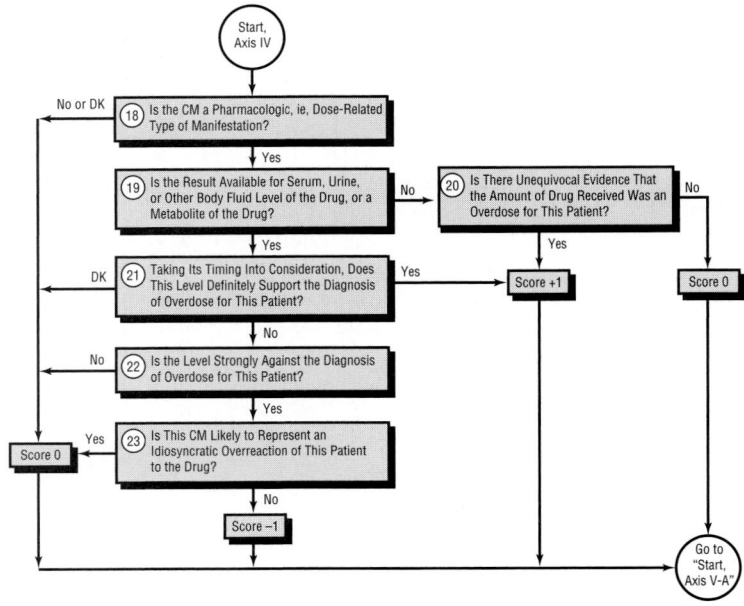

Figure 4. Axis IV. Drug levels and evidence of overdose. For explanation of abbreviations, see Axis I.

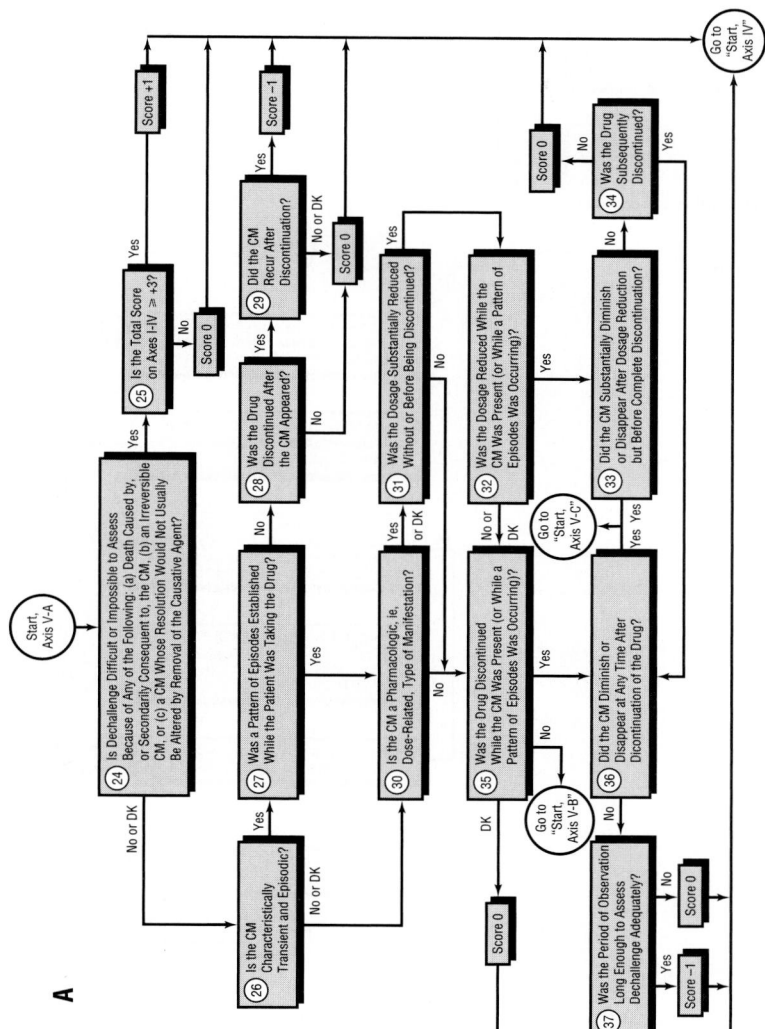

Figure 5A. Axis V-A. Dechallenge: Difficult assessments. For explanation of abbreviations, see Axis I.

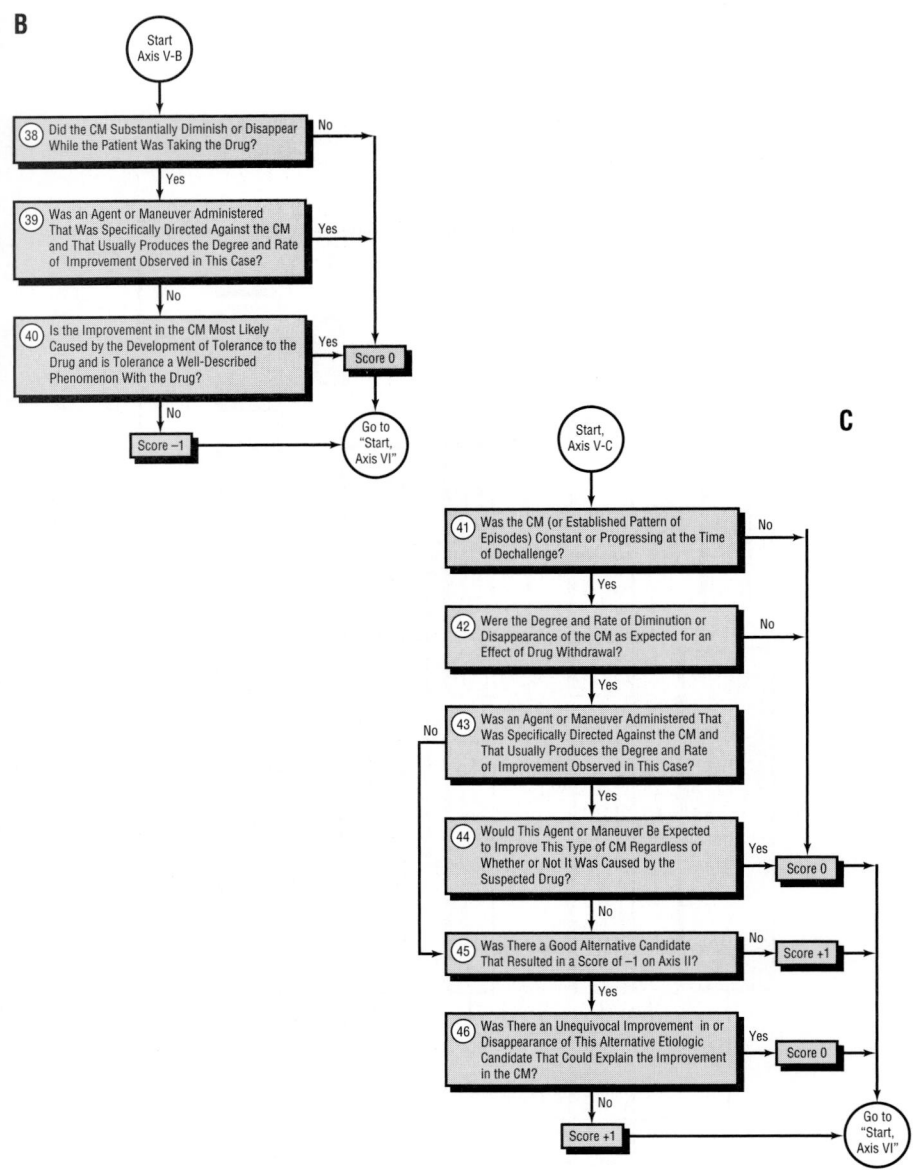

Figure 5B. Axis V-B. Dechallenge: Absence of dechallenge. For explanation of abbreviations, see Axis I.
C. Axis V-C. Dechallenge: Improvement after dechallenge. For explanation of abbreviations, see Axis I.

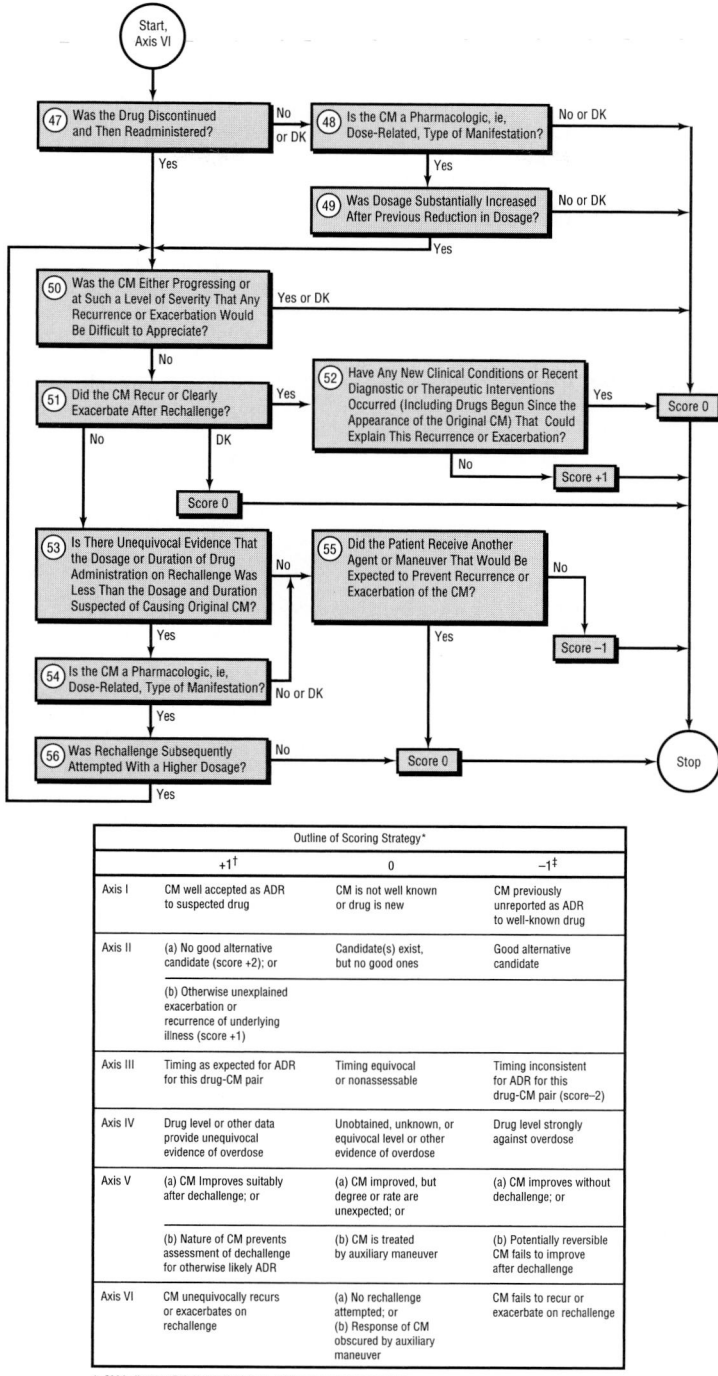

Figure 6. Axis VI. Rechallenge. For explanation of abbreviations, see Axis I.

Appendix 16–2

Naranjo Algorithm*

To assess the adverse drug reaction, please answer the following questionnaire and give the pertinent score.

	Yes	No	Don't Know	Score
1. Are there previous *conclusive* reports on this reaction?	+1	0	0	
2. Did the adverse event appear after the suspected drug was administered?	+2	–1	0	
3. Did the adverse reaction improve when the drug was discontinued or a *specific* antagonist was administered?	+1	0	0	
4. Did the adverse reaction reappear when the drug was readministered?	+2	–1	0	
5. Are there alternative causes (other than the drug) that could on their own have caused the reaction?	–1	+2	0	
6. Did the reaction reappear when a placebo was given?	–1	+1	0	
7. Was the drug detected in the blood (or other fluids) in concentrations known to be toxic?	+1	0	0	
8. Was the reaction more severe when the dose was increased, or less severe when the dose was decreased?	+1	0	0	
9. Did the patient have a similar reaction to the same or similar drugs in *any* previous exposure?	+1	0	0	
10. Was the adverse event confirmed by any objective evidence?	+1	0	0	

Total Score_____

Score Interpretation
__Definite = ≥9
__Probable = 5–8
__Possible = 1–4
__Doubtful = ≤0

*Naranjo CA, Busto U, Sellers EM, Sandor P, Ruiz I, Roberts EA, et al. A method of estimating the probability of adverse drug reactions. Clin Pharmacol Ther 1981; 30(2):239–45.

16-3

Jones Algorithm*

START HERE:**

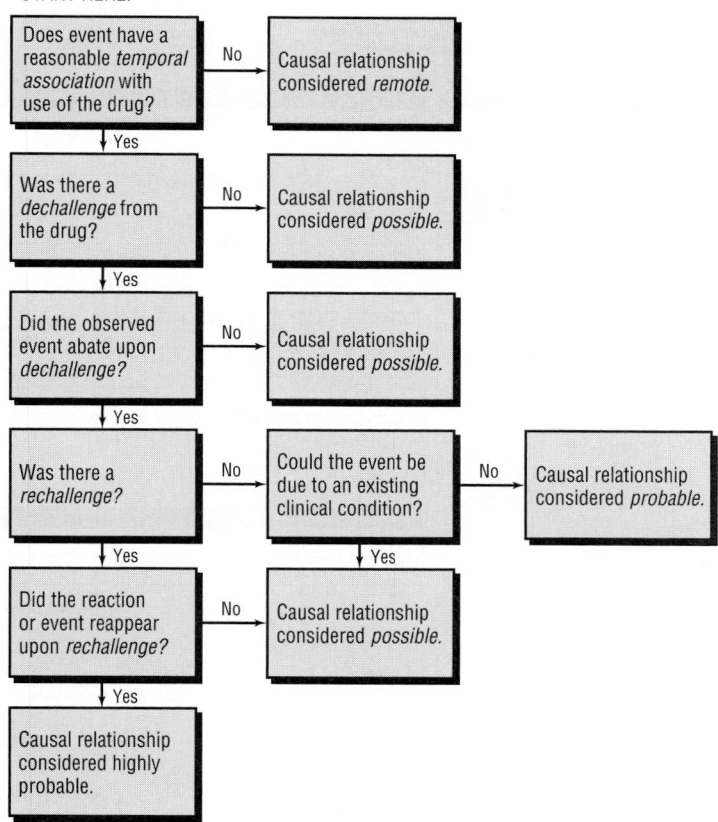

**Each drug is carried through independently; if > 1 drug was dechallenged or rechallenged simultaneously causality for all is ≤ possible.

QUESTIONS:

1. Did the reaction follow a reasonable temporal sequence?
2. Did the patient improve after stopping the drug?
3. Did the reaction reappear on repeated exposure (rechallenge)?
4. Could the reaction be reasonably explained by the known characteristics of the patient's *clinical state?*

*Jones JK. Adverse drug reactions in the community health setting: approaches to recognizing, counseling, and reporting. Clin Comm Health 1982; 5(2):58–67.

16-4

Appendix 16-4

MedWatch Form

MEDWATCH

THE FDA MEDICAL PRODUCTS REPORTING PROGRAM

For **VOLUNTARY** reporting by health professionals of adverse events and product problems

Page ___ of ___

Form Approved: OMB No. 0910-0291 Expires: 11/30/00
See OMB statement on reverse

FDA Use Only

Triage unit
sequence #

PLEASE TYPE OR USE BLACK INK

A. Patient information

1. Patient identifier

In confidence

2. Age at time of event:

or ___

Date of birth:

3. Sex
- [ ] female
- [ ] male

4. Weight
___ lbs
or
___ kgs

B. Adverse event or product problem

1. [ ] Adverse event   and/or   [ ] Product problem (e.g., defects/malfunctions)

2. Outcomes attributed to adverse event (check all that apply)
- [ ] death ___ (mo/day/yr)
- [ ] life-threatening
- [ ] hospitalization – initial or prolonged
- [ ] disability
- [ ] congenital anomaly
- [ ] required intervention to prevent permanent impairment/damage
- [ ] other:

3. Date of event (mo/day/yr)

4. Date of this report (mo/day/yr)

5. Describe event or problem

6. Relevant tests/laboratory data, including dates

7. Other relevant history, including preexisting medical conditions (e.g., allergies, race, pregnancy, smoking and alcohol use, hepatic/renal dysfunction, etc.)

C. Suspect medication(s)

1. Name (give labeled strength & mfr/labeler, if known)

#1

#2

2. Dose, frequency & route used

#1

#2

3. Therapy dates (if unknown, give duration) from/to (or best estimate)

#1

#2

4. Diagnosis for use (indication)

#1

#2

5. Event abated after use stopped or dose reduced

#1 [ ] yes [ ] no [ ] doesn't apply

#2 [ ] yes [ ] no [ ] doesn't apply

6. Lot # (if known)

#1

#2

7. Exp. date (if known)

#1

#2

8. Event reappeared after reintroduction

#1 [ ] yes [ ] no [ ] doesn't apply

#2 [ ] yes [ ] no [ ] doesn't apply

9. NDC # (for product problems only)
___ – ___ – ___

10. Concomitant medical products and therapy dates (exclude treatment of event)

D. Suspect medical device

1. Brand name

2. Type of device

3. Manufacturer name & address

4. Operator of device
- [ ] health professional
- [ ] lay user/patient
- [ ] other:

5. Expiration date (mo/day/yr)

6.
model # ___
catalog # ___
serial # ___
lot # ___
other # ___

7. If implanted, give date (mo/day/yr)

8. If explanted, give date (mo/day/yr)

9. Device available for evaluation? (Do not send to FDA)
- [ ] yes
- [ ] no
- [ ] returned to manufacturer on ___ (mo/day/yr)

10. Concomitant medical products and therapy dates (exclude treatment of event)

E. Reporter (see confidentiality section on back)

1. Name & address   phone #

2. Health professional? [ ] yes [ ] no

3. Occupation

4. Also reported to
- [ ] manufacturer
- [ ] user facility
- [ ] distributor

5. If you do NOT want your identity disclosed to the manufacturer, place an " X " in this box. [ ]

FDA

Mail to: MEDWATCH
5600 Fishers Lane
Rockville, MD 20852-9787

or FAX to:
1-800-FDA-0178

FDA Form 3500

Submission of a report does not constitute an admission that medical personnel or the product caused or contributed to the event.

ADVICE ABOUT VOLUNTARY REPORTING

Report experiences with:
- medications (drugs or biologics)
- medical devices (including in-vitro diagnostics)
- special nutritional products (dietary supplements, medical foods, infant formulas)
- other products regulated by FDA

Report SERIOUS adverse events. An event is serious when the patient outcome is:
- death
- life-threatening (real risk of dying)
- hospitalization (initial or prolonged)
- disability (significant, persistent or permanent)
- congenital anomaly
- required intervention to prevent permanent impairment or damage

Report even if:
- you're not certain the product caused the event
- you don't have all the details

Report product problems – quality, performance or safety concerns such as:
- suspected contamination
- questionable stability
- defective components
- poor packaging or labeling
- therapeutic failures

How to report:
- just fill in the sections that apply to your report
- use section C for all products except medical devices
- attach additional blank pages if needed
- use a separate form for each patient
- report either to FDA or the manufacturer (or both)

Important numbers:
- 1-800-FDA-0178   to FAX report
- 1-800-FDA-7737   to report by modem
- 1-800-FDA-1088   to report by phone or for more information
- 1-800-822-7967   for a VAERS form for vaccines

If your report involves a serious adverse event with a device and it occurred in a facility outside a doctor's office, that facility may be legally required to report to FDA and/or the manufacturer. Please notify the person in that facility who would handle such reporting.

Confidentiality: The patient's identity is held in strict confidence by FDA and protected to the fullest extent of the law. The reporter's identity, including the identity of a self-reporter, may be shared with the manufacturer unless requested otherwise. However, FDA will not disclose the reporter's identity in response to a request from the public, pursuant to the Freedom of Information Act.

The public reporting burden for this collection of information has been estimated to average 30 minutes per response, including the time for reviewing instructions, searching existing data sources, gathering and maintaining the data needed, and completing and reviewing the collection of information. Send comments regarding this burden estimate or any other aspect of this collection of information, including suggestions for reducing this burden to:

DHHS Reports Clearance Office
Paperwork Reduction Project (0910-0291)
Hubert H. Humphrey Building, Room 531-H
200 Independence Avenue, S.W.
Washington, DC 20201

"An agency may not conduct or sponsor, and a person is not required to respond to, a collection of information unless it displays a currently valid OMB control number."

Please DO NOT RETURN this form to this address.

U.S. DEPARTMENT OF HEALTH AND HUMAN SERVICES
Public Health Service • Food and Drug Administration

FDA Form 3500-back   **Please Use Address Provided Below – Just Fold In Thirds, Tape and Mail**

- -

**Department of
Health and Human Services**
Public Health Service
Food and Drug Administration
Rockville, MD 20857

Official Business
Penalty for Private Use $300

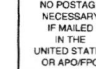

NO POSTAGE
NECESSARY
IF MAILED
IN THE
UNITED STATES
OR APO/FPO

BUSINESS REPLY MAIL
FIRST CLASS MAIL   PERMIT NO. 946   ROCKVILLE, MD

POSTAGE WILL BE PAID BY FOOD AND DRUG ADMINISTRATION

MEDWATCH
The FDA Medical Products Reporting Program
Food and Drug Administration
5600 Fishers Lane
Rockville, MD 20852-9787

Appendix 16-5

USP-ISMP Medication Error Reporting Program (MERP) Form

MEDI-CATION ERRORS

REPORTING PROGRAM

USP MEDICATION ERRORS REPORTING PROGRAM
Presented in cooperation with the Institute for Safe Medication Practices
The USP Practitioners' Reporting Network℠ is an FDA MEDWATCH partner

☐ ACTUAL ERROR ☐ POTENTIAL ERROR

Please describe the error. Include sequence of events, personnel involved, and work environment (e.g., code situation, change of shift, short staffing, no 24-hr. pharmacy, floor stock). If more space is needed, please attach separate page.

Was the medication administered to or used by the patient? ☐ No ☐ Yes   Date and time of event:_____

What type of staff or health care practitioner made the initial error? _____

Describe outcome (e.g., death, type of injury, adverse reaction). _____

If the medication did not reach the patient, describe the intervention. _____

Who discovered the error? _____

When and how was error discovered? _____

Where did the error occur (e.g., hospital, outpatient or retail pharmacy, nursing home, patient's home)? _____

Was another practitioner involved in the error ? ☐ No ☐ Yes If yes, what type of practitioner? _____

Was patient counseling provided? ☐ No ☐ Yes If yes, before or after error was discovered?_____

If a product was involved, please complete the following:

	Product #1	Product #2
Brand name of product involved		
Generic name		
Manufacturer		
Labeler (if different from mfr.)		
Dosage form		
Strength/concentration		
Type and size of container		
NDC number		

If available, please provide relevant patient information (age, gender, diagnosis, etc.). Patient identification not required.

Reports are most useful when relevant materials such as product label, copy of prescription/order, etc. can be reviewed.
Can these materials be provided? ☐ No ☐ Yes If yes, please specify. _____

Suggest any recommendations you have to prevent recurrence of this error or describe policies or procedures you have instituted to prevent future similar errors.

A copy of this report is routinely sent to the Institute for Safe Medication Practices (ISMP), to the manufacturer/labeler, and to the Food and Drug Administration (FDA). **USP may release my identity to: (check boxes that apply)**
☐ ISMP ☐ The manufacturer and/or labeler as listed above ☐ FDA ☐ Other persons requesting a copy of this report ☐ Anonymous to all

Your name and title

Your facility name, address, and ZIP

Telephone number
(include area code)

Signature

Date

Return to the attention of:
Diane D. Cousins, R.Ph.
USP PRN
12601 Twinbrook Parkway
Rockville, MD 20852-1790

Call Toll Free: 800-23-ERROR (800-233-7767)
or FAX 301-816-8532
USP home page: http://www.usp.org/prn

Date Received by USP:

File Access Number:

C-194
WEB pdf
10/14/97

Additional forms can be found in the *USP DI Vol. I* and *Vol. III* and in all monthly *Updates.*

MEDICATION ERRORS REPORTING PROGRAM

Medication Errors Do Occur

Medication errors can occur anywhere, any time along the drug therapy course, from prescribing through transcribing, dispensing, administering, and monitoring. An error can cause confusion, alarm, and frustration for the health care provider and for the patient. And YES, an error can even cause a death or injury to your patient. The causes of errors are many; for example, lack of product knowledge or training; poor communication; ambiguities in product names, directions for use, medical abbreviations, handwriting, or labeling; job stress; poor procedures or techniques; or patient misuse. Along this continuum, any health care professional may be the cause of or contribute to an actual or potential error.

A Safer Environment for Your Patients

It is important to recognize that health care providers learn from medication errors. By sharing your experience through the nationwide USP Medication Errors Reporting (MER) Program you help your colleagues to gain an understanding of why errors occur and how to prevent them. You can also have a positive impact on the quality of patient care and influence drug standards and information. When others are informed about an error, the chance of recurrence may be lessened. Education regarding medication errors assists health care professionals to avoid errors by recognizing the circumstances and causes of actual and potential errors.

Easy Access

Just call 800-233-7767 to reach a USP health care professional, who will take your report and respond to your concerns. Reports may also be submitted in writing or faxed. All reports are forwarded to the Food and Drug Administration, the product manufacturer/labeler when appropriate, the ISMP, and the USP Divisions of Standards and Information Development. If you wish to remain anonymous to any of these sources, the USP will act as your intermediary in all correspondence. While including your identity is optional, it does allow for appropriate follow-up with you to discuss your observations or provide feedback.

USP: A Partner in MEDWATCH

The USP Practitioners' Reporting Network is a partner in MEDWATCH, the FDA's medical products reporting program. As a partner, USP PRN contributes to the FDA's efforts to protect the public health by helping to identify serious adverse events for the agency. This means that your reported information is shared with the FDA on a daily basis, or immediately if necessary.

 The USP PRN® is designed to collect experiences and observations from health care providers through four separate reporting programs:

- The USP Drug Product Problem Reporting Program
- The USP Medication Errors Reporting Program
- The USP Drug Product Problem Reporting Program for Radiopharmaceuticals
- The USP Veterinary Practitioners' Reporting Program

The Institute for Safe Medication Practices, the Society of Nuclear Medicine, and the American Veterinary Medical Association cooperate in presenting the USP PRN.

Your Input Could Make the Difference!

USP PRN...CALL US WHEN YOU NEED US.

SINCE 1820
U.S. Pharmacopeia
12601 Twinbrook Parkway,
Rockville, MD 20852-1790

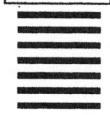
NO POSTAGE
NECESSARY
IF MAILED
IN THE
UNITED STATES

BUSINESS REPLY MAIL
FIRST-CLASS MAIL PERMIT NO 39 ROCKVILLE MD
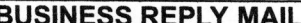
POSTAGE WILL BE PAID BY ADDRESSEE:

DIANE D COUSINS RPh
THE USP PRACTITIONERS' REPORTING NETWORK
12601 TWINBROOK PARKWAY
ROCKVILLE MD 20897-5211

Reprinted with permission of the United States Pharmacopeia. ©1999 The United States Pharmacopeial Convention, Inc.

17-1

Appendix 17-1

Investigational New Drug Application

<table>
<tr><td colspan="2">DEPARTMENT OF HEALTH AND HUMAN SERVICES
PUBLIC HEALTH SERVICE
FOOD AND DRUG ADMINISTRATION
INVESTIGATIONAL NEW DRUG APPLICATION (IND)
(TITLE 21, CODE OF FEDERAL REGULATIONS (CFR) PART 312)</td><td>Form Approved: OMB No. 0910-0014.
Expiration Date: September 30, 2002
See OMB Statement on Reverse.

NOTE: No drug may be shipped or clinical investigation begun until an IND for that investigation is in effect (21 CFR 312.40).</td></tr>
</table>

1. NAME OF SPONSOR

2. DATE OF SUBMISSION

3. ADDRESS *(Number, Street, City, State and Zip Code)*

4. TELEPHONE NUMBER *(Include Area Code)*

5. NAME(S) OF DRUG *(Include all available names: Trade, Generic, Chemical, Code)*

6. IND NUMBER *(If previously assigned)*

7. INDICATION(S) *(Covered by this submission)*

8. PHASE(S) OF CLINICAL INVESTIGATION TO BE CONDUCTED:
☐ PHASE 1 ☐ PHASE 2 ☐ PHASE 3 ☐ OTHER_____ *(Specify)*

9. LIST NUMBERS OF ALL INVESTIGATIONAL NEW DRUG APPLICATIONS (21 CFR Part 312), NEW DRUG OR ANTIBIOTIC APPLICATIONS *(21 CFR Part 314)*, DRUG MASTER FILES *(21 CFR Part 314.420)*, AND PRODUCT LICENSE APPLICATIONS (21 CFR Part 601) REFERRED TO IN THIS APPLICATION.

10. **IND submission should be consecutively numbered. The initial IND should be numbered "Serial number: 000." The next submission (e.g., amendment, report, or correspondence) should be numbered "Serial Number: 001." Subsequent submissions should be numbered consecutively in the order in which they are submitted.**

SERIAL NUMBER

___ ___ ___

11. THIS SUBMISSION CONTAINS THE FOLLOWING: *(Check all that apply)*
☐ INITIAL INVESTIGATIONAL NEW DRUG APPLICATION (IND)   ☐ RESPONSE TO CLINICAL HOLD

PROTOCOL AMENDMENT(S):	INFORMATION AMENDMENT(S):	IND SAFETY REPORT(S):
☐ NEW PROTOCOL	☐ CHEMISTRY/MICROBIOLOGY	☐ INITIAL WRITTEN REPORT
☐ CHANGE IN PROTOCOL	☐ PHARMACOLOGY/TOXICOLOGY	☐ FOLLOW-UP TO A WRITTEN REPORT
☐ NEW INVESTIGATOR	☐ CLINICAL	

☐ RESPONSE TO FDA REQUEST FOR INFORMATION   ☐ ANNUAL REPORT   ☐ GENERAL CORRESPONDENCE

☐ REQUEST FOR REINSTATEMENT OF IND THAT IS WITHDRAWN, INACTIVATED, TERMINATED OR DISCONTINUED   ☐ OTHER _____ *(Specify)*

CHECK ONLY IF APPLICABLE

JUSTIFICATION STATEMENT MUST BE SUBMITTED WITH APPLICATION FOR ANY CHECKED BELOW. REFER TO THE CITED CFR SECTION FOR FURTHER INFORMATION.

☐ TREATMENT IND 21 CFR 312.35(b)   ☐ TREATMENT PROTOCOL 21 CFR 312.35(a)   ☐ CHARGE REQUEST/NOTIFICATION 21 CFR312.7(d)

FOR FDA USE ONLY

CDR/DBIND/DGD RECEIPT STAMP	DDR RECEIPT STAMP	DIVISION ASSIGNMENT:
		IND NUMBER ASSIGNED:

FORM FDA 1571 (10/99)   PREVIOUS EDITION IS OBSOLETE.   **PAGE 1 OF 2**   EF

Created by Electronic Document Services/USDHHS: (301) 443-2454

12.

CONTENTS OF APPLICATION
This application contains the following items: *(Check all that apply)*

☐ 1. Form FDA 1571 *[21 CFR 312.23(a)(1)]*

☐ 2. Table of Contents *[21 CFR 312.23(a)(2)]*

☐ 3. Introductory statement *[21 CFR 312.23(a)(3)]*

☐ 4. General Investigational plan *[21 CFR 312.23(a)(3)]*

☐ 5. Investigator's brochure *[21 CFR 312.23(a)(5)]*

☐ 6. Protocol(s) *[21 CFR 312.23(a)(6)]*

    ☐ a. Study protocol(s) *[21 CFR 312.23(a)(6)]*

    ☐ b. Investigator data *[21 CFR 312.23(a)(6)(iii)(b)]* or completed Form(s) FDA 1572

    ☐ c. Facilities data *[21 CFR 312.23(a)(6)(iii)(b)]* or completed Form(s) FDA 1572

    ☐ d. Institutional Review Board data *[21 CFR 312.23(a)(6)(iii)(b)]* or completed Form(s) FDA 1572

☐ 7. Chemistry, manufacturing, and control data *[21 CFR 312.23(a)(7)]*

    ☐ Environmental assessment or claim for exclusion *[21 CFR 312.23(a)(7)(iv)(e)]*

☐ 8. Pharmacology and toxicology data *[21 CFR 312.23(a)(8)]*

☐ 9. Previous human experience *[21 CFR 312.23(a)(9)]*

☐ 10. Additional information *[21 CFR 312.23(a)(10)]*

13. IS ANY PART OF THE CLINICAL STUDY TO BE CONDUCTED BY A CONTRACT RESEARCH ORGANIZATION? ☐ YES ☐ NO

    IF YES, WILL ANY SPONSOR OBLIGATIONS BE TRANSFERRED TO THE CONTRACT RESEARCH ORGANIZATION? ☐ YES ☐ NO

    IF YES, ATTACH A STATEMENT CONTAINING THE NAME AND ADDRESS OF THE CONTRACT RESEARCH ORGANIZATION, IDENTIFICATION OF THE CLINICAL STUDY, AND A LISTING OF THE OBLIGATIONS TRANSFERRED.

14. NAME AND TITLE OF THE PERSON RESPONSIBLE FOR MONITORING THE CONDUCT AND PROGRESS OF THE CLINICAL INVESTIGATIONS

15. NAME(S) AND TITLE(S) OF THE PERSON(S) RESPONSIBLE FOR REVIEW AND EVALUATION OF INFORMATION RELEVANT TO THE SAFETY OF THE DRUG

I agree not to begin clinical investigations until 30 days after FDA's receipt of the IND unless I receive earlier notification by FDA that the studies may begin. I also agree not to begin or continue clinical investigations covered by the IND if those studies are placed on clinical hold. I agree that an Institutional Review Board (IRB) that complies with the requirements set fourth in 21 CFR Part 56 will be responsible for initial and continuing review and approval of each of the studies in the proposed clinical investigation. I agree to conduct the investigation in accordance with all other applicable regulatory requirements.

16. NAME OF SPONSOR OR SPONSOR'S AUTHORIZED REPRESENTATIVE	17. SIGNATURE OF SPONSOR OR SPONSOR'S AUTHORIZED REPRESENTATIVE	
18. ADDRESS *(Number, Street, City, State and Zip Code)*	19. TELEPHONE NUMBER *(Include Area Code)*	20. DATE

(**WARNING:** A willfully false statement is a criminal offense. U.S.C. Title 18, Sec. 1001.)

Public reporting burden for this collection of information is estimated to average 100 hours per response, including the time for reviewing instructions, searching existing data sources, gathering and maintaining the data needed, and completing reviewing the collection of information. Send comments regarding this burden estimate or any other aspect of this collection of information, including suggestions for reducing this burden to:

Food and Drug Administration CBER (HFM-99) 1401 Rockville Pike Rockville, MD 20852-1448	Food and Drug Administration CDER (HFD-94) 5516 Nicholson Lane Kensington, MD 20895	"An agency may not conduct or sponsor, and a person is not required to respond to, a collection of information unless it displays a currently valid OMB control number."

Please **DO NOT RETURN** this application to this address.

FORM FDA 1571 (10/99)   PAGE 2 OF 2

Appendix 17-2

Statement of Investigator

DEPARTMENT OF HEALTH AND HUMAN SERVICES PUBLIC HEALTH SERVICE FOOD AND DRUG ADMINISTRATION **STATEMENT OF INVESTIGATOR** *(TITLE 21, CODE OF FEDERAL REGULATIONS (CFR) PART 312)* (See instructions on reverse side.)	Form Approved: OMB No. 0910-0014. Expiration Date: **September 30, 2002** *See OMB Statement on Reverse.*
	NOTE: No investigator may participate in an investigation until he/she provides the sponsor with a completed, signed Statement of Investigator, Form FDA 1572 (21 CFR 312.53(c)).

1. NAME AND ADDRESS OF INVESTIGATOR

2. EDUCATION, TRAINING, AND EXPERIENCE THAT QUALIFIES THE INVESTIGATOR AS AN EXPERT IN THE CLINICAL INVESTIGATION OF THE DRUG FOR THE USE UNDER INVESTIGATION. ONE OF THE FOLLOWING IS ATTACHED.

☐ CURRICULUM VITAE ☐ OTHER STATEMENT OF QUALIFICATIONS

3. NAME AND ADDRESS OF ANY MEDICAL SCHOOL, HOSPITAL OR OTHER RESEARCH FACILITY WHERE THE CLINICAL INVESTIGATION(S) WILL BE CONDUCTED.

4. NAME AND ADDRESS OF ANY CLINICAL LABORATORY FACILITIES TO BE USED IN THE STUDY.

5. NAME AND ADDRESS OF THE INSTITUTIONAL REVIEW BOARD (IRB) THAT IS RESPONSIBLE FOR REVIEW AND APPROVAL OF THE STUDY(IES).

6. NAMES OF THE SUBINVESTIGATORS *(e.g., research fellows, residents, associates)* WHO WILL BE ASSISTING THE INVESTIGATOR IN THE CONDUCT OF THE INVESTIGATION(S).

7. NAME AND CODE NUMBER, IF ANY, OF THE PROTOCOL(S) IN THE IND FOR THE STUDY(IES) TO BE CONDUCTED BY THE INVESTIGATOR.

FORM FDA 1572 (10/99) PREVIOUS EDITION IS OBSOLETE. **PAGE 1 OF 2**

Created by: PCS Media Arts
Branch (301) 443-2454 EF

8. ATTACH THE FOLLOWING CLINICAL PROTOCOL INFORMATION:

☐ FOR PHASE 1 INVESTIGATIONS, A GENERAL OUTLINE OF THE PLANNED INVESTIGATION INCLUDING THE ESTIMATED DURATION OF THE STUDY AND THE MAXIMUM NUMBER OF SUBJECTS THAT WILL BE INVOLVED.

☐ FOR PHASE 2 OR 3 INVESTIGATIONS, AN OUTLINE OF THE STUDY PROTOCOL INCLUDING AN APPROXIMATION OF THE NUMBER OF SUBJECTS TO BE TREATED WITH THE DRUG AND THE NUMBER TO BE EMPLOYED AS CONTROLS, IF ANY; THE CLINICAL USES TO BE INVESTIGATED; CHARACTERISTICS OF SUBJECTS BY AGE, SEX, AND CONDITION; THE KIND OF CLINICAL OBSERVATIONS AND LABORATORY TESTS TO BE CONDUCTED; THE ESTIMATED DURATION OF THE STUDY; AND COPIES OR A DESCRIPTION OF CASE REPORT FORMS TO BE USED.

9. COMMITMENTS:

I agree to conduct the study(ies) in accordance with the relevant, current protocol(s) and will only make changes in a protocol after notifying the sponsor, except when necessary to protect the safety, rights, or welfare of subjects.

I agree to personally conduct or supervise the described investigation(s).

I agree to inform any patients, or any persons used as controls, that the drugs are being used for investigational purposes and I will ensure that the requirements relating to obtaining informed consent in 21 CFR Part 50 and institutional review board (IRB) review and approval in 21 CFR Part 56 are met.

I agree to report to the sponsor adverse experiences that occur in the course of the investigation(s) in accordance with 21 CFR 312.64.

I have read and understand the information in the investigator's brochure, including the potential risks and side effects of the drug.

I agree to ensure that all associates, colleagues, and employees assisting in the conduct of the study(ies) are informed about their obligations in meeting the above commitments.

I agree to maintain adequate and accurate records in accordance with 21 CFR 312.62 and to make those records available for inspection in accordance with 21 CFR 312.68.

I will ensure that an IRB that complies with the requirements of 21 CFR Part 56 will be responsible for the initial and continuing review and approval of the clinical investigation. I also agree to promptly report to the IRB all changes in the research activity and all unanticipated problems involving risks to human subjects or others. Additionally, I will not make any changes in the research without IRB approval, except where necessary to eliminate apparent immediate hazards to human subjects.

I agree to comply with all other requirements regarding the obligations of clinical investigators and all other pertinent requirements in 21 CFR Part 312.

INSTRUCTIONS FOR COMPLETING FORM FDA 1572
STATEMENT OF INVESTIGATOR:

1. Complete all sections. Attach a separate page if additional space is needed.

2. Attach curriculum vitae or other statement of qualifications as described in Section 2.

3. Attach protocol outline as described in Section 8.

4. Sign and date below.

5. FORWARD THE COMPLETED FORM AND ATTACHMENTS TO THE SPONSOR. The sponsor will incorporate this information along with other technical data into an Investigational New Drug Application (IND).

10. SIGNATURE OF INVESTIGATOR

11. DATE

(**WARNING:** A willfully false statement is a criminal offense. U.S.C. Title 18, Sec. 1001.)

Public reporting burden for this collection of information is estimated to average 84 hours per response, including the time for reviewing instructions, searching existing data sources, gathering and maintaining the data needed, and completing reviewing the collection of information. Send comments regarding this burden estimate or any other aspect of this collection of information, including suggestions for reducing this burden to:

Food and Drug Administration
CBER (HFM-99)
1401 Rockville Pike
Rockville, MD 20852-1448

Food and Drug Administration
CDER (HFD-94)
5516 Nicholson Lane
Kensington, MD 20895

"An agency may not conduct or sponsor, and a person is not required to respond to, a collection of information unless it displays a currently valid OMB control number."

Please DO NOT RETURN this application to this address.

FORM FDA 1572 (10/99)   PAGE 2 OF 2

Appendix 17–3

Protocol Medication Economic Analysis

Date:
Protocol title:
Study chairperson:

Hospital Cost Analysis

Drug	Hospital Cost per Cycle*	Number of Cycles	Total Cost per Patient	Number of Patients	Total Protocol Cost	Annual Cost
Primary Therapy						
Supportive Care						

*When applicable, doses calculated on 1.7 m² or 70 kg at initial dose level and costs include infusion fluids, administration sets, and tubing.

Patient Charge Analysis

Drug	Patient Charge per Cycle*	Number of Cycles	Total Charge per Patient	Number of Patients	Total Patient Billing
Primary Therapy					
Supportive Care					

*When applicable, charges include infusion fluids, administration sets, and tubing.

Reimbursement Risk

Drug	FDA Labeled	Compendium

Comments

SUMMARY

17-4

Appendix 17-4

Investigational Drug Accountability Record

Form approved.
OMB No. 0925-0240
Expires. 6/30/91

National Institutes of Health
National Cancer Institute

PAGE NO. _____

CONTROL RECORD ☐

Investigational Drug Accountability Record

SATELLITE RECORD ☐

Name of Institution   Protocol No. (NCI)

Drug Name, Dose Form and Strength

Protocol Title   Dispensing Area

Investigator

Line No.	Date	Patient's Initials	Patient's I.D. Number	Dose	Quantity Dispensed or Received	Balance Forward / Balance	Manufacturer and Lot No.	Recorder's Initials
1.								
2.								
3.								
4.								
5.								
6.								
7.								
8.								
9.								
10.								
11.								
12.								
13.								
14.								
15.								
16.								
17.								
18.								
19.								
20.								
21.								
22.								
23.								
24.								

NIH-2564
9-85

Glossary

Abstracting service. A database that provides abstracts and citations for journal articles.

Abstracts. A synopsis (usually of 250 words or less) of the most important aspect(s) of an article.

Action guides. A term coined by Beauchamp and Childress to refer to a hierarchical approach to analysis of an ethical issue when forming particular judgments about the issue.

Adverse drug event (ADE). Any injury caused by a medicine. This includes adverse drug reactions and medication errors.

Adverse drug reaction (ADR). The Food and Drug Administration's (FDA) definition of ADRs is "any adverse event associated with the use of a drug in humans, whether or not considered drug related, including the following: adverse event occurring in the course of the use of a drug product in professional practice; an adverse event occurring from drug overdose, whether accidental or intentional; an adverse event occurring from drug abuse; an adverse event occurring from drug withdrawal; and any significant failure of expected pharmacologic action." Adverse drug reactions also include drug interactions. Several other definitions are available; many of those are discussed in Chap. 16.

Agenda for change. An initiative adopted by the JCAHO in 1986 intended to improve standards by focusing on key functions of quality of care, to monitor the performance of health care organizations using indicators, to improve the relevance and quality of the survey process, and to enhance the accuracy and value of JCAHO accreditation.

Alpha (level of significance). The probability of a false positive result in a study.

Analytic research. Quantitative research conducted in a controlled environment to determine cause and effect relationships.

A priori. In reference to clinical trials, to do something prior to initiation of the study.

Article proposal. A letter asking the publisher whether he or she would be interested in possibly publishing something on a particular topic written by the person(s) who are inquiring.

Aspect of care. A term used in quality assurance programs to indicate the title that describes the area being evaluated.

Attributable risk. A statistical technique used in follow-up studies to determine the risk associated with exposure to a certain factor on disease state development. Attributable risk estimates the number of disease cases per number of exposures to the factor.

Beta. The probability of a false negative result in a study.

Bioequivalence studies. Research that evaluates whether products are similar in rate and extent of absorption.

Bibliography. A list of references, usually seen at the end of a piece of professional writing.

"Black letter rules." Principles of law that are known generally to all and are free from doubt and ambiguity. Also known as hornbook law, because they are in a format that would probably be enunciated in a hornbook.

Blinding. The procedures used in a clinical study to ensure that the investigator, subject, or both are unaware of which treatment is being administered. In a single-blind study, either the investigator or the subject does not know the treatment being received and in a double-blind study both the investigator and the subject are unaware of the treatment being received.

Body area network (BAN). A multidevice, interconnected computer system carried on a person. Sometimes referred to as a wearable computer.

Boolean operators (logical operators). Words used to combine search terms (i.e., AND, OR, and NOT) when using computerized databases.

Case law. The aggregate of reported cases; the law pertaining to a particular subject as formed by adjudged cases.

Case-control study. A study where a group of subjects (i.e., cases) with a particular characteristic (e.g., disease) is compared to a group (i.e., controls) without the characteristic to determine the influence of certain factors on development of the characteristic. Also called a trohoc study.

CD-ROM (compact disc–read only memory). A storage and retrieval system for large quantities of computerized data. Data located on the compact disc can be accessed, but not added to or changed (i.e., read only memory). Use of CD-ROMs generally requires availability of a multimedia computer.

Clinical investigation. Any experiment in which a drug is administered or dispensed to one or more human subjects. Relating to investigational drugs, an experiment is any use of a drug (except for the use of a marketed drug) in the course of medical practice. Although there are many other definitions, this is the FDA's definition and would seem the appropriate one to use given the nature of this topic. Please note that the FDA does not regulate the practice of medicine and prescribers are (as far as the agency is concerned) free to use any marketed drug for "off-label use."

Clinical practice guidelines. The United States Department of Health and Human Services, Public Health Service, Agency for Health Care Policy and Research (AHCPR) defined clinical practice guidelines as "systematically developed statements to assist practitioner and patient decisions about appropriate healthcare for specific clinical circumstances."

Clinical safety officer (CSO). Also known as the Regulatory Management Officer (RMO). This will be the sponsor's FDA contact person. Generally the CSO/RMO assigned to a drug's Investigational New Drug application will also be assigned to the New Drug Application.

Clinical significance. The clinical importance of data generated in a study, irrespective of statistical results.

Closed formulary. A drug formulary that restricts the drugs available within an institution or available under a third-party plan.

Co-author. Any individual who writes a portion of an article, chapter, book, and so on. This includes individuals other than the primary author, whose name is normally listed first on a publication.

Cohort study. *See* follow-up study.

Comparative negligence. The allocation of responsibility for damages incurred between the plaintiff and defendant, based on relative negligence of the two; the reduction of the damages to be recovered by the negligent plaintiff in proportion to his fault.

Compliance. A measure of how well instructions are followed. In a study, compliance refers to how well a patient follows instructions for medication administration and how well the investigator follows the study protocol.

Computer network. An interconnection of computers and computer-related devices (e.g., printers, modems, etc.) that allows the computers to interchange data, electronic mail, programs, and other files. In addition, a network allows sharing of peripheral devices, such as printers, modems, fax boards, etc. Normally, this interconnection is via a dedicated wiring system (other than telephone/modem communication); however, wireless connections are possible.

Concurrent indicator. An indicator used in any quality assurance program that determines whether quality is acceptable while an action is being taken or care is being given.

Confidence intervals. A measurement of the variability of study data. A 95% confidence interval is a numerical range that contains the true value for the population 95% of the time.

Consequentialist theories. Those moral theories that describe actions or decisions as morally right or wrong based on their consequences.

Continuous quality improvement (CQI). The term given to the methodologies used in the process of total quality management. Efforts to improve quality are part of each participant's responsibilities on an ongoing basis.

Contract research organization (CRO). An individual or organization, who sponsors an investigational new drug (IND) or new drug application (NDA), and assumes one or more of the obligations of the sponsor through an independent contractual agreement.

Control group. The group of test animals or humans that receive a placebo or active control. For most preclinical and clinical trials, the FDA will require that this group receive placebo (commonly referred to as the placebo control). However, some studies may have an "active" control that generally consists of an available (standard of care) treatment modality. An active control may, with the concurrence of the FDA, be used in studies where it would be considered unethical to use a placebo. A historical control is one in which a group of previous patients is compared to a "matched" set of patients receiving the new therapy. A historical control might be used in cases where the disease is consistently fatal (e.g., AIDS).

Controls. A treatment (placebo, active, historical) used for comparison in a study. The investigator usually wishes to determine superiority of a new treatment over the control in terms of efficacy and safety.

Cost-benefit study. A study where monetary value is given for both costs and benefits associated with a drug or service. The results are expressed as a ratio (benefit to cost) and the ratio is used to determine the economic value of the drug or service.

Cost-effectiveness study. A study where the cost of a drug or service is compared to its therapeutic impact. Cost-effectiveness studies determine the relative efficiency of various drugs or services in achieving desired therapeutic outcomes.

Cost-minimization study. A study that compares costs of drugs or services that have been determined to have equivalent therapeutic outcomes.

Cost-utility study. A study that relates therapeutic outcomes to both costs of drugs or services and patient preferences and measures cost per unit of utility. Utility is the amount of satisfaction obtained from a drug or service.

Coverage error. Error that occurs when there is a discrepancy between the target population and the population from which the sample was derived. Also called sampling error.

Criteria. A statement of the activity to be measured and evaluated. *Also see* indicator.

Cross-over study. A study where each subject receives all study treatments, and end points during the various treatments are compared.

Cross-sectional study. A study where measurements are taken at a single point in time.

Dechallenge. In relation to adverse drug reactions (ADRs), this occurs when the drug is taken away and the patient is monitored to determine if the ADR abates or decreases in intensity.

Deep pocket. Practical consideration that involves the naming of additional co-defendants in personal injury lawsuits to provide assurance to the plaintiff that there will be sufficient assets to pay the judgment.

Delta. The amount of difference that the investigators wish to detect between treatment groups in a study.

Deontological theories. Moral theories that propose that the intrinsic qualities of an act or decision assert its moral rightness or wrongness rather than consequences.

Descriptive research. Quantitative research that describes naturally occurring events.

Descriptive statistics. Statistics that describe data such as medians, modes, and standard deviations.

Drug formularies. *See* formulary.

Drug formulary system. *See* formulary system.

Drug informatics. A technologically advanced version of drug information. This often denotes the electronic management of drug information.

Drug information (DI). The provision of unbiased, well-referenced, and critically evaluated information on any aspect of pharmacy practice.

Drug information center (DIC). A physical location where pharmacists have the resources (e.g., books, journals, computer systems, etc.) to provide drug information. This area is generally staffed by a pharmacist specializing in drug information, but may be used by a variety of the pharmacy staff or other individuals.

Drug information service. A professional service providing drug information. This service is normally located in a drug information center.

Drug interaction. The FDA defines this as "a pharmacologic response that cannot be explained by the action of a simple drug, but is due to two or more drugs acting simultaneously."

Drug master file (DMF). Reference on file with the FDA that contains information regarding the drug. There are five different types of DMF. The one that is most commonly used when filing an IND is the CMC-DMF (Chemistry, Manufacturing, and Controls-Drug Master File), which contains information regarding the chemistry, manufacturing, and controls of the drug.

Drug product. The final dosage form. Prepared from the drug substance.

Drug regimen review (DRR). The monthly evaluation of nursing home charts by pharmacists.

Drug substance. Bulk compound from which the drug product is prepared.

Drug use/usage evaluation (DUE). *See* medication use evaluation.

Drug utilization review (DUR). A program often related to outpatient pharmacy services designed to educate physicians and pharmacists in identifying and reducing the frequency and patterns of fraud, abuse, gross overuse, or inappropriate or medically unnecessary care. DUR is typically retrospective in nature and utilizes claims data as its primary source of information.

Duty. A moral or legal obligation.

Electronic mail (e-mail). Brief messages sent from one computer to another, similar in use to interoffice memos. This serves as a quick, informal method of written communication. Also, e-mail may be used to send other items, such as word processing files, graphics, video, and so on to others.

End point. A parameter measured in a clinical study. The primary end point is the major variable analyzed and reflects the main objective of the study. Secondary end points are additional variables of interest monitored during clinical studies.

Ethical theories. Integrated bodies of principles and rules that may include mediating rules that govern cases of conflicts.

Ethics (defined by AACP). Philosophical inquiry into the moral dimensions of human conduct.

Ethics (defined by Beauchamp and Childress). A generic term for several ways of examining the moral life.

Exclusion criteria. Characteristics of subjects that prohibit entrance into the study, if present.

Extemporaneous compounding. The practice of compounding prescriptions from a list of several ingredients, usually performed by a pharmacist.

False negatives. Individuals with the disease that were incorrectly identified as being disease free by the test.

False positives. Individuals without the disease that were incorrectly identified as having the disease by the test.

File transfer protocol (FTP). A method to transfer files from one computer to another.

Follow-up study. A study where subjects exposed to a factor and those not exposed to the factor are followed forward in time and compared to determine the factor's influence on disease state development. Also called a cohort study.

Food and Drug Administration (FDA). The agency of the U.S. government that is responsible for ensuring the safety and efficacy of all drugs on the market. This agency will approve drugs for marketing.

Formulary. A continually revised list of medications that are readily available for use within an institution or from a third-party payer (e.g., insurance company, government) that reflects the current clinical judgment of the medical staff or the payer.

Formulary system. A method used to develop a drug formulary. It is sometimes even thought of as a philosophy.

Galley proofs. A copy of a written work as it is to be published. The purpose of this document is to allow the author(s) to make a final check to ensure everything is correct before actual publication.

Health Plan Employer Data and Information Set (HEDIS). A set of performance measures used to compare managed health care plans.

Health-related quality of life (HR-QOL). A general term for the impact of many dimensions of health status (such as physical, social, and cognitive functioning; mental health; symptom tolerance; overall well-being, etc.) on quality of life.

Historical data. Data used in research that was collected prior to the decision to conduct the study (e.g., medical records, insurance information, MEDICAID databases).

Homogenicity tests. Tests used when conducting a meta-analysis to determine the similarity of studies whose results were combined for the analysis.

Hypothesis. The researchers' assumptions regarding probable study results. The research hypothesis or alternative hypothesis (H_A) is the expectation of the researchers in terms of study results. The null hypothesis (H_0) is the no difference hypothesis, which assumes equality amongst study treatments. The null hypothesis is the basis for all statistical tests and must be rejected in order to accept the research hypothesis.

http (hypertext transfer protocol). A method by which information is encoded and transmitted on the World Wide Web.

https. A secure form of http, used to transmit confidential information, such as credit card numbers.

Incidence rate. Measures the probability that a healthy person will develop a disease within a specified period of time. It is the number of new cases of disease in the population over a specific time period.

Inclusion criteria. Characteristics of subjects that must be present for subjects to be entered into the study.

Indexing service. A database of biomedical journal citations.

Indicator. A statement of a measurable item in the area being evaluated that signals whether the area being evaluated is or is not of sufficient quality.

Indicator drug. A drug that, when prescribed, may offer evidence that an adverse effect to a drug may have occurred. Pharmacists can then investigate further to determine whether there really was an adverse effect. Examples are found in Table 16–1.

Inferential statistics. Statistics (i.e., parametric and nonparametric tests) that determine the statistical importance of differences between groups and allow conclusions to be drawn from the data.

Informed consent. The document signed by a subject, or the subject's representative, entering into a trial that informs him or her of the potential benefits and risks of the trial. This document indicates that the person is willing to participate in the study.

Inherent drug risks. Risks that are unique to the drug and usually identified in the package insert, but do not include probable or common side effects.

Institutional review board (IRB). A group of individuals from various disciplines (e.g., lay people, physicians, pharmacists, nurses, clergy) who evaluate protocols for clinical studies to assess risks to patients and benefits to society.

Intention-to-treat analysis. Analysis of all subjects in a study regardless of whether they completed or dropped out of the study.

Interim analysis. Evaluation of data at specified time points before scheduled termination or completion of a study.

Internet. A worldwide computer network.

Interval data. Data in which each measurement has an equal distance between points, but an arbitrary zero (e.g., temperature in Fahrenheit).

Investigational new drug. A drug, antibiotic, or biological that is used in a clinical investigation. The label of an investigational drug must bear the statement: "Caution: New Drug—Limited by Federal (or United States) law to investigational use."

Investigational new drug application (IND). A submission to the FDA containing chemical information, preclinical data, and a detailed description of the planned clinical trials. Thirty days after submission of this document to the FDA by the sponsor, clinical trials may be initiated in humans (unless a clinical hold is placed by the FDA). When the FDA allows the studies to proceed, this document allows unapproved drugs to be shipped in interstate commerce.

Investigator. The individual responsible for initiating the clinical trial at the study site. This individual must treat the patients, ensure that the protocol is followed, evaluate responses and adverse reactions, solve problems as they arise, and ensure proper conduct of the study.

JCAHO. Joint Commission on Accreditation of Healthcare Organizations.

Joint and several liability. Refers to the sharing of liabilities among a group of people collectively and also individually. If the defendants are "jointly and severally" liable, the injured party may sue some or all of the defendants together, or each one separately, and may collect equal or unequal amounts from each.

Kurtosis. Refers to how flat or peaked the curve appears. A curve with a flat or board top is referred to as platykurtic while a peaked distribution is described as leptokurtic.

Law. Written rules set by the whole society, or its representatives, that address the responsibilities of that society's members.

Listserver. A service offered by some e-mail systems that allows a member of the listserver to send an e-mail message to one particular Internet address where it will be sent to all members of the listserver. This acts as a dynamic distribution list for e-mail messages.

Local area network (LAN). A group of computers connected in a way that they may share data, programs, and or equipment over a small geographic area (e.g., building, department).

Locality rule. Legal doctrine created in the latter part of the nineteenth century that stated that the local defendant practitioner would have his or her standard of performance evaluated in light of the performance of other peers in the same or similar communities. Also known as community rule.

Logical operator. A term such as AND, OR, NOT, NEAR, or WITH that can be used in searching a computer database. See Chap. 5 for more detailed information.

Mainframe computer. A large centralized computer that is used via computer terminals or other devices. This term is becoming blurred as smaller computer systems gain greater capabilities.

Mean (arithmetic mean). The most common measure of central tendency for data measured on an interval or ratio scale that is best described as the average numerical value for the data set. Calculated as the sum of the observations divided by the number of observations.

Measurement error. Error that occurs when the interviewer influences the collection of data or when the survey item itself is unclear from the respondent's point of view. Also called response bias.

Median. The middle value in a set of ranked data. In other words, the value such that half of the data points fall above it and half fall below it. In terms of percentiles, it is the value at the 50th percentile.

Medical executive committee. A committee that acts as the administrative body of a medical staff in an institution. It is responsible for overseeing all aspects of care within the institution. This committee may be known by other names at specific institutions.

Medical subject headings (MeSH terms). A thesaurus of official indexing terms used when searching some of the databases of the National Library of Medicine (e.g., MEDLINE, TOX-LINE).

Medication error. Any preventable event that has the potential to lead to inappropriate medication use or patient harm.

Medication misadventure. Any iatrogenic hazard or incident associated with medications. It includes adverse drug events, adverse drug reactions, and medication errors.

Medication use evaluation (MUE). The component of a health care organization's quality improvement program that should examine all aspects of medication use including prescribing, dispensing, administration, and monitoring of medication use. Prior to 1986, this function was commonly referred to as Drug use (or usage) evaluation.

MedLARS. *See* Medical Literature Analysis and Retrieval System

Medical Literature Analysis and Retrieval System (MedLARS). The computerized information retrieval system at the National Library of Medicine.

MedWatch. The FDA Medical Products Reporting Program that monitors clinically significant adverse drug events and problems with medical products. Information is found at <<http://www.fda.gov/medwatch>>.

Meta-analysis. A type of review where conclusions are based on the summarization of results obtained from combining and statistically evaluating data from previously conducted studies. Also called a quantitative systematic review.

Middle technical style. A writing style used by professionals addressing professionals in other fields. It tends to be formal and avoids use of the first person (e.g., I, us). Technical jargon is avoided in this writing style.

Mode. The most frequently occurring value or category in the set of data. A data set can have more than one mode.

Modified systematic approach. A seven-step approach to answering drug information requests that includes (1) securing demographics of requestor, (2) obtaining background information, (3) determining and categorizing the ultimate question, (4) developing strategies and conducting searches, (5) performing evaluation, analysis, and synthesis, (6) formulating and providing responses, and (7) conducting follow-up and documentation.

Morbidity. Detrimental consequences (other than death) related to a treatment, exposure, or disease state.

Narrative review. *See* nonsystematic review.

N-of-1 study. A controlled study conducted in a single subject where periods of exposure to a treatment are compared to periods of exposure to a placebo to determine the effects of the treatment on various variables and outcomes in the subject.

National Committee for Quality Assurance (NCQA). An organization dedicated to assessing and reporting on the quality of managed care plans; it surveys and accredits managed care organizations much like JCAHO accredits hospitals.

Negative formulary. A drug formulary that starts out with every marketed drug product and specifically eliminates products that are considered inferior, unnecessary, unsafe, too expensive, and so forth.

Negligence. Failure to exercise that degree of care that a person of ordinary prudence or a reasonable person would exercise under the same circumstances. Elements of a negligence case include (1) duty breached, (2) damages, (3) direct causation, and (4) defenses absent.

New drug application (NDA). The application to the FDA requesting approval to market a new drug for human use. The NDA contains data supporting the safety and efficacy of the drug for its intended use.

Nominal data. Data that are categorical (e.g., yes/no; male/female).

Noninherent drug risks. Risks that are created by the particular drug in combination with some extrinsic factor that the pharmacist should reasonably know about.

Nonparametric statistics. Statistical tests used to analyze data that are not normally distributed such as nominal and ordinal data.

Nonresponse bias. *See* nonresponse error.

Nonresponse error. Error that occurs when a significant number of subjects in the sample do not respond to the survey and when responders differ from nonresponders in a way that influences, or could influence, the results. Also called nonresponse bias.

Nonsystematic review. A review article that summarizes previously conducted research, but does not provide a description of the systematic methods used to identify the research included in the article. Also called a narrative review.

Null hypothesis. *See* hypothesis.

Number needed to treat (NNT). The number of patients who need to be treated for every one patient who benefits from a treatment. NNT is calculated as the reciprocal of absolute risk reduction.

OBRA '90. *See* Omnibus Budget Reconciliation Act of 1990.

Odds ratios. A statistical technique used in case-control studies to determine the risk of exposure to a factor on development of a certain characteristic or disease state. Odds ratios estimate relative risk.

Omnibus Budget Reconciliation Act of 1990 (OBRA '90). A statute (Public Law 101-508) focused on drug benefits provided under Medicaid. The statute requires pharmacists to conduct drug utilization review, including prescription screening, patient counseling, and documentation of interventions.

On-line. The process of connecting to a remote computer via modem or network.

Open formulary. A formulary that allows any marketed drug to be ordered in an institution or under a third-party plan. Can be considered an oxymoron.

Ordinal data. Data measured on an arbitrary scale that reflects a ranking (e.g., 1+, 2+ edema).

ORYX™. A JCAHO initiative to mandate the use of performance measurement tools to monitor outcomes and to integrate this data into the accreditation process.

Outcome indicators. Quality assurance indicators that review whether the final desired result was obtained from whatever action was being reviewed.

Overview. A general term for a summary of the literature. Includes nonsystematic (narrative), systematic (qualitative), and qualitative (meta analyses) reviews.

***p*-value.** A number that is generated during use of inferential statistics. The *p*-value indicates whether a statistical difference exists between groups. If the *p*-value is less than or equal to alpha or the level of significance, the difference is statistically significant. If the *p*-value is greater than alpha, the difference is not statistically significant.

Parallel study. A study where two or more groups receive different treatments and the outcomes are compared.

Parameter. A measurement that describes part of the population.

Parametric statistics. Statistical tests used to analyze data with a normal (e.g., bell-shaped) distribution. Commonly used to analyze ratio and interval data.

Parenteral admixtures. Solutions containing drug products for intravenous administration.

Peer review. A quality assurance program that centers on the evaluation of specific individuals by other similar professionals. Also, the process where a group of experts review a manuscript for accuracy and appropriateness for publication in a biomedical journal.

Pharmaceutical care. The responsible provision of drug therapy for the purpose of achieving definite outcomes that improve a patient's quality of life.

Pharmacoeconomics. The study of the economic impact of drug therapies or services.

Pharmacy and Therapeutics (P&T) Committee. A group in an institution or company that oversees any and/or all aspects of drug therapy for that institution or company. In hospitals, it is usually a subcommittee of the medical staff. May be known by a variety of similar names, such as Pharmacy and Formulary Committee, Drug and Therapeutics Committee (DTC), or Formulary Committee.

Placebo. A pharmaceutical preparation that does not contain a pharmacologically active ingredient, but is otherwise identical to the active drug preparation in terms of appearance, taste, and smell.

Poison information. A specialized area of drug information. By definition, it is the provision of information on the toxic effects of an extensive range of chemicals, as well as plant and animal exposures.

Poison information center. A place that specializes in research, management, and dissemination of toxicity information. A physician usually directs it, although a pharmacist directs many on a day-to-day basis. Often, pharmacists and nurses provide staffing of these centers.

Policy. A broad general statement that takes into consideration and describes the goals and purposes of a policy and procedure document.

Popular technical style. A writing style used by professionals addressing laypeople. This is less formal than writing addressed to professionals.

Population. Every individual in the entire universe with the characteristics or disease states under investigation. Because entire populations are generally very large, a sample representative of the population is usually selected for an investigation.

Positive formulary. A drug formulary that starts out with no drug products and specifically adds products, after appropriate evaluation, that are needed by the institution or company.

Postmarketing surveillance study. A study designed to examine drug use and frequency of side effects following approval by the FDA.

Power. The ability to detect a statistical difference between study groups. Power is dependent on sample size and mathematically is calculated as 1-beta.

Prescribability. The ability of a drug to be prescribed for the first time.

Prevalence. Measures the number of people in the population who have the disease at a given time.

Primary author. The author listed first on a publication. Sometimes referred to as the "first author."

Primary literature. Original research published in biomedical journals.

Principles. In ethical analysis, a principle is relatively broad and fundamental in scope, and guides ethical decision making or actions.

Procedures. Specific actions to be taken.

Process indicators. Quality assurance indicators based on the presence or absence of policies and procedures. These assume that if policies and procedures are appropriate they will be effective and be properly performed.

Professional ethics. Rules of conduct or standards by which a particular group in society regulates its actions and sets standards for its members.

Professional writing. Any written communication prepared in the fulfillment of the practice of a profession.

Programmatic research. Research focused on the impact and economic value of programs and services provided by pharmacists in community and institutional settings.

Prospective indicator. An indicator used in any quality assurance program that determines whether quality is acceptable before an action is taken or care is given.

Prospective study. A study where data are collected forward in time from date of study initiation.

Publication bias. The situation where research demonstrating favorable results is more likely to be published than that showing negative results.

Pure technical style. A writing style used by professionals addressing other professionals in the same field. It tends to be formal and avoids use of the first person (e.g., I, us). Technical jargon can be used in this writing style.

Push technology. Method by which information is actively sent to users' computers with little, if any, effort required by the user. The information may be displayed as a screen saver or the computer may in some way let the user know that the information is available to be displayed (e.g., pop-up notification).

Qualitative systematic review. *See* systematic review.

Quality. A degree or grade of excellence that can be applied to goods, services, processes, or even people.

Quality Assessment and Assurance Committee. A committee found in long-term care facilities to evaluate quality of care, including drug usage evaluation.

Quality assurance. A process used to ensure that something is done or made well enough. It is usually retrospective and focuses only on a particular component within a process, not the entire process.

Quality of life. This is an evaluation of a patient's living situation based on the patient's environment, family life, financial situation, education, and health. It is used in quality assurance programs when developing indicators. In some cases, quality of life aspects will take precedence over the absolute best treatment. For example, a quick cure to a disease state may not be desirable when it costs so much that a family is bankrupted in the process.

Quantitative systematic review. *See* meta-analysis.

Random error. *See* sampling error.

Randomization. The process used to ensure that subjects in a study have an equal and independent chance of being assigned to any of the treatment groups in a study.

Range. The difference between the highest data value and the lowest data value.

Ratio data. Data in which each measurement has an equal distance between points and also an absolute zero (e.g., temperature in Kelvin).

Rechallenge. In relation to adverse drug reactions, this indicates that the drug was taken away and, after the adverse drug reaction abates, the patient is given the same medication in an attempt to elicit the same response a second time.

Referee. An expert in a particular area who reviews a written document to determine whether it is appropriate for publication.

Refereed publication. A publication in which the editors have experts in the appropriate field review items submitted for possible publication to determine whether those items are of suitable quality.

Relative risk. A statistical technique used in follow-up studies to determine the risk associated with exposure to a certain factor on disease state development. Relative risk estimates how many times greater the risk of disease state development is in patients exposed to a certain factor compared to those who are not exposed.

Research hypothesis. *See* hypothesis.

Response bias. *See* measurement error.

Respondeat superior. Refers to the proposition that the employer is responsible for the negligent acts of its agents or employees.

Restatement (second) of torts. "An attempt by the American Law Institute to present an orderly statement of the general common law of the United States, including in that term not only the law developed solely by judicial decision, but also the law that has grown from the application by the courts of statutes. . . ." It takes into account other factors, such as the modern trend of the law according to influential jurisdictions and well-thought out opinions.

Retrospective indicator. An indicator used in any quality assurance program that determines whether quality was acceptable after an action was taken or care was given.

Retrospective study. A study that analyzes historical data (e.g., previously collected data such as medical records or insurance information).

Rule. In ethical analysis, a rule guides ethical decision making or actions, but is relatively specific in context and restricted in scope.

Sample. A group of subjects chosen as representatives of a population to participate in a study.

Sample size. The number of subjects in a study.

Sampling bias. *See* coverage error.

Sampling error. Error that occurs when the research surveys only a subset (sample) of all possible subjects within the population of interest.

Secondary literature. Resources that index and/or abstract literature from biomedical journals.

Sensitivity. The probability that a diseased individual will have a positive test result. It is the true positive rate of the test.

Sensitivity analysis. Tests that are undertaken to determine the influence of various criteria or conditions on study results. Sensitivity analyses are commonly used in meta-analyses and pharmacoeconomic research.

Skewness. The measure of symmetry of a curve.

Specificity. The probability that a disease-free individual will have a negative test result. Specificity is the true negative rate of the test.

Sponsor. An organization (or individual) that takes responsibility for and initiates a clinical investigation. The sponsor may be an individual or pharmaceutical company, government agency, academic institution, private organization, or other organization.

Sponsor-investigator. An individual who both initiates and conducts a clinical investigation (i.e., submits the IND and directly supervises administration of the drug) as well as performing other investigator responsibilities.

Stability study. A study designed to determine the stability of drugs in various preparations.

Standard. A term used in quality assurance program that indicates how often a indicator must be complied with. The level of compliance will be set at either 0% (i.e., never done) or 100% (i.e., always done). A threshold, which allows compliance of between 0% and 100%, has sometimes been used instead of a standard.

Standard deviation (SD). (1) A measurement of the range of data values (i.e., variability) around the mean. (2) The measure of the average amount by which each observation in a series of data points differs from the mean. In other words, how far away is each data point from the mean (dispersion or variability) or the average deviation from the mean.

Standard error of the mean (SEM). An estimate of the true mean of the population from the mean of the sample. Mathematically SEM is calculated as the standard deviation divided by the square root of the sample size. Ninety-five percent of the time, true mean of the population lies within ± 2 standard errors of the sample mean.

Statistic. A measurement that describes part of a sample.

Statistical significance. The impact of a study in terms of the outcome of statistical tests conducted on the data. A study is said to be statistically significant when statistical tests demonstrate a difference between treatment groups.

Statute. Written law enacted by a legislature other than that of a municipality.

Strict liability. Liability without fault. Defendant is liable even though not lacking in care. Negligence despite proof of prudence.

Structure indicators. Quality assurance indicators based on the presence or absence of items, such as staffing patterns, available space, equipment, resources, or administrative organization.

Study objective. A brief statement of the goals and purpose of a research study.

Subgroup analysis. Evaluation of subsets of subjects within the study sample.

Subject. An individual who participates in a clinical investigation (either as the recipient of the investigational drug or as a member of the control group).

Survey research. Research where responses to questions asked of subjects are analyzed to determine the incidence, distribution, and relationships of sociological and psychological variables.

Switchability. The ability to exchange one drug for another.

Symposium. A meeting focused on a particular topic.

Systematic review. A summary of previously conducted studies where the research to be included in the review is systematically identified; however, the results are not statistically combined as would occur with a quantitative systematic review or meta-analysis. Also called a qualitative systematic review.

Target drug program. A program that evaluates the use of a medication or group of medications on an ongoing basis. Within these programs, interventions are usually made at the time of discovery based on established criteria or guidelines.

Telnet. A program for microcomputers that causes the computer to mimic a dumb terminal, so that it can run programs on other computers (usually minicomputers or mainframes) over Internet or other computer networks.

Teratogenicity. Toxicity of drugs to the unborn fetus.

Tertiary literature. Textbooks and drug compendia (includes full text computer databases).

Third-party plan. A method of reimbursement for medical care in which neither the care provider or patient are charged. Third-party payers include insurance plans, health maintenance organizations, and government entities.

Threshold. A term used in quality assurance program that indicates how often an indicator must be complied with. Unlike standards, thresholds can be set at any level of compliance from 0% to 100%.

Total quality management (TQM). A management concept dealing with the implementation of continuous quality improvement.

Trohoc study. *See* case-control study.

True experiment. A study where researchers apply a treatment and determine its effects on subjects.

True negatives. Individuals without the disease that were correctly identified as being disease free by the test.

True positives. Individuals with the disease that were correctly identified as diseased by the test.

Type I error. The probability of a false positive result. The probability of a type I error is equal to alpha and occurs when the null hypothesis is rejected when it is in fact true.

Type II error. The probability of a false negative result. The probability of a type II error is equal to beta and occurs when the null hypothesis is accepted when it is in fact false.

Unexpected drug reaction. The FDA defines this as "one that is not listed in the current labeling for the drug as having been reported or associated with the use of the drug. This includes an ADR that may be symptomatically or pathophysiologically related to an ADR listed in the labeling but may differ from the labeled ADR because of greater severity or specificity (e.g., abnormal liver function vs. hepatic necrosis)."

Uniform resource locator (URL). An Internet address (e.g., <<http://druginfo.creighton.edu>>).

USENET news. A large number of discussion groups that are replicated in numerous places on the Internet. Users can read items posted on a topic and can contribute their own items to be posted. In many ways, this can be thought of as a large electronic bulletin board service on the Internet.

Validity. The truthfulness of study results. Internal validity refers to the extent to which the study results reflect what actually happened in the study. External validity is the degree to which the study results can be applied to patients routinely encountered in clinical practice.

Variables. Factors (characteristics that are being observed or measured) that are the focus of a study. The independent variable (e.g., treatment) causes change in the dependent variable (e.g., outcome).

Variance. A measurement of the range of data values (i.e., variability) about the mean. Variance is the square of the standard deviation.

Virtual private network (VPN). A method to connect computers over a distance; for example, over the Internet, that allows secure transmission of confidential data.

Warranty. An assurance by one party to a contract of the existence of a fact upon which the other party may rely, intended to relieve the promisee of any duty to ascertain the fact for himself or herself. Amounts to a promise to indemnify the promisee for any loss if the fact warranted proves untrue. Warranties may be express (made overtly) or implied (by implication).

Web browser. A computer program used to access information on the World Wide Web. The most popular programs are Microsoft Internet Explorer and Netscape Navigator/Communicator.

Web portal. A web site that acts as an interface to the Internet for users. Many Internet search engines are considered to be web portals. A variation on this, the enterprise portal, can also be used by an institution to help guide employees to necessary information within the institution or out on the Internet.

Web site. A group of web pages that will provide information to the person requesting that information. These pages are generally grouped under one main Internet address (URL).

Wide area network (WAN). A group of computers connected in a way that they may share data, programs, and or equipment over a distance (e.g., connection between computers owned by an institution that are scattered in clinics around a city).

World Wide Web. Computers connected to the Internet that provide a graphical interface to a variety of information that is available as text, pictures, sounds, databases, and other electronic files. Generally accessed using a Web Browser, such as Internet Explorer or Netscape.

XHTML (extensible HTML). A combination of HTML and extensible markup language.

XML (extensible markup language). A superset of HTML that provides information on the content of a web page, presentation of the information (how it looks), and semantics (what it means). This is designed to make it easier to find more relevant information using search engines.

Index